Annual Update in Intensive Care and Emergency Medicine 2014

The series *Annual Update in Intensive Care and Emergency Medicine* is the continuation of the series entitled *Yearbook of Intensive Care Medicine* in Europe and *Intensive Care Medicine: Annual Update* in the United States.

Jean-Louis Vincent
Editor

Annual Update in Intensive Care and Emergency Medicine 2014

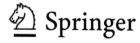 Springer

Editor

Prof. Jean-Louis Vincent
Erasme Hospital
Université libre de Bruxelles
Brussels, Belgium
jlvincen@ulb.ac.be

ISSN 2191-5709
ISBN 978-3-319-03745-5   ISBN 978-3-319-03746-2 (eBook)
DOI 10.1007/978-3-319-03746-2
Springer Cham Heidelberg New York Dordrecht London

Cover design: WMXDesign GmbH, Heidelberg

Printed on acid-free paper

Springer is part of Springer Science+Business Media
www.springer.com

Contents

Common Abbreviations

ALI	Acute lung injury
ARDS	Acute respiratory distress syndrome
BAL	Bronchoalveolar lavage
COPD	Chronic obstructive pulmonary disease
CPAP	Continuous positive airway pressure
CPB	Cardiopulmonary bypass
CT	Computed tomography
CVP	Central venous pressure
DO_2	Oxygen delivery
EKG	Electrocardiogram
EVLW	Extravascular lung water
FiO_2	Inspired fraction of oxygen
GEDV	Global end-diastolic volume
ICU	Intensive care unit
IL	Interleukin
LV	Left ventricular
MAP	Mean arterial pressure
MRI	Magnetic resonance imaging
NF-κB	Nuclear factor kappa-B
NO	Nitric oxide
OR	Odds ratio
PAC	Pulmonary artery cather
PAOP	Pulmonary artery occlusion pressure
PEEP	Positive end-expiratory pressure
PET	Positron emission tomography
RBC	Red blood cell
RCT	Randomized controlled trial
ROS	Reactive oxygen species
RRT	Renal replacement therapy
RV	Right ventricular
$ScvO_2$	Central venous oxygen saturation
SIRS	Systemic inflammatory response syndrome
SOFA	Sequential organ failure assessment
TNF	Tumor necrosis factor
VAP	Ventilator-associated pneumonia
VILI	Ventilator-induced lung injury
V_T	Tidal volume

Part I
Infections and Sepsis

Fever Management in Intensive Care Patients with Infections

P. Young and M. Saxena

Introduction

'Humanity has but three great enemies: fever, famine and war; of these by far the greatest, by far the most terrible, is fever' [1].

Fever is one of the cardinal signs of infection and, nearly 120 years after William Osler's statement in his address to the 47th annual meeting of the American Medical Association [1], infectious diseases remain a major cause of morbidity and mortality. Despite this, it is unclear whether fever itself is truly the enemy or whether, in fact, the febrile response represents an important means to help the body fight infection. Furthermore, it is unclear whether the administration of antipyretic medications or physical cooling measures to patients with fever and infection is beneficial or harmful [2, 3]. Here, we review the biology of fever, the significance of the febrile response in animals and humans, and the current evidence-base regarding the utility of treating fever in intensive care patients with infectious diseases.

The Biology of Fever

Regulation of Normal Body Temperature

Thermoregulation is a fundamental homeostatic mechanism that maintains body temperature within a tightly regulated range. The ability to internally regulate body temperature is known as endothermy and is a characteristic of all mammals and birds. The thermoregulatory system consists of an afferent sensory limb, a central

P. Young ✉
Intensive Care Unit, Wellington Regional Hospital, Wellington, New Zealand
e-mail: paul.young@ccdhb.org.nz

M. Saxena
Department of Intensive Care Medicine, St. George Hospital, Kogarah, Australia

J.-L. Vincent (Ed.), *Annual Update in Intensive Care and Emergency Medicine 2014*,
DOI 10.1007/978-3-319-03746-2_1, © Springer International Publishing Switzerland
and BioMed Central Ltd. 2014

processing center, and an efferent response limb. In humans, the central processing center controlling the thermoregulatory set-point is the hypothalamus. Both warm-sensitive and cold-sensitive thermoreceptors are involved in the afferent limb. Stimulation of the cold-sensitive receptors activates efferent responses relayed via the hypothalamus that reduce heat loss and increase heat production. These responses include reducing blood flow to the peripheries and increasing heat production by mechanisms including shivering. Conversely, stimulation of warm-sensitive receptors ultimately increases heat loss through peripheral vasodilation and evaporative cooling caused by sweating.

The Cellular and Molecular Basis of the Febrile Response

Upward adjustment of the normal hypothalamic thermoregulatory set-point leading to fever is typically part of a cytokine-mediated systemic inflammatory response syndrome that can be triggered by various infectious etiologies including bacterial, viral, and parasitic infections as well as by a range of non-infectious etiologies including severe pancreatitis and major surgery.

In patients with sepsis, the febrile response involves innate immune system activation via Toll-like receptor 4 (TLR-4). This activation leads to production of pyrogenic cytokines including interleukin (IL)-1β, IL-6, and tumor necrosis factor (TNF)-α. These pyrogenic cytokines act on an area of the brain known as the organum vasculosum of the laminae terminalis (OVLT) leading to the release of prostaglandin E_2 (PGE_2) via activation of the enzyme cyclo-oxygenase-2 (COX-2). PGE_2 binds to receptors in the hypothalamus leading to an increase in heat production and a decrease in heat loss until the temperature in the hypothalamus reaches a new, elevated, set-point. Once the new set-point is attained, the hypothalamus maintains homeostasis around this new set-point by the same mechanisms involved in the regulation of normal body temperature. However, in addition, there are a number of important specific negative feedback systems in place that prevent excessive elevation of body temperature. One key system is the glucocorticoid system, which acts via nuclear factor-kappa B (NF-κB) and activator protein-1 (AP-1). Both these mediators have anti-inflammatory properties and downregulate the production of pyrogenic cytokines, such as IL-1β, IL-6, and TNF-α. The febrile response is further modulated by specific antipyretic cytokines including IL-1 receptor antagonist (IL-1RA), IL-10, and TNF-α binding protein.

Heat Shock Proteins and the Febrile Response

The negative feedback systems outlined above are not the only mechanisms that exist to protect cells from being damaged by the febrile response. In addition, the heat shock proteins (HSPs) provide intrinsic resistance to thermal damage. Genes encoding the HSPs probably first evolved more than 2.5 billion years ago. They represent an important system providing protection to cells, not only against extremes of temperature, but also against other potentially lethal stresses including toxic chemicals and radiation injury. During heat-stress, transcription and translation of HSPs is upregulated. HSPs can then trigger refolding of heat-damaged proteins preserving them until heat-stress has passed or, if necessary, can transport denatured proteins to organelles for intracellular degradation. As well as providing protection against cellular damage from the thermal stress induced by fever, the HSPs may themselves be important regulators of the febrile response. For example, HSP 70 inhibits pyrogenic cytokine production via NF-κB. HSPs also inhibit programmed cell death, which might otherwise be induced by an invading pathogen.

The Physiological Consequences of Fever

The febrile response leads to a marked increase in metabolic rate. In humans, generating fever through shivering increases the metabolic rate above basal levels by six-fold [4]. In critically ill patients with fever, cooling reduces oxygen consumption by about 10 % per °C decrease in core temperature and significantly reduces cardiac output and minute ventilation [5]. Any potential benefit of the febrile response needs to be weighed against this substantial metabolic cost.

The Immunological Consequences of Fever

Temperatures in the physiological febrile range stimulate the maturation of murine dendritic cells. This is potentially important because dendritic cells act as the key antigen presenting cells in the immune system. Human neutrophil cell motility and phagocytosis are enhanced by temperatures in the febrile range, and growth of intracellular bacteria in human macrophages *in vitro* is reduced by temperatures in the febrile range compared to normal temperatures. Murine macrophages demonstrate a range of enhanced functions at temperatures in the febrile range. These effects include enhanced expression of the Fc receptors that are involved in mediating antibody responses, and enhanced phagocytosis. Temperatures in the physiological febrile range enhance binding of human lymphocytes to the vascular endothelium. This L-selectin-mediated binding is important in facilitating lymphocyte migration to sites of tissue inflammation or infection. In mice, T lymphocyte-mediated killing of virus-infected cells is increased by temperatures in the febrile range and helper T-cell potentiation of antibody responses is enhanced. In contrast to other cells of the immune system, the cytotoxic activity of natural killer cells is reduced by temperatures in the febrile range compared to normal body temperature. Although their functions are enhanced by temperatures in the physiological febrile range (38–40 °C), neutrophils and macrophages have substantially reduced function at temperatures of ≥ 41 °C.

The Effects of Fever on the Viability of Microbial Pathogens

Temperatures in the human physiological febrile range cause direct inhibition of some viral and bacterial organisms such as influenza virus [6], *Streptococcus pneumonia* [7, 8], and *Neisseria meningitides* [9] which can all cause life-threatening illnesses. For influenza, the degree of heat sensitivity appears to be a determinant of virulence, such that strains with a shut-off temperature of $\leq 38\,^\circ C$ cause mild symptoms, whereas strains with a shut-off temperature of $\geq 39\,^\circ C$ cause severe symptoms [6]. The susceptibility of a pathogen to heat may have significance in terms of its pathogenicity in a particular host. For example, *Campylobacter jejuni* is not pathogenic in birds (body temperature $42\,^\circ C$) but is pathogenic in humans (body temperature $37\,^\circ C$) and the growth and chemotactic ability of *C. jejuni in vitro* are greater at $37\,^\circ C$ than at $42\,^\circ C$ [10].

The Significance of Fever in Animals with Infections

The febrile response to infection is seen in a range of animal species including not only endotherms, such as mammals and birds, but also ectotherms, including reptiles, amphibians, and fish. The febrile response can be blocked by inhibition of COX in a diverse range of species including desert iguanas [11] and bluegill sunfish [12], as well as higher animals like humans. As COX catalyzes the generation of prostaglandins from arachidonic acid, this suggests that the pivotal role of PGE_2 in the regulation of the thermostatic set-point may be preserved in these species as well as in higher animals. Such a common biochemical mechanism to regulate fever across such a diverse group of animals raises the possibility that the febrile response may have evolved in a common ancestor. If this is the case, then fever probably emerged as an evolutionary response more than 350 million years ago [13]. As the febrile response comes at a significant metabolic cost [4, 5], its persistence across such a broad range of species provides strong circumstantial evidence that the response has some evolutionary advantage. Furthermore, given that the response appears ubiquitous, it logically follows that the components of the immune system would have evolved to function optimally in the physiological febrile range.

In experimental models in mammals, the febrile response appears to offer a survival advantage across a range of viral infections. Newborn mice infected with coxsackie virus, which are allowed to develop a fever have a much lower mortality than mice which are prevented from developing a fever [14]. Similarly, increasing the environmental temperature from 23–$26\,^\circ C$ to $38\,^\circ C$ increases the core temperature of *Herpes simplex*-infected mice by about $2\,^\circ C$ and increases their survival from $0\,\%$ to $85\,\%$ [15]. A meta-analysis of the effect of antipyretic medications on mortality in animal models of influenza infection demonstrated that antipyretic treatment was associated with an increased mortality risk [OR 1.34 (95 % CI 1.04-1.73)] [16].

Studies in mammalian models of bacterial infections have generally yielded similar results. In rabbits infected with *Pasteurella multocida*, the presence of a mild fever of up to 2.25 °C above normal was correlated with the greatest chance of survival compared to either normothermia or fever of > 2.25 °C above normal [17]. Although mice are predominantly endothermic, they appear to require external sources of heat to generate a fever. If mice are allowed to position themselves in a cage with a temperature gradient, they increase their ambient temperature preference and elevate their core temperature by 1.1 °C after a lipopolysaccharide (LPS) challenge [18]. Housing mice at 35.5 °C rather than 23 °C increases their core body temperature by about 2.5 °C, alters cytokine expression, and improves survival in *Klebsiella pneumoniae* peritonitis [19]. In this model, the elevated body temperature seen with increased ambient temperature was associated with a 100,000-fold reduction in the intraperitoneal bacterial load [19]. A recently published systematic review and meta-analysis of the effects of antipyretic medications on mortality in *S. pneumoniae* infection identified four animal studies comparing aspirin to placebo and demonstrated that the administration of aspirin was associated with an increased risk of death [OR 1.97 (95 %CI 1.22-3.19)] [20].

The Significance of Fever in Humans with Infection

Fever, Hyperthermia, and Antipyresis in Non-ICU Patients with Infections

Viral infections

Two double blind randomized placebo-controlled trials in 45 volunteers inoculated with either rhinovirus type 21 (study one) or rhinovirus type 25 (study two) demonstrated that administration of aspirin did not alter the proportion of patients who developed clinical illness or significantly alter the frequency or severity of symptoms [21]. Although the administration of aspirin significantly increased the shedding of rhinovirus in these trials, only one of the 45 patients developed fever so this increase in shedding was probably not attributable to the antipyretic effect of aspirin [21]. A similar study of 60 volunteers inoculated with rhinovirus and randomized to aspirin, paracetamol, ibuprofen, or placebo showed that the use of either aspirin or paracetamol was associated with suppression of the serum antibody response and a rise in circulating monocytes [22]. There were no significant differences in viral shedding among the four groups. However, the subjects treated with aspirin or paracetamol had a significant increase in nasal symptoms and signs compared to the placebo group [22]. In rhinovirus-infected volunteers treated with pseudoephedrine, the addition of ibuprofen had no effect on symptoms or on viral shedding or viral titers [23]. Again, only two of the 58 subjects developed a fever. A randomized controlled trial of children aged six months to six years with presumed non-bacterial infection and a fever of ≥ 38 °C demonstrated that administration of paracetamol increased the children's activity but not their mood, comfort or appetite [24].

Overall, the data from clinical studies in non-ICU patients do not support the hypothesis that antipyresis has a clinically significant beneficial or detrimental impact on the course or severity of minor viral illnesses. Although antipyretic medicines may increase the duration of rhinovirus shedding and time until crusting of chicken pox lesions, these effects seems unlikely to be attributable to antipyresis and are of uncertain clinical importance.

Bacterial infections

There are no randomized controlled trial data examining strategies of fever management on patient-centered outcomes in non-ICU patients with bacterial infections. However, there are historical examples of dramatic responses to treatment with therapeutic hyperthermia in some infectious diseases. It has been known since the time of Hippocrates that progressive paralysis due to neurosyphilis sometimes resolves after an illness associated with high fever. This observation led Julius Wagner-Jauregg to propose, in 1887, that inoculation of malaria might be a justifiable therapy for patients with 'progressive paralysis'. His rationale was that one could substitute an untreatable condition for a treatable one – malaria being treatable with quinine. In 1917, he tested his hypothesis in nine patients with paralysis due to syphilis by injecting them with blood from patients suffering from malaria. Three of the patients had remission of their paralysis. This led to further experiments and clinical observations on more than a thousand patients with remission occurring in 30 % of patients with neurosyphilis-related progressive paralysis 'treated' with fever induced by malaria compared to spontaneous remission rates of only 1 %. This work on fever therapy led to Julius Wagner-Jauregg being awarded the Nobel Prize in Physiology or Medicine in 1927 [25]. Subsequently, fever therapy was shown to be effective in treating gonorrhea. Inducing a hyperthermia of 41.7 °C for six hours in the 'Kettering hypertherm chamber' led to cure in 81 % of cases [26].

A number of observational studies have examined the association between body temperature and outcome in patients with various bacterial infections, including pneumonia [27], spontaneous bacterial peritonitis [28], and Gram-negative bacteremia [29]. These studies show that the absence of fever is a sign of poor prognosis in patients with bacterial infections. Overall, the design of these studies does not allow one to distinguish between the absence of fever as a marked of disease severity or impaired host resilience rather than the presence of fever as a protective response.

Fever in ICU Patients with Infections

Observational studies of fever and fever management in ICU patients

The epidemiology of fever in ICU patients and the frequency and utility of antipyretic use in ICU patients has been evaluated in a number of observational studies. The most important of the studies are summarized in Table 1.

The incidence of fever attributable to infection in observational studies in various critical care settings varies from 8 % to 37 % [31, 34, 36–41]. These studies use a variety of definitions of fever and a range of methods to record temperature, mak-

Table 1 Summary of key observational studies of fever and fever management in ICU patients

	Design, Setting, and Participants	Key Findings
Laupland et al. 2008 [30]	Retrospective cohort study of patients admitted to four ICUs in Calgary between 2000 and 2006; $n = 24,204$ ICU admissions in 20,466 patients	• Fever of $\geq 38.3\,°C$ developed during 44 % of ICU admissions and high fever $\geq 39.3\,°C$ during 8 % of admissions • Fever was not associated with increased ICU mortality but high fever was associated with a significantly increased risk of death
Young et al. 2011 [31]	Inception cohort study in three tertiary ICUs in Australia and New Zealand over six weeks in 2010 identifying patients with fever $\geq 38\,°C$ and known or suspected infection; $n = 565$	• 9 % of patients admitted to ICU had or developed a fever and known or suspected infection • Paracetamol was administered to about $^2/_3$ of patients with fever and known or suspected infection on any given day
Selladu-rai et al. 2011 [32]	Retrospective cohort study of patients admitted to a single tertiary ICU in Australia with sepsis between December 2009 and August 2010; $n = 106$	• 69 % of septic patients received paracetamol at least once during their first seven days in ICU • 88 % of septic patients with a fever $> 38\,°C$ received paracetamol during their first seven days in ICU • Septic patients with a fever $> 38\,°C$ were 6.8 times (95 % CI 1.9-24.7) more likely to receive paracetamol than septic patients who were not febrile
Lee et al. 2012 [33]	Inception cohort study of consecutive patients admitted to 25 ICUs in Japan and Korea for more than 48 hours over three months in 2009; $n = 1,425$	• NSAID use independently associated with increased 28-day mortality in patients with sepsis (adjusted OR 2.61; 95 % CI 1.11-6.11; p = 0.03) but with a trend towards a decreased 28-day mortality in patients without sepsis (adjusted OR 0.22; 95 % 0.03-1.74; p = 0.15) • Paracetamol use independently associated with increased 28-day mortality in patients with sepsis (adjusted OR 2.05; 95 % CI 1.19-3.55; p = 0.01) but with a trend towards a decreased 28-day mortality in patients without sepsis (adjusted OR 0.58; 95 % 0.06-5.26; p = 0.63)
Laupland et al. 2012 [34]	Inception cohort study of patients admitted to French ICUs contributing to the Outcomerea database between April 2000 and November 2010; $n = 10,962$	• 25.7 % of patients had a fever of $\geq 38.3\,°C$ at ICU presentation • Fever was not associated with increased mortality but hypothermia was an independent predictor of death in medical patients
Young et al. 2012 [35]	Retrospective cohort study of 636,051 patients in Australia, New Zealand and the UK admitted to the ICU between 2005 until 2009	• Elevated body temperature in the first 24 hours in ICU was associated with an increased risk of mortality in patients without infections and a decreased risk of mortality in patients with infections
Niven et al. 2012 [36]	Interrupted time series analysis of cumulative fever incidence in ICUs in Calgary from 2004–2009	• The cumulative incidence of fever ≥ 38.3 during ICU admission decreased from 50.1 % to 25.5 % over the 5.5 years of the study

CI: confidence interval; ICU: intensive care unit; NSAIDs: non-steroidal anti-inflammatory drugs; OR: odds ratio

ing comparisons between studies difficult. In these studies, the presence of fever was associated with either an increased risk of death [30, 39–41] or no difference in mortality risk compared to a normal temperature [34]. Only two studies have evaluated the mortality risk of patients with sepsis separately from patients without sepsis [33, 35]. In the first study, fever was associated with an increased 28-day mortality risk in patients without sepsis but not in patients with sepsis [33] raising the possibility that the presence of infection might be an important determinant of the significance of the febrile response in ICU patients. Similarly, in a retrospective cohort study [35] ($n = 636,051$) using two independent, multicenter, geographically distinct and representative databases we found that peak temperatures above 39.0 °C in the first 24 hours after ICU admission were generally associated with a reduced risk of in-hospital mortality in patients with an admission diagnosis of infection. Conversely, higher peak temperatures were associated with an increased risk of in-hospital mortality in patients with a non-infection diagnosis.

Overall, although one recent study suggests that the incidence of fever is decreasing over time [36], existing observational data suggest that fever is a commonly encountered abnormal physical sign in ICU patients. Unfortunately, because of the potential for unmeasured confounding factors, it is impossible to establish whether treating fever in ICU patients with an infection is beneficial or harmful on the basis of observational studies.

Interventional studies of fever management in ICU patients

Two recently published meta-analyses found no evidence that antipyretic therapy was either beneficial or harmful in non-neurologically injured ICU patients [2, 3]. Nearly all of the patients included in these meta-analyses had known or suspected sepsis and one of the meta-analyses only included patients with infection [3]. In both meta-analyses, the authors noted that existing studies lacked adequate statistical power to detect clinically important differences and recommended that large randomized controlled trials were urgently needed. The details of published interventional studies of fever management strategies in ICU patients are summarized in Table 2.

The largest published randomized controlled trial evaluated the use of ibuprofen in critically ill patients with sepsis [43]. Patients with severe sepsis were randomized to receive 10 mg/kg of ibuprofen or placebo every six hours for a total of eight doses. Although the use of ibuprofen significantly reduced body temperature, it did not alter 30-day mortality, which was 37 % in the ibuprofen-treated group and 40 % in the placebo group. This study was designed to evaluate the use of ibuprofen as an anti-inflammatory rather than as an anti-pyretic and, while the use of ibuprofen significantly reduced temperature compared to placebo, the study included patients who were hypothermic as well as patients who were febrile. An additional confounding factor was that patients assigned to the ibuprofen group were treated with paracetamol more often than those assigned to the control group. On the basis of this [43] and other smaller studies [45, 46] of non-steroidal anti-inflammatory drugs (NSAIDs) in critically ill patients, it is clear that NSAIDs are effective at reducing temperature in febrile ICU patients. However, there is no consistent mortality

Table 2 Summary of randomized controlled trials investigating the management of fever in critically ill adults

	Design, Setting, and Participants	Key Findings
Bernard et al. 1991 [42]	Double blind placebo-controlled trial of ibuprofen in patients with severe sepsis; $n = 30$	• Ibuprofen significantly reduced temperature, heart rate, and peak airway pressure • There was no significant difference between ibuprofen and placebo in terms of in-hospital mortality rate (18.8 % ibuprofen-treated group vs. 42.9 % placebo-treated group)
Bernard et al. 1997 [43]	Double blind placebo-controlled trial of ibuprofen in patients with severe sepsis in seven centers in North America; $n = 455$	• Ibuprofen significantly reduced temperature, heart rate, oxygen consumption, and lactic acidosis in patients with severe sepsis • Ibuprofen did not alter the incidence or duration of shock or ARDS and had no significant effect on 30-day mortality (37 % ibuprofen-treated group vs. 40 % placebo-treated group)
Memis et al. 2004 [44]	Double blind placebo-controlled trial of lornoxicam in patients with severe sepsis in one center in Turkey; $n = 40$	• No significant difference between lornoxicam and placebo was demonstrated in terms of hemodynamic parameters, biochemical parameters, cytokine levels, or ICU mortality (35 % lornoxicam-treated group vs. 40 % placebo-treated group)
Morris et al. 2011 [45]	Multicenter, randomized trial comparing the antipyretic efficacy of a single dose of placebo, 100 mg, 200 mg, or 400 mg of i. v. ibuprofen in hospitalized patients of whom > 90 % had infections; $n = 120$ (53 critically ill)	• All doses of ibuprofen tested were effective in lowering temperature • There were no significant difference between treatment groups with respect to ventilation requirements, length of stay or in-hospital mortality (4 % placebo, 3 % 100 mg ibuprofen, 7 % 200 mg ibuprofen, 6 % 400 mg ibuprofen)
Haupt et al. 1991 [46]	Multicenter, placebo-controlled randomized trial of ibuprofen in patients with severe sepsis; $n = 29$	• Ibuprofen significantly reduced body temperature • There was no significant difference between the treatment groups in terms of in-hospital mortality (30.8 % in the placebo group vs. 56.3 % in the ibuprofen group)
Schulman et al. 2006 [47]	Single center, unblinded, randomized trial of aggressive vs. permissive temperature management in febrile patients in a trauma ICU; $n = 82$	• There was no significant difference between the treatment arms in terms of the number of new infections • The in-hospital mortality was 15.9 % in the aggressive treatment group and 2.6 % in the permissive treatment group (p = 0.06)
Niven et al. 2012 [48]	Multicenter, unblinded randomized trial of aggressive vs. permissive temperature management in febrile ICU patients; $n = 26$	• The mean daily temperature was lower in the patients assigned to aggressive fever management • The in-hospital mortality was 21 % in the aggressive treatment group and 17 % in the permissive treatment group (p = 1.0)

Continuation see next page

Table 2 *Continued*

	Design, Setting, and Participants	Key Findings
Schortgen et al. 2012 [49]	Multicenter, randomized controlled trial of external cooling in patients with fever and septic shock receiving mechanical ventilation in seven centers in France; $n = 200$	• External cooling significantly reduced body temperature • External cooling did not alter the proportion of patients who had a 50 % reduction in vasopressor dose after 48 hours • Day-14 mortality was significantly lower in the patients assigned to external cooling but there was no significant difference between the groups in terms of ICU or in-hospital mortality

ARDS: acute respiratory distress syndrome; ICU: intensive care unit.

signal from the existing studies of NSAIDs. Some studies show trends towards benefit [42–44] with the use of NSAIDs and others show trends towards harm [45, 46].

The second largest published study of temperature management in febrile ICU patients evaluated the use of external cooling [49]. This study randomized 200 febrile patients with septic shock requiring vasopressors, mechanical ventilation, and sedation to external cooling to normothermia (36.5-37 °C) for 48 hours or no external cooling. The primary endpoint was the proportion of patients with a 50 % decrease in vasopressor use at 48 hours after randomization. There was no significant difference between the treatment groups for the primary endpoint, which was achieved in 72 % of the patients assigned to external cooling and 61 % of the patients assigned to standard care. This study had a large number of secondary endpoints including mean body temperature, the proportion of patients who achieved 50 % reduction in vasopressors at 2 hours, 12 hours, 24 hours, and 36 hours as well as day-14, ICU, and hospital mortality. The secondary endpoints generally favored external cooling and day-14 mortality was noted to be significantly lower in the external cooling group (19 % vs. 34 %; p = 0.0013). This difference in mortality was not evident by the time of ICU or hospital discharge and caution should be exerted in interpreting these endpoints as it is possible that they were affected by a type 1 error due to a lack of statistical power.

Another trial compared temperature control strategies in a tertiary trauma ICU and randomized patients to either aggressive temperature control or a permissive strategy [47]. Patients assigned to the aggressive treatment arm received regular paracetamol once the temperature exceeded 38.5 °C and physical cooling was added when the temperature exceeded 39.5 °C. Patients assigned to the permissive treatment arm received paracetamol and cooling when the temperature reached 40 °C. This trial originally aimed to enroll 672 patients; however, it was stopped by the Data Safety Monitoring Board after enrolment of 82 patients due to a trend towards increased mortality in the aggressive treatment group. While all deaths were attributed to septic causes, conventional stopping rules were not used and differences between the study treatment arms could be due to chance. This study had other major limitations including a lack of blinding or placebo-control, and potential confounding from the uncontrolled use of other antipyretic drugs and per-protocol use of external cooling. A similar open-label randomized study enrolled 26 febrile ICU patients and assigned them to aggressive or permissive temperature management [48]. In this study, the aggressive fever control group received paracetamol 650 mg enterally every 6 hours when the temperature was $\geq 38.3\,°C$ and received physical cooling for temperature $\geq 39.5\,°C$. The permissive group did not receive paracetamol until the temperature was $\geq 40\,°C$ and did not receive physical cooling until the temperature reached $\geq 40.5\,°C$. All patients assigned to aggressive temperature management had an infectious etiology of fever and 75 % of patients assigned to the permissive management arm had an infectious etiology at baseline. The 28-day all cause mortality was not significantly different between the two groups.

The safety and efficacy of using paracetamol to treat fever in ICU patients with infections is being evaluated in a 700-patient phase IIb, multicenter, randomized placebo-controlled trial (the HEAT trial), which is due to complete enrolment in November 2014 [50].

Conclusion

There is a significant body of animal data demonstrating that fever is an important component of the host response to infection and confers a survival advantage in a number of animal species. The conservation of a metabolically costly response across a broad range of animal species suggests that the response probably has an evolutionary advantage. There are some interesting historical examples of hyperthermia being employed to treat infectious diseases. However, in the modern era the relevance of these examples is questionable. Furthermore, arguments based on the evolutionary importance of the febrile response do not necessarily apply to critically ill patients who are, by definition, supported beyond the limits of normal physiological homeostasis. Humans are not adapted to critical illness. In the absence of modern medicine and intensive care, most critically ill patients with fever and infection would presumably die. Among critically ill patients, it is biologically plausible that there is a balance to be struck between the potential benefits of reducing metabolic rate that come with fever control and the potential risks of a deleterious effect on host defense mechanisms. Remarkably, at present, we do not know what effect treating fever in critically ill patients with infections has on patient-centered outcomes. These treatments include commonly used interventions such as paracetamol and physical cooling. This area of research is of high priority given the global epidemiology of fever in critically ill patients and the generalizability of the candidate interventions.

References

1. Osler W (1896) The study of the fevers of the south. JAMA XXVI:1001–1004
2. Niven DJ, Stelfox HT, Laupland KB (2013) Antipyretic therapy in febrile critically ill adults: A systematic review and meta-analysis. J Crit Care 28:303–310

3. Jefferies S, Weatherall M, Young P, Eyers S, Perrin KG, Beasley CR (2011) The effect of antipyretic medications on mortality in critically ill patients with infection: a systematic review and meta-analysis. Crit Care Resus 13:125–131
4. Horvath SM, Spurr GB, Hutt BK, Hamilton LH (1956) Metabolic cost of shivering. J Appl Physiol 8:595–602
5. Manthous CA, Hall JB, Olson D et al (1995) Effect of cooling on oxygen consumption in febrile critically ill patients. Am J Respir Crit Care Med 151:10–14
6. Chu CM, Tian SF, Ren GF, Zhang YM, Zhang LX, Liu GQ (1982) Occurrence of temperature-sensitive influenza A viruses in nature. J Virol 41:353–359
7. Small PM, Tauber MG, Hackbarth CJ, Sande MA (1986) Influence of body temperature on bacterial growth rates in experimental pneumococcal meningitis in rabbits. Infect Immun 52:484–487
8. Enders JF, Wu CJ, Shaffer MF (1936) Studies on natural immunity to pneumococcus type III: IV. Observations on a non-type specific humoral factor involved in resistance to pneumococcus type III. J Exp Med 64:425–438
9. Moench M (1926) A study of the heat sensitivity of the meningococcus in vitro within the range of therapeutic temperatures. J Lab Clin Med 57:665–676
10. Khanna MR, Bhavsar SP, Kapadnis BP (2006) Effect of temperature on growth and chemotactic behaviour of Campylobacter jejuni. Lett Appl Microbiol 43:84–90
11. Bernheim HA, Kluger MJ (1976) Fever: effect of drug-induced antipyresis on survival. Science 193:237–239
12. Reynolds WW (1977) Fever and antipyresis in the bluegill sunfish, Lepomis macrochirus. Comparative biochemistry and physiology. Comp Biochem Physiol C 57:165–167
13. Kluger M (1979) The evolution of fever. In: Kluger M (ed) Fever: Its Biology, Evolution, and Function, 1st edn. Princeton University Press, New Jersey, pp 106–127
14. Strouse S (1909) Experimental Studies on Pneumococcus Infections. J Exp Med 11:743–761
15. Armstrong C (1942) Some recent research in the field of neurotropic viruses with especial reference to lymphocytic choriomeningitis and herpes simplex. Mil Surg 91:129–145
16. Eyers S, Weatherall M, Shirtcliffe P, Perrin K, Beasley R (2010) The effect on mortality of antipyretics in the treatment of influenza infection: systematic review and meta-analysis. J R Soc Med 103:403–411
17. Kluger MJ, Vaughn LK (1978) Fever and survival in rabbits infected with Pasteurella multocida. J Physiol 282:243–251
18. Akins C, Thiessen D, Cocke R (1991) Lipopolysaccharide increases ambient temperature preference in C57BL/6J adult mice. Physiol Behav 50:461–463
19. Jiang Q, Cross AS, Singh IS, Chen TT, Viscardi RM, Hasday JD (2000) Febrile core temperature is essential for optimal host defense in bacterial peritonitis. Infect Immun 68:1265–1270
20. Jefferies S, Weatherall M, Young P, Eyers S, Beasley R (2012) Systematic review and meta-analysis of the effects of antipyretic medications on mortality in Streptococcus pneumoniae infections. Postgrad Med J 88:21–27
21. Stanley ED, Jackson GG, Panusarn C, Rubenis M, Dirda V (1975) Increased virus shedding with aspirin treatment of rhinovirus infection. JAMA 231:1248–1251
22. Graham NM, Burrell CJ, Douglas RM, Debelle P, Davies L (1990) Adverse effects of aspirin, acetaminophen, and ibuprofen on immune function, viral shedding, and clinical status in rhinovirus-infected volunteers. J Infect Dis 162:1277–1282
23. Sperber SJ, Sorrentino JV, Riker DK, Hayden FG (1989) Evaluation of an alpha agonist alone and in combination with a nonsteroidal antiinflammatory agent in the treatment of experimental rhinovirus colds. Bull N Y Acad Med 65:145–160
24. Kramer MS, Naimark LE, Roberts-Brauer R, McDougall A, Leduc DG (1991) Risks and benefits of paracetamol antipyresis in young children with fever of presumed viral origin. Lancet 337:591–594

25. Wagner-Jauregg J (1927) The treatment of dementia paralytica by malaria innoculation. Nobel Lectures: Physiology or Medicine 1922–1941. Elsevier, New York, pp 159–169

26. Owens C (1936) The value of fever therapy for gonorrhea. JAMA 107:1942–1946

27. Ahkee S, Srinath L, Ramirez J (1997) Community-acquired pneumonia in the elderly: association of mortality with lack of fever and leukocytosis. South Med J 90:296–298

28. Weinstein MP, Iannini PB, Stratton CW, Eickhoff TC (1978) Spontaneous bacterial peritonitis. A review of 28 cases with emphasis on improved survival and factors influencing prognosis. Am J Med 64:592–598

29. Bryant RE, Hood AF, Hood CE, Koenig MG (1971) Factors affecting mortality of gram-negative rod bacteremia. Arch Intern Med 127:120–128

30. Laupland KB, Shahpori R, Kirkpatrick AW, Ross T, Gregson DB, Stelfox HT (2008) Occurrence and outcome of fever in critically ill adults. Crit Care Med 36:1531–1535

31. Young P, Saxena M, Eastwood GM, Bellomo R, Beasley R (2011) Fever and fever management among intensive care patients with known or suspected infection: a multicentre prospective cohort study. Crit Care Med 13:97–102

32. Selladurai S, Eastwood GM, Bailey M, Bellomo R (2011) Paracetamol therapy for septic critically ill patients: a retrospective observational study. Crit Care Resus 13:181–186

33. Lee BH, Inui D, Suh GY et al (2012) Association of body temperature and antipyretic treatments with mortality of critically ill patients with and without sepsis: multi-centered prospective observational study. Crit Care 16:R33

34. Laupland KB, Zahar JR, Adrie C et al (2012) Determinants of temperature abnormalities and influence on outcome of critical illness. Crit Care Med 40:145–151

35. Young PJ, Saxena M, Beasley R et al (2012) Early peak temperature and mortality in critically ill patients with or without infection. Intensive Care Med 38:437–444

36. Niven DJ, Stelfox HT, Shahpori R, Laupland KB (2013) Fever in adult ICUs: An interrupted time series analysis. Crit Care Med 41:1863–1869

37. Kiekkas P, Velissaris D, Karanikolas M et al (2010) Peak body temperature predicts mortality in critically ill patients without cerebral damage. Heart Lung 39:208–216

38. Moran JL, Peter JV, Solomon PJ et al (2007) Tympanic temperature measurements: are they reliable in the critically ill? A clinical study of measures of agreement. Crit Care Med 35:155–164

39. Circiumaru B, Baldock G, Cohen J (1999) A prospective study of fever in the intensive care unit. Intensive Care Med 25:668–673

40. Peres Bota D, Lopes Ferreira F, Melot C, Vincent JL (2004) Body temperature alterations in the critically ill. Intensive Care Med 30:811–816

41. Barie PS, Hydo LJ, Eachempati SR (2004) Causes and consequences of fever complicating critical surgical illness. Surg Infect (Larchmt) 5:145–159

42. Bernard GR, Reines HD, Halushka PV et al (1991) Prostacyclin and thromboxane A2 formation is increased in human sepsis syndrome. Effects of cyclooxygenase inhibition. Am Rev Respir Dis 144:1095–1101

43. Bernard GR, Wheeler AP, Russell JA et al (1997) The effects of ibuprofen on the physiology and survival of patients with sepsis. The Ibuprofen in Sepsis Study Group. N Engl J Med 336:912–918

44. Memis D, Karamanlioglu B, Turan A, Koyuncu O, Pamukcu Z (2004) Effects of lornoxicam on the physiology of severe sepsis. Crit Care 8:R474–R482

45. Morris PE, Promes JT, Guntupalli KK, Wright PE, Arons MM (2010) A multi-center, randomized, double-blind, parallel, placebo-controlled trial to evaluate the efficacy, safety, and pharmacokinetics of intravenous ibuprofen for the treatment of fever in critically ill and non-critically ill adults. Crit Care 14:R125

46. Haupt MT, Jastremski MS, Clemmer TP, Metz CA, Goris GB (1991) Effect of ibuprofen in patients with severe sepsis: a randomized, double-blind, multicenter study. The Ibuprofen Study Group. Crit Care Med 19:1339–1347

47. Schulman CI, Namias N, Doherty J et al (2005) The effect of antipyretic therapy upon out-comes in critically ill patients: a randomized, prospective study. Surg Infect (Larchmt) 6:369–375
48. Niven DJ, Stelfox HT, Leger C, Kubes P, Laupland KB (2013) Assessment of the safety and feasibility of administering antipyretic therapy in critically ill adults: A pilot randomized clinical trial. J Crit Care 28:296–302
49. Schortgen F, Clabault K, Katsahian S et al (2012) Fever control using external cooling in septic shock: a randomized controlled trial. Am J Respir Crit Care Med 185:1088–1095
50. Young PJ, Saxena MK, Bellomo R et al (2012) The HEAT trial: a protocol for a multicentre randomised placebo-controlled trial of IV paracetamol in ICU patients with fever and infection. Crit Care Resus 14:290–296

Review on Iron, Immunity and Intensive Care

L. T. van Eijk, D. W. Swinkels, and P. Pickkers

Introduction

Critically ill patients represent a heterogeneous group of patients with a broad array of (co)morbidities. Although highly diverse, one characteristic that applies to practically all critically ill patients is a greatly disturbed iron homeostasis. Iron redistribution is one of the key factors contributing to the development of anemia, which is common on the intensive care unit (ICU). Nearly all patients develop anemia during their ICU stay [1, 2]. Although blood transfusions are independently associated with worse outcome, 40 to 50 % of patients receive one or more transfusions during their ICU stay [1]. This underscores the need to understand ICU-related anemia and find alternative therapies. The field of iron biology has experienced an enormous surge of interest since the discovery of hepcidin in 2001, the key regulator of iron homeostasis [3]. Since then, many investigations have focused on iron homeostasis and its interactions with inflammation, which are numerous. Although most of the pathophysiological mechanisms have been clarified in animal models and chronically inflamed patients, studies in the critically ill are limited. However, although anemia on the intensive care is frequently encountered, awareness of the changes in iron balance that accompany or underlie this anemia is low. This review provides an overview of iron biology during inflammation, and clarifies its relation with microbial virulence, immunity, and oxidative stress reactions. In addition, consequences for the critically ill patient are discussed.

L. T. van Eijk · P. Pickkers ✉
Department of Intensive Care Medicine, Radboud University Nijmegen Medical Centre,
Nijmegen, Netherlands
e-mail: p.pickkers@ic.umcn.nl

D. W. Swinkels
Department of Laboratory Medicine, Laboratory of Genetic, Endocrine and Metabolic Diseases,
Radboud University Nijmegen Medical Centre, Nijmegen, Netherlands

J.-L. Vincent (Ed.), *Annual Update in Intensive Care and Emergency Medicine 2014*, 17
DOI 10.1007/978-3-319-03746-2_2, © Springer International Publishing Switzerland
2014

Iron Biology

Undeniably, iron is essential to vertebrate life. It is the fourth most abundant element in the earth's crust, and many species depend on its constant availability, because iron is needed for many basic cellular processes like respiration and DNA replication. Although the role of iron in physiological processes is evident, iron is considered a double-edged sword, because iron management is also difficult and dangerous. Difficult because iron is practically insoluble, both in and outside the body, being readily oxidized in physiological conditions to the insoluble ferric (Fe^{3+}) form, and dangerous because most microbes thrive well on iron, as they need it for replication and growth. In addition, because iron can catalyze oxidative stress reactions that can cause harm to cells and organelles, the host may be harmed by iron; on the other hand, oxidative stress reactions are necessary to kill invading microorganisms. To overcome these problems, humans and most other species have evolved in a way that enables them to take-up iron and utilize it safely by making use of specific protein complexes, such as transferrin, lactoferrin, ferritin and heme proteins, while keeping iron away from microbes and not letting it take part in oxidative stress reactions. In addition, the major iron transporting molecule, transferrin, is normally only partly saturated (30–40 %), so that iron is readily bound to transferrin once it appears in the plasma. As a consequence, although as much as 20–25 mg of iron is transported through the blood to the bone marrow every day, the iron freely available in plasma is extremely low, in the order of magnitude of 10^{-18} M [4].

Within the body, most of the iron is stored intracellularly. The total quantity of iron in the human body is normally maintained at approximately 50 mg/kg body weight in males and approximately 40 mg/kg in females, distributed among functional, transport, and storage compartments. The largest amount of iron is present in the erythrocytes, where approximately two-thirds of the total body iron supply is built into heme proteins. Another 300–500 mg of iron is carried by erythroid progenitor cells of the bone marrow. The other major iron storage protein is ferritin, accounting for approximately 500 mg of iron, being primarily deposited in hepatocytes and macrophages of the reticuloendothelial system. Normally, not more than 0.1 % of the body's iron (approximately 3 mg) can be found in the plasma compartment, where almost all iron is bound to transferrin while it is transported to cells in need of iron, primarily erythroid progenitor cells.

As iron is a transition metal, it can exist in either a ferric form (Fe^{3+}) or a ferrous form (Fe^{2+}). In general, iron within the body exists as ferric iron, bound to molecules that ensure its solubility. Free ferrous iron can be found in small amounts within the cytosol, which is referred to as the 'labile iron pool'. In the plasma, iron can also be bound to other molecules, including citrate and albumin. These molecules generally have a much lower affinity for iron and, therefore, iron that is not bound to transferrin, i. e., non-transferrin-bound-iron (NTBI), is more likely to participate in chemical reactions [5]. This is especially the case for 'labile plasma iron' (LPI), a fraction of NTBI that is involved in oxidative stress reactions, and which will be discussed separately.

Regulation of Iron Homeostasis

Hepcidin Controls Iron Homeostasis

The uptake of iron is tightly regulated to meet systemic iron requirements. Because humans have no physiological mechanism for the active elimination of iron, total body iron is controlled almost exclusively by the rate of iron absorption from the duodenum. Two major sources exist via which iron can enter the bloodstream (Fig. 1). A small quantity of iron (approximately 1–2 mg per day) is taken up from duodenal enterocytes, which absorb iron from the gut. More importantly, most of the iron (20–25 mg per day) is recycled by macrophages of the reticuloendothelial system that retrieve iron from phagocytosed senescent red blood cells (RBCs) [6]. Iron enters the cytosol of enterocytes and macrophages through divalent metal transporter 1 (DMT1), from where it can either be stored in ferritin, or gets exported through the iron exporter, ferroportin. Once in the plasma, iron is bound primarily to transferrin and is taken up by cells expressing the type 1 transferrin receptor (TfR1). Most of the iron is transported to the bone marrow, but practically all cell types, including immune cells, carry TfR1, because they are all dependent on iron to some extent.

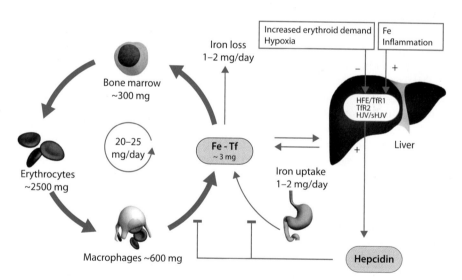

Fig. 1 System iron regulation. Iron can enter the plasma from duodenal enterocytes and from macrophages of the reticuloendothelial system that recycle iron from senescent erythrocytes. From the plasma, iron is mainly transported to the bone marrow, where it is used for the production of new red blood cells. Hepcidin attenuates the release of iron from macrophages, and the uptake of iron from the gut, thereby leading to decreased serum iron levels. Hepcidin is produced in the liver and is induced by increased iron supply and inflammation, whereas it is downregulated by low iron supply, hypoxia and increased erythropoiesis. TfR: transferrin receptor; HJV: hemojuvelin. Adapted from [50] with permission of the authors

The expression of ferroportin on the cell surface of macrophages and duodenal enterocytes is strictly controlled by the peptide hormone, hepcidin, which is produced in the liver in response to a wide range of signals. By binding to ferroportin, hepcidin induces the internalization and degradation of ferroportin [7], thereby downregulating iron efflux. In circumstances of increased iron demands, hepcidin production is decreased, leading to higher expression of ferroportin and an increase in circulating iron.

Hepcidin Regulation

Four main factors exist that regulate hepcidin expression by hepatocytes: Iron status, oxygen tension, erythropoietic activity and inflammation (reviewed by Fleming and Ponka [8] and Zhao et al. [9] among others).

Iron status regulates hepcidin both through liver iron stores and circulating transferrin-bound iron. Increased liver iron stores stimulate the hepatic expression of bone morphogenetic protein 6 (BMP-6). Binding of BMP to its receptor on hepatocytes together with the co-receptor hemojuvelin, leads to activation of the transcription factor, SMAD4 (sons of mothers against decapentaplegic homologue protein 4), thereby stimulating hepcidin transcription. Circulating iron-transferrin complexes lead to the dissociation of the iron sensing molecule, HFE, from TfR1, after which it complexes with TfR2, leading to hepcidin transcription through a signaling cascade that is not yet entirely elucidated, but may involve hemojuvelin-induced hepcidin expression via SMAD signaling.

Decreased oxygen tension leads to increased intracellular levels of the transcription factor, hypoxia-inducible factor-1α (HIF 1α), which prevents BMP-induced hepcidin production through the upregulation of matriptase-2, which cleaves the BMP-co-receptor, hemojuvelin, from the hepatocellular surface. Increased erythropoietic activity markedly decreases hepcidin through a mechanism that is not entirely clarified, but probably requires one or more soluble signaling molecules. Growth differentiation factor 15 (GDF15) and twisted gastrulation protein homolog 1 (TWSG1), may be two of these factors, but others have yet to be discovered. Inflammation-induced hepcidin production is mediated through pro-inflammatory cytokines, mainly interleukin (IL)-6, that lead to activation of signal transducer and activator of transcription 3 (STAT3) through the IL-6 receptor, thereby activating hepcidin transcription. In addition the hepatic expression of activin B, a cytokine of the transforming growth factor-β (TGF-β) superfamily, is increased by inflammation, and also activates the BMP receptor pathway and increases hepcidin expression.

In summary, hepcidin is induced by increased iron supply and inflammation, and downregulated by iron deficiency, hypoxia and erythropoietic activity.

Inflammation-induced Changes in Iron Homeostasis

A profound change in body iron distribution is one of the key features of anemia of critical illness, diverting iron from the circulation to storage sites. Iron is shifted from the extracellular to the intracellular compartment as a result of inflammation by induction of hepcidin production in the liver. This leads to the subsequent internalization and degradation of ferroportin on iron exporting cells, especially macrophages of the reticuloendothelial system. The resultant iron restriction leads to attenuation of erythropoiesis, a process which is already hampered by the inflammatory process through the downregulation of transferrin receptors on erythroid progenitor cells, and the decreased production of erythropoietin (EPO), either as a direct effect of inflammatory cytokines or as a consequence of impaired renal function. These mechanism are identical to those that cause anemia of chronic disease, and therefore 'anemia of inflammation' has been suggested as a better name for anemia that develops in both chronic and acute systemic inflammatory diseases [10].

Typical laboratory changes during anemia of inflammation are a lowered serum iron and transferrin saturation, and an increased ferritin level. As ferritin may be elevated in a variety of conditions, including infection, inflammation and malnutrition, normal or high ferritin levels do not exclude iron deficiency. Low transferrin saturation in combination with high ferritin levels may indicate functional iron deficiency. Reticulocyte counts are typically low compared to the grade of anemia and the reticulocyte hemoglobin content is also diminished. Less common laboratory parameters include zinc-protoporpherin, which is elevated in the case of iron-restricted erythropoiesis, and hepcidin, which is usually increased in the case of inflammation, whereas suppression of hepcidin during inflammation is indicative of absolute iron deficiency. Interestingly, iron deficiency can also exist without anemia. However, the relevance of this for critically ill patients is currently not known.

Effects of Iron on Microbes

Iron Affects Virulence of Pathogens

It is theorized that the shifts in iron distribution during inflammation contribute to innate immunity by withholding iron from pathogens. Iron acquisition is a major determinant for survival and replication of microbes within the host. Human plasma is normally a hostile environment for pathogens. As the antibacterial effect of plasma *in vitro* can be attenuated by adding iron, whereas it can be mimicked *in vitro* by transferrin and lactoferrin, iron binding molecules within the plasma are held responsible for its anti-microbial effect [11].

In vivo experiments have demonstrated that animals injected with various forms of iron are much more susceptible to infection. The clinical relevance of this finding is substantiated by the observation that patients suffering from iron overload are more likely to become infected and have a worse outcome [12]. In addition, iron supplementation during malaria infection has been related to increased mortality [13].

The importance of iron for microbes is further illustrated by the fact that many bacteria and fungal strains possess mechanisms for the acquisition of iron. Three main strategies of microbes to attain iron are:

1) expression of receptors for host iron-binding proteins, such as transferrin, lactoferrin and heme;
2) reductive elemental uptake of iron through cell surface reductases; and
3) utilization of siderophores, which act as high affinity iron chelators to scavenge iron from host iron-carrying molecules. Several hundreds of microbial siderophores have been identified. By exploiting these strategies, microbes can survive in the host even at sites where iron concentrations are quite low.

Animal studies have shown that iron loading worsens experimental sepsis [14]. This is not only related to the fact that microbes can utilize this iron for growth, but mainly because iron can contribute to oxidative stress-induced organ damage. In contrast, iron chelation has been shown to protect against bacterial growth as well as oxidative stress-induced organ damage, and has proven beneficial in animal models of sepsis [15].

Intracellular Versus Extracellular Pathogens

As explained above, infection and inflammation lead to intracellular iron sequestration which is considered part of innate immunity. However, intracellularly living and dividing pathogens might benefit from increased intracellular iron. Indeed, blocking iron efflux by hepcidin or a mutation of ferroportin has a promoting effect on the growth of intracellular pathogens, such as *Salmonella typhimurium*, *Mycobacterium tuberculosis*, *Chlamydia psittaci*, *Chlamydia trachomatis* and *Legionella pneumophila*, whereas lowering cellular iron levels by the expression of ferroportin has the opposite effect [16]. Another striking observation is that iron chelators can inhibit malaria growth *in vitro* and *in vivo* [17] and iron deficiency in patients may protect against malaria probably because the intracellular labile iron pool is significantly reduced during iron deficiency. Hence, in contrast to the beneficial effect of decreased plasma iron in most infections, in case of intracellular infections the opposite may be true. In this context, the local transcriptional upregulation of ferroportin that occurs following infection with *S. typhimurium* or *M. tuberculosis* could be considered as an innate anti-microbial defense mechanism based on iron deprivation [18].

Effects of Iron on the Host

Innate Immunity

Much effort has been put into elucidating the effects of iron on the different aspects of immunity. Many observations seem conflicting, illustrating the complexity of the effects of iron. With regard to innate immunity, it has been shown that elevated intracellular iron promotes nuclear factor-kappa B (NF-κB)-mediated cytokine production [19], while it inhibits expression of the important anti-microbial molecule, inducible nitric oxide synthase (iNOS) [20]. On the other hand, low intracellular iron inhibits NF-κB activity, and iron chelation increases iNOS. Another important transcription factor that is affected by iron status is HIF-1α, a molecule that gets degraded swiftly under physiologic conditions [21]. When intracellular iron concentrations are low, HIF-1α is spared from degradation, so it can act as a transcription factor for several pro-inflammatory cytokines. Therefore, it seems that both iron overload and iron deficiency can lead to enhanced inflammatory signaling, either through NF-κB or HIF-1α.

The fact that intracellular iron concentrations affect the transcription of inflammatory cytokines suggests that ferroportin and hepcidin could also have immune modulating effects. For hepcidin, both pro-inflammatory and anti-inflammatory effects have been reported *in vitro* and *in vivo* [22, 23]. However, as these findings have not yet been reproduced, the immune modulating effects of hepcidin are still the subject of debate.

Less is known about the influence of iron overload on innate immunity. Macrophages from HFE-knockout mice, which have high ferroportin levels and therefore low intracellular iron levels due to a lack of hepcidin, produced lower amounts of tumor necrosis factor (TNF)-α and IL-6 compared to wild-type mice in response to *S. typhimurium* infections. *In vivo* this effect was associated with attenuated inflammation, but increased pathogen burden [24], which could be corrected by administration of hepcidin or ferrous sulfate.

Evidence also is available from animal data showing an aggravated immune response and associated mortality in murine models of sepsis after iron loading [14], whereas iron chelation appears to attenuate inflammation and improve outcome [15]. Direct effects of iron loading and iron chelation therapy on innate immunity in humans are still unknown.

Adaptive Immunity

In contrast to innate immunity, activation of the adaptive immune response is characterized by an extensive proliferation of B and T lymphocytes, which rely on their ability to acquire iron through TfR1. Polyclonal proliferation of human B and T lymphocytes can be inhibited by antibodies against TfR1 [25]. Absence of TfR1 results in the complete arrest of T cell differentiation, whereas the development of IgM positive B cells is severely attenuated [26]. Nutritional iron deficiency is associated with impaired lymphocyte function [27]. Furthermore, the profile of cytokine expression by lymphocytes may be altered by iron deficiency [28] and iron overload [29].

Oxidative Stress

Labile plasma iron and poorly liganded iron have the potential to catalyze Haber-Weiss and Fenton reactions [30], whereby superoxide radical and hydrogen peroxide yield the highly reactive hydroxyl radical, causing damage to cells and organelles. These reactive oxygen intermediates are inevitable byproducts of aerobic respiration and are also generated during several enzymatic reactions. In addition, they are produced by the membrane-bound NADPH oxidase complex, which is primarily expressed in phagocytic neutrophils and macrophages, serving as a tool for antimicrobial defense [31]. During infection this compound is used to generate high levels of superoxide in a 'respiratory burst' in which several species of potent oxidants are formed that enhance microbial killing.

An increase in the steady state levels of reactive oxygen (and nitrogen) species beyond the antioxidant capacity of the organism, called oxidative (and nitrosative) stress, is encountered in many pathological conditions, such as systemic inflammation. Although the respiratory burst is needed for effective pathogen eradication, oxidative stress causes damage to vital organs and may contribute to the development of multiple organ failure. The kidney may be especially vulnerable as an acid environment, such as tubular urine, enhances the formation of reactive hydroxyl radicals. In support of this suggestion, iron and heme-induced oxidative stress caused by cardiopulmonary bypass during cardiac surgery was associated with the development of acute kidney injury [32].

The role of NTBI and labile plasma iron in critical illness and their putative roles in oxidative stress-induced organ injury need to be further investigated. A practical problem in these investigations is that the methods currently available for the measurement of NTBI and labile plasma iron have not yet been analytically and clinically validated.

Consequences for Critical Care

Anemia on the ICU

Anemia is highly prevalent in critically ill and injured patients. Two-thirds of patients are already anemic on admission to the ICU [1], increasing to 97 % of patients by day 8 [1, 2]. ICU-related anemia is not only very frequent among critically ill patients, it is also associated with increased transfusion rates and worse outcome, including weaning failure [33], myocardial infarction [34] and increased risk of death [35]. More than one-third of all ICU patients receive transfusions sometime during their ICU stay, increasing to more than 70 % when ICU stay exceeds one week [1]. Moreover, the number of transfusions is independently associated with longer ICU stay, increased risk of complications and increased mortality [1], stressing the importance of understanding the pathophysiology of ICU-related anemia and finding alternative therapies. In addition, the problem of anemia extends far beyond ICU admission, as approximately 50 % of patients with anemia at ICU discharge were still anemic 6 months later [36].

The development of anemia can be attributed to two main reasons: First, erythrocyte lifespan is extensively shortened due to hemolysis, the increased clearance of erythrocytes by macrophages, diagnostic phlebotomy, tissue injury, invasive procedures and gastrointestinal bleeding. Second, red cell production is attenuated during inflammation, due to decreased EPO production and signaling and the aforementioned alterations in iron metabolism.

Decreased Erythrocyte Lifespan

Blood loss due to tissue injury, invasive procedures (drainage, catheter placement, renal replacement therapy), gastrointestinal bleeding and systemic inflammation-associated hemolysis are obvious reasons for reduced RBC survival in ICU patients. Less obvious is the loss of blood through diagnostic phlebotomy, which represents a mean daily loss of 40 to 70 ml of blood, while under physiological conditions only 2–3 ml of new erythrocytes are formed per day. This phenomenon, termed the "anemia of chronic investigation" [37], has been reported to account for 30 % of required blood transfusions. Including other reasons for blood loss, the median total loss of blood for critically ill patients has been calculated to be as high as 128 ml per day [38], representing a daily iron loss of 64 mg, exceeding normal iron intake more than 20-fold. Considering that during inflammatory states hardly any iron is absorbed due to the actions of hepcidin, the imbalance in iron uptake and iron loss is even greater.

An increased clearance of erythrocytes by macrophages during the inflammatory process has attracted attention over the last decade. It seems that inflammation leads to stress on erythrocytes that may be mediated through cytokines, hypoxia, disturbances in acid-base balance, endothelial damage, oxidative stress or alterations in lipid metabolism, resulting in damage to the red cells and increased phosphatidylserine expression on RBC membranes, flagging them for removal by macrophages of the reticuloendothelial system [39]. In addition, a sudden and continued decrease in EPO production, as can be observed during acute inflammatory states, may promote the clearance of a subset of young erythrocytes by macrophages [40].

Attenuation of RBC Production During Inflammation

Decreased erythrocyte production during inflammatory states is the result of three main mechanisms [41]. First, EPO concentrations decrease quickly and remain inappropriately low during inflammation, probably as a result of a combination of decreased renal function and pro-inflammatory cytokine inhibition. Second, the response of erythroid progenitor cells to EPO is attenuated as well, as a result of direct effects of cytokines and downregulation of EPO receptors. Third, as described earlier, several cytokines, including IL-1β, IL-6 and TNF-α, induce hepcidin production, leading to less serum iron available for the bone marrow. This limits iron availability for erythroid progenitor cells and impairs heme biosynthesis, leading to iron restricted erythropoiesis [41]. This pathway has indeed been shown to be relevant for the anemia observed in sepsis patients [42] as hepcidin levels correlated with the extent of anemia and blood transfusions needed. Impaired iron homeostasis and EPO signaling are worsened by medication often used on the ICU. Norepinephrine and phenylephrine directly inhibit hematopoietic precursor maturation; furthermore, EPO release is suppressed by ACE inhibitors, angiotensin receptor blockers, calcium channel blockers, theophylline, and β-adrenergic blockers.

Erythropoiesis-Stimulating Agents

As the impaired production of EPO and the blunted response to EPO together with iron restriction are central to the anemia of inflammation, some studies have attempted to stimulate erythropoiesis with exogenously administered EPO in critically ill patients. In a meta-analysis, the odds of a patient receiving a blood transfusion were significantly reduced and the number of units of blood transfused per patient was decreased; however, there was no statistically significant effect on length of stay in the ICU or hospital or on overall mortality [43].

Iron Supplementation for the Critically Ill

Low serum iron and high ferritin levels constitute the typical iron profile of critically ill patients and are indicative of an inflammatory iron profile. Despite generally high ferritin levels, iron deficiency often coexists with inflammation and may concern up to 40 % of critically ill patients. Therefore, it has been suggested that iron supplementation, alone or in combination with erythropoiesis-stimulating agents, may also be beneficial in the ICU setting. As mentioned earlier, iron has been shown to promote the growth and virulence of a number of microbes responsible for nosocomial infections. As a result, concern exists related to greater infection rates and (oxidative stress induced) organ injury with iron supplementation. Although this outcome is biologically plausible, evidence from human studies is lacking. Multiple studies have failed to show any increased risk of infection associated with iron therapy in chronic hemodialysis patients [44]. Few studies have examined iron supplementation in the critical care population. Available observational studies in postoperative or critically ill patients show no association between intravenous iron administration and risk of infection [45]. In 863 patients undergoing cardiopulmonary bypass surgery who were subsequently treated with both intravenous iron and EPO or with blood transfusions, there was no difference in subsequent infection rate [46]. In a trial of 200 patients receiving care in a surgical ICU [47], it was shown that enteral iron supplementation (ferrous sulfate 325 mg three times daily) reduced transfusion rate in patients with baseline iron deficiency. Finally, intravenous iron therapy with and without EPO administration reduces allogeneic blood transfusions in surgical patients [48]. Iron appears to be effective in correcting anemia, despite inflammation. Moreover, none of these studies has shown a clear adverse effect on infection rates, which is compatible with the notion that the NTBI fraction in particular is important for the risk of infection, whereas this fraction is usually low in iron-deficient patients even after iron treatment. A multicenter randomized clinical trial of intravenous iron for the treatment of anemia in critically ill trauma patients is currently being performed (ClinicalTrials.gov identifier NCT01180894).

In addition to the lack of clear evidence that iron administration is harmful to the iron-deficient critically ill patient, iron deficiency is also associated with impaired immunity and increased susceptibility to infection, as well as being associated with increased length of stay in the ICU [49], providing an extra reason to further examine the possible role of iron administration in the setting of intensive care medicine.

Future Perspectives

Although iron homeostasis is complicated, it is clear that iron can play a crucial role during infection or inflammation in critically ill patients. However, although the discovery of several novel players in iron metabolism, including hepcidin and its interaction with ferroportin, has resulted in an enormous surge in research on iron biology, a lot still needs to be learned, especially with regard to the ICU setting. Future research should clarify whether iron plays a detrimental role in the development of organ failure or not. Most notably, the occurrence of labile plasma iron during operative procedures and during the ICU stay and its relation with the occurrence of organ dysfunction should be investigated. In addition, iron may play a decisive role in infections, in which for some reason pathogens are not fully eradicated despite optimal antimicrobial treatment, and hold potential for therapeutic intervention.

In the case of iron deficiency, the possibility of treating anemia with intravenous iron supplementation in critically ill patients should be further examined, either in combination with erythropoiesis-stimulating agents or not. In elective major surgical procedures, such as coronary artery surgery, early iron fortification can probably accelerate recovery and prevent complications from anemia. Finally, therapies directed against the action of hepcidin are being developed, which may be useful in the future treatment of anemia of critical illness.

Conclusion

Profound changes in iron metabolism occur in critically ill patients. These changes are predominantly the result of both blood loss and the inflammatory process, and are relevant to the intensive care patient for three reasons:

1) anemia is frequently observed in critically ill patients, is associated with impaired immunity and worse outcome, and cannot be adequately compensated by transfusions or erythropoiesis – stimulating agents, whereas there might be an additive role for iron supplementation;
2) iron homeostasis may determine the fate of an infection, as iron is an essential nutrient for pathogens, and future research should, therefore, clarify the exact role of bound and unbound iron in critically ill infected patients;
3) iron can catalyze oxidative stress reactions that cause organ damage, especially when non-transferrin-bound or labile iron exists. This latter observation is especially relevant to the critically ill patient as they are likely to suffer from oxidative stress and organ failure, whereas at the same time increased labile iron concentrations are more likely to be present.

Future studies should further clarify the role of iron in critical illness and organ dysfunction, as the prevention of non-transferrin-bound or labile iron may contribute to the prevention of organ dysfunction, whereas at the same time, iron supplementation or counteracting the actions of hepcidin may represent an adjuvant therapy to prevent anemia of critical illness.

References

1. Corwin HL, Gettinger A, Pearl RG et al (2004) The CRIT Study: Anemia and blood transfusion in the critically ill-current clinical practice in the United States. Crit Care Med 32:39–52
2. Thomas J, Jensen L, Nahirniak S, Gibney RT (2010) Anemia and blood transfusion practices in the critically ill: a prospective cohort review. Heart Lung 39:217–225
3. Ganz T (2003) Hepcidin, a key regulator of iron metabolism and mediator of anemia of inflammation. Blood 102:783–788
4. Bullen JJ, Rogers HJ, Griffiths E (1978) Role of iron in bacterial infection. Curr Top Microbiol Immunol 80:1–35
5. Brissot P, Ropert M, Le Lan C, Loréal O (2012) Non-transferrin bound iron: a key role in iron overload and iron toxicity. Biochim Biophys Acta 1820:403–410
6. Andrews NC, Schmidt PJ (2007) Iron homeostasis. Annu Rev Physiol 69:69–85
7. Nemeth E, Tuttle MS, Powelson J (2004) Hepcidin regulates cellular iron efflux by binding to ferroportin and inducing its internalization. Science 306:2090–2093
8. Fleming RE, Ponka P (2012) Iron overload in human disease. N Engl J Med 366:348–359
9. Zhao N, Zhang AS, Enns CA (2013) Iron regulation by hepcidin. J Clin Invest 123:2337–2343
10. Corwin HL, Krantz SB (2000) Anemia of the critically ill: "acute" anemia of chronic disease. Crit Care Med 28:3098–3099
11. Kochan I (1973) The role of iron in bacterial infections, with special consideration of host-tubercle bacillus interaction. Curr Top Microbiol Immunol 60:1–30
12. Bullen JJ, Rogers HJ, Spalding PB, Ward CG (2006) Natural resistance, iron and infection: a challenge for clinical medicine. J Med Microbiol 55:251–258

13. Sazawal S, Black RE, Ramsan M et al (2006) Effects of routine prophylactic supplementation with iron and folic acid on admission to hospital and mortality in preschool children in a high malaria transmission setting: community-based, randomised, placebo-controlled trial. Lancet 367:133–143

14. Zager RA (2005) Parenteral iron treatment induces MCP-1 accumulation in plasma, normal kidneys, and in experimental nephropathy. Kidney Int 68:1533–1542

15. Messaris E, Antonakis PT, Memos N, Chatzigianni E, Leandros E, Konstadoulakis MM (2004) Deferoxamine administration in septic animals: improved survival and altered apoptotic gene expression. Int Immunopharmacol 4:455–459

16. Paradkar PN, De Domenico I, Durchfort N, Zohn I, Kaplan J, Ward DM (2008) Iron depletion limits intracellular bacterial growth in macrophages. Blood 112:866–874

17. Hershko C, Peto TE (1988) Deferoxamine inhibition of malaria is independent of host iron status. J Exp Med 168:375–387

18. Cherayil BJ (2010) Iron and immunity: immunological consequences of iron deficiency and overload. Arch Immunol Ther Exp (Warsz) 58:407–415

19. Bubici C, Papa S, Dean K, Franzoso G (2006) Mutual cross-talk between reactive oxygen species and nuclear factor-kappa B: molecular basis and biological significance. Oncogene 25:6731–6748

20. Weiss G, Werner-Felmayer G, Werner ER, Grünewald K, Wachter H, Hentze MW (1994) Iron regulates nitric oxide synthase activity by controlling nuclear transcription. J Exp Med 180:969–976

21. Kaelin WG, Ratcliffe PJ Jr. (2008) Oxygen sensing by metazoans: the central role of the HIF hydroxylase pathway. Mol Cell 30:393–402

22. De Domenico I, Koening CL, Zhang TY et al (2010) Hepcidin mediates transcriptional changes that modulate acute cytokine-induced inflammatory responses in mice. J Clin Invest 120:2395–2405

23. Pagani A, Nai A, Corna G et al (2011) Low hepcidin accounts for the proinflammatory status associated with iron deficiency. Blood 118:736–746

24. Wang L, Johnson EE, Shi HN, Walker WA, Wessling-Resnick M, Cherayil BJ (2008) Attenuated inflammatory responses in hemochromatosis reveal a role for iron in the regulation of macrophage cytokine translation. J Immunol 181:2723–2731

25. Kemp JD, Thorson JA, Gomez F, Smith KM, Cowdery JS, Ballas ZK (1989) Inhibition of lymphocyte activation with anti-transferrin receptor Mabs: a comparison of three reagents and further studies of their range of effects and mechanism of action. Cell Immunol 122:218–230

26. Ned RM, Swat W, Andrews NC (2003) Transferrin receptor 1 is differentially required in lymphocyte development. Blood 102:3711–3718

27. Oppenheimer SJ (2001) Iron and its relation to immunity and infectious disease. J Nutr 131:616S–633S

28. Jason J, Archibald LK, Nwanyanwu OC et al (2001) The effects of iron deficiency on lymphocyte cytokine production and activation: preservation of hepatic iron but not at all cost. Clin Exp Immunol 126:466–473

29. Melo RA, Garcia AB, Viana SR, Falcão RP (1997) Lymphocyte subsets in experimental hemochromatosis. Acta Haematol 98:72–75

30. Gutteridge JM (1986) Iron promoters of the Fenton reaction and lipid peroxidation can be released from haemoglobin by peroxides. FEBS Lett 201:291–295

31. Hampton MB, Kettle AJ, Winterbourn CC (1998) Inside the neutrophil phagosome: oxidants, myeloperoxidase, and bacterial killing. Blood 92:3007–3017

32. Haase M, Bellomo R, Haase-Fielitz A (2010) Novel biomarkers, oxidative stress, and the role of labile iron toxicity in cardiopulmonary bypass-associated acute kidney injury. J Am Coll Cardiol 55:2024–2033

33. Khamiees M, Raju P, DeGirolamo A, Amoateng-Adjepong Y, Manthous CA (2001) Predictors of extubation outcome in patients who have successfully completed a spontaneous breathing trial. Chest 120:1262–1270

34. Thygesen K, Alpert JS, White HD et al (2007) Universal definition of myocardial infarction. Eur Heart J 28:2525–2538
35. Rasmussen L, Christensen S, Lenler-Petersen P, Johnsen SP (2011) Anemia and 90-day mortality in COPD patients requiring invasive mechanical ventilation. Clin Epidemiol 3:1–5
36. Bateman AP, McArdle F, Walsh TS (2009) Time course of anemia during six months follow up following intensive care discharge and factors associated with impaired recovery of erythropoiesis. Crit Care Med 37:1906–1912
37. Barie PS (2004) Phlebotomy in the intensive care unit: strategies for blood conservation. Crit Care 8:34–36
38. von Ahnsen N, Muller C, Serke S, Frei U, Eckardt KU (1999) Important role of nondiagnostic blood loss and blunted erythropoietic response in the anemia of medical intensive care patients. Crit Care Med 27:2630–2639
39. Reggiori G, Occhipinti G, De Gasperi A, Vincent JL, Piagnerelli M (2009) Early alterations of red blood cell rheology in critically ill patients. Crit Care Med 37:3041–3046
40. Rice L, Alfrey CP (2005) The negative regulation of red cell mass by neocytolysis: physiologic and pathophysiologic manifestations. Cell Physiol Biochem 15:245–250
41. Weiss G, Goodnough LT (2005) Anemia of chronic disease. N Engl J Med 352:1011–1023
42. van Eijk LT, Kroot JJ, van der Hoeven JG, Swinkels DW, Pickkers P (2011) Inflammation-induced hepcidin-25 is associated with the development of anemia in septic patients: an observational study. Crit Care 15:R9
43. Zarychanski R, Turgeon AF, McIntyre L, Fergusson DA (2007) Erythropoietin-receptor agonists in critically ill patients: a meta-analysis of randomized controlled trials. CMAJ 177:725–734
44. Hayat A (2008) Safety issues with intravenous iron products in the management of anemia in chronic kidney disease. Clin Med Res 6:93–102
45. Hoen B, Paul-Dauphin A, Kessler M (2002) Intravenous iron administration does not significantly increase the risk of bacteremia in chronic hemodialysis patients. Clin Nephrol 57:457–461
46. Torres S, Kuo YH, Morris K, Neibart R, Holtz JB, Davis JM (2006) Intravenous iron following cardiac surgery does not increase the infection rate. Surg Infect (Larchmt) 7:361–366
47. Pieracci FM, Henderson P, Rodney JR et al (2009) Randomized, double-blind, placebo-controlled trial of effects of enteral iron supplementation on anemia and risk of infection during surgical critical illness. Surg Infect (Larchmt) 10:9–19
48. Shander A, Spence RK, Auerbach M (2010) Can intravenous iron therapy meet the unmet needs created by the new restrictions on erythropoietic stimulating agents? Transfusion 50:719–732
49. Bellamy MC, Gedney JA (1998) Unrecognised iron deficiency in critical illness. Lancet 352:1903
50. Swinkels DW, Janssen MC, Bergmans J, Marx JJ (2006) Hereditary hemochromatosis: genetic complexity and new diagnostic approaches. Clin Chem 52:950–968

Sepsis Guideline Implementation: Benefits, Pitfalls and Possible Solutions

N. Kissoon

Introduction

Clinical practice guidelines are useful in improving quality of care and outcomes, reducing inappropriate variation in practice, promoting efficient use of resources, informing and empowering patients and informing public policy. However, difficulties arise when guidelines are poorly introduced into routine daily practice and, as a consequence, many patients do not receive the care intended or receive harmful or unnecessary care [1].

Many guidelines have been formulated for the treatment of sepsis in children and adults [2–6]. These guidelines emphasize early recognition and aggressive treatment of the patient with sepsis in order to improve outcomes. However, the context in which a guideline is to be used is important and to a large extent determines whether it will be implemented successfully [2, 3, 6–8]. Thus, in an attempt to make sepsis guidelines relevant in both resource-poor and resource-rich environments, the level of resources in various settings have been taken into account and guidelines have been formulated to suit both resource rich and poor regions of the world [2–4]. Sepsis guidelines for children have also been designed to accommodate both resource and skill sets for countries with varying under-five mortality rates (Fig. 1) and to accommodate resources for monitoring and treatment from district clinics to tertiary care facilities [2] (Fig. 2), while guidelines for sepsis management of both adults and children have been proposed by the Global Intensive Care Working Group of the European Society of Intensive Care Medicine [3]. In addition, tremendous effort has been expended in revising the Surviving Sepsis Campaign guidelines to include new evidence since its previous iteration in 2008 [4]. Although these efforts are laudable, adherence to these guidelines has met with mixed results in both resource poor and rich regions. Therefore, while resources to im-

N. Kissoon ✉
British Columbia Childrens Hospital, BC V6H 3V4 Vancouver, Canada
e-mail: nkissoon@cw.bc.ca

J.-L. Vincent (Ed.), *Annual Update in Intensive Care and Emergency Medicine 2014*,
DOI 10.1007/978-3-319-03746-2_3, © Springer International Publishing Switzerland
and BioMed Central Ltd. 2014

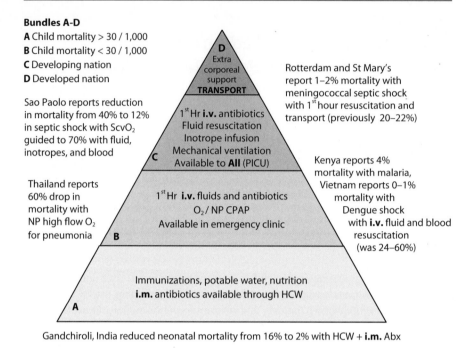

Bundles A-D

A Child mortality > 30 / 1,000
B Child mortality < 30 / 1,000
C Developing nation
D Developed nation

Sao Paolo reports reduction in mortality from 40% to 12% in septic shock with ScvO$_2$ guided to 70% with fluid, inotropes, and blood

Thailand reports 60% drop in mortality with NP high flow O$_2$ for pneumonia

Rotterdam and St Mary's report 1–2% mortality with meningococcal septic shock with 1st hour resuscitation and transport (previously 20–22%)

Kenya reports 4% mortality with malaria, Vietnam reports 0–1% mortality with Dengue shock with **i.v.** fluid and blood resuscitation (was 24–60%)

D Extra corporeal support **TRANSPORT**

1st Hr **i.v.** antibiotics
Fluid resuscitation
Inotrope infusion
Mechanical ventilation
Available to **All** (PICU)

1st Hr **i.v.** fluids and antibiotics
O$_2$ / NP CPAP
Available in emergency clinic

Immunizations, potable water, nutrition
i.m. antibiotics available through HCW

Gandchiroli, India reduced neonatal mortality from 16% to 2% with HCW + **i.m.** Abx

Fig. 1 Global Newborn and Child Sepsis guidelines: Proposed Bundles A-D align with local resources. CPAP: continuous positive airway pressure; i.v.: intravenous; i.m.: intramuscular; ScvO$_2$: central venous oxygen saturation; Abx: antibiotics; pRBCs: packed red blood cells; PICU: pediatric intensive care unit; HCW: healthcare worker

plement guidelines are important, other factors beyond resources may also mitigate against successful adoption. This manuscript will address some of these issues. It will outline the benefits of compliance with sepsis guidelines, the published experience with compliance, possible reasons for poor compliance and offer some possible solutions to improve compliance and ultimately patient outcomes.

Benefits of Compliance with Sepsis Guidelines

There is no doubt that adherence with guidelines is associated with better outcomes. Indeed, adherence to the American College of Critical Care Medicine (ACCM) guidelines for children has led to a 30 % decrease in mortality when the guidelines for initial resuscitation were followed by physicians in community hospitals [9]. Moreover, a decrease of 27 % in mortality was seen in children managed according to ACCM guidelines, including central venous oxygen saturation (ScvO$_2$)-directed therapy, in an intensive care unit [10]. Adherence to sepsis guidelines in a pediatric emergency department in Texas resulted in a decrease in the need for mechanical ventilation and vasoactive agents and a decrease in mortality from 4 to 2.5 % [11].

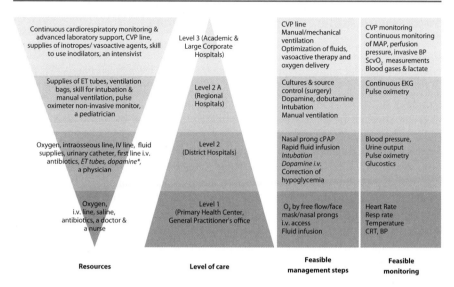

Resources	Level of care	Feasible management steps	Feasible monitoring
Continuous cardiorespiratory monitoring & advanced laboratory support, CVP line, supplies of inotropes/ vasoactive agents, skill to use inodilators, an intensivist	Level 3 (Academic & Large Corporate Hospitals)	CVP line Manual/mechanical ventilation Optimization of fluids, vasoactive therapy and oxygen delivery	CVP monitoring Continuous monitoring of MAP, perfusion pressure, invasive BP ScvO₂ measurements Blood gases & lactate
Supplies of ET tubes, ventilation bags, skill for intubation & manual ventilation, pulse oximeter non-invasive monitor, a pediatrician	Level 2 A (Regional Hospitals)	Cultures & source control (surgery) Dopamine, dobutamine Intubation Manual ventilation	Continuous EKG Pulse oximetry
Oxygen, intraosseous line, IV line, fluid supplies, urinary catheter, first line i.v. antibiotics, ET tubes, dopamine*, a physician	Level 2 (District Hospitals)	Nasal prong cPAP Rapid fluid infusion Intubation Dopamine i.v. Correction of hypoglycemia	Blood pressure, Urine output Pulse oximetry Glucostics
Oxygen, i.v. line, saline, antibiotics, a doctor & a nurse	Level 1 (Primary Health Center, General Practitioner's office)	O₂ by free flow/face mask/nasal prongs i.v. access Fluid infusion	Heart Rate Resp rate Temperature CRT, BP

Fig. 2 Resources and interventions expected to be made available at different levels of health care facilities in resource-poor economies. CVP: central venous pressure; MAP: mean arterial pressure; ScvO₂: central venous oxygen saturation; BP: blood pressure; ET: endotracheal * *Not available universally at all level 2 facilities*

Guideline adherence in children with sepsis resulted in a 57 % reduction in pediatric intensive care unit (PICU) hospital length of stay in Boston [12], while in Utah increasing compliance with sepsis guidelines resulted in a decrease in mortality from 8.4 to 3.5 % [13]. In all these instances, although outcomes improved with compliance, adherence to some elements of the guideline was less than optimal and in many instances the entire bundle was provided to few patients. Similar findings have been seen in adults in the Surviving Sepsis Campaign in which there was a significant decrease in mortality with adherence to resuscitation and management bundles [14]. Unadjusted hospital mortality decreased from 37 % to 30.8 % over 2 years (p = 0.001), offering optimism for further improvement in outcomes [14]. The experience of the World Federation of Pediatric Intensive and Critical Care Societies (WFPICCS) initiative in children is similar with significant decreases in mortality with compliance with the resuscitation bundle (OR 0.40, 95 % CI 0.19-0.72 p < 0.004) and compliance with the management bundle was also associated with a decrease in mortality (OR 0.30, 95 % CI 0.10-0.80, p < 0.018) [2]. These benefits applied to children in both the developed and the developing world. In addition, although outcomes improved as resources increased, adherence did not differ markedly suggesting that resources, while important, are not the only determinant of compliance.

Success with Adherence to Sepsis Guidelines

In the WFPICCS endeavor, resuscitation bundle compliance ranged from 24–52 % while management bundle compliance range from 10–25 % across centers [2]. Similarly, in the Surviving Sepsis Campaign, compliance with the entire management bundle started at 18 % and increased to approximately 36 % at the end of two years [14]. In children in areas that were adequately resourced, the news is no better. Indeed, there was 19 % adherence to the resuscitation bundle at Boston Children's Hospital with significant delays in intravenous fluid administration and inotrope administration [13]. In Utah and Texas, while intense efforts achieved an increase in compliance, this was still suboptimal, with the highest compliance – 80 % – for intravenous fluids, antibiotic administration and lactate evaluation [11, 12]. Delayed recognition and delayed intravenous fluids and inotropes were also reported, along with a 36 % adherence to pre-PICU care, in a follow-up assessment of treatment guidelines for meningococcemia in the UK [15]. In India, a survey reported 12 % adherence to the ACCM guidelines among physicians; this low adherence was attributed mostly to lack of skills and knowledge [16]. Adherence to guidelines has also been poor in other parts of the world, including in Africa, where less than 50 % of the Surviving Sepsis Campaign guidelines were implemented; the predominant reasons were resource-limitations and lack of education [7]. In Asia (China, Hong Kong, India, Malaysia, Singapore and South Korea) adherence to Surviving Sepsis Campaign guidelines ranged from 5–15 % [17]. Low adherence to sepsis guidelines was also found in Germany, where there was a perception reality gap; physicians perceived that adherence to low tidal volume ventilation was 80 %, whereas in reality it was 2.6–17 %. Similarly, the perception of adherence to glycemic control was 66 % whereas the reality was 6 % [18]. Suboptimal management related to lack of adherence to sepsis guidelines has also been reported in children in France, England, and Australia [19–21]. In most cases, suboptimal management resulted from underestimation of disease severity, physician delay in administrating antibiotics or fluids, insufficient fluid administration and inadequate inotropic support.

Reasons for Poor Adherence

Major contributors to poor adherence to guidelines are many fold and include failure to recognize sepsis, lack of familiarity or lack of awareness of the sepsis guideline, lack of agreement with the specific guideline, or lack of agreement with guidelines in general, as well as lack of motivation [22, 23]. In addition there are many external barriers to guideline implementation. For instance, the characteristics of the guidelines may render them impractical to implement – in some cases they are too detailed and try to address all eventualities, whereas in others they may suggest resources, such as laboratory tests, methods of monitoring and treatment options, that are not available locally [3, 6, 7]. Environmental factors, such as lack of time, lack of resources, lack of reimbursement and organizational constraints, may also preclude adoption of guidelines. For instance, in areas where there are critical staff

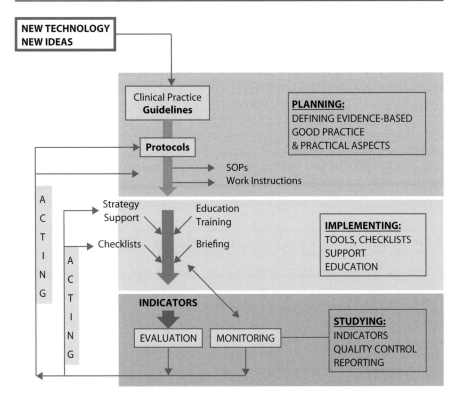

Fig. 3 Clinical practice guidelines: Preparation, implementation, evaluation and revision are all important for successful adoption

shortages, it is unreasonable to place further burdens, such as frequent monitoring and documentation, which are the standard of care in areas with substantially more resources. In many areas of the world, white blood cell counts to determine systemic inflammatory response syndrome (SIRS) criteria, laboratory capabilities for blood culture and pulse oximetry or supplemental oxygen are not readily available [6, 7].

Poor guideline adoption may also be due to the fact that incentives may not be aligned to the behavior. There are also concerns which lead to skepticism that guidelines may be subject to biases (used as a financial and marketing tool). Doubts about the evidence on which a guideline is based stems from skepticism of the composition of the panels of experts that mold these judgments. While guideline users could sometimes adjust for these biases, in some cases the values and goals and conflicts are not explicit to allow for any adjustments. Moreover, some have argued that there are too many sepsis guidelines and some are out of date and present conflicting information. A major concern in the United States is the fact that these guidelines may be turned into performance measures to critique the quality of physician care and even dictate hospital accreditation.

In our local experience, clinicians were skeptical when a sepsis guideline was introduced because they felt that screening for sepsis in the emergency department was not necessary because their triage system was robust enough to detect sepsis. Others felt their pediatric early warning systems served the same purpose on the wards, and still others felt that introduction of the sepsis guideline implied that they were managing sepsis incorrectly beforehand. These reasons for skepticism are not unique to any single institution or any particular guideline and imply that crafting a resource-appropriate guideline is an important process but without attention to cultural issues, implementation and adoption are likely to be less than optimal (Fig. 3 [24]). Another area that has hindered adoption and sustainability is the failure to measure meaningful outcomes and share the information widely with team members.

A Framework for Crafting a Sepsis Guideline

In order to circumvent some of the barriers outlined above, as a first step, the guideline writing process should be rigorous and transparent. It is important that appropriate clinicians and policy makers be involved early in the discussion pertaining either to crafting a guideline *de novo* or to adapting an existing guideline, such as the WFPICCS society or Surviving Sepsis Campaign guidelines. This is important because failure to invite the appropriate broad representation to the table will likely lead to frustration, suspicion and ultimately failure. For example, in our institution an oversight on our part was failure to involve pharmacy representatives at the start of the process even though they are involved in stocking unit doses of antibiotics in the emergency room and ICUs.

The AGREE tool is an example of a tool that provides a roadmap to either create or evaluate a guideline (http://www.agreetrust.org). Strict adherence to the elements included in such a roadmap will enable all stages to be conducted without missing any important steps, will insure the appropriate team members are involved, and will insure transparency and literature review. It will also allow evaluation of the necessary resources and outcome measures as well as opportunities for revising the guideline. The AGREE tool consists of 6 domains (Table 1) that address all aspects of implementation. Each of these domains controls a series of items (total 23) that guide every step of guideline development and address factors that may preclude adoption. AGREE is not the only tool that serves to assist in guideline development but it is validated, easy to use, widely accepted and comes with an easily accessible training manual.

Barriers to successful guideline implementation are summarized in Fig. 4. Poor adherence can be due to inherent flaws in the process used in preparing the guidelines as outlined above, but just as important are the strategies used in implementation. Moreover, if quality control indicators for evaluation and monitoring are not appropriate and agreed on, monitoring will be haphazard and inadequate and provide meaningless information. This poses a problem in that if outcome measures are not monitored diligently, it is very difficult to determine the effectiveness of

Table 1 The Appraisal of Guidelines for Research and Evaluation (AGREE)

Domain 1. *Scope and Purpose*:	The overall aim of the guideline, the specific health questions, and the target population.
Domain 2. *Stakeholder Involvement*:	The extent to which the guideline was developed by the appropriate stakeholders and represents the views of its intended users.
Domain 3. *Rigor of Development*:	The process used to gather and synthesize the evidence, the methods to formulate the recommendations, and to update them.
Domain 4. *Clarity of Presentation*:	The language, structure, and format of the guideline.
Domain 5. *Applicability*:	The likely barriers and facilitators to implementation, strategies to improve uptake, and resource implications of applying the guideline.
Domain 6. *Editorial Independence*:	The formulation of recommendations not being unduly biased with competing interests.
Overall assessment:	Includes the rating of the overall quality of the guideline and whether the guideline would be recommended for use in practice.

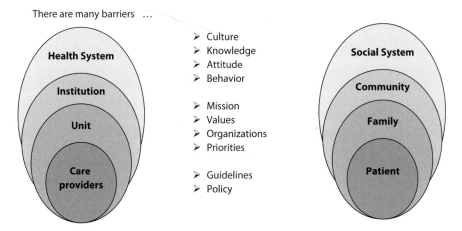

Fig. 4 Barriers to successful guideline implementation: All must be addressed for successful adoption of guidelines

the guideline and to act to revise the guideline and protocol or address deficiencies in guideline implementation. Feedback loops using rapid PDSA (Plan, Do, Study, Act) cycles are important to continuously improve the guideline itself as well as to address cultural, resource and care process issues. In addition, with the advent of new technology, the framework used should include processes to incorporate these new facets to improve the care processes (Fig. 3).

Obstacles and Solutions in Implementation

In many parts of the developing world, poor guideline adherence is due to a lack of resources such that those who are responsible for implementation of the guideline are unable to do so. The obstacles in sepsis guideline implementation are unique to the local environment and hence an environmental scan is important to highlight the deficiencies that need to be addressed [7]. In some areas, the deficiencies are obvious and mostly relate to a lack of personnel and supplies. For example, in many areas of the world, human resources and equipment and supplies, such as antimicrobials, fluids and oxygen, are lacking or sporadically available. Essential staff, equipment and supplies, therefore, need to be provided for successful implementation [25, 26]. Deficiencies such as these should be brought to the attention of clinicians in positions of authority and policymakers so that they can be addressed. There are limits to the resources that can be invested and this also highlights the importance of crafting guidelines that are realistic to the local context. For example, expectations regarding laboratory monitoring for diagnosis and response to therapy are context dependent; in many areas of the world, blood counts are rarely available and monitoring may involve vital signs and pulse oximetry only.

Overcoming some of the major challenges also requires creativity especially when resources are limited. For example, lack of time and staff is a major barrier that can be somewhat circumvented by creating standard operating procedures [5, 9, 10–13, 27]. Sepsis screening, for example, should be incorporated into the triage process in emergency departments rather than be done separately. In as much as possible, sepsis screening and treatment must be standard work and hence also be congruent with early warning scores and systems [28]. In addition, creating sepsis carts and standard flow sheets can also assist in standardizing and avoiding duplication of work. Prepacked kits consisting of intravenous cannulas and fluid administration sets as well as readily accessible essential drugs and fluids may also encourage greater compliance. Specialized training and equipment is also an issue but in resource limited environments less invasive monitoring, use of peripheral inotropes and procedural training may be needed.

Lack of education, including recognition of signs and symptoms of sepsis, is an issue that may lend to poor compliance and needs to be addressed. With little training, even patients and families, village health workers and non-physician clinicians, such as anesthetic assistants and nurses, can be taught to recognize and treat sepsis, as reported from Malawi [25, 26]. Familiarity with the guideline should be insured as well as insuring that several versions are not in circulation. Courses that are sanctioned by the World Health Organization, such as the Emergency Triage Assessment and Treatment and the Integrated Management of Adolescent and Adult Illness, are useful in resource poor areas and address critical illness as well as sepsis [6, 29].

What poses greater difficulty is attitudinal and cultural aversion to guideline adoption and adherence (Fig. 2). To overcome this barrier, advocacy, leadership and support is necessary from clinicians and policy makers alike to address all facets of process and structure (Fig. 5). We have found that involvement of an anthropologist to assist in identifying causes of aversion and to facilitate change can enable

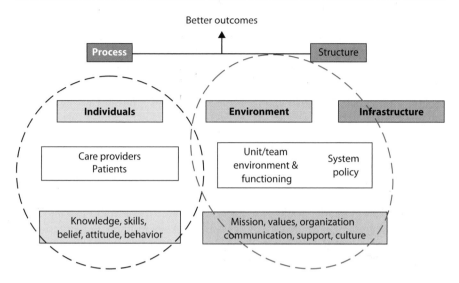

Fig. 5 Improving performance in sepsis management requires attention to both process and structure. Individuals, the environment and infrastructure must be conducive to successful guideline adoption

dramatic positive gains. Attempts at building a community of practice emphasizing shared values and goals and shared learning experiences can also be a useful robust enabler. A community of practice may generate innovative ideas to circumvent resource limitations, ensure staff engagement and advance educational efforts [30, 31]. A community of practice can foster collaboration among medical specialties, such as the emergency department and the ICU, through standard operating practices. A team model is associated with an increase in compliance with guideline of 80 % versus 40 % in the non-team model [8]. The community can also foster early referral to the ICU and involvement of sepsis crash teams and rapid response teams in the care of patients with sepsis. A stewardship program can enable a robust quality assurance program and the designation of an ambassador and feedback systems can facilitate sustainability [30, 32]. Ultimately, ensuring guideline adherence requires a gargantuan effort from those in leadership such that the culture of the organization changes to embrace guidelines as part of standard work. Moreover, commitment has to be ongoing because a decline in vigilance is likely to result in loss of previous gains [5]. The rewards for sustained dogged effort can be improved guideline adherence both in resource-rich and resource-poor environments.

Conclusion

Guidelines are useful in improving the quality of care and outcomes, reducing inappropriate variation in practice and promoting efficient use of resources. However, the benefits are hampered by poor adoption in both resource-rich and resource-poor environments. Adoption and adherence to guidelines is hampered by many factors, including the very nature of the process used in preparing the guidelines, as well as clinicians' skepticism, cultural aversion to guidelines and resource limitations that preclude implementation.

In order to circumvent these issues it is suggested that a uniform and transparent inclusive process be used to craft the guidelines. The AGREE tool is one example of a system to insure that guideline development is rigorous. Strict adherence to its elements will enable *all* steps of the guideline process to be conducted, will involve the appropriate team members, and will insure transparency and literature review. Such tools also include systems to allow evaluation of resources needed and outcome measures as well as opportunities for revising the guideline. The guidelines should also be crafted with a knowledge of the context they would be employed. An environmental scan to identify the possible barriers to implementation in any setting is important. The most common barriers are lack of personnel and resources for carrying out the steps required for guideline adherence. These barriers should be addressed early in the implementation stage for guideline adoption to be successful. Rigorous attention should be paid to outcome measures to determine adherence to guidelines as well as relevance to patient care. Many of the barriers to guideline adherence can be overcome by close adherence to the culture of the environment in which the guideline will be adopted. Developing a community of practice in which all clinicians are involved in the development and promotion of the guidelines may ensure their success. Ensuring that a guideline is successfully adopted requires a tremendous investment of resources and effort. However, the favorable outcomes associated with guideline adherence far outweigh the effort that is needed for successful implementation.

References

1. Grol R, Grimshaw J (2003) From best evidence to best practice: effective implementation of change in patients' care. Lancet 36:1225–1230
2. Kissoon N, Carcillo JA, Espinosa V et al (2011) World Federation of Pediatric and Intensive Care Societies: Global Sepsis Initiative. Pediatr Crit Care Med 12:494–503
3. Dunser MW, Festic E, Dondorp A et al (2012) Recommendations for sepsis management in resource-limited settings. Intensive Care Med 38:557–574
4. Dellinger RP, Levy MM, Rhodes A et al (2013) Surviving Sepsis Campaign: international guidelines for management of severe sepsis and septic shock 2012. Intensive Care Med 39:165–228
5. Plambech MZ, Lurie AI, Ipsen HL (2012) Initial successful implementation of sepsis guidelines in an emergency department. Dan Med J 59:A4545
6. Jacob ST, Lim M, Banura P et al (2013) Integrating sepsis management recommendations into clinical care guidelines for district hospitals in resource-limited settings: the necessity to augment new guidelines with future research. BMC Med 11:107
7. Baelani I, Jochberger S, Laimer T et al (2012) Identifying resource needs for sepsis care and guideline implementation in the Democratic Republic of the Congo: a cluster survey of 66 hospitals in four eastern provinces. Middle East J Anesthesiol 21:559–575

8. Na S, Kuan WS, Mahadevan M et al (2012) Implementation of early goal-directed therapy and the surviving sepsis campaign resuscitation bundle in Asia. Int J Qual Health Care 24(5):452–462

9. Han YY, Carcillo JA, Dragotta MA et al (2003) Early reversal of pediatric-neonatal septic shock by community physicians is associated with improved outcome. Pediatrics 112:793–799

10. De Oliveira CF, deOliveira DS, Gottschald AF et al (2008) ACCM/PALS hemodynamic support guidelines for paediatric septic shock: an outcomes comparison with and without monitoring central venous oxygen saturation. Intensive Care Med 34:1065–1075

11. Cruz AT, Perry AM, Williams EA et al (2011) Implementation of goal-directed therapy for children with suspected sepsis in the emergency department. Pediatrics 127:e758–e766

12. Larsen GY, Mecham N, Greenbert R (2011) An emergency department septic shock protocol and care guideline for children initiated at triage. Pediatrics 127:e1585–e1592

13. Paul R, Neuman MI, Monuteaux MC, Melendez E (2012) Adherence to PALS sepsis guidelines and hospital length of stay. Pediatrics 130:e273–e280

14. Levy MM, Dellinger RP, Townsend SR et al (2010) The Surviving Sepsis Campaign: results of an international guideline-based performance improvement program targeting severe sepsis. Crit Care Med 38:367–374

15. Ninis N, Phillips C, Bailey L et al (2005) The role of healthcare delivery in the outcomes of meningococcal disease in children: case-control study of fatal and non-fatal cases. BMJ 330:1475

16. Santhanam I, Kissoon N, Kamath SR, Ranjit S, Ramesh J, Shankar J (2009) GAP between knowledge and skills for the implementation of the ACCM/PALS septic shock guidelines in India: is the bridge too far? Indian J Crit Care Med 13:54–58

17. Phua J, Koh Y, Du B et al (2011) Management of severe sepsis in patients admitted to Asian intensive care units: prospective cohort study. BMJ 13:342:d3245

18. Brunkhorst FM, Engel C, Ragaller M et al (2008) Practice and perception – a nationwide survey of therapy habits in sepsis. Crit Care Med 36(27):199–125

19. Launay E, Gras-Le Guen C, Martinot A et al (2010) Suboptimal care in the initial management of children who died from severe bacterial infection: a population-based confidential inquiry. Pediatr Crit Care Med 11:469–474

20. Inwalds DP, Tasker RC, Peters MJ, Nadel S (2009) Emergency management of children with severe sepsis in the United Kingdom: the results of the Paediatric Intensive Care Society sepsis audit. Arch Dis Child 94:348–353

21. McIntyre PB, Macintyre CR, Gilmour R et al (2005) A population based study of the impact of corticosteroid therapy and delayed diagnosis on the outcome of childhood pneumococcal meningitis. Arch Dis Child 90:391–396

22. Cabana MD, Rand CS, Powe NR et al (1999) Why don't physicians follow clinical practice guidelines: A framework for improvement. JAMA 282:1458–1465

23. Shaneyfelt TM, Centor RM (2009) Reassessment of clinical practice guidelines: go gently into that good night. JAMA 301:868–869

24. Leone M, Ragonnet B, Alonso S et al (2012) Variable compliance with clinical practice guidelines identified in a 1-day audit at 66 French adult intensive care units. Crit Care Med 40:3189–3195

25. Pollach G, Namboya F (2013) Preventing intensive care admissions for sepsis in tropical Africa (PICASTA): and extension of the international pediatric global sepsis initiative: and African perspective. Pediatr Crit Care Med 14:561–570

26. Kissoon N (2013) Preventing intensive care admissions for sepsis in tropical Africa: PICASTA – food for thought. Pediatr Crit Care Med 14:644–645

27. Barochia AV, Cui X, Vitberg D et al (2010) Bundled care for septic shock: an analysis of clinical trials. Crit Care Med 39:668–678

28. Nguyen HB, Corbett SW, Steele R et al (2007) Implementation of a bundle of quality indica-
    tors for the early management of severe sepsis and septic shock is associated with decreased
    mortality. Crit Care Med 35:1105–1112
29. Irimu GW, Gathara D, Zurovac D et al (2012) Performance of health workers in the man-
    agement of seriously sick children at a Kenyan tertiary hospital: before and after a training
    intervention. PLoS One 7:e39964
30. Schramm GE, Kashyap R, Mullon JJ et al (2011) Septic shock: a multidisciplinary response
    team and weekly feedback to clinicians improve the process of care and mortality. Crit Care
    Med 39:252–258
31. Wenger E (2000) Communities of practice and social learning systems. Organization 7:225–
    246
32. Shorr AF, Micek ST, Jackson WL et al (2007) Economic implications of an evidence-based
    sepsis protocol: can we improve outcomes and lower costs? Crit Care Med 35:1257–1262

Antimicrobial Dosing during Extracorporeal Membrane Oxygenation

P. M. Honoré, R. Jacobs, and H.D. Spapen

Introduction

Extracorporeal membrane oxygenation (ECMO) is increasingly used to support cardiac and respiratory function in critically ill patients [1]. As in continuous renal replacement therapy (CRRT), antimicrobial dose adaptation during ECMO has been completely neglected for decades [2, 3]. However, ECMO has been shown to enhance the already profound physiologic derangements in critically ill patients, thereby significantly altering drug pharmacokinetics (PK) [4].

Common mechanisms that influence PK during ECMO are sequestration in the circuit, increased volume of distribution (V_d), decreased drug elimination and, in analogy with CRRT [5, 6], direct adsorption to the membrane [7]. Lipophilic highly protein-bound antimicrobials with a large V_d (e. g., voriconazole) are markedly sequestered in the circuit [4, 8–11]. In contrast, hydrophilic antimicrobials with a small V_d (e. g., β-lactams and glycopeptides) are more prone to hemodilution and direct adsorption by the membrane [4, 8–12].

Clinical PK data obtained during ECMO are scarce and mainly originate from studies in neonates [4, 13]. The physiologic processes that influence absorption, distribution, metabolism, and excretion in the newly born are, however, still immature and poorly match those of adults [4, 13]. Current recommendations for adjustment of antimicrobial dosing during ECMO are also only available for neonates [13]. The purpose of this chapter is, therefore, to identify and review published data on antimicrobial PK behavior during ECMO and its potential implications in adult intensive care unit (ICU) patients [8–11]. We then propose a 'framework' to facilitate antimicrobial dose decisions during ECMO in this population. Obviously, these recommendations will need further refinement once more robust data emerge from ongoing large controlled studies [14].

P. M. Honoré ✉ · R. Jacobs · H.D. Spapen
Intensive Care Dept, University Hospital, Vrije Universiteit Brussel, Brussels, Belgium
e-mail: Patrick.Honore@uzbrussel.be

J.-L. Vincent (Ed.), *Annual Update in Intensive Care and Emergency Medicine 2014*,
DOI 10.1007/978-3-319-03746-2_4, © Springer International Publishing Switzerland
2014

Mechanisms of Altered Antimicrobial Pharmacokinetics During ECMO

Sequestration in the Circuit

Some antimicrobials are markedly sequestrated in the ECMO circuit [4, 8, 10]. The extent of loss depends primarily on the physicochemical properties of the drugs, but also on type, age, and functioning of the circuit [9, 15]. Because of the high bleeding risk, most ICUs run ECMO without anticoagulation (i. e., the Heparin Free ECMO Protocol) accepting a shorter oxygenator lifespan [15]. We and others use heparin-coated tubing and oxygenators and perform ECMO without heparin in all patients. This approach does not increase thrombosis risk and results in a 5 to 8 day oxygenator lifespan.

PK studies in neonates and adults [4, 8, 10, 13] have consistently demonstrated increased V_d and decreased drug clearance (CL) during ECMO. PK alterations, however, may be multifactorial [16]. For example, sequestration of lipophilic antimicrobials in the circuit is not only related to an increased V_d but also depends on 'third space' formation and membrane adsorption [8, 10, 13].

Effects of Hemodilution

Hemodilution mathematically increases the body's plasma proportion and thus decreases the concentration of water-soluble agents [4–11]. Hemodilution may also alter protein binding capacity [4, 8–10]. Taken together, hemodilution will affect, in particular, the PK of hydrophilic antimicrobials [4, 8–12].

Direct Adsorption on Oxygenator Membranes

Large amounts of hydrophilic antimicrobials are adsorbed by the new generation of oxygenator membranes (i. e., mostly methacrylate, but also acrylonitrile and polymethylmethacrylate membranes in selected oxygenators). Adsorption occurs directly onto the surface but also into the bulk of the membrane. This effect reduces the speed of the saturation process, which develops mainly at the surface [5–7].

Impact of ECMO on Specific Antibiotics and Antifungals

Aminoglycosides

Animal experiments and studies in neonates have shown that an increased V_d is responsible for lower plasma aminoglycoside concentrations during ECMO. Aminoglycoside adsorption on methacrylate membrane oxygenators has not been thoroughly evaluated [4–6]. Preliminary results in veno-venous ECMO (VV-ECMO) encourage the use of higher than usually recommended loading doses [13, 16]. For example, an initial dose of amikacin as high as 30–35 mg/kg has been suggested to obtain effective bactericidal peak levels [17]. Severe pulmonary infections are more frequently noticed in patients undergoing veno-arterial ECMO (VA-ECMO). One explanation might be that VA-ECMO decreases pulmonary blood flow and amikacin availability in the lungs. However, therapeutic pulmonary vein concentrations were detected early after amikacin injection in pigs [18], although were not monitored over time. Awaiting more conclusive data, it also seems reasonable to infuse an amikacin loading dose of 30 to 35 mg/kg in patients receiving VA-ECMO.

Carbapenems

Carbapenems are time-dependent bactericidal antibiotics. Optimal activity is reached at concentrations that remain above the minimum inhibitory concentration (MIC) of the pathogen for at least 40 % of the dosing interval. Meropenem is degraded and significantly sequestered in the ECMO circuit after 4 to 6 h of treatment. A study in surgical patients revealed extreme interindividual variability of meropenem PK between the 1st and 4th day of treatment [19]. This finding was recently corroborated by Taccone et al. [20], who found that predefined PK targets after an initial dose of 1 g meropenem were reached in only 75 % of patients with severe sepsis and septic shock (22 % among them with untreated acute kidney injury [AKI]!). The authors concluded that PK changes induced by sepsis were largely unpredictable and usual variables, such as age, disease severity, presence of shock, vasopressor requirements and need for mechanical ventilation, were not predictive of PK adequacy. Roberts et al. showed great V_d variability in severe sepsis both in the same patient (especially the central compartment [± 45 %]) and between patients (almost 27 %) [21]. Although all patients had serum creatinine values below 1.36 mg/dl, variability of individual and inter-patient meropenem CL ranged between 10 % and 20 %. Furthermore, ECMO induces a systemic inflammatory response syndrome (SIRS). Independently from underlying sepsis, this ECMO-induced SIRS impairs meropenem CL and augments V_d [4,16]. The duration of meropenem infusion has also been shown to influence time above the MIC. In patients with ventilator-associated pneumonia (VAP) [22], a 30-min infusion of 1 g meropenem tid resulted in an adequate time above an MIC of 1 mg/l in only 74.7 % of the patients. When MIC increased to 16 mg/l, only an extended 3 h infusion of 2 g meropenem tid could reach the 40 % "time above the MIC" target [22].

Optimization of meropenem treatment during ECMO thus requires either more frequent dosing, a dose increase, or prolonged infusion [23, 24]. Ideally, meropenem should be infused continuously over 24 h but, due to its relative instability at room temperature, only a 3 h infusion is feasible [25]. We, therefore, suggest that a 3 h infusion of 2 g meropenem every 4 to 6 h should be administered. However, possible adaptations have to be anticipated since new, in particular crystalloid-primed, circuits, may increase meropenem sequestration by allowing new sites to bind [4, 7–11]. Future studies should focus on more stable carbapenems, such as doripenem [26].

Goncalves-Pereira and Paiva recently proposed the concept of antibiotic dose modulation in critically ill patients [27]. This revolutionary approach aims to adapt antibiotic therapy as a function of bacterial load and clinical response. In practice, the largest antibiotic dose is administered upfront when microbial load and PK "swings" are highest in an attempt to lower the risk of drug underdosing and subsequent treatment failure. Antibiotic dose is then progressively tempered under PK guidance when sepsis or SIRS is subsiding. With regard to meropenem therapy in ECMO patients, this implies additional administration of a 4 g loading dose on top of an increased daily maintenance dose.

Piperacillin-tazobactam

Treatment with piperacillin-tazobactam in conditions of increased V_d and CL (e. g., severe burns, CRRT and ECMO) is challenging [16]. Piperacillin-tazobactam remains stable for at least 24 h at room temperature, making it suitable for continuous infusion. Such an approach allowed higher steady-state concentrations and a longer timespan above the MIC even at a lower daily dose [28, 29]. A recent study in septic patients showed that a 24 h infusion containing as low a dose as 8 g piperacillin-tazobactam resulted in significantly longer times above a MIC of 16 mg/l (100 % vs. 62 %) as compared with administration of a 4 g tid bolus [30]. Mortality rate in both groups was similar [30]. In VAP patients, piperacillin-tazobactam penetrated relatively well into bronchial secretions [31], yet was poorly secreted in epithelial lining fluid (ELF). For example, in patients with severe nosocomial *Pseudomonas aeruginosa* pneumonia, steady-state concentrations of piperacillin-tazobactam in ELF after infusion of 4 g/0.5 g tid remained substantially lower than the MIC [32]. Continuous infusion also increased intrapulmonary concentration up to around threefold in patients with moderate kidney injury as compared to patients with preserved renal function [32]. The relationship between piperacillin-tazobactam concentrations in ELF and clinical outcome has been questioned. However, Boselli et al. demonstrated that a continuous 24 h infusion of 16 g/2 g piperacillin-tazobactam produced higher alveolar concentrations and better outcome than a 12 g/1.5 g infusion in patients with VAP [33]. Whether a similar strategy is also applicable for patients with VAP who are treated with ECMO remains unknown.

In conclusion, we may assume that the classical 4 g loading dose is insufficient. Rather, a piperacillin-tazobactam loading dose of up to 6 g/0.75 g or 8 g/1 g should be given, followed by a continuous infusion of 16 g/2 g [33].

Glycopeptides

Vancomycin

Vancomycin is a hydrophilic antibiotic. PK studies in a heterogeneous population receiving ECMO confirmed decreased CL and increased V_d [34]. A vancomycin loading dose (30 mg/kg) to account for this enlarged V_d followed by therapeutic drug monitoring to keep maintenance doses around 30 mg/kg/day has been suggested. Such a high loading dose in ECMO patients is in line with the current recommended loading (35 mg/kg over 4 h) [35] and maintenance (30 mg/kg) doses administered in patients receiving CRRT [36].

Teicoplanin

Teicoplanin is also a hydrophilic antibiotic. PK behavior is influenced by increased V_d during ECMO. Because of its high protein binding, teicoplanin dosing during extracorporeal treatment is even more challenging. This issue becomes particularly obvious in the presence of hypoalbuminemia [37], when a higher CL of unbound drug fraction can be expected. In this condition, a supplemental or higher teicoplanin dose can be safely administered [16, 38, 39]. Treatment should aim to achieve serum trough levels of 20–60 mg/l for patients with severe Gram-positive infection [39, 40]. Therefore, a regimen consisting of three loading doses of 15 mg/kg every 12 h followed by 600 mg once daily has been suggested [40, 41]. This proposed regimen requires confirmation in ECMO patients because a recent study showed massive adsorption of teicoplanin on polysulfone acrylonitrile oxygenator membranes [41].

Linezolid

Linezolid is a hydrophilic antibiotic and thus also subject to an increased V_d in patients undergoing ECMO. Recent investigations are in favor of higher linezolid doses (600 mg tid) during ECMO [42]. However, potential adverse effects, which may occur more often at the proposed dose (e. g., severe thrombocytopenia), should not be neglected.

Ciprofloxacin

Being strongly lipophilic, ciprofloxacin has a very large V_d in critically ill patients. Because sequestration occurs during ECMO, a high loading dose of 800 mg followed by 400 mg tid has been suggested [4, 5, 13]. Future PK studies in ECMO patients must focus on both loading and maintenance doses, since quinolones are both concentration- and time-dependent antibiotics [16].

Tigecycline

Tigecycline is lipophilic and has a high (± 5 l/kg) V_d in critically ill patients [43]. It is unlikely that ECMO-induced hemodilution enhances this V_d, yet the drug is sequestrated in the ECMO circuit. Veinstein et al. investigated tigecycline PK in ECMO patients and found no modification of plasma tigecycline levels at the currently advocated dose [43]. However, these investigators did not measure drug levels in the ELF. It remains unclear whether the excellent tissue penetration of tigecycline is not challenged by an ECMO-related increase in renal elimination and adsorption of the drug. Still, the 'classical' 100 mg loading dose followed by 50 mg bid as maintenance treatment is considered sufficient for treating most infections [43]. However, concerns about risks of selecting resistant microorganisms have incited some authors to suggest higher tigecycline doses (up to 150 mg loading, followed by 100 mg bid) [44, 45].

Colistin

Colistin has recently reemerged as an ultimate therapeutic 'rescue' agent for multidrug-resistant Gram-negative organisms. Dose recommendations exist for colistimethate sodium, which is the parenteral formulation of colistin. Colistin is a large cationic molecule with a molecular weight of 1750 Da and is tightly bound to cell membrane lipids. In addition to being a lipophilic drug characterized by a huge V_d in critically ill patients, colistin was also found to be adsorbed on the dialysis membrane during CRRT [6]. Moreover, colistin is a concentration-dependent antibiotic. Given the highly resistant nature of the bacteria treated with colistin, maintenance of levels above the MIC is thus crucial. In accordance to dose adjustments in CRRT [6, 46] and burn patients [46, 47], a loading dose of 9 million international units (MIU) followed by 4.5 MIU tid is proposed when starting ECMO.

Antifungals

Voriconazole

Voriconazole is a second generation broad-spectrum triazole. It is lipophilic and its antifungal activity is concentration-dependent. Mehta et al. described dramatic sequestration (up to $\geq 70\%$!) in the ECMO circuit resulting in drug concentrations largely below the MIC [48]. During the first 96 h of ECMO, the dose of voriconazole should, therefore, be increased to 6 mg/kg bid [49]. Close monitoring of drug levels and liver function is required when this dose is applied.

Fluconazole

Up to 80 % of fluconazole is reabsorbed by the kidney. Thus, monitoring of renal function is imperative to avoid underdosing [2]. The incidence of AKI in patients undergoing ECMO is very high [50]. Moreover, ECMO initiation often necessitates urgent administration or adjustment of vasoactive drug therapy, resulting in substantial hemodynamic fluctuations that may alter renal blood flow [50]. In addition to this ischemia/reperfusion-associated disorder, other ECMO-related factors, such as systemic inflammation due to interaction between blood and artificial surfaces, a hypercoagulable state, and the occurrence of hemolysis/hemoglobinuria, may also predispose patients to (exacerbation of) AKI [50]. As in CRRT, the dose of fluconazole should be increased to 600 mg bid [2], preferentially under monitoring of drug levels and liver function.

Conclusions

Antibiotic dosing and eventual dose adaptation in critically ill patients undergoing ECMO has long been a 'blind spot'. It has now been convincingly demonstrated that some antibiotics and antifungals are sequestered from the circulation during ECMO. The mechanism of sequestration is multifactorial and differs between hydrophilic and lipophilic agents. This ECMO-related impact on antimicrobial PK behavior is clinically relevant because inadequate antimicrobial coverage is associated with treatment failure, development of resistance and worse outcome. In analogy with the so-called "dialysis/CRRT trauma" – a term used to describe 'collateral damage' encountered in patients undergoing RRT in the ICU [3] – this unwarranted effect of ECMO on antimicrobial efficacy could be regarded as part of an 'ECMO trauma'. Awareness of this previously unrecognized 'antimicrobial-ECMO dilemma' could allow timely adjustments to minimize its consequences. As such, all proposed dose modifications of relevant antibiotics and antifungals have been summarized in Table 1. ECMO will increasingly become part of ICU treatment in various populations

Table 1 Suggested loading and maintenance doses for relevant antimicrobial agents in ECMO-treated patients

Antibiotic/Antifungal	Loading dose	Maintenance dose
Amikacin	30–35 mg/kg	TDM
Meropenem	4 g	2 g over 3 h every 4–6 h (qid)
Piperacillin-tazobactam	6 g/0.75 g to 8 g/1 g	16 g/2 g (CI)
Vancomycin	35 mg/kg over 4 h	30 mg/kg (TDM)
Teicoplanin	15 mg/kg 3x every 12 h	600 mg od
Linezolid		600 mg tid
Ciprofloxacin	800 mg	400 mg tid
Tigecycline	150 mg	100 mg bid
Colistin	9 MIU	4.5 MIU tid
Voriconazole		6 mg/kg bid
Fluconazole		600 mg bid

TDM: therapeutic drug monitoring; CI: continuous infusion; MIU: million international units; od: once daily; bid: twice daily; tid: three times daily; qid: four times daily

of critically ill patients. Because the outcome of most of these patients will ultimately depend on an adequate antimicrobial approach, it is imperative to establish guidelines for optimal initial and maintenance antimicrobial dosing.

References

1. Bartlett RH, Gattinoni L (2010) Current status of extracorporeal life support (ECMO) for cardiopulmonary failure. Minerva Anestesiol 76:534–540
2. Honore PM, Jacobs R, Spapen HD (2012) Use of antifungal drugs during continuous hemofiltration therapies. In: Vincent JL (ed) Annual Update in Intensive Care and Emergency Medicine. Springer, Heidelberg, pp 337–347
3. Maynar JM, Honore PM, Sanchez-Izquierdo JA, Herrera M, Spapen HD (2012) Handling RRT-related adverse effects in ICU patients: the Dialytrauma concept. Blood Purif 34:177–176
4. Shekar K, Fraser JF, Smith MT, Roberts JA (2012) Pharmacokinetic changes in patients receiving extracorporeal membrane oxygenation. J Crit Care 27:e9–18
5. Honore PM, Jacobs R, Spapen HD (2013) Antibiotic Adsorption on CRRT Membranes. Relevance and impact on antibiotic dosing in critically ill patients. In: Vincent JL (ed) Annual Update in Intensive Care and Emergency Medicine. Springer, Heidelberg, pp 123–135
6. Honore PM, Jacobs R, Lochy S et al (2013) Acute respiratory muscle weakness and apnea in a critically ill patient induced by colistin neurotoxicity: key potential role of hemoadsorption elimination during continuous venovenous hemofiltration. Int J Nephrol Renovasc Dis 6:107–111
7. Nakabayashi N, Iwasaki Y (2004) Copolymers of 2-methacryloyloxyethyl phosphorylcholine (MPC) as biomaterials. Biomed Mater Eng 14:345–354
8. Shekar K, Mullany DV, Corley A et al (2012) Increased sedation requirements in patients receiving extracorporeal life support for respiratory and cardio-respiratory failure. Anaesth Intensive Care 40:648–655
9. MacLaren G, Combes A, Bartlett RH (2012) Contemporary extracorporeal membrane oxygenation for adult respiratory failure: life support in the new era. Intensive Care Med 38:210–220
10. Shekar K, Roberts JA, McDonald CI et al (2012) Sequestration of drugs in the circuit may lead to therapeutic failure during extracorporeal membrane oxygenation. Crit Care 16:R194
11. Shekar K, Roberts JA, Ghassabian S et al (2013) Altered antibiotic pharmacokinetics during extracorporeal membrane oxygenation: cause for concern? J Antimicrob Chemother 68:726–727
12. Wildschut ED, Ahsman MJ, Allegaert K, Mathot RA, Tibboel D (2010) Determinants of drug absorption in different ECMO circuits. Intensive Care Med 36:2109–2116
13. Mousavi S, Levcovich B, Mojtahedzadeh M (2011) A systematic review on pharmacokinetic changes in critically ill patients: role of extracorporeal membrane oxygenation. Daru 19:312–321
14. Shekar K, Roberts JA, Welch S et al (2012) ASAP ECMO: Antibiotic, sedative and analgesic pharmacokinetics during extracorporeal membrane oxygenation: a multi-centre study to optimise drug therapy during ECMO. BMC Anesthesiol 12:29
15. Muellenbach RM, Kredel M, Kranke P, Kunze E et al (2012) Prolonged heparin-free extracorporeal membrane oxygenation in multiple injured acute respiratory distress syndrome patients with traumatic brain injury. J Trauma Acute Care Surg 72:1444–1447
16. Jamal JA, Economou CJ, Lipman J, Roberts JA (2012) Improving antibiotic dosing in special situations in the ICU: burns, renal replacement therapy and extracorporeal membrane oxygenation. Curr Opin Crit Care 18:460–471

17. Taccone FS, Laterre PF, Spapen H et al (2010) Revisiting the loading dose of amikacin for patients with severe sepsis and septic shock. Crit Care 14:R53
18. Bělohlávek J, Springer D, Mlček M, et al (2013) Early vancomycin, amikacin and gentamicin concentrations in pulmonary artery and pulmonary tissue are not affected by VA ECMO (venoarterial extracorporeal membrane oxygenation) in a pig model of prolonged cardiac arrest. Pulm Pharmacol Ther 26:655–660
19. Lovering AM, Vickery CJ, Watkin DS et al (1995) The pharmacokinetics of meropenem in surgical patients with moderate or severe infections. J Antimicrob Chemother 36:165–172
20. Taccone FS, Laterre PF, Dugernier T et al (2010) Insufficient β-lactam concentrations in the early phase of severe sepsis and septic shock. Crit Care 14:R126
21. Roberts JA, Kirkpatrick CM, Roberts MS, Robertson TA, Dalley AJ, Lipman J (2009) Meropenem dosing in critically ill patients with sepsis and without renal dysfunction: intermittent bolus versus continuous administration? Monte Carlo dosing simulations and subcutaneous tissue distribution. J Antimicrob Chemother 64:142–150
22. Jaruratanasirikul S, Sriwiriyajan S, Punyo J (2005) Comparison of the pharmacodynamics of meropenem in patients with ventilator-associated pneumonia following administration by 3-hour infusion or bolus injection. Antimicrob Agents Chemother 49:1337–1339
23. Varghese JM, Roberts JA, Lipman J (2010) Pharmacokinetics and pharmacodynamics in critically ill patients. Curr Opin Anaesthesiol 23:472–478
24. Gonçalves-Pereira J, Póvoa P (2011) Antibiotics in critically ill patients: a systematic review of the pharmacokinetics of β-lactams. Crit Care 15:R206
25. Berthoin K, Le Duff CS, Marchand-Brynaert J, Carryn S, Tulkens PM (2010) Stability of meropenem and doripenem solutions for administration by continuous infusion. J Antimicrob Chemother 65:1073
26. Hsaiky L, Murray KP, Kokoska L, Desai N, Cha R (2013) Standard versus prolonged doripenem infusion for treatment of gram-negative infections. Ann Pharmacother 47:999–1006
27. Goncalves-Pereira J, Paiva JA (2013) Dose modulation: a new concept of antibiotic therapy in the critically ill patient ? J Crit Care 28:341–346
28. Roberts JA, Webb S, Paterson D, Ho KM, Lipman J (2009) A systematic review on clinical benefits of continuous administration of beta-lactam antibiotics. Crit Care Med 37:2071–2078
29. Lorente L, Jimenez A, Martin MM et al (2009) Clinical cure of ventilator-associated pneumonia treated with piperacillin/tazobactam administered by continuous or intermittent infusion. Int J Antimicrob Agents 33:464–468
30. Rafati MR, Rouini MR, Mojtahedzadeh M et al (2006) Clinical efficacy of continuous infusion of piperacillin compared with intermittent dosing in septic critically ill patients. Int J Antimicrob Agents 28:122–127
31. Jehl F, Muller-Serieys C, de Larminat V, Monteil H, Bergogne-Berezin E (1994) Penetration of piperacillin-tazobactam into bronchial secretions after multiple doses to intensive care patients. Antimicrob Agents Chemother 38:2780–2784
32. Boselli E, Breilh D, Cannesson M et al (2004) Steady-state plasma and intrapulmonary concentrations of piperacillin/tazobactam 4 g/0.5 g administered to critically ill patients with severe nosocomial pneumonia. Intensive Care Med 30:976–979
33. Boselli E, Breilh D, Rimmelé T et al (2008) Alveolar concentrations of piperacillin/tazobactam administered in continuous infusion to patients with ventilator-associated pneumonia. Crit Care Med 36:1500–1506
34. Mulla H, Pooboni S (2005) Population pharmacokinetics of vancomycin in patients receiving extracorporeal membrane oxygenation. Br J Clin Pharmacol 60:265–275
35. Beumier M, Roberts JA, Kabtouri H, et al (2013) A new regimen for continuous infusion of vancomycin during continuous renal replacement therapy. J Antimicrob Chemother 68:2859–2865

36. Spapen HD, van Janssen Doorn K, Diltoer M et al (2011) Retrospective evaluation of possible renal toxicity associated with continuous infusion of vancomycin in critically ill patients. Ann Intensive Care 1:26
37. Ulldemolins M, Roberts JA, Rello J et al (2011) The effects of hypoalbuminaemia on optimizing antibacterial dosing in critically ill patients. Clin Pharmacokinet 50:99–110
38. Wolter K, Claus M, Wagner K, Fritschka E (1994) Teicoplanin pharmacokinetics and dosage recommendations in chronic hemodialysis patients and in patients undergoing continuous veno-venous hemodialysis. Clin Nephrol 42:389–397
39. Matthews PC, Chue AL, Wyllie D et al (2014) Increased teicoplanin doses are associated with improved serum levels but not drug toxicity. J Infect 68:43–49
40. Matsumoto K, Kanazawa N, Watanabe E et al (2013) Development of initial loading procedure for teicoplanin in critically ill patients with severe infections. Biol Pharm Bull 36:1024–1026
41. Shiraishi Y, Okajima M, Sai Y, Miyamoto K, Inaba H (2012) Elimination of teicoplanin by adsorption to the filter membrane during haemodiafiltration: screening experiments for linezolid, teicoplanin and vancomycin followed by in vitro haemodiafiltration models for teicoplanin. Anaesth Intensive Care 40:442–449
42. De Rosa FG, Corcione S, Baietto L et al (2013) Pharmacokinetics of linezolid during extracorporeal membrane oxygenation. Int J Antimicrob Agents 41:590–591
43. Veinstein A, Debouverie O, Gregoire N et al (2012) Lack of effect of extracorporeal membrane oxygenation on tigecycline pharmacokinetics. J Antimicrob Chemother 67:1047–1048
44. Muralidharan G, Micalizzi M, Speth J, Raible D, Troy S (2005) Pharmacokinetics of tigecycline after single and multiple doses in healthy subjects. Antimicrob Agents Chemother 44(49):220–229
45. Ramirez J, Dartois N, Gandjini H, Yan JL, Korth-Bradley J, McGovern PC (2013) Randomized phase 2 trial to evaluate the clinical efficacy of two high-dosage tigecycline regimens versus imipenem-cilastatin for treatment of hospital-acquired pneumonia. Antimicrob Agents Chemother 57:1756–1762
46. Markou N, Fousteri M, Markantonis SL et al (2012) Colistin pharmacokinetics in intensive care unit patients on continuous venovenous haemodiafiltration: an observational study. J Antimicrob Chemother 67:2459–2462
47. Dudhani RV, Turnidge JD, Coulthard K et al (2010) Elucidation of the pharmacokinetic/pharmacodynamic determinant of colistin activity against Pseudomonas aeruginosa in murine thigh and lung infection models. Antimicrob Agents Chemother 54:1117–1124
48. Mehta NM, Halwick DR, Dodson BL et al (2007) Potential drug sequestration during extracorporeal membrane oxygenation: results from an ex vivo experiment. Intensive Care Med 33:1018–1024
49. Spriet I, Annaert P, Meersseman P et al (2009) Pharmacokinetics of caspofungin and voriconazole in critically ill patients during extracorporeal membrane oxygenation. J Antimicrob Chemother 63:767–770
50. Askenazi DJ, Selewski DT, Paden ML et al (2012) Renal replacement therapy in critically ill patients receiving extracorporeal membrane oxygenation. Clin. J Am Soc Nephrol 7:1328–1336

Corticosteroids as Adjunctive Treatment in Community-Acquired Pneumonia

O. Sibila, M. Ferrer, and A. Torres

Introduction

Community-acquired pneumonia (CAP) is the leading cause of morbidity and mortality from infectious diseases in developed countries. It affects more than 5 million adults and accounts for more than 1 million admissions each year in the United States. Pneumonia is the sixth leading cause of death worldwide, and age-adjusted mortality is increasing. Despite effective antibiotic therapy, about 12–36 % patients admitted to the intensive care unit (ICU) with severe CAP die within a short period of time. Development of an efficacious adjunctive treatment, therefore, has important implications for reducing this high attributable mortality.

During infectious pneumonia, the arrival of pathogens in the lung creates a complex inflammatory response, with the interaction of several defense mechanisms and the production of a number of inflammatory mediators and acute phase proteins. The aim of this inflammatory response is to control progression of the infection. If the reaction is over proportioned, various systemic consequences can negatively influence the clinical progression of the infection. On the other hand, an excessive host inflammatory response is related to poor outcomes in CAP. Elevated cytokine release has been linked to treatment failure, ICU admission and mortality.

Corticosteroids exert an anti-inflammatory and immunosuppressive effect that may affect pneumonia pathogenesis [1]. The use of corticosteroids is considered a risk factor for opportunistic or highly resistant bacterial pneumonia because of their immunosuppressive effects [2, 3]. However, corticosteroids have also been postulated as adjunctive therapy for CAP based on the rationale of their anti-inflammatory effect. Experimental studies have demonstrated that corticosteroid

O. Sibila
Servei de Pneumologia, Hospital de la Santa Creu i Sant Pau, Barcelona, Spain

M. Ferrer · A. Torres ✉
Servei de Pneumologia, Insitut Clinic del Torax, Barcelona, Spain
e-mail: atorres@clinic.ub.es

J.-L. Vincent (Ed.), *Annual Update in Intensive Care and Emergency Medicine 2014*,
DOI 10.1007/978-3-319-03746-2_5, © Springer International Publishing Switzerland
2014

treatment attenuates pneumonia-associated inflammatory responses [4–6], with a decreased pulmonary bacterial burden [5] and an improvement in histopathological severity scores [6]. Some clinical trials testing the usefulness of systemic corticosteroids as adjunctive therapy for CAP have described some benefit [7–12], whereas others showed no benefit or even an increase in related adverse effects [13, 14].

The main purpose of this report is to review the efficacy and safety of corticosteroids as adjunctive therapy in the treatment of CAP in adults. For this purpose, we performed a review of published articles in the English language with the following search terms: Corticosteroids and community-acquired pneumonia.

Corticosteroids: Mechanisms of Action

Corticosteroids are the most effective and widely used anti-inflammatory drugs. The most relevant systemic corticoids available on the market are prednisolone, cortisone, dexamethasone, hydrocortisone, methylprednisolone, prednisone, and triamcinolone. Corticosteroids are involved in a wide range of physiological processes, including regulation of inflammation, immune response, stress response, protein catabolism, carbohydrate metabolism and blood electrolyte levels. In CAP pathogenesis, corticosteroids may regulate the expression and action of many cytokines involved in the inflammatory response associated with pneumonia. In short, corticosteroids can switch off genes that encode pro-inflammatory molecules and can switch on genes that encode anti-inflammatory molecules. This anti-inflammatory effect may be beneficial if it modulates the associated inflammatory response. However, corticosteroids also exert a decisive influence on the immune function of different host defenses against bacteria. An excessive immunosuppressive effect may be harmful for the host.

Corticosteroids are transported in the blood bound to transcortin and albumin, although a small portion is free and acts in a metabolically active state. The free corticosteroid molecules readily cross the plasma membrane into the cytoplasm. To exert their effects, corticosteroids need to bind to a specific cytoplasmic glucocorticoid receptor (GR) [15]. Once activated, the drug–receptor complex moves into the nucleus of the cell and binds to the DNA and directly or indirectly regulates the transcription of important inflammatory target genes [16]. In fact, the anti-inflammatory effects of corticosteroids are due to three different molecular mechanisms [1]. First, the activated GR binds as a homodimer to specific DNA sequences located in the promoter regions of target genes to induce transcription of several anti-inflammatory molecules, such as lipocortin 1, interleukin (IL)-10 or phospholipase A2 inhibitor (transactivation). Second, an indirect negative regulation of gene expression is achieved by GR-protein interaction (transrepression). In brief, the ligand activated receptor binds as a monomer to key pro-inflammatory transcription factors, such as activator protein (AP)-1 and nuclear factor (NF)-κB. The resulting complex inhibits the initiation of transcription of relevant genes that play a central role in inflammation such as inflammatory cytokines (IL-1, IL-6, tu-

Table 1 Effect of corticosteroids on gene transcription

Enhanced molecules	Lipocortin 1
	β2-receptors
	IL-10
	IL-1 receptor
	Inhibitor of nuclear factor-κB
	Phospholipase A2 inhibitor
Decreased molecules	Cytokines (IL-1, IL-2, IL-3, IL-4, IL-5, IL-6, IL-8, IL-11, IL-13, TNF-α)
	Chemokines (exotoxin, MIP-1α, monocyte chemotactic protein)
	Receptors (IL-2 receptor, neurokinin-1 receptor)
	Adhesion molecules (intercellular adhesion molecule-1 and vascular cell adhesion molecule-1)
	Enzymes (nitric oxide synthase, cyclooxygenase 2, phospholipase A2)

IL: interleukin; TNF: tumor necrosis factor

mor necrosis factor [TNF]-α), chemokines or adhesion molecules [1] (Table 1). The third mechanism is corticosteroid signaling through membrane-associated receptors and second messengers (so-called non genomic pathways). The best-described non-genomic mechanism involves the activation of endothelial nitric oxide synthase (eNOS), which is responsible for a rapid vasorelaxation effect.

Experimental studies confirmed these anti-inflammatory effects in pneumonia [4–6]. Li et al. [4] found that hydrocortisone decreased the inflammatory response significantly in a mouse model of *Escherichia coli* pneumonia, reducing the risk of death. Another experimental study in severe pneumonia induced by *Pseudomonas aeruginosa* in piglets demonstrated that the association of methylprednisolone with antibiotics attenuated local inflammatory response and decreased bacterial burden in the lungs [5]. Meduri et al. [17] demonstrated that methylprednisolone may suppress bacterial replication and intracellular bacterial growth in an *in vitro* study using human monocytic cells. Tagliabue et al. [6] showed in experimental *Mycoplasma pneumonia* respiratory infection in mice that steroids given with macrolide therapy reduced lung histopathology scores.

Use of Corticosteroids in CAP

Respiratory diseases are the most common indication for corticosteroids. Corticosteroids are currently recommended in most case of acute exacerbation of chronic respiratory diseases where bronchospasm is present, such as chronic obstructive pulmonary disease (COPD), asthma or bronchiectasis. Epidemiological studies have demonstrated that chronic respiratory diseases, mainly COPD, are risk factors for CAP [18]. COPD is a common disease and the third leading cause of morbidity and mortality in the United States [19, 20]. The Copenhagen City Heart Study reported that COPD patients had a two-fold risk of hospitalization for CAP compared with patients without COPD. In addition, worsening severity of COPD, as demonstrated by worsening forced expiratory volume in one second (FEV_1), was associated with a higher risk of hospitalization and mortality due to CAP. Sliedrecht et al. [18] reported similar results in a very old population (>85 years of age), in which patients with COPD had a three-fold higher risk of CAP compared with non-COPD patients.

Despite the high use of corticosteroids in clinical practice, few studies have evaluated the impact of prior corticosteroid use in patients with CAP. Malave et al. [21] studied the impact of prior systemic corticosteroid use on clinical outcomes in a cohort of 787 hospitalized CAP patients. In this study, prior corticosteroid use was not associated with poor outcomes such as increased 30-day mortality, higher severity of illness at the time of presentation or in the presence of the resistant or opportunistic pathogens. However, there was no information regarding the indication, dose, duration and stopping of corticosteroids in these CAP patients. Patients with corticosteroid use had a higher rate of COPD, which was the most common comorbid condition [21]. Polverino et al. [22] recently published the reasons for acute use of systemic corticosteroids in a large cohort of 3,257 patients admitted for CAP. In this study, 260 patients (8 %) received corticosteroids at admission. The main reasons for administering acute corticosteroids were the presence of chronic respiratory conditions and severe clinical presentation. However, systemic corticosteroid use did not influence mortality or clinical stability as was expected according to the initial severity of illness score [22]. In contrast, corticosteroids were significantly associated with a longer length of stay.

It is not clear that COPD patients with CAP have worse outcomes than those without COPD. Recent studies have shown that COPD patients who develop pneumonia have higher mortality compared to CAP patients without COPD [23–25], but other studies reported a protective effect [26] or no effect [27, 28] on mortality. In addition, in the development of the Pneumonia Severity Index (PSI), the best-validated risk adjustment tool for CAP, COPD was not associated with worse severity of illness at presentation [29]. These differences in mortality may be associated with adjunctive therapies, such as corticosteroids, rather than the pneumonia itself [30]. In the Spanish multicenter Neumofail study [26], which searched for factors related to lack of response to antimicrobial treatment in CAP, COPD was detected as a protective factor. The authors hypothesized that the routine use of corticosteroids in COPD may justify this finding.

Role of Corticosteroids as Adjunctive Therapy

The use of corticosteroids as adjunctive therapy in CAP remains controversial [31]. The best evidence of benefit of corticosteroids comes from studies in specific groups of CAP patients caused by less common pathogens, such as *Pneumocystis jirovecii*, *Varicella* or fungal pneumonia. Randomized controlled trials (RCTs) have shown that corticosteroids reduce mortality in acquired immunodeficiency syndrome (AIDS) patients with *P. jirovecii* and significant hypoxia [32, 33]. Different cohort studies have suggested that corticosteroids may also improve the outcome of severe *Varicella* pneumonia [34, 35]. Anecdotally, corticosteroids

Table 2 Main results from randomized controlled trials (RCTs) in the last 10 years evaluating the effects of corticosteroids as adjuvant therapy in community-acquired pneumonia (CAP)

Author/year [ref]	Study design	No of patients	Disease	Main Effect
Confalonieri et al., 2005 [7]	DB RCT	46	CAP requiring ICU	Decreased mortality
Mikami et al., 2007 [9]	Open-label RCT	31	Hospitalized CAP	Early stabilization of vital signs
Snijders et al., 2010 [13]	DB RCT	213	Hospitalized CAP	Increased late failure
Meijvis et al., 2011 [10]	DB RCT	304	Hospitalized CAP	Reduced length of stay
Fernandez-Serrano et al., 2011 [11]	DB RCT	56	Hospitalized CAP	Decreased length of stay
Sabry et al., 2011 [12]	DB RCT	80	Hospitalized CAP	Decreased duration MV

DB: double-blind; MV: mechanical ventilation

are frequently used in the setting of severe fungal pneumonia, particularly due to histoplasmosis [36] and blastomycosis [37].

A few retrospective studies have evaluated the impact of corticosteroid treatment as adjuvant therapy in CAP patients. Garcia-Vidal et al. [8] performed an observational study of a cohort of 308 hospitalized patients with severe CAP, in which 77 % were treated with standard antimicrobial therapy and 23 % received both antibiotic and systemic corticosteroids. Clinical characteristics were similar among groups except prevalence of COPD, which was higher in the steroid group. In this study, mortality decreased in patients who received simultaneous administration of corticosteroids with antibiotic treatment (odds ratio [OR] 0.28, 95 % CI 0.113-0.732) [8]. Another retrospective study presented data on 111 severe CAP patients requiring invasive mechanical ventilation, in which corticosteroids were prescribed in 55 % of patients [14]. The main indications for corticosteroid use were bronchospasm and septic shock. These authors showed that the administration of adjunctive corticosteroid therapy did not influence mortality, withdrawal of vasopressors or organ failure recovery in this cohort of ICU patients [14].

Several RCTs have evaluated the effect of corticosteroids in CAP in the last ten years with conflicting results (Table 2). Confalonieri et al. [7] assessed the efficacy and safety of hydrocortisone in 46 patients with severe CAP requiring ICU admission. These authors demonstrated a mortality reduction in the group treated with hydrocortisone, a better modulation of the systemic inflammatory response (determined by serum C-reactive protein [CRP]) and significant improvement in clinical endpoints, such as chest x-ray score, multiple organ dysfunction syndrome (MODS) severity scale, PaO_2/FiO_2 ratio, delayed septic shock and ICU and hospital stay [7]. However, the small sample size and differences among groups at admission limited the generalizability of the results. Other RCTs performed in less severe patients with CAP who required hospitalization gave conflicting results. Mikami et al. [9] performed an open-label RCT in 31 CAP hospitalized patients in Japan. In this study, patients treated with prednisone had an earlier stabilization of vital signs and a shorter duration of intravenous antibiotic administration. However, there were no differences among groups in the other clinical outcomes evaluated [9]. Snijders et al. [13] studied the impact of prednisolone compared to placebo among 213 hospitalized patients with CAP. The authors found no differences regarding the rate of 30-day mortality, time to clinically stability or length of hospital stay among groups. In addition, patients treated with corticosteroids had a faster decline in serum CRP levels compared to placebo. In contrast, late clinical failure (defined as >72 hours from admission) was more common in the corticosteroid group. However, there were no differences among groups when a subanalysis was performed in the most severe CAP populations [13]. Meijvis et al. [10] evaluated the effect of intravenous dexamethasone versus placebo in the first 4 days after admission in 304 CAP hospitalized patients. There were no differences between groups in the main outcomes evaluated, including in-hospital mortality, ICU admission and severe adverse events. However, corticosteroid-treated patients had a shorter length of hospital stay compared to the placebo group. In addition, a faster decline of the associated inflammatory response (measured by CRP and IL-6) was observed in the corticosteroid arm [10]. Fernandez-Serrano et al. [11] reported that in 56 hospitalized CAP patients, those treated with antibiotics in combination with methylprednisolone experienced an improvement in respiratory failure rates and a faster time to clinical resolution. A quicker decrease after 24 hours of treatment of CRP and IL-6 was also observed in the corticosteroid group. However, there were no differences among groups in mortality, ICU admission, need for mechanical ventilation or LOS [11]. Sabry et al. [12] randomized 80 CAP hospitalized patients in Egypt to receive hydrocortisone for 7 days or placebo. At day 8, those patients treated with corticosteroid showed a significant improvement in the PaO_2/FiO_2 ratio, chest radiography score and a significant reduction in CRP levels, sequential organ failure assessment (SOFA) score, and delayed septic shock compared to the control group. In addition, hydrocortisone treatment was associated with a significant reduction in the duration of mechanical ventilation. However, there were no differences in ICU mortality between groups [12].

Although most of these results seem to point towards a beneficial effect of corticosteroids in pneumonia, a recent meta-analysis evaluating all RCTs that used corticosteroids as adjunctive therapy in hospitalized patients with CAP between 1956 and 2011 (nine trials involving 1,001 patients) did not suggest a benefit of corticosteroid treatment in terms of reducing mortality (Peto OR 0.62, 95 % CI 0.37-1.04, p=0.07) [38]. However, when only the most severely ill population was considered, the use of corticosteroids was associated with improved mortality (Peto OR 0.26, 95 % CI 0.11-0.64, p=0.03) [38]. Another meta-analysis, in which the previous data were expanded by including patients with CAP recruited in trials investigating prolonged low-dose glucocorticoid treatment in septic shock and/or early acute respiratory distress syndrome (ARDS) (n=1,206) confirmed the previous result. Again, corticosteroid treatment was associated with a survival advantage for the severe CAP population (relative risk [RR] 0.66, 95 % CI 0.51-0.84, p = 0.001) [39].

Duration of Treatment

Duration and termination of corticosteroid treatment are important points to consider. There is evidence that rapid tapering of corticosteroids can induce a hemodynamic and immunological rebound effect if pro-inflammatory cytokine levels increase and their receptors continue being suppressed [40]. Studies in sepsis showed that hydrocortisone infusion produces a significant decrease in circulating levels of different molecules depending on the transcription factor, NF-κB, such as IL-6 or E-selectin. The suppression of steroid treatment caused a rebound effect in most of these mediators [41]. However, prolonged corticosteroid treatment is associated with downregulation of corticosteroid levels and a suppression of the hypothalamic-pituitary-adrenal (HPA) axis, affecting systemic inflammation after treatment [42].

Different durations of corticosteroid treatment were used in the most recent RCTs in CAP patients (Table 3). The largest trial was conducted over 9 days, and was the only study in which gradual corticosteroid withdrawal was conducted [11]. No rebound of inflammation was reported in any of these studies [7, 9–13]. Furthermore, a recent meta-analysis found that when a subgroup analysis by duration of corticosteroid treatment was performed, patients with prolonged corticosteroid treatment, defined as 5 or more days of treatment, had significantly reduced mortality (Peto OR 0.51, 95 % CI 0.26-0.97, p = 0.04) [38].

Table 3 Type of corticosteroid, duration of treatment and main adverse effects from randomized controlled trials evaluating the effects of corticosteroids as adjuvant therapy in community-acquired pneumonia in the last 10 years

Author/year [ref]	Type of corticosteroid, dosage	Duration of treatment	Gradual withdrawal	Adverse effects
Confalonieri et al., 2005 [7]	Hydrocortisone 240 mg/d	7 days	no	none
Mikami et al., 2007 [9]	Prednisolone 40 mg/d	3 days	no	none
Snijders et al., 2010 [13]	Prednisolone 40 mg/d	7 days	no	none
Meijvis et al., 2011 [10]	Dexamethasone 5 mg/d	4 days	no	Hyperglycemia
Fernandez-Serrano et al., 2011 [11]	Methylprednisolone 620 mg	9 days	yes	none
Sabry et al., 2011 [12]	Hydrocortisone 300 mg/d	7 days	no	none

Adverse Effects

Potential adverse effects of corticosteroid use in CAP are another important issue that should be clarified. Different studies performed in patients with septic shock and ARDS have demonstrated that corticosteroids may favor the onset of metabolic disorders, superinfection, and muscle weakness. Recent studies in sepsis found that corticosteroids increased the risk of hyperglycemia and hypernatremia [43]. Table 3 shows the most important adverse effects detected in recent RCTs using corticosteroids in CAP. Meijvis et al. [10] reported increased levels of glycemia in CAP patients treated with dexamethasone. Although other RCTs performed in CAP patients did not make the same observation [7, 9, 11–13], corticosteroid treatment was detected as a risk factor for hyperglycemia in a meta-analysis conducted by Nie et al. (Peto OR 2.64, 95 % CI 1.68-4.15, p < 0.0001) [38]. Van den Berghe et al. [44] demonstrated that intensive blood glucose control reduces morbidity and mortality among critically ill patients. Therefore, strict control of blood glucose levels is systematically recommended in these patients in current guidelines [45].

Several studies involving patients with sepsis and ARDS have suggested that corticosteroid use increases the risk of secondary infections [46–48]. The prolonged use of corticosteroids can alter the phagocytic action of macrophages and alveolar granulocytes, which can facilitate the acquisition of severe bacterial and opportunistic infections. Several studies have identified an increased incidence of potentially highly resistant bacteria [3] and opportunistic infections of the lung, such as *Aspergillus* spp, *P. jirovecci* and *Nocardia* spp in patients taking corticosteroids for prolonged periods of time. However, no reports of superinfection have been associated with corticosteroid treatment as an adjunctive therapy in CAP [7–14, 38].

Another concerning issue is the influence of corticosteroids on muscle function. Several studies in critically ill patients receiving mechanically ventilation found a strong association between corticosteroid treatment and muscle weakness [49]. However, in studies conducted in hospitalized CAP patients, the association between corticosteroid treatment and neuromuscular weakness has not been described [7–14].

Conclusions

The immunoregulatory effect of corticosteroids is able to decrease the associated inflammatory response in pneumonia, which is related to poor outcomes when it is excessive. Observational studies have suggested a corticosteroid benefit in patients with pneumonia and concomitant corticosteroid administration, most of them with chronic lung disease. Several RCTs have been performed in recent years evaluating the use of corticosteroids as adjunctive therapy in CAP with conflicting results, although differences in severity of illness and duration of treatment limit the generalizability of the results. Recent meta-analyses demonstrated improvements in mortality rates in patients with severe CAP. Further, adequately powered randomized trials, especially in the most severe population with high associated inflammatory responses, are needed to confirm this potentially beneficial effect.

References

1. Rhen T, Cidlowsky JA (2005) Antiinflammatory action of glucocorticoids – new mechanisms for old drugs. N Engl J Med 353:1711–1723
2. Stuck AE, Minder CE, Frey FJ (1989) Risk of infectious complications in patients taking glucocorticoids. Rev Infect Dis 11:954–963
3. Falguera M, Carratala J, Ruiz-Gonzalez A et al (2009) Risk factors and outcome of community-acquired pneumonia due to Gram-negative bacilli. Respirology 14:105–111
4. Li Y, Cui X, Li X et al (2008) Risk of death does not alter the efficacy of hydrocortisone therapy in a mouse E. coli pneumonia model: risk and corticosteroids in sepsis. Intensive Care Med 34:568–577
5. Sibila O, Luna CM, Agusti C et al (2008) Effects of glucocorticoids in ventilated piglets with severe pneumonia. Eur Respir J 32:1037–1046
6. Tagliabue C, Salvatore CM, Techasaensiri C et al (2008) The impact of steroids given with macrolide therapy on experimental Mycoplasma pneumoniae respiratory infection. J Infect Dis 198:1180–1188
7. Confalonieri R, Rubino G, Carbone A et al (2005) Hydrocortisone infusion for severe community-acquired pneumonia: a preliminary randomized study. Am J Respir Crit Care Med 171:242–248
8. Garcia-Vidal C, Calbo E, Pascual V et al (2007) Effects of systemic steroids in patients with severe community-acquired pneumonia. Eur Respir J 30:951–956
9. Mikami K, Suzuki M, Kitagawa H et al (2007) Efficacy of corticosteroids in the treatment of community-acquired pneumonia requiring hospitalization. Lung 185:249–255
10. Meijvis S, Hardeman H, Remmelts H et al (2011) Dexamethasone and length of hospital stay in patients with community-acquired pneumonia: a randomised, double-blind, placebo-controlled triall. Lancet 377:2023–2030
11. Fernandez-Serrano S, Dorca J, Garcia-Vidal C et al (2011) Effect of corticosteroids on the clinical course of community-acquired pneumonia: a randomized controlled trial. Crit Care 15:R96
12. Sabry NA, Omar EED (2011) Corticosteroids and ICU course of community acquired pneumonia in Egyptian settings. Pharmacol Pharm 2:73–81
13. Snijders D, Daniels JM, de Graaff CS, van der Werf TS, Boersma WG (2010) Efficacy of corticosteroids in community-acquired pneumonia: a randomized double-blinded clinical trial. Am J Respir Crit Care Med 181:975–982
14. Salluh JI, Soares M, Coelho LM et al (2011) Impact of systemic corticosteroids on the clinical course and outcomes of patients with severe community-acquired pneumonia: a cohort study. J Crit Care 26:193–200
15. De Bosscher K, Vanden Berghe W, Haegeman G (2003) The interplay between the glucocorticoid receptor and nuclear factor-kappaB or activator protein-1: molecular mechanisms for gene repression. Endocr Rev 24:488–522
16. Barnes PJ (2006) Corticosteroid effects on cell signaling. Eur Respir J 27:413–426
17. Meduri GU, Kanagat S, Bronze M et al (2001) Effects of methylprednisolone on intracellular bacterial growth. Clin Diagn Lab Immunol 8:1156–1163
18. Sliedrecht A, den Elzen WP, Verheij TJ et al (2008) Incidence and predictive factors of lower respiratory tract infections among the very elderly in the general population. The Leiden 85-plus Study. Thorax 63:817–822
19. Mannino DM, Homa DM, Akinbami LJ, Ford ES, Redd SC (2002) Chronic obstructive pulmonary disease surveillance-United States. MMWR Surveill Summ 51:1–16

20. Minino AM, Murphy SL, Xu J, Kochanek KD (2011) Deaths: final data for 2008. Natl Vital Stat Rep 7:1–126

21. Malave A, Laserna E, Sibila O, Mortensen EM, Anzueto A, Restrepo MI (2012) Impact of prior systemic corticosteroid use in patients admitted with community-acquired pneumonia. Ther Adv Respir Dis 6:323–330

22. Polverino E, Cilloniz C, Dambrava P et al (2013) Systemic corticosteroids for community-acquired pneumonia: Reasons for use and lack of benefits on outcome. Respirology 18:263–271

23. Restrepo MI, Mortensen EM, Pugh JA, Anzueto A (2006) COPD is associated with increased mortality and severity scoring in community-acquired pneumonia. Eur Respir J 28:346–351

24. Rello J, Rodriguez A, Torres A et al (2006) Implications of COPD in patients admitted to the intensive care unit by community-acquired pneumonia. Eur Respir J 27:1210–1216

25. Molinos L, Clemente MG, Miranda B et al (2009) Community-acquired pneumonia in patients with and without chronic obstructive pulmonary disease. J Infect 58:417–424

26. Menéndez R, Torres A, Zalacaín R et al (2004) Risk factors of treatment failure in community acquired pneumonia: implications for disease outcome. Thorax 59:960–965

27. Torres A, Dorca J, Zalacaín R et al (1996) Community-acquired pneumonia in chronic obstructive pulmonary disease. Am J Respir Crit Care Med 154:1456–1461

28. Liapikou A, Polverino E, Ewig S et al (2012) Severity and outcomes of hospitalised community-acquired pneumonia in COPD patients. Eur Respir J 39:855–856

29. Fine MJ, Auble TE, Yealy DM et al (1997) A prediction rule to identify low-risk patients with community-acquired pneumonia. N Engl J Med 336:243–250

30. Torres A, Menendez R (2006) Mortality in COPD patients with community-acquired pneumonia: who is the third partner? Eur Respir J 28:262–263

31. Wunderink RG, Mandell LA (2012) Adjunctive therapy in community-acquired pneumonia. Semin Respir Crit Care Med 33:311–318

32. Gagnon S, Boota AM, Fischl MA et al (1990) Corticosteroids as adjunctive therapy for severe Pneumocystis carinii pneumonia in the acquired immunodeficiency syndrome: a double-blind, placebo-controlled trial. N Engl J Med 323:1444–1450

33. Bozzette SA, Sattler FR, Chiu J et al (1990) A controlled trial of early adjunctive treatment with corticosteroids for Pneumocystis carinii pneumonia in the acquired immunodeficiency syndrome. California Collaborative Treatment Group. N Engl J Med 323:1451–1457

34. Mer M, Richards GA (1998) Corticosteroids in life-threatening varicella pneumonia. Chest 114:426–431

35. Adhami N, Arabi Y, Raees A et al (2006) Effect of corticosteroids on adult varicella pneumonia: cohort study and literature review. Respirology 11:437–441

36. Goldman M, Johnson PC, Sarosi GA (1999) Fungal pneumonias: the endemic mycoses. Clin Chest Med 20:507–519

37. Lahm T, Neese S, Thornburg AT et al (2008) Corticosteroids for blastomycosis-induced ARDS: a report of two patients and review of the literature. Chest 133:1478–1480

38. Nie W, Zhang Y, Cheng J, Xiu Q (2012) Corticosteroids in the treatment of community-acquired pneumonia in adults: A meta-analysis. Plos ONE 7:e47926

39. Confalonieri M, Annane D, Antonaglia C, Santagiuliana M, Borriello EM, Meduri GU (2013) Is prolongued low-dose glucocorticoid treatment beneficial in community-acquired pneumonia. Curr Infect Dis Rep 15:158–166

40. Barber AE, Coyle SM, Fischer E et al (1995) Influence of hypercortisolemia on soluble tumor necrosis factor receptor II and interleukin-1 receptor antagonist responses to endotoxin in human beings. Surgery 118:406–410

41. Keh D, Boenkhe T, Weber-Cartens S et al (2003) Immunologic and hemodynamic effects of "low-dose" hydrocortisone in septic shock. A double blind, randomised, placebo-controlled, crossover study. Am J Respir Crit Care Med 167:512–520

42. Barber AE, Coyle SM, Marano MA et al (1993) Glucocorticoid therapy alters hormonal and cytokine responses to endotoxin in man. J Immunol 150:1999–2006

43. Annane D, Bellisant E, Bollaert PE et al (2009) Corticosteroids in the treatment of severe sepsis and septic shock in adults: a systematic review. JAMA 301:2362–2375

44. Van den Berghe G, Wouters P, Weekers F et al (2001) Intensin insulin therapy in the critically ill patients. N Engl J Med 345:1359–1367

45. Mandell LA, Wunderink RG, Anzueto A et al (2007) Infectious Diseases Society of America/American Thoracic Society consensus guidelines on the management of community-acquired pneumonia in adults. Clin Infect Dis 44(2):27–72

46. Sprung CL, Caralis PV, Marcial EH et al (1984) The effects of high-dose corticosteroids in patients with septic shock. A prospective, controlled study. N Engl J Med 311:1137–1143

47. Sprung CL, Annane D, Keh D et al (2008) Hydrocortisone therapy for patients with septic shock. N Engl J Med 358:111–124

48. Bernard GR, Luce JM, Sprung CL et al (1987) High-dose corticosteroids in patients with the adult respiratory distress syndrome. N Engl J Med 317:1565–1570

49. Meduri GU, Headley AS, Golden E et al (1998) Effect of prolonged methylprednisolone therapy in unresolving acute respiratory distress syndrome. A randomized controlled trial. JAMA 280:159–165

Ventilator-associated Pneumonia in the ICU

A. A. Kalanuria, M. Mirski, and W. Ziai

Introduction

Ventilator-associated pneumonia (VAP) is defined as pneumonia that occurs 48–72 hours or thereafter following endotracheal intubation, characterized by the presence of a new or progressive infiltrate, signs of systemic infection (fever, altered white blood cell count), changes in sputum characteristics, and detection of a causative agent [1]. VAP contributes to approximately half of all cases of hospital-acquired pneumonia [1, 2]. VAP is estimated to occur in 9–27 % of all mechanically ventilated patients, with the highest risk being early in the course of hospitalization [1, 3]. It is the second most common nosocomial infection in the intensive care unit (ICU) and the most common in mechanically ventilated patients [4, 5]. VAP rates range from 1.2 to 8.5 per 1,000 ventilator days and are reliant on the definition used for diagnosis [6]. Risk for VAP is greatest during the first 5 days of mechanical ventilation (3 %) with the mean duration between intubation and development of VAP being 3.3 days [1, 7]. This risk declines to 2 %/day between days 5 to 10 of ventilation, and 1 %/day thereafter [1, 8]. Earlier studies placed the attributable mortality for VAP at between 33–50 %, but this rate is variable and relies heavily on the underlying medical illness [1]. Over the years, the attributable risk of death has decreased and is more recently estimated at 9–13 % [9, 10], largely because of implementation of preventive strategies. Approximately 50 % of all antibiotics administered in ICUs are for treatment of VAP [2, 4]. Early onset VAP is defined as

A. A. Kalanuria
Department of Neurology, University of Maryland School of Medicine, Baltimore, MD 21201, USA

M. Mirski · W. Ziai ✉
Department of Anesthesiology/Critical Care Medicine, Johns Hopkins University School of Medicine, Baltimore, MD 21287, USA
e-mail: weziai@jhmi.edu

J.-L. Vincent (Ed.), *Annual Update in Intensive Care and Emergency Medicine 2014*,
DOI 10.1007/978-3-319-03746-2_6, © Springer International Publishing Switzerland
and BioMed Central Ltd. 2014

pneumonia that occurs within 4 days and this is usually attributed to antibiotic sensitive pathogens whereas late onset VAP is more likely caused by multidrug resistant (MDR) bacteria and emerges after 4 days of intubation [1, 4]. Thus, VAP poses grave implications in endotracheally intubated adult patients in ICUs worldwide and leads to increased adverse outcomes and healthcare costs. Independent risk factors for development of VAP are male sex, admission for trauma and intermediate underlying disease severity, with odds ratios (OR) of 1.58, 1.75 and 1.47–1.70, respectively [7].

Pathogenesis

The complex interplay between the endotracheal tube, presence of risk factors, virulence of the invading bacteria and host immunity largely determine the development of VAP. The presence of an endotracheal tube is by far the most important risk factor, resulting in a violation of natural defense mechanisms (the cough reflex of glottis and larynx) against microaspiration around the cuff of the tube [4, 11]. Infectious bacteria obtain direct access to the lower respiratory tract via: (1) microaspiration, which can occur during intubation itself; (2) development of a biofilm laden with bacteria (typically Gram-negative bacteria and fungal species) within the endotracheal tube; (3) pooling and trickling of secretions around the cuff; and (4) impairment of mucociliary clearance of secretions with gravity dependence of mucus flow within the airways [11–13]. Pathogenic material can also collect in surrounding anatomic structures, such as the stomach, sinuses, nasopharynx and oropharynx, with replacement of normal flora by more virulent strains [11, 12, 14]. This bacterium-enriched material is also constantly thrust forward by the positive pressure exerted by the ventilator. Whereas reintubation following extubation increases VAP rates, the use of non-invasive positive pressure ventilation has been associated with significantly lower VAP rates [4]. Host factors such as the severity of underlying disease, previous surgery and antibiotic exposure have all been implicated as risk factors for development of VAP [1].

In addition, it has recently been noted that critically ill patients may have impaired phagocytosis and behave as functionally immunosuppressed even prior to emergence of nosocomial infection [4, 15, 16]. This effect is attributed to the detrimental actions of the anaphylatoxin, C5a, which impairs neutrophil phagocytic activity and impairs phagocytosis by neutrophils [15]. More recently, a combined dysfunction of T-cells, monocytes, and neutrophils has been noted to predict acquisition of nosocomial infection [16]. For example, elevation of regulatory T-cells (Tregs), monocyte deactivation (measured by monocyte HLA-DR expression) and neutrophil dysfunction (measured by CD88 expression), have cumulatively shown promise in predicting infection in the critically ill population, as compared to healthy controls [16].

Microbiology

The type of organism that causes VAP usually depends on the duration of mechanical ventilation. In general, early VAP is caused by pathogens that are sensitive to antibiotics, whereas late onset VAP is caused by multi-drug resistant and more difficult to treat bacteria. However, this is by no means a rule and merely a guide to initiate antibiotic therapy until further clinical information is available.

Typically, bacteria causing early-onset VAP include *Streptococcus pneumoniae* (as well as other streptococcus species), *Hemophilus influenzae*, methicillin-sensitive *Staphylococcus aureus* (MSSA), antibiotic-sensitive enteric Gram-negative bacilli, *Escherichia coli*, *Klebsiella pneumonia*, *Enterobacter* species, *Proteus* species and *Serratia marcescens*. Culprits of late VAP are typically MDR bacteria, such as methicillin-resistant *S. aureus* (MRSA), *Acinetobacter*, *Pseudomonas aeruginosa*, and extended-spectrum beta-lactamase producing bacteria (ESBL) [4]. The exact prevalence of MDR organisms is variable between institutions and also within institutions [1]. Patients with a history of hospital admission for ≥ 2 days in the past 90 days, nursing home residents, patients receiving chemotherapy or antibiotics in the last 30 days and patients undergoing hemodialysis at outpatient centers are susceptible to drug resistant bacteria [1, 4]. Commonly found bacteria in the oropharynx can attain clinically significant numbers in the lower airways. These bacteria include *Streptococcus viridans*, *Corynebacterium*, coagulase-negative staphylococcus (CNS) and *Neisseria* species. Frequently, VAP is due to polymicrobial infection. VAP from fungal and viral causes has a very low incidence, especially in the immunocompetent host [1].

Pathogens causing VAP, their frequency (in parenthesis) and their possible mode of multi-drug resistance, if any, are listed below [1–3]:
1. *Pseudomonas* (24.4 %): Upregulation of efflux pumps, decreased expression of outer membrane porin channel, acquisition of plasmid-mediated metallo-beta-lactamases.
2. *S. aureus* (20.4 %, of which > 50 % MRSA): Production of a penicillin-binding protein (PBP) with reduced affinity for beta-lactam antibiotics. Encoded by the mecA gene.
3. Enterobacteriaceae (14.1 % – includes *Klebsiella* spp., *E. coli*, *Proteus* spp., *Enterobacter* spp., *Serratia* spp., *Citrobacter* spp.): Plasmid mediated production of ESBLs, plasmid-mediated AmpC-type enzyme.
4. *Streptococcus* species (12.1 %).
5. *Hemophilus* species (9.8 %).
6. *Acinetobacter* species (7.9 %): Production of metalloenzymes or carbapenemases.
7. *Neisseria* species (2.6 %).
8. *Stenotrophomonas maltophilia* (1.7 %).
9. Coagulase-negative staphylococcus (1.4 %).
10. Others (4.7 % – includes *Corynebacterium*, *Moraxella*, *Enterococcus*, fungi).

Diagnosis

At the present time, there is no universally accepted, gold standard diagnostic criterion for VAP. Several clinical methods have been recommended but none have the needed sensitivity or specificity to accurately identify this disease [17]. Daily bedside evaluation in conjunction with chest radiography can only be suggestive of the presence or absence of VAP, but not define it [18]. Clinical diagnosis of VAP can still miss about a third of VAPs in the ICU compared to autopsy findings and can incorrectly diagnose more than half of patients, likely due to poor interobserver agreement between clinical criteria [8, 18, 19]. Postmortem studies comparing VAP diagnosis with clinical criteria showed 69 % sensitivity and 75 % specificity, in comparison to autopsy findings [20].

The American Thoracic Society (ATS) and the Infectious Diseases Society of America (IDSA) guidelines recommend obtaining lower respiratory tract samples for culture and microbiology [1]. Analysis of these samples can be quantitative or qualitative. This guideline also allows use of tracheal aspirates for their negative predictive value (94 % for VAP). Johanson et al. described clinical criteria for diagnosis of VAP as follows [21]:

1. New or progressive radiographic consolidation or infiltrate. In addition, at least 2 of the following:
2. Temperature > 38 °C
3. Leukocytosis (white blood cell count $\geq$ 12,000 cells/mm^3) or leukopenia (white blood cell count < 4,000 cells/mm^3)

   Presence of purulent secretions

The clinical pulmonary infection score (CPIS) takes into account clinical, physiological, microbiological and radiographic evidence to allow a numerical value to predict the presence or absence of VAP (Table 1) [18, 22]. Scores can range between zero and 12 with a score of $\geq$ 6 showing good correlation with the presence of VAP [22]. Despite the clinical popularity of the CPIS, debate continues regarding its diagnostic validity. One meta-analysis of 13 studies evaluating the accuracy of CPIS in diagnosing VAP reported pooled estimates for sensitivity and specificity for CPIS as 65 % (95 % CI 61–69 %) and 64 % (95 % CI 60–67 %), respectively [23]. Despite its apparent straightforward calculation, the inter-observer variability in CPIS calculation remains substantial, jeopardizing its routine use in clinical trials [24]. Of all the criteria used to calculate the CPIS, only time-dependent changes in the PaO_2/FiO_2 ratio early in VAP may provide some predictive power for VAP outcomes in clinical trials, namely clinical failure and mortality [25]. However, a trial by Singh and colleagues [26] demonstrated that the CPIS is an effective clinical tool for determining whether to stop or continue antibiotics for longer than 3 days. In that study, antibiotics were discontinued at day 3 for patients who had been randomized to receive ciprofloxacin instead of standard of care, if their CPIS remained $\leq$ 6. Mortality and length of ICU stay did not differ despite a shorter duration (p = 0.0001) and lower cost (p = 0.003) of antimicrobial therapy in the experimental as compared with the standard therapy arm, and the development of antimicrobial

Table 1 The clinical pulmonary infection score (CPIS)

Assessed Parameter	Result	Score
Temperature (°Celsius)	36.5–38.4 °C	0
	38.5–38.9 °C	1
	≤ 36 or ≥ 39 °C	2
Leukocytes in blood (cells/mm^3)	4,000–11,000/mm^3	0
	< 4,000 or > 11,000/mm^3	1
	≥ 500 Band cells	2
Tracheal secretions (subjective visual scale)	None	0
	Mild/non-purulent	1
	Purulent	2
Radiographic findings (on chest radiography, excluding CHF and ARDS)	No infiltrate	0
	Diffuse/patchy infiltrate	1
	Localized infiltrate	2
Culture results (endotracheal aspirate)	No or mild growth	0
	Moderate or florid growth	1
	Moderate or florid growth AND pathogen consistent with Gram stain	2
Oxygenation status (defined by PaO$_2$:FiO$_2$)	> 240 or ARDS	0
	≤ 240 and absence of ARDS	2

ARDS: acute respiratory distress syndrome; CHF: congestive heart failure

resistance was lower among patients whose antibiotics were discontinued compared to those who received standard of care.

Respiratory samples can be obtained using several techniques:
1. Endotracheal aspirate: Easiest to obtain, does not require provider involvement.
2. Bronchoalveolar lavage (BAL): Requires bronchoscopic guidance.
3. Mini-bronchoalveolar lavage (mini-BAL): Performed 'blind', i. e., without bronchoscopic guidance.
4. Protected specimen brush (PSB): Utilizes a brush at the tip of the catheter which is rubbed against the bronchial wall.

The ATS/IDSA guidelines note that use of a bronchoscopic bacteriologic strategy has been shown to reduce 14-day mortality when compared with a clinical strategy (16.2 % vs. 25.8 %, p = 0.02) [1]. When samples are obtained by BAL techniques (BAL, mini-BAL or PSB), the diagnostic threshold is 10^3 colony forming units (cfu)/ml for protected specimen brushing and 10^4 cfu/ml for BAL. In one multicenter study, BAL- and PSB-based diagnosis was associated with significantly more antibiotic-free days (11.5 ± 9.0 vs. 7.5 ± 7.6, p < 0.001) compared to guideline-based clinical diagnosis alone [27]. This study also demonstrated short-term mortality benefit in the BAL/PSB group. More recent evidence from the Canadian Clinical Trials study of 740 suspected VAP patients randomized to BAL or tracheal suctioning suggests that (excluding patients known to be colonized/infected with pseudomonas species or MRSA) similar clinical outcomes and overall use of antibiotics is observed when either BAL with quantitative culture or endotracheal aspiration with non-quantitative culture is used for diagnosis [28]. This finding was confirmed by a Cochrane meta-analysis of 1,367 patients which again found no difference in mortality in the invasive vs. non-invasive groups (26.6 % and 24.7 %, respectively), in quantitative versus qualitative cultures (relative risk 1.53, 95 % CI 0.54–4.39) or in antibiotic use [29].

Once specimens are obtained, the sample is sent for Gram stain, culture and sensitivity. The Gram stain can provide crucial initial clues to the type of organism(s) and whether or not the material is purulent (defined as ≥ 25 neutrophils and ≤ 10 squamous epithelial cells per low power field) [1,12]. Culture results can be reported as semi-quantitative and/or quantitative values. Semi-quantitative values obtained by endotracheal sampling are considered positive when the agar growth is moderate (+++) or heavy (++++), while quantitative positivity is defined as ≥ 10^5 cfu/ml. Exact speciation of pathogen bacteria and their sensitivity to antibiotics can take a few days, but provides invaluable information.

Mechanically ventilated patients in the ICU receive frequent chest X-rays and presence of infiltrate(s) and/or consolidation is considered part of diagnostic criteria and is widely used. However, there are several clinical conditions that have radiographic appearances similar to VAP. These conditions are commonly encountered in mechanically ventilated patients and include aspiration and chemical pneumonitis, atelectasis, congestive heart failure, acute respiratory distress syndrome (ARDS), pleural effusion and intra-alveolar hemorrhage to name a few. Hence, reliance on chest radiography for the diagnosis of VAP is not advisable. There is poor correlation between radiographic signs (alveolar infiltrates, air bronchograms) and histopathological diagnosis of pneumonia [12]. The sensitivity and specificity of presence of infiltrates on chest X-ray is also not encouraging [12]. On the flip-side, the negative predictive value of infiltrates may have clinical utility. In a meta-analysis by Klompas, the presence or absence of fever, elevated white blood cell count, or purulent secretions did not substantively predict the probability of infection; however, the absence of a new infiltrate on a plain radiograph lowered the likelihood of VAP [18].

VAP must be distinguished from tracheo-bronchitis. Clinical features of these diseases can overlap, but only VAP will demonstrate the presence of hypoxia and the presence of infiltrate/consolidation on chest radiography [12].

Recently, the Centers for Disease Control and Prevention (CDC) rolled out new surveillance criteria for possible or probable VAP [17]. The goals were to capture other common complications of ventilator care, to improve objectivity of surveillance to allow comparability across centers for public reporting, and to minimize gaming [30]. Per these new criteria, a period of at least 2 days of stable or decreasing ventilator settings (daily minimum positive end-expiratory pressure [PEEP] or fraction of inspired oxygen [FiO$_2$]) followed by consistently higher settings for at least 2 additional calendar days is required before a patient can be said to have a ventilator-associated condition (VAC). Most VACs are attributable to pneumonia, pulmonary edema, atelectasis, or ARDS, conditions which all have well researched prevention and management strategies [31]. Signs of infection/inflammation (abnormal temperature or white-cell count and administration of one or more new antibiotics for at least 4 days) classify the patient as an "infection-related ventilator-associated complication," or IVAC. Presence of purulent secretions (according to quantitative Gram staining criteria) and pathogenic culture data will label the patient as possible or probable VAP. Patients with an IVAC and purulent secretions alone or pathogenic cultures alone have "possible pneumonia"; those with both purulent secretions and positive quantitative or semiquantitative cultures have "probable pneumonia". Probable pneumonia is also defined by suggestive histopathological features, positive pleural-fluid cultures, or diagnostic tests for legionella and selected viruses. Chest radiograph findings have been excluded in the new criteria because of their subjectivity without increased accuracy. This is not intended to reduce the role of radiography in clinical care. At the present time, the new CDC algorithm is for surveillance purposes only.

In the United States, VAP has been proposed as an indicator of quality of care in public reporting, and its prevention is a national patient safety goal. The threat of non-reimbursement and financial penalties for this diagnosis has put pressure on hospitals to minimize VAP rates [13]. This has resulted in potential artifacts in surveillance with more than 50 % of non-teaching medical ICUs in the United States reporting VAP rates close to zero [30, 32]. These rates are an order of magnitude lower than those in European centers, which utilize similar preventive and treatment strategies suggesting that reductions in VAP rates may not reflect improvements in prevention so much as subjective surveillance biases. It is anticipated that the new CDC surveillance paradigm for ventilator-associated events will help achieve a more realistic VAP rate.

Treatment

Selecting the appropriate antibiotic depends on the duration of mechanical ventilation. Late onset VAP (> 4 days) requires broad spectrum antibiotics whereas early onset (≤ 4 days) can be treated with limited spectrum antibiotics [1]. An updated local antibiogram for each hospital and each ICU based on local bacteriological patterns and susceptibilities is essential to guide optimally dosed initial empiric therapy [1]. With any empiric antibiotic regimen, de-escalation is the key to reduce emergence of resistance [33]. Delays in initiation of antibiotic treatment may add to the excess mortality risk with VAP [1]. Tables 2 and 3 highlight the recommended treatment regimens for VAP.

Owing to the high rate of resistance to monotherapy observed with *P. aeruginosa*, combination therapy is always recommended. Acinetobacter species respond best to carbapenems (also active against ESBL positive Enterobacteriaceae), colistin, polymyxin B and ampicillin/sulbactam [36, 37]. Although MDR organisms are usually associated with late-onset VAP, recent evidence suggests that they are increasingly associated with early-onset VAP as well [37, 38]. The role of inhaled antibiotics in the setting of failure of systemic antibiotics is unclear [1]. The usual duration of treatment for early-onset VAP is 8 days and longer in the case of late-onset VAP or if MDR organisms are suspected or identified [39–41].

Despite therapy, if no response is observed, it may be prudent to reconsider the diagnosis, reassess the organism being treated or search for other reasons for signs

Table 2 Comparison of recommended initial empiric therapy for ventilator-associated pneumonia (VAP) according to time of onset [1, 34, 41]

Early-onset VAP	Late-onset VAP
Second or third generation cephalosporin: e. g., ceftriaxone: 2 g daily; cefuroxime: 1.5 g every 8 hours; cefotaxime: 2 g every 8 hours	Cephalosporin e. g., cefepime: 1–2 g every 8 hours; ceftazidime 2 g every 8 hours
OR	OR
Fluoroquinolones e. g., levofloxacin: 750 mg daily; moxifloxacin: 400 mg daily	Carbepenem e. g., imipenem + cilastin: 500 mg every 6 hours or 1 g every 8 hours; meropenem: 1 g every 8 hours
OR	OR
Aminopenicillin + beta-lactamase inhibitor e. g., ampicillin + sulbactam: 3 g every 8 hours	Beta-lactam/beta-lactamase inhibitor e. g., piperacillin + tazobactam: 4.5 g every 6 hours
OR	PLUS
Ertapenem 1 g daily	Aminoglycoside e. g., amikacin: 20 mg/kg/day; gentamicin: 7 mg/kg/day; tobramycin: 7 mg/kg/day
	OR
	Antipseudomonal fluoroquinolone e. g., ciprofloxacin 400 mg every 8 hours; levofloxacin 750 mg daily
	PLUS Coverage for MRSA e. g., vancomycin: 15 mg/kg every 12 hours
	OR
	linezolid: 600 mg every 12 hours

Optimal dosage includes adjusting for hepatic and renal failure. Trough levels for vancomycin (15–20 mcg/ml), amikacin (< 5 mcg/ml), gentamicin (< 1 mcg/ml) and tobramycin (< 1 mcg/ml) should be measured frequently to avoid untoward systemic side effects. All recommended doses are for intravenous infusion. Usual duration of therapy is 8 days unless treatment is for multidrug resistant organisms, in which case treatment will be for 14 days.

and symptoms. Because of the challenges associated with diagnosing VAP, especially early in the course, the IDSA/ATS guidelines highlight the importance of reassessing patients at 48–72 hours once pertinent data are available to determine whether the patient should continue antibiotic therapy for VAP or whether an alternative diagnosis should be pursued. In one study, Swoboda et al. [42] found that half of the empiric antibiotic use for VAP in two surgical ICUs was prescribed for patients without pneumonia.

Prevention

There are multiple recommended measures for prevention of VAP. These measures are summarized in Table 4 [43–46]. Institutions or ICUs may observe a reduction

Table 3 Recommended therapy for suspected or confirmed multidrug resistant organisms and fungal VAP [1, 34, 35, 41]

Pathogen	Treatment
Methicillin-resistant *Staphylococcus aureus* (MRSA)	See Table 2
Pseudomonas aeruginosa	Double coverage recommended. See Table 2
Acinetobacter species	Carbapenem e. g., imipenem + cilastin; 1 g every 8 hours; meropenem 1 g every 8 hours OR Beta-Lactam/beta-lactamase inhibitor e. g., ampicillin + sulbactam: 3 g every 8 hours OR Tigecycline: 100 mg loading dose, then 50 mg every 12 hours
Extended-spectrum beta-lactamase (ESBL) positive enterobacteriaceae	Carbepenem e. g., imipenem + cilastin: 1 g every 8 hours; meropenem: 1 g every 8 hours
Fungi	Fluconazole: 800 mg every 12 hours; caspofungin: 70 mg loading dose, then 50 mg daily; voriconazole (for aspergillus species): 4 mg/kg every 12 hours
Legionella	Macrolides (e. g., azithromycin) OR Fluoroquinolones (e. g., levofloxacin)

in VAP rates by utilizing a 'VAP-bundle' approach [44, 47] using elements depicted in Table 4. The 5-element Institute of Healthcare Improvement (IHI) VAP bundle [47] includes: Head of bed elevation, oral care with chlorhexidine, stress ulcer prophylaxis, deep venous thrombosis prophylaxis, and daily sedation assessment and spontaneous breathing trials. Each of these elements has been shown to reduce the incidence of VAP although the quality of evidence supporting the effectiveness and importance of each intervention has been questioned. Even studies using VAP bundles have been criticized as failing to demonstrate clinical and cost effectiveness [48]. A before-after study which systematically implemented a VAP prevention bundle using IHI methodology showed a significant reduction in VAP rates, antibiotic use and MRSA acquisition [43]. There was no reduction, however, in duration of mechanical ventilation or ICU admission. The IHI emphasizes the need for high (95 %) overall compliance rates with VAP bundles although this particular study reported overall bundle compliance rates of 70 %. Issues with completeness of documentation may underestimate compliance, which remains an important feature of VAP bundle prevention strategies. Another important contribution towards VAP prevention and shortening periods of antibiotic exposure was a recent prospective study (n = 129), which concluded that a single-dose of antibiotics within 4 h of intubation may be effective in preventing early onset VAP in

Table 4 Suggested measures for prevention of ventilator-associated pneumonia (VAP) [41, 42, 49]

ICU focused measures	Institution focused measures
Alcohol-based hand washing policy	Surveillance program for pathogen profiling and creation of "antibiogram"
Early discontinuation of invasive devices	Frequent educational programs to reduce unnecessary antibiotic prescription
Reduce reintubation rates	Propagate use of non-invasive positive pressure ventilation (NIPPV)
Use of oropharyngeal vs. nasopharyngeal feeding tubes	Endotracheal tubes (ETTs) with potential benefit: Polyurethane-cuffed ETT Silver/antibiotic coated ETT Aspiration of subglottic secretions (HI-LO ETT)
Semi-recumbent patient positioning (30–45°)	Maintain policy for oral decontamination Selective digestive decontamination (SDD)
Endotracheal tube cuff pressure ~ 20 cm H_2O	Early weaning and extubation
Early tracheostomy	Daily sedation holds
Small bowel feeding instead of gastric feeding	Preference on using heat-moisture exchangers over heater humidifiers
Prophylactic probiotics	Mechanical removal of the biofilm (e. g., the mucus shaver)

a cohort of comatose patients [49]. A randomized clinical trial is needed to address this question.

Conclusion

VAP occurs frequently and is associated with significant morbidity in critically ill patients. The primary obstacle in diagnosing VAP is the absence of gold standard criteria and, therefore, VAP continues to be an inconspicuous clinical syndrome. There is enough evidence to indicate that VAP is preventable and that hospitals can decrease VAP rates, a factor that the new CDC VAP definitions are poised to demonstrate more objectively. The diagnostic challenge of VAP has multiple implications for therapy. Although a CPIS score > 6 may correlate with VAP, the sensitivity, specificity and inter-rater agreement of this criterion alone are not encouraging. Microbiological data should be used for tailoring antibiotic therapy and not be restricted only to diagnosis. The pitfall in using empiric antibiotics for suspicion of VAP is the potential for antibiotic overuse, emergence of resistance, unnecessary adverse effects and potential toxicity. The major goals of VAP management are early, appropriate antibiotics in adequate doses followed by de-escalation based on microbiological culture results and the clinical response of the patient. Antimicrobial stewardship programs involving pharmacists, physicians and other healthcare providers optimize antibiotic selection, dose, and duration to increase efficacy in targeting causative pathogens and allow the best clinical outcome.

References

1. American Thoracic Society, Infectious Diseases Society of America (2005) Guidelines for the management of adults with hospital-acquired, ventilator-associated, and healthcare-associated pneumonia. Am J Respir Crit Care Med 171:388–416
2. Vincent JL, Bihari DJ, Suter PM et al (1995) The prevalence of nosocomial infection in intensive care units in Europe. JAMA 274:639–644
3. Chastre J, Fagon JY (2002) State of the art: ventilator-associated pneumonia. Am J Respir Crit Care Med 165:867–903
4. Hunter JD (2012) Ventilator associated pneumonia. BMJ 344(e3325):e3325
5. Afshari A, Pagani L, Harbarth S (2012) Year in review 2011: Critical care – infection. Crit Care 16:242–247
6. Skrupky LP, McConnell K, Dallas J, Kollef MH (2012) A comparison of ventilator-associated pneumonia rates as identified according to the National Healthcare Safety Network and American College of Chest Physicians Criteria. Crit Care Med 40:281–284
7. Rello J, Ollendorf D, Oster G et al (2002) Epidemiology and outcomes of ventilator-associated pneumonia in a large US database. Chest 122:2115–2121
8. Cook DJ, Walter SD, Cook RJ et al (1998) Incidence of and risk factors for ventilator-associated pneumonia in critically ill patients. Ann Int Med 129:433–440
9. Melsen WG, Rovers MM, Koeman M, Bonten MJM (2011) Estimating the attributable mortality of ventilator-associated pneumonia from randomized prevention studies. Crit Care Med 39:2736–2742
10. Melsen WG, Rovers MM, Groenwold RH et al (2013) Attributable mortality of ventilator-associated pneumonia: a meta-analysis of individual patient data from randomised prevention studies. Lancet Infect Dis 13:665–671
11. Zolfaghari PS, Wyncoll DL (2011) The tracheal tube: gateway to ventilator-associated pneumonia. Crit Care 15:310–317
12. Grgurich PE, Hudcova J, Lei Y, Sarwar A, Craven DE (2013) Diagnosis of ventilator-associated pneumonia: controversies and working toward a gold standard. Curr Opin Infect Dis 26:140–150
13. Mietto C, Pinciroli R, Patel N, Berra L (2013) Ventilator associated pneumonia: evolving definitions and preventive strategies. Respir Care 58:990–1007
14. Rocha LA, Marques Ribas R, da Costa Darini AL, Gontijo Filho PP (2013) Relationship between nasal colonization and ventilator-associated pneumonia and the role of the environment in transmission of Staphylococcus aureus in intensive care units. Am J Infect Control 41:1236–1240
15. Morris AC, Brittan M, Wilkinson TS et al (2011) C5a-mediated neutrophil dysfunction is RhoA-dependent and predicts infection in critically ill patients. Blood 117:5178–5188
16. Conway Morris A, Anderson N, Brittan M et al (2013) Combined dysfunctions of immune cells predict nosocomial infection in critically ill patients. Br J Anaesth 3:1–10
17. National Healthcare Safety Network (NHSN) (2013) July 2013 CDC/NHSN Protocol Clarifications Available at: http://www.cdc.gov/nhsn/PDFs/pscManual/10-VAE_FINAL.pdf Accessed Oct 2013
18. Klompas M (2013) Clinician's Corner: Does this patient have ventilator-associated pneumonia? JAMA 297:1583–1593
19. Petersen IS, Aru A, Skødt V et al (1999) Evaluation of pneumonia diagnosis in intensive care patients. Scand J Infect Dis 31:299–303
20. Fàbregas N, Ewig S, Torres A et al (1999) Clinical diagnosis of ventilator associated pneumonia revisited: comparative validation using immediate post-mortem lung biopsies. Thorax 54:867–873
21. Johanson WG, Pierce AK, Sanford JP, Thomas GD (1972) Nosocomial respiratory infections with gram-negative bacilli. The significance of colonization of the respiratory tract. Ann Int Med 77:701–706

22. Pugin J, Auckenthaler R, Mili N, Janssens JP, Lew PD, Suter PM (1991) Diagnosis of ventilator-associated pneumonia by bacteriologic analysis of bronchoscopic and nonbroncho-scopic "blind" bronchoalveolar lavage fluid. Am Rev Respir Dis 143:1121–1129
23. Shan J, Chen HL, Zhu JH (2011) Diagnostic accuracy of clinical pulmonary infection score for ventilator-associated pneumonia: a meta-analysis. Respir Care 56:1087–1094
24. Zilberberg MD, Shorr AF (2010) Ventilator-associated pneumonia: the clinical pulmonary infection score as a surrogate for diagnostics and outcome. Clin Infect Dis 1:S131–S135
25. Shorr AF, Cook D, Jiang X, Muscedere J, Heyland D (2008) Correlates of clinical failure in ventilator-associated pneumonia: insights from a large, randomized trial. J Crit Care 23:64–73
26. Singh N, Rogers P, Atwood CW, Wagener MM, Yu VL (2000) Short-course empiric antibiotic therapy for patients with pulmonary infiltrates in the intensive care unit. A proposed solution for indiscriminate antibiotic prescription. Am J Respir Crit Care Med 162:505–511
27. Fagon JY, Chastre J, Wolff M et al (2000) Invasive and noninvasive strategies for management of suspected ventilator-associated pneumonia. A randomized trial. Ann Intern Med 132:621–630
28. Canadian Critical Care Trials Group (2013) A randomized trial of diagnostic techniques for ventilator-associated pneumonia. N Engl J Med 355:2619–2630
29. Berton DC, Kalil AC, Cavalcanti M, Teixeira PJ (2012) Quantitative versus qualitative cultures of respiratory secretions for clinical outcomes in patients with ventilator-associated pneumonia Chocrane Database Syst Rev CD006482
30. Klompas M (2013) Complications of mechanical ventilation – the CDC's new surveillance paradigm. N Engl J Med 368:1472–1475
31. Hayashi Y, Morisawa K, Klompas M et al (2013) Toward improved surveillance: the impact of ventilator-associated complications on length of stay and antibiotic use in patients in intensive care units. Clin Infect Dis 56:471–477
32. Dudeck MA, Horan TC, Peterson KD et al (2011) National Healthcare Safety Network (NHSN) Report, data summary for 2010, device-associated module. Am J Infect Control 39:798–816
33. Masterton RG (2011) Antibiotic de-escalation. Crit Care Clin 27:149–162
34. Torres A, Ewig S, Lode H, Carlet J (2009) Defining, treating and preventing hospital acquired pneumonia: European perspective. Intensive Care Med 35:9–29
35. Walkey AJ, O'Donnell MR, Wiener RS (2011) Linezolid vs glycopeptide antibiotics for the treatment of suspected methicillin-resistant Staphylococcus aureus nosocomial pneumonia: a meta-analysis of randomized controlled trials. Chest 139:1148–1155
36. Munoz-Price LS, Weinstein RA (2008) Acinetobacter Infection. N Engl J Med 358:1271–1281
37. Martin-Loeches I, Deja M, Koulenti D et al (2013) Potentially resistant microorganisms in intubated patients with hospital-acquired pneumonia: the interaction of ecology, shock and risk factors. Intensive Care Med 39:672–681
38. Pasquale TR, Jabrocki B, Salstrom SJ et al (2013) Emergence of methicillin-resistant Staphy-lococcus aureus USA300 genotype as a major cause of late-onset nosocomial pneumonia in intensive care patients in the USA. Int J Infect Dis 17:e398–e403
39. Capellier G, Mockly H, Charpentier C et al (2012) Early-onset ventilator-associated pneumo-nia in adults randomized clinical trial: comparison of 8 versus 15 days of antibiotic treatment. PloS one 7:e41290
40. Chastre J, Wolff M, Fagon J-Y et al (2003) Comparison of 8 vs 15 days of antibiotic therapy for ventilator-associated pneumonia in adults: a randomized trial. JAMA 290:2588–2598
41. Dimopoulos G, Poulakou G, Pneumatikos IA, Armaganidis A, Kollef MH, Matthaiou DK (2013) Short- versus long-duration antibiotic regimens for ventilator-associated pneumonia: a systematic review and meta-analysis. Chest 144:1759–1767
42. Swoboda SM, Dixon T, Lipsett PA (2006) Can the clinical pulmonary infection score impact ICU antibiotic days? Surg Infect (Larchmt) 7:331–339
43. Morris AC, Hay AW, Swann DG et al (2011) Reducing ventilator-associated pneumonia in intensive care: impact of implementing a care bundle. Crit Care Med 39:2218–2224

44. Alhazzani W, Almasoud A, Jaeschke R et al (2013) Small bowel feeding and risk of pneumonia in adult critically ill patients: a systematic review and meta-analysis of randomized trials. Crit Care 17:R127
45. Muscedere J, Rewa O, McKechnie K, Jiang X, Laporta D, Heyland DK (2011) Subglottic secretion drainage for the prevention of ventilator-associated pneumonia: a systematic review and meta-analysis. Crit Care Med 39:1985–1991
46. Morrow LE, Kollef MH (2010) Recognition and prevention of nosocomial pneumonia in the intensive care unit and infection control in mechanical ventilation. Crit Care Med 38:S352–S362
47. Youngquist P, Carroll M, Farber M et al (2007) Implementing a ventilator bundle in a community hospital. Jt Comm J Qual Patient Saf 33:219–225
48. Zilberberg MD, Shorr AF, Kollef MH (2009) Implementing quality improvements in the intensive care unit: Ventilator bundle as an example. Crit Care Med 37:305–309
49. Vallés J, Peredo R, Burgueño MJ et al (2013) Efficacy of single-dose antibiotic against early-onset pneumonia in comatose patients who are ventilated. Chest 143:1219–1225

Part II
Optimal Oxygen Therapy

A Re-evaluation of Oxygen Therapy and Hyperoxemia in Critical Care

S. Suzuki, G. M. Eastwood, and R. Bellomo

Introduction

Oxygen therapy is universally administered to acutely ill patients. Most of these patients require a higher than normal fraction of inspired oxygen (FiO_2) in order to maintain an adequate arterial oxygen concentration (PaO_2). Despite the ubiquitous use of oxygen therapy in critical care, relatively little is known about the benefits and risks associated with oxygen therapy in adult critical illness and the correct dosing of such therapy in different subgroups of acutely ill patients. In this chapter, we discuss the rationale for oxygen therapy, recent insights into the risks associated with hyperoxemia, and the imperative to re-evaluate our oxygen therapy practice and targets for critically ill patients.

Rationale for Oxygen Therapy

Oxygen is a physiologic requirement for normal cellular function and is essential to sustaining human life. Under normal conditions, the human body has adapted to the oxygen concentration of ambient air (21 %) with the normal PaO_2 at atmospheric pressure (760 mmHg) at 80–100 mmHg [1]. This corresponds to an oxygen saturation of 95–96 % when measured by arterial blood gas sampling (SaO_2) or via pulse oximetry (SpO_2). A failure to maintain adequate blood oxygen concentrations can lead to cellular hypoxia, organ dysfunction and death. Hypoxemia is a common finding among critically ill patients irrespective of their underlying diagnosis [2]. Hypoxemia is believed to carry significant risk and in most cases is generally carefully avoided. Conversely, although hyperoxemia is believed to provide a buffer of

S. Suzuki · G. M. Eastwood · R. Bellomo ✉
Department of Intensive Care, Austin Hospital, 3084 Heidelberg, Melbourne, Australia
e-mail: rinaldo.bellomo@austin.org.au

J.-L. Vincent (Ed.), *Annual Update in Intensive Care and Emergency Medicine 2014*,   81
DOI 10.1007/978-3-319-03746-2_7, © Springer International Publishing Switzerland
2014

safety in some high risk patients, it may also be injurious to lung tissue and other organs.

Oxygen Therapy

Oxygen therapy is the therapeutic administration of supplemental oxygen to patients, primarily for the treatment or prevention of hypoxemia. A wide range of oxygen delivery devices are available for use in practice ranging from nasal cannulas, high-flow nasal cannulas through to invasive mechanical ventilation with an endotracheal tube. Indeed, oxygen therapy is often believed to be a simpler method of increasing tissue oxygenation in acute care compared to manipulating cardiac preload (fluid loading), contractility or afterload (infusion of inotropes and other vasoactive drugs) and improving oxygen-carrying capacity (transfusing blood) [3].

Oxygen Toxicity

Molecular Effects

Although the damage associated with severe hypoxemia appears obvious, injury associated with hyperoxemia is less well understood. Common explanations offered for hyperoxemic damage typically focus on the production of reactive oxygen species (ROS) and reactive nitrogen species, leading to cellular dysfunction or death [4–7]. ROS are free, negatively charged molecules containing an unpaired electron, which can cause death and lysis of oxygen-sensitive cells by oxidizing DNA, proteins and lipids, resulting in the microvascular and alveolar cell injury typical of oxygen toxicity [7, 8]. While production of ROS is physiological and necessary for energy production and innate immunity, in tissue hyperoxia, ROS and subsequent reaction products formed by mitochondria and other intracellular organelles may exceed the capacity of the antioxidant enzymes to detoxify them [8] and cause tissue injury.

Pulmonary Toxicity

Lung tissue is particularly susceptible to oxygen-related damage when exposed to supranormal oxygen concentrations. Prolonged exposure to FiO_2 of 0.6 leads to alveolar septal injury in baboons [9]. Sinclair and colleagues reported that 4 hours exposure to FiO_2 of 0.5 enhanced the severity of lung injury induced by high-stretch ventilation in rabbits, as determined by histopathology changes [10]. Additionally, ventilation with oxygen (6 hours) even at ambient air level (21 %), but not without oxygen (100 % nitrogen) increases tissue volumes, myofibroblast differentiation and apoptosis in sheep lung [11]. Even in the healthy human lung, exposure to high FiO_2 of 0.95 for a short period of time (17 hours) will cause increased alveolar capillary leak, as well as evidence of fibrotic changes [12]. Supplemental oxygen has also been associated with absorption atelectasis, an increase in ventilation/perfusion (V/Q) mismatch [13], impaired alveolar macrophages and promotion of pulmonary infection [14].

Extrapulmonary Toxicity

Animal studies have also shown that supranormal oxygen concentrations (hyperoxemia) can reduce heart rate and cardiac output and increase systemic vascular resistance [15, 16]. These findings have been confirmed in healthy volunteers [17] and patients with congestive heart failure, in whom the effect is more pronounced [18]. In addition, hyperoxemia has been shown to decrease cerebral blood flow by 11 to 33 % in healthy adults [19, 20]. The mechanism for the decrease in cerebral blood flow is presumably partly due to direct increase in cerebrovascular resistance as a result of increased vasoconstriction, whereas the accompanying small decrease in end-expiratory carbon dioxide may also influence cerebral blood flow [19, 21].

Current Oxygen Saturation Recommendations

At the present time, despite concerns related to hyperoxemia and high FiO_2, oxygen therapy is commonly and liberally used in the management of acute conditions, such as ischemic heart disease, sepsis, pneumonia, stroke, and cardiac arrest [22–24]. Supplemental oxygen is regarded as safe and, because of fear of giving too little, there has been almost no concern about giving too much [25]. In particular, in emergency situations, 100 % oxygen is always provided until the emergent period is over. Once the patient is past the acute period, oxygen saturation targets should be established and oxygen therapy modified. However, the timeliness and targets of such adjustments remain unknown and, in many patients, high FiO_2 therapy with associated hyperoxemia is continued for much longer than required after the initial emergency, resulting in prolonged hyperoxemia.

The British Thoracic Society (BTS) guidelines for the emergency use of oxygen in adults [6] and a recent review [22] recommend oxygen saturation (SpO_2) targets of 94 % to 98 % for most acutely ill patients or 88 % to 92 % for those at risk of hypercapnic respiratory failure. The Acute Respiratory Distress Syndrome (ARDS) Network protocols recommended maintaining an SpO_2 of 88 % to 95 % (PaO_2 55–80 mmHg) [25]. However, evidence supporting such recommendations is lacking and these recommendations are essentially based on expert opinion, observational data and inductive physiological reasoning. Thus, for patients admitted to the intensive care unit (ICU), the optimal SpO_2 target levels remain unclear. Moreover, it is unclear whether there is compliance with such targets in daily practice, given the weakness of the evidence to support them and the all-abiding concern about avoiding hypoxemia. Nonetheless, there are many aspects of the physiological and clinical effects of hyperoxemia and high FiO_2 therapy, which raise concern (Box 1).

Box 1:
Reported adverse events potentially the result of or associated with hyperoxemia
Cardiovascular system
- Decreased stroke volume
- Increased systemic vascular resistance
- Coronary artery vasoconstriction
- Decreased cardiac output in congestive heart failure
- Increased left ventricular end-diastolic pressure

Pulmonary system
- Hypercapnia in chronic obstructive pulmonary disease
- Increased mortality in chronic obstructive pulmonary disease

Cerebrovascular system
- Increased stroke severity
- Increased stroke-related mortality
- Increased release of neuron-specific enolase after cardiac arrest
- Increased mortality after resuscitation from cardiac arrest

Oxygen Therapy in Acute Illness

Chronic Obstructive Pulmonary Disease

The level of evidence supporting the view that giving oxygen can lead to clinically important adverse effects is strongest in the management of acute exacerbations of chronic obstructive pulmonary disease (COPD). A well-designed randomized trial of high-concentration versus titrated-oxygen treatment (target SpO_2 88–92 %) in the pre-hospital treatment of suspected acute exacerbation of COPD was recently conducted in Australia [26]. In an intention-to-treat analysis of 405 patients, the risk of death was significantly reduced by 58 % with titrated oxygen treatment. In the subgroup of patients with confirmed COPD, the risk of death was reduced by 78 % with titrated oxygen treatment. Thus, controlled oxygen therapy titrated to achieve oxygen saturations of 88–92 % can be considered the correct therapeutic regimen in patients with acute exacerbations of COPD, as recommended in the BTS guidelines [6]. It is unclear whether this should be the target for all patients with acute respiratory illness or only those on mechanical ventilation.

Perioperative Care

Several trials have reported that perioperative use of 80 % oxygen decreases the rate of surgical site infection after abdominal surgery as compared with 30 % oxygen [5]. However, the largest and arguably the best designed trial conducted to date, the PeRioperative OXygen Fraction (PROXI) trial, found no significant difference in surgical site infections when 1,400 patients were randomized to receive 80 or 30 % oxygen during and 2 hours after acute or elective laparotomy [27]. Additionally, a recent follow-up study of the PROXI trial revealed that patients randomized to 80 % perioperative oxygen administration were more likely to have died at long term follow-up compared with those randomized to 30 % oxygen [28]. This observation raises concerns about the use of high FiO_2, and the pursuit or maintenance of hyperoxemia during and after major surgery.

Stroke

Ronning and Guldvog showed that survival at 1 year for patients with mild or moderate stroke was significantly greater in those given air than in those given 100 % oxygen for the first 24 hours after the event [29]. A very small ($n = 16$) study of short term high flow oxygen treatment (45 l/min for 8 hours) after acute stroke showed transient early improvements in neurological performance and infarct size but no long-term clinical benefit at three months [30]. This study was followed by a larger trial of the same intervention, which was stopped after 85 patients were enrolled because of an imbalance of deaths in favor of the control group (40 % mortality on oxygen vs. 17 % mortality on room air) [31]. Observational data in 2,643 critically ill, mechanically ventilated stroke patients found that hyperoxemia was common but that there was no relationship between worst oxygen level on day of admission and subsequent outcome [32]. Finally, a recent, randomized controlled pilot study showed routine oxygen supplementation at a low flow rate (2–3 l/min via nasal cannula) for 72 hours after acute stroke led to a small, but statistically significant, improvement in neurological recovery at 1 week [33] but none of the key outcomes differed at six months between the groups [34]. Following this pilot study, a large multicenter, prospective, randomized, open, blinded-endpoint study is now ongoing [35]. Until the results of this trial are reported, it is unclear whether giving supplemental oxygen to stroke patients is beneficial.

Acute Myocardial Infarction

Concerns have been raised about the role of supplemental oxygen in the management of acute myocardial infarction (AMI) [36]. Current evidence is suggestive of several harmful effects associated with supplemental oxygen, yet published studies are underpowered or lack the ability to draw a causal relationship [36, 37]. To date, four randomized controlled clinical trials have studied the effect of oxygen in AMI patients. In a double-blind, randomized in-hospital study, 200 patients with AMI were allocated to receive air or face mask supplemental oxygen for the initial 24 hours of hospitalization [38]. Findings revealed no significant difference in mortality, incidence of arrhythmias or use of analgesics between the groups. However, the oxygen group had higher serum aspartate aminotransferase levels and a greater incidence of sinus tachycardia. In a second study, 50 patients were allocated to either room air or face mask supplemental oxygen [39]. The incidence of hypoxemia ($SpO_2 < 90\%$) was 70% and that of severe hypoxemia ($SpO_2 < 80\%$) 35% in patients who were not treated with oxygen, compared with 27% and 4% in those who were administered oxygen. The requirement for analgesia or presence of ST-segment change, however, did not differ with oxygen use. This study did not report mortality rate. In the third study, 137 patients were allocated to either supplemental oxygen (4–6 l/min) or air [40]. Complications including heart failure, pericarditis and rhythm disorders occurred less frequently in the oxygen group (relative risk 0.45, 95% CI 0.22-0.94). One patient out of 58 died in the oxygen group and none of 79 participants in the air group. Finally, the most recent trial compared routine oxygen use versus titrated oxygen therapy [41]. There was only 1 death in the 68 patients treated with routine oxygen and 2 in 68 of those treated with the titrated oxygen therapy in this study (relative risk 0.5; 95% CI 0.05-5.4). The investigators found no evidence of benefit or harm from high-concentration compared with titrated oxygen in initially uncomplicated ST-segment elevation myocardial infarction and concluded that large randomized controlled trials are required to resolve this clinical uncertainty.

Cardiac Arrest

Animal experiments using a model of cardiac arrest provide strong evidence that hyperoxemia aggravates neurological injury [42] and justify concerns that similar injury might occur in humans. There is emerging evidence to support early goal-directed oxygenation targets during the immediate post-resuscitation care of cardiac arrest patients. Kilgannon and colleagues reported the results of a multicenter observational trial comparing outcomes in patients after non-traumatic cardiac arrest based on PaO_2. These authors found that hyperoxemia ($PaO_2 \geq 300$ mmHg) within 24 hours following ICU arrival was independently associated with increased mortality compared to both the normoxemic and the hypoxemic group [43]. Additionally, they identified a dose-dependent association between supranormal oxygen tension and risk of in-hospital death [44]. Another recent observational study is consistent with these findings [45]. In contrast, a large, multicenter, observational cohort study in Australia and New Zealand using the same oxygenation thresholds did not show any correlation between arterial hyperoxia and outcome following cardiac arrest [46]. This lack of correlation was confirmed by a study in 957 patients from a cardiac registry in Australia [47]. Several studies are under way to assess the feasibility and safety of delivering conservative oxygen therapy to patients experiencing an out-of-hospital cardiac arrest.

Mechanically Ventilated Patients

Mechanical ventilation is a life-saving intervention commonly applied to acutely ill patients. In order to determine the association between hyperoxemia and mortality in mechanically ventilated patients, two large cohort observational studies have recently been conducted. In the first study, de Jonge and colleagues performed a retrospective audit of 36,307 patients from 50 ICUs in The Netherlands and reported that high FiO_2 and high PaO_2 in the first 24 hours after admission were independently associated with increased in-hospital mortality in ventilated ICU patients [48]. However, a bi-national multicenter observational study in Australia and New Zealand involving 152,680 patients from 150 ICUs found no independent relationship between hyperoxemia in the first 24 hours in ICU and mortality in ventilated patients [49]. Given the discrepancy related to the impact of early hyperoxemia on mortality for mechanically ventilated patients, the widespread use of oxygen, the uncertainty over therapeutic targets and the observational nature of the above studies, more investigations appear desirable.

Re-evaluating Oxygen Therapy and Oxygen Targets in Acute Illness

Although there is increasing awareness of the potential harms of hyperoxemia, these concerns have not translated into changes to more conservative routine practice. In large observational studies in patients after cardiac arrest, hyperoxemia (defined as $PaO_2 \geq 300$ mmHg) occurred in 18 % of patients in a US cohort [43] and in 10.6 % of patients in a cohort from Australia and New Zealand [43]. Of 126,778 arterial blood gas measurements from 5,498 mechanically ventilated ICU patients, 22 % had a PaO_2 above 120 mmHg and in most cases such hyperoxemic levels did not lead to adjustment of ventilator settings if the FiO_2 was < 0.41 [50]. This lack of attention to careful oxygen therapy titration has been confirmed by detailed observational studies.

Two recent observational studies have described in detail current oxygen therapy in mechanically ventilated ICU patients who required ventilation for > 48 hours. In the first study, a time-weighted average FiO_2 of 0.42 was applied to achieve a time-weighted average SpO_2 of 97.1 % for the initial 7 days of mechanical ventilation [51] (Figs. 1 and 2). In the second prospective observational study, patients spent most of their time with an FiO_2 between 0.3 and 0.5 and had a relatively high SpO_2 and PaO_2, implying that further decreases in FiO_2 could likely be easily and safely implemented [52] (Figs. 1 and 2). The authors concluded that an interventional study comparing current liberal oxygen practice to more conservative oxygen targets (PaO_2 of between 60 to 65 mmHg and/or SpO_2 of between 90 to 92 %) was possible.

Fortunately, a pilot study in mechanically ventilated ICU patients (NCT 01684124), and a randomized controlled trial in ICU patients (NCT01319643), and studies in patients with AMI [49], stroke [35] and traumatic brain injury (NCT01201291) are all currently underway. These studies will provide clinical information on the safety, feasibility and/or efficacy of a more conservative approach to oxygen therapy in several acute care settings.

Fig. 1 Graphic display of time weighted average (TWA) for SpO$_2$, FiO$_2$, PaO$_2$ in mechanically ventilated patients from two recent observational studies [51, 52]. Seemingly unnecessarily high FiO$_2$ levels despite relative hyperoxemia appear common

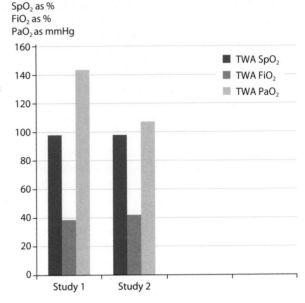

Fig. 2 Graphic representation of mean PaO$_2$ in critically ill mechanically ventilated patients from two recent observational studies [51, 52]. Over the first 5 days of mechanical ventilation, despite moderate levels of FiO$_2$, the average PaO$_2$ was in the hyperoxemic range

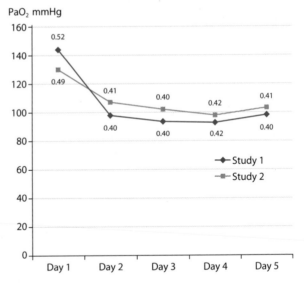

Conclusions

Intensive care clinicians make decisions every day regarding the management of oxygen therapy for acutely ill patients. Despite mounting concern over the clinical risks of supplemental oxygen therapy, current oxygen management remains liberal, excess oxygen is routinely delivered, hyperoxemia is common and guidelines are not based on high quality evidence. Given the ubiquitous use and the possible harmful effects of excessive oxygen administration, it is time to re-evaluate our therapeutic targets and obtain higher level evidence to guide the selection of therapeutic targets for oxygen therapy in critical illness.

References

1. Considine J (2005) The reliability of clinical indicators of oxygenation: a literature review. Contemp Nurse 18:258–267
2. Martin DS, Grocott MP (2012) Oxygen therapy in critical illness: Precise control of arterial oxygenation and permissive hypoxemia. Crit Care Med 4:423–432
3. Lavery GG, Corris PA (2012) Should we be giving high concentration oxygen to all patients treated in an ambulance? J R Coll Physicians Edinb 42:36–42
4. Budinger GR, Mutlu GM (2013) Balancing the risks and benefits of oxygen therapy in critically iii adults. Chest 143:1151–1162
5. Meyhoff CS, Staehr AK, Rasmussen LS (2012) Rational use of oxygen in medical disease and anesthesia. Curr Opin Anaesthesiol 25:363–370
6. O'Driscoll BR, Howard LS, Davison AG (2008) BTS guideline for emergency oxygen use in adult patients. Thorax 63:vi1–68
7. Hayes RA, Shekar K, Fraser JF (2013) Is hyperoxaemia helping or hurting patients during extracorporeal membrane oxygenation? Review of a complex problem. Perfusion 28:184–193
8. Jackson RM (1985) Pulmonary oxygen toxicity. Chest 88:900–905
9. Crapo JD, Hayatdavoudi G, Knapp MJ, Fracica PJ, Wolfe WG, Piantadosi CA (1994) Progressive alveolar septal injury in primates exposed to 60 % oxygen for 14 days. Am J Physiol 267:L797–L806
10. Sinclair SE, Altemeier WA, Matute-Bello G, Chi EY (2004) Augmented lung injury due to interaction between hyperoxia and mechanical ventilation. Crit Care Med 32:2496–2501
11. Allison BJ, Crossley KJ, Flecknoe SJ, Davis PG, Morley CJ, Hooper SB (2010) Ventilation and oxygen: dose-related effects of oxygen on ventilation-induced lung injury. Pediatr Res 67:238–243
12. Davis WB, Rennard SI, Bitterman PB, Crystal RG (1983) Pulmonary oxygen toxicity. Early reversible changes in human alveolar structures induced by hyperoxia. N Engl J Med 309:878–883
13. Downs JB (2003) Has oxygen administration delayed appropriate respiratory care? Fallacies regarding oxygen therapy. Respir Care 48:611–620
14. Baleeiro CE, Wilcoxen SE, Morris SB, Standiford TJ, Paine R 3rd (2003) Sublethal hyperoxia impairs pulmonary innate immunity. J Immunol 171:955–963
15. Lodato RF (1989) Decreased O2 consumption and cardiac output during normobaric hyperoxia in conscious dogs. J Appl Physiol 67:1551–1559
16. Fracica PJ, Knapp MJ, Piantadosi CA et al (1991) Responses of baboons to prolonged hyperoxia: physiology and qualitative pathology. J Appl Physiol 71:2352–2362
17. Harten JM, Anderson KJ, Angerson WJ, Booth MG, Kinsella J (2003) The effect of normobaric hyperoxia on cardiac index in healthy awake volunteers. Anaesthesia 58:885–888
18. Haque WA, Boehmer J, Clemson BS, Leuenberger UA, Silber DH, Sinoway LI (1996) Hemodynamic effects of supplemental oxygen administration in congestive heart failure. J Am Coll Cardiol 27:353–357
19. Johnston AJ, Steiner LA, Gupta AK, Menon DK (2003) Cerebral oxygen vasoreactivity and cerebral tissue oxygen reactivity. Br J Anaesth 90:774–786
20. Floyd TF, Clark JM, Gelfand R et al (2003) Independent cerebral vasoconstrictive effects of hyperoxia and accompanying arterial hypocapnia at 1 ATA. J Appl Physiol 95:2453–2461

21. Watson NA, Beards SC, Altaf N, Kassner A, Jackson A (2000) The effect of hyperoxia on cerebral blood flow: a study in healthy volunteers using magnetic resonance phase-contrast angiography. Eur J Anesthesiol 17:152–159
22. Decalmer S, O'Driscoll BR (2013) Oxygen: friend or foe in peri-operative care? Anaesthesia 68:8–12
23. Iscoe S, Beasley R, Fisher JA (2011) Supplementary oxygen for nonhypoxemic patients: O(2) much of a good thing? Crit Care 15:305
24. Cornet AD, Kooter AJ, Peters MJ, Smulders YM (2012) Supplemental oxygen therapy in medical emergencies: more harm than benefit? Arch Intern Med 172:289–290
25. The Acute Respiratory Distress Syndrome Network (2000) Ventilation with lower tidal volumes as compared with traditional tidal volumes for acute lung injury and the acute respiratory distress syndrome. N Engl J Med 342:1301–1308
26. Austin MA, Wills KE, Blizzard L, Walters EH, Wood-Baker R (2010) Effect of high flow oxygen on mortality in chronic obstructive pulmonary disease patients in prehospital setting: randomised controlled trial. BMJ 341:c5462
27. Meyhoff CS, Wetterslev J, Jorgensen LN et al (2009) Effect of high perioperative oxygen fraction on surgical site infection and pulmonary complications after abdominal surgery: the PROXI randomized clinical trial. JAMA 302:1543–1550
28. Meyhoff CS, Jorgensen LN, Wetterslev J, Christensen KB, Rasmussen LS (2012) Increased long-term mortality after a high perioperative inspiratory oxygen fraction during abdominal surgery: follow-up of a randomized clinical trial. Anesth Analg 115(4):849–854
29. Ronning OM, Guldvog B (1999) Should stroke victims routinely receive supplemental oxygen? A quasi-randomized controlled trial. Stroke 30:2033–2037
30. Singhal AB, Benner T, Roccatagliata L et al (2005) A pilot study of normobaric oxygen therapy in acute ischemic stroke. Stroke 36:797–802
31. Normobaric Oxygen Therapy in Acute Ischemic Stroke Trial. Available at http://www.clinicaltrials.gov/ct2/show/NCT00414726. Accessed August 2013.
32. Young P, Beasley R, Bailey M et al (2012) Study of Oxygen in Critical Care (SOCC) Group: The association between early arterial oxygenation and mortality in ventilated pateints with acute ischaemic stroke. Crit Care Resusc 14:14–19
33. Roffe C, Ali K, Warusevitane A et al (2011) The SOS pilot study: a RCT of routine oxygen supplementation early after acute stroke-effect on recovery of neurological function at one week. PloS one 6:e19113
34. Ali K, Warusevitane A, Lally F et al (2013) The stroke oxygen pilot study: a randomized controlled trial of the effects of routine oxygen supplementation early after acute stroke-effect on key outcomes at six months. PloS one 8:e59274
35. The Stroke Oxygen Study: a multi-centre, prospective, randomised, open, blinded-endpoint study of routine oxygen treatment in the first 72 hours after a stroke. Available at http://www.so2s.co.uk Accessed August 2013.
36. Stub D, Smith K, Bernard S et al (2012) A randomized controlled trial of oxygen therapy in acute myocardial infarction Air Verses Oxygen In myocarDial infarction study (AVOID Study). Am Heart J 163:339–345
37. Burls A, Cabello JB, Emparanza JI, Bayliss S, Quinn T (2011) Oxygen therapy for acute myocardial infarction: a systematic review and meta-analysis. Emerg Med J 28:8–12
38. Rawles JM, Kenmure AC (1976) Controlled trial of oxygen in uncomplicated myocardial infarction. BMJ 1:1121–1123
39. Wilson AT, Channer KS (1997) Hypoxaemia and supplemental oxygen therapy in the first 24 hours after myocardial infarction: the role of pulse oximetry. J R Coll Physicians Lond 31:657–661
40. Ukholkina GB, Kostianov I, Kuchkina NV, Grendo EP, Gofman I (2005) Effect of oxygenotherapy used in combination with reperfusion in patients with acute myocardial infarction. Kardiologiia 45:59

41. Ranchord AM, Argyle R, Beynon R et al (2012) High-concentration versus titrated oxygen therapy in ST-elevation myocardial infarction: a pilot randomized controlled trial. Am Heart J 163:168–175

42. Pilcher J, Weatherall M, Shirtcliffe P, Bellomo R, Young P, Beasley R (2012) The effect of hyperoxia following cardiac arrest – A systematic review and meta-analysis of animal trials. Resuscitation 83:417–422

43. Kilgannon JH, Jones AE, Shapiro NI et al (2010) Association between arterial hyperoxia following resuscitation from cardiac arrest and in-hospital mortality. JAMA 303:2165–2171

44. Kilgannon JH, Jones AE, Parrillo JE et al (2011) Relationship between supranormal oxygen tension and outcome after resuscitation from cardiac arrest. Circulation 123:2717–2722

45. Janz DR, Hollenbeck RD, Pollock JS, McPherson JA, Rice TW (2012) Hyperoxia is associated with increased mortality in patients treated with mild therapeutic hypothermia after sudden cardiac arrest. Crit Care Med 40:3135–3139

46. Bellomo R, Bailey M, Eastwood GM et al (2011) Arterial hyperoxia and in-hospital mortality after resuscitation from cardiac arrest. Crit Care 15:R90

47. Ihle JF, Bernard S, Bailey MJ, Pilcher D, Smith K, Scheinkestel CD (2013) Hyperoxia in the intensive care unit and outcome after out-of-hospital ventricular fibrillation cardiac arrest. Crit Care Resusc 15:186–190

48. de Jonge E, Peelen L, Keijzers PJ et al (2008) Association between administered oxygen, arterial partial oxygen pressure and mortality in mechanically ventilated intensive care unit patients. Crit Care 12:R156

49. Eastwood G, Bellomo R, Bailey M et al (2012) Arterial oxygen tension and mortality in mechanically ventilated patients. Intensive Care Med 38:91–98

50. de Graaff AE, Dongelmans DA, Binnekade JM, de Jonge E (2011) Clinicians' response to hyperoxia in ventilated patients in a Dutch ICU depends on the level of FiO2. Intensive Care Med 37:46–51

51. Panwar R, Capellier G, Schmutz N et al (2013) Current oxygenation practice in ventilated patients-an observational cohort study. Anaesth Intensive Care 41:505–514

52. Suzuki S, Eastwood GM, Peck L, Glassford NJ, Bellomo R (2013) Current oxygen management in mechanically ventilated patients: A prospective observational cohort study. J Crit Care 28:647–654

Normoxia and Hyperoxia in Neuroprotection

P. Le Roux

Introduction

Oxygen (O_2) is one of the commonest therapeutic agents used in hospitals and the outpatient setting. It is a drug in the true sense of the word with specific biochemical properties, specific physiologic actions, a range of effective doses, and known adverse effects at high doses. Oxygen is widely available and commonly prescribed and the cost of a single use of O_2 is low. However, there are few evidence-based data on its use in many clinical conditions. This is particularly important for neuroprotection, because the human brain weighs about 2 % of total body mass yet consumes 20 % of the O_2 and 25 % of the glucose used by the whole body at rest. The O_2 and energy reserves in the brain are very limited, and its survival and function depend on a constant supply of O_2 and energy-rich substrate. Consequently there is interest in the role of O_2 in neuroprotection, including: 1) avoidance of hypoxia, 2) hyperoxic resuscitation, 3) hyperbaric oxygen (HBO), 4) normobaric hyperoxia (NBO), and 5) correction of brain oxygen (PbtO$_2$). However, the margin of safety between effective and potentially toxic O_2 doses is relatively narrow and hence O_2 use in neuroprotection requires a full understanding of the balance between its benefits and potentially deleterious effects. Here, we will review the role of normoxia or hyperoxia in neuroprotection for acute neurological disorders. The role of HBO or NBO to potentiate recovery after concussion or for post-traumatic stress disorder, and its role in infection, wound healing, high altitude sickness and diving will not be reviewed.

P. Le Roux ✉
Department of Neurosurgery, Thomas Jefferson University, Philadelphia, PA USA
e-mail: LeRouxP@MLHS.ORG

J.-L. Vincent (Ed.), *Annual Update in Intensive Care and Emergency Medicine 2014*,   93
DOI 10.1007/978-3-319-03746-2_8, © Springer International Publishing Switzerland
2014

Benefits of Hyperoxia

There are many potential beneficial effects of hyperoxia in the brain, e. g., it increases $PbtO_2$, restores brain mitochondrial redox potential, decreases intracranial pressure (ICP), restores aerobic metabolism, and improves pressure autoregulation [1–6]. Systemically, hyperoxia has several effects including:

1) a temporary increase in blood pressure through an increase in total peripheral vascular resistance secondary to systemic peripheral vasoconstriction;
2) inhibition of neutrophil adherence;
3) reduction in expression of the endothelial adhesion molecules, E-selectin and intercellular adhesion molecule (ICAM)-1;
4) induction of endothelial nitric oxide synthase (eNOS) production;
5) it influences macrophage and T-cell function; and
6) it provokes anti-inflammatory responses in macrophages among others [7].

Oxygen Toxicity

The benefits of O_2 therapy and its potential toxicity have been known since the late 18th century. However, the concept of O_2 toxicity and the toxic threshold (exposure length and level) remain debated although it is known that healthy individuals can breathe 55 % fraction of inspired oxygen (FiO_2) for 7 days [8]. There are three major concerns: 1) lung toxicity (including the airway); 2) central nervous system (CNS) toxicity; and 3) altered cerebral blood flow (CBF) [9].

Our knowledge comes mostly from animal HBO studies and from the diving and aviation industry, and suggests that CNS toxicity may occur when O_2 partial pressure is > 2.0 atmosphere absolute (ATA). In addition the effects of hyperoxia have been well studied in very premature infants (< 28 weeks gestation) with longitudinal studies establishing a relationship between hyperoxia and development of retinopathy of prematurity, chronic lung disease, and brain injury [10]. In adults, acute tracheobronchitis is the earliest clinical syndrome. This condition does not develop in humans breathing O_2 at partial pressures < 0.05 MPa (0.5 ATA or 50 % O_2 at normal atmospheric pressure). In healthy humans breathing > 95 % O_2 at normal atmospheric pressure (1 ATA), tracheobronchitis develops after a latent period of 4 to 22 hours, but as early as 3 hours while breathing O_2 at 3 ATA. The symptoms subside within a few hours of termination of hyperoxia, with complete resolution within a few days. Other pulmonary concerns important in neuroprotection include absorption atelectasis, hypoxic pulmonary vasoconstriction (HPV), and hyperoxia-induced lung injury. At different O_2 doses, different mechanisms may underlie pulmonary toxicity: At 1 or 1.5 ATA, an inflammatory response and destruction of the alveolar-capillary barrier leading to edema, impaired gas exchange, and respiratory failure evolves over time, whereas at 2–3 ATA, pulmonary injury is accelerated but less inflammatory in character, and events in the brain often are a prelude to lung pathology. The CNS-mediated component of this lung injury can be attenuated by selective inhibition of neuronal NOS (nNOS) or by unilateral vagus nerve transection [11]. In many acute neurologic disorders, e. g., traumatic brain injury (TBI) and subarachnoid hemorrhage (SAH), lung injury is common and whether the pulmonary toxicity is from the disease or the treatment can be difficult to elucidate. Recently, Rockswold et al. [2, 3] examined bronchoalveolar lavage (BAL) interleukin (IL)-8 and IL-6 assays in TBI patients who received HBO (1.5 ATA) and NBO. No increase in these inflammatory markers was observed suggesting no toxic effects of the treatment.

Many factors can influence CNS O_2 toxicity, e. g., carbon dioxide (CO_2), physical activity, circadian rhythm, gender, and fluid status [8]. Minor symptoms of O_2 toxicity include nausea, dizziness, headache, disorientation, and blurred vision. Seizures may develop at higher O_2 concentrations. Breathing 100 % O_2 at 1 atm, may reduce CBF by vasoconstriction in normal individuals. In select patients this effect may be beneficial since it can reduce ICP. When breathing hyperoxic mixtures, reactive oxygen species (ROS), including O_2 free radicals, can be generated at a rate exceeding the body's antioxidant capacity and can subsequently initiate lipid peroxidation and cellular destruction [12]. Brain tissue is especially vulnerable to lipid peroxidation and ROS. This observation may be true in ischemia and reperfusion but the role of hyperoxic-induced ROS in TBI is less clear. Indeed several clinical studies in severe TBI using microdialysis or cerebrospinal fluid (CSF) analysis during HBO or NBO found no evidence of oxidative stress [2, 3, 13]; instead markers of lipid peroxidation, phospholipid degradation, and inflammation, e. g., F2-isoprostanes and glycerol actually decreased, suggesting a biochemical benefit. Individually tailored O_2 treatment regimens specific to the disease are likely important; nevertheless there are various therapies that have been shown to reduce O_2 toxicity, e. g., minocycline, topiramate, sildenafil, pentoxifylline, omeprazole, omega-3 fatty acid supplementation, estradiol, colchicine and caffeine among many others [14–17].

Hyperbaric Oxygen

HBO can increase $PbtO_2$. In animal ischemia or cardiac arrest models, or clinical stroke studies, HBO can reduce infarct volume, blood brain barrier disruption, edema and neurologic deficits [18–23]. In experimental TBI, HBO can ameliorate neuron injury and reduce edema [25–27]. In severe TBI patients, HBO improves metabolism measured by microdialysis, decreases ICP and reduces mortality, particularly when there is cerebral edema and elevated ICP [2, 3, 28, 29]. However, administering HBO is a formidable undertaking and patients must be moved out of the intensive care unit (ICU) to the HBO chamber. Furthermore, its feasibility remains limited because HBO chambers are expensive and available at only a few centers.

Normobaric Hyperoxia

Although HBO has a more robust treatment effect than NBO on oxidative cerebral metabolism [2], NBO (100 % FiO_2 at 1 ATA) has several advantages over HBO: it is simple to administer, non-invasive, inexpensive, widely available, and can be started promptly after TBI or stroke (e. g., by paramedics). Many possible mechanisms have been reported to describe the neuroprotective effects of NBO, such as improved tissue oxygenation, increased CBF, reduced oxidative stress, maintaining penumbral oxygenation and protecting the blood brain barrier [24]. However, the end result may depend on what the predominant mechanism of cell injury is, because experimental studies suggest that NBO may reduce excitotoxin-induced injury but aggravate O_2 and glucose deprivation-induced cell injury [30]. In animal models, NBO administered during transient ischemia attenuated magnetic resonance imaging (MRI) abnormalities, stroke lesion volumes, and the frequency of peri-infarct depolarizations (PIDs) and improved outcome without increasing markers of oxidative stress [31–35]. These effects could be seen despite complete flow arrest [36]. These experimental observations, i. e., increased FiO_2 can ameliorate brain injury during ischemia, have been confirmed in clinical studies. In particular, in a small, randomized trial in humans, Singhal et al. [37] observed that high-flow O_2 was associated with reduced clinical deficits and MRI abnormalities in select patients with acute ischemic stroke, supporting the importance of dissolved O_2 in salvaging vulnerable tissue.

In TBI, hypoxia is a significant adverse factor and aerobic metabolism and mitochondrial function are disturbed. Hence, there is interest in NBO as a treatment in patients with TBI. In experimental TBI models, NBO can reduce the severity and extent of secondary brain damage, the volume of contusions and morbidity [27, 38, 39]. Following moderate or severe TBI, brain glucose is decreased and lactate increased; these changes are attenuated by breathing 100 % O_2, i. e., hyperoxia restores 'normal' metabolism [40, 41]. However, care is needed in extrapolating these biochemical results, because there is evidence that in some circumstances elevated brain lactate may be protective [42]. Several groups have studied NBO (100 % FiO_2) in TBI patients using microdialysis, near-infrared spectroscopy (NIRS) and $PbtO_2$ monitors; the results are mixed and depend in part on methodology [4–6, 41, 43–48]. In general, they show that NBO increases $PbtO_2$ and reduces lactate and glutamate levels particularly during the first 24 hours after TBI. The 'beneficial' effects on the lactate/pyruvate ratio or $PbtO_2$ depend on baseline values and in patients with normal baseline levels a significant change in metabolic variables may not occur [46, 47]. The effects are most noticeable in patients who have elevated baseline brain lactate levels. Interestingly, a greater $PbtO_2$ response appears to be associated with worse outcome [47]. Together, these data suggest that there is a narrow effective dose and that NBO may only be effective in a specific group of patients. It should be remembered that the monitors used in these various studies are local monitors. More global measures, e. g., using positron emission tomography (PET), may provide better insight. However, PET studies provide conflicting data with some studies suggesting that NBO does not improve the cerebral metabolic rate for oxygen [48] and others showing an effect only in "at-risk" tissue [5].

Correction of Brain Oxygen

Many factors can influence oxygen levels in the brain (Box 1) and rather than delivering high O_2 doses, simple correction of $PbtO_2$ using a variety of therapies may suffice, thus avoiding the potentially deleterious effects associated with hyperoxia. Brain oxygen monitors have been used in the clinical environment since 1993 and were first included in the treatment guidelines for severe TBI in 2007 and their use and physiology has been described in several reviews [49–51]. Decreases in $PbtO_2$ are not benign and are associated with independent chemical markers of brain ischemia [52] in microdialysis studies. The number, duration, and intensity of brain hypoxic episodes ($PbtO_2 < 15$ mmHg), and any $PbtO_2$ value < 5 mmHg are associated with poor outcome after TBI [53–60]. Indeed, a $PbtO_2 < 10$ mmHg after TBI is associated with a significant increase in both mortality and unfavorable outcome [58]. Furthermore, the burden of brain hypoxia is an independent factor associated with poor outcome [60]. The exact relationship with outcome, however, may vary depending on where the probe is placed (i. e., in normal white matter, in the penumbra, or in a contusion [61, 62]). Similar but less robust relationships between reduced $PbtO_2$ and poor outcome are observed in SAH [63, 64].

Box 1:

Factors that may influence oxygen levels in the brain ($PbtO_2$)

Local factors of major influence on $PbtO_2$	Systemic factors of major influence on $PbtO_2$
1. Oxygen consumption of neurons and glial cells	1. Intracranial pressure
2. Oxygen diffusion conditions/gradients in tissue	2. Arterial blood pressure and cerebral perfusion pressure
3. Number of perfused capillaries per tissue volume	3. PaO_2, $PaCO_2$, pH,
4. Length and diameter of perfused capillaries	4. Temperature
5. Capillary perfusion rate and microflow pattern	5. Blood hemoglobin content, P50, viscosity, and hematocrit
6. Hemoglobin oxygen release in microcirculation	

Brain oxygen monitoring is useful in a variety of clinical situations in which secondary brain injury may occur [65, 66], and some studies suggest that $PbtO_2$ complements ICP monitoring. Episodes of brain hypoxia are common and may occur even when ICP and cerebral perfusion pressure (CPP) are normal [60, 67–69], emphasizing the potential value of multimodal monitoring that integrates data from several physiologic monitors. A strong relationship is observed between $PbtO_2$ and several drivers of brain perfusion, such as mean arterial pressure (MAP), CPP, and end-tidal CO_2 [70–72]. This observation can help clinicians to better understand the complex pathophysiology of the brain after an acute insult, evaluate autoregulation, and identify optimal physiologic targets and the utility of therapeutic interventions [73–79]. Some, but not all, observational series suggest that the addition of $PbtO_2$-based care to conventional ICP- and CPP-based care is associated with improved outcome after severe TBI [80–83]; this question is now being evaluated in a multicenter clinical trial.

What is the Optimal Oxygen Level During Resuscitation?

An association between hypoxia and poor outcome from TBI, ischemic stroke, and SAH is well documented. Hence, avoidance of hypoxia is central to management guidelines for all these conditions. However, it is unclear whether hyperoxygenation is beneficial and the concept of hyperoxic resuscitation is controversial. Hyperoxic resuscitation has been studied most in reperfusion and cardiac arrest. In animal models of global cerebral ischemia or ventricular fibrillation, cardiac arrest hyperoxic reperfusion increases hippocampal neuronal death and induces behavioral deficits [84] and impairs oxidative energy metabolism [85]. In the last decade, moderate hypothermia has become the mainstay of treatment in the post-resuscitation period after clinical cardiac arrest. However, for the damaged brain, optimal O_2 transport, including arterial oxygenation, may also be important; international guidelines recommend a target arterial O_2 saturation of 94 % to 98 % [86]. There are, however, conflicting data on hyperoxia in the immediate post-resuscitation period with some studies finding a dose-dependent association between supranormal O_2 tension and risk of in-hospital death [87], and others reporting that hyperoxia did not have a robust or consistently reproducible association with mortality [88]. In these studies, the relationship with cerebral outcomes and neurologic function was not well studied.

In observational clinical studies of severe TBI, both hyperoxia and hypoxia are equally detrimental to short-term outcomes [89, 90]. These conflicting results may depend on the mechanism of cellular injury and highlight the pathophysiological complexity of acute neurologic disorders. Several studies suggest that hyperoxia (or NBO) reduces excitotoxin-induced calcium influx and subsequent neuronal degeneration but favors ischemia-induced (oxygen-glucose deprivation) brain damage and neuronal death [30, 91]. Although there may be deleterious effects with hyperoxia, some experimental studies suggest that benefits of enhanced O_2 delivery during TBI resuscitation may outweigh detrimental increases in oxidative stress and neuroinflammation and reduce fluid requirements [92, 93]. The implication of these observations is that there is no 'one size fits all' and use of a narrower, targeted therapeutic window for oxygenation may improve outcomes. Consistent with this observation, Balan et al. [94], in a clinically applicable protocol designed to reduce post-resuscitative hyperoxia in dogs by using oximetry and aiming for an O_2 saturation of 95 %, observed reduced CA1 neuron injury and improved outcome.

Conclusions

Hypoxia is a known risk factor for adverse outcome in a variety of acute neurologic disorders but whether increasing the O_2 supply to supraphysiological levels has beneficial or detrimental effects on patients has been a matter of debate for decades. In part, the effects may depend on the disease and the dose, e. g., amount and time of exposure [95]. Clinical physiologic studies demonstrate that HBO and NBO improve brain oxidative metabolism; for some investigators this is important but for others it represents only a biological epiphenomena. However, it appears that O_2 treatment is not an all or nothing phenomenon but has a graduated effect. Several studies suggest that $PbtO_2$-directed therapy may contribute to reduced mortality and improved outcome of TBI patients but there is clinical equipoise. What is clear is that any injury to the brain triggers a battery of damaging events, some of which may benefit from a specific therapy (O_2) and some that will not. The challenge is to identify the patient who will benefit.

Oxygen therapy – especially NBO – guided by measures of brain metabolism and function, may offer a simple and effective therapeutic strategy. Combining NBO with other agents or treatments that target multiple mechanisms of injury may achieve better outcomes than an individual treatment alone. More importantly, correcting abnormal oxygenation or metabolism in the brain rather than using O_2 therapy in all may be the most effective approach. The success of any O_2 therapy will depend on recognizing that the margin of safety between effective and potentially toxic O_2 doses is relatively narrow, on the ability to carefully control its dose, on careful adherence to therapeutic protocols, and on individually tailored treatment regimens.

References

1. Rangel-Castilla L, Lara LR, Gopinath S, Swank PR, Valadka A, Robertson C (2010) Cerebral hemodynamic effects of acute hyperoxia and hyperventilation after severe traumatic brain injury. J Neurotrauma 27:1853–1863
2. Rockswold SB, Rockswold GL, Zaun DA, Liu J (2013) A prospective, randomized Phase II clinical trial to evaluate the effect of combined hyperbaric and normobaric hyperoxia on cerebral metabolism, intracranial pressure, oxygen toxicity, and clinical outcome in severe traumatic brain injury. J Neurosurg 118:1317–1328
3. Rockswold SB, Rockswold GL, Zaun DA et al (2010) A prospective, randomized clinical trial to compare the effect of hyperbaric to normobaric hyperoxia on cerebral metabolism, intracranial pressure, and oxygen toxicity in severe traumatic brain injury. J Neurosurg 112:1080–1094
4. Tolias CM, Reinert M, Seiler R, Gilman C, Scharf A, Bullock MR (2004) Normobaric hyperoxia-induced improvement in cerebral metabolism and reduction in intracranial pressure

in patients with severe head injury: a prospective historical cohort-matched study. J Neurosurg 101:435–444

5. Nortje J, Coles JP, Timofeev I et al (2008) Effect of hyperoxia on regional oxygenation and metabolism after severe traumatic brain injury: preliminary findings. Crit Care Med 36:273–281

6. Tisdall MM, Tachtsidis I, Leung TS, Elwell CE, Smith M (2008) Increase in cerebral aerobic metabolism by normobaric hyperoxia after traumatic brain injury. J Neurosurg 109:424–432

7. Bitterman H (2009) Bench-to-bedside review: oxygen as a drug. Crit Care 13:205

8. Bitterman N (2004) CNS oxygen toxicity. Undersea Hyperbar Med 31:63–72

9. Lambertsen CJ, Kough R, Cooper D, Emmel G, Loeschcke H, Schmidt C (1953) Oxygen toxicity: effects in man of oxygen inhalation at 1 and 3.5 atmospheres upon blood gas transport, cerebral circulation, and cerebral metabolism. J Appl Physiol 5:471–485

10. Deuber C, Terhaar M (2011) Hyperoxia in very preterm infants: a systematic review of the literature. J Perinat Neonatal Nurs 25:268–274

11. Demchenko IT, Welty-Wolf KE, Allen BW, Piantadosi CA (2007) Similar but not the same: normobaric and hyperbaric pulmonary oxygen toxicity, the role of nitric oxide. Am J Physiol Lung Cell Mol Physiol 293:L229–L238

12. Halliwell B, Gutteridge JMC (1984) Oxygen toxicity, oxygen radicals, transition metals and disease. Biochem J 219:1–14

13. Puccio AM, Hoffman LA, Bayir H et al (2009) Effect of short periods of normobaric hyperoxia on local brain tissue oxygenation and cerebrospinal fluid oxidative stress markers in severe traumatic brain injury. J Neurotrauma 26:1241–1249

14. Jin X, Liu J, Liu KJ, Rosenberg GA, Yang Y, Liu W (2013) Normobaric hyperoxia combined with minocycline provides greater neuroprotection than either alone in transient focal cerebral ischemia. Exp Neurol 240:9–16

15. de Visser YP, Walther FJ, Laghmani el H, Boersma H, van der Laarse A, Wagenaar GT (2009) Sildenafil attenuates pulmonary inflammation and fibrin deposition, mortality and right ventricular hypertrophy in neonatal hyperoxic lung injury. Respir Res 10:30

16. Kurul SH, Yiş U, Kumral A et al (2009) Protective effects of topiramate against hyperoxic brain injury in the developing brain. Neuropediatrics 40:22–27

17. Gerstner B, Sifringer M, Dzietko M et al (2007) Estradiol attenuates hyperoxia-induced cell death in the developing white matter. Ann Neurol 61:562–573

18. Schabitz WR, Schade H, Heiland S et al (2004) Neuroprotection by hyperbaric oxygenation after experimental focal cerebral ischemia monitored by MRI. Stroke 35:1175–1179

19. Yang ZJ, Camporesi C, Yang X et al (2002) Hyperbaric oxygenation mitigates focal cerebral injury and reduces striatal dopamine release in a rat model of transient middle cerebral artery occlusion. Eur J Appl Physiol 87:101–107

20. Miljkovic-Lolic M, Silbergleit R, Fiskum G, Rosenthal RE (2003) Neuroprotective effects of hyperbaric oxygen treatment in experimental focal cerebral ischemia are associated with reduced brain leukocyte myeloperoxidase activity. Brain Res 971:90–94

21. Chang CF, Niu KC, Hoffer BJ, Wang Y, Borlongan CV (2000) Hyperbaric oxygen therapy for treatment of postischemic stroke in adult rats. Exp Neurol 166:298–306

22. Rosenthal RE, Silbergleit R, Hof PR, Haywood Y, Fiskum G (2003) Hyperbaric oxygen reduces neuronal death and improves neurological outcome after canine cardiac arrest. Stroke 34:1311–1316

23. Veltkamp R, Siebing DA, Sun L et al (2005) Hyperbaric oxygen reduces blood-brain barrier damage and edema after transient focal cerebral ischemia. Stroke 36:1679–1683

24. Qi Z, Liu W, Luo Y, Ji X, Liu KJ (2013) Normobaric hyperoxia-based neuroprotective therapies in ischemic stroke. Med Gas Res 3:2

25. Vlodavsky E, Palzur E, Soustiel JF (2006) Hyperbaric oxygen therapy reduces neuroinflammation and expression of matrix metalloproteinase-9 in the rat model of traumatic brain injury. Neuropathol Appl Neurobiol 32:40–50

26. Niklas A, Brock D, Schober R et al (2004) Continuous measurements of cerebral tissue oxygen pressure during hyperbaric oxygenation-HBO effects on brain edema and necrosis after severe brain trauma in rabbits. J Neurol Sci 219:77–82

27. Palzur E, Vlodavsky E, Mulla H, Arieli R, Feinsod M, Soustiel JF (2004) Hyperbaric oxygen therapy for reduction of secondary brain damage in head injury: an animal model of brain contusion. J Neurotrauma 21:41–48

28. Rockswold SB, Rockswold GL, Vargo JM et al (2001) Effects of hyperbaric oxygenation therapy on cerebral metabolism and intracranial pressure in severely brain injured patients. J Neurosurg 94:403–411

29. Rockswold GL, Ford SE, Anderson DC et al (1992) Results of a prospective randomized trial of treatment of severely brain-injured patients with hyperbaric oxygen. J Neurosurg 76:929–934

30. Haelewyn B, Chazalviel L, Nicole O, Lecocq M, Risso JJ, Abraini JH (2011) Moderately delayed post-insult treatment with normobaric hyperoxia reduces excitotoxin-induced neuronal degeneration but increases ischemia-induced brain damage. Med Gas Res 1:2

31. Singhal AB, Dijkhuizen RM, Rosen BR et al (2002) Normobaric hyperoxia reduces MRI diffusion abnormalities and infarct size in experimental stroke. Neurology 58:945–952

32. Singhal AB, Wang X, Sumii T, Mori T, Lo EH (2002) Effects of normobaric hyperoxia in a rat model of focal cerebral ischemia-reperfusion. J Cereb Blood Flow Metab 22:861–868

33. Flynn EP, Auer RN (2002) Eubaric hyperoxemia and experimental cerebral infarction. Ann Neurol 52:566–572

34. Miyamoto O, Auer RN (2000) Hypoxia, hyperoxia, ischemia, and brain necrosis. Neurology 54:362–371

35. Shin HK, Dunn AK, Jones PB et al (2007) Normobaric hyperoxia improves cerebral blood flow and oxygenation, and inhibits peri-infarct depolarizations in experimental focal ischaemia. Brain 130:1631–1642

36. Veltkamp R, Warner DS, Domoki F, Brinkhous AD, Toole JF, Busija DW (2000) Hyperbaric oxygen decreases infarct size and behavioral deficit after transient focal cerebral ischemia in rats. Brain Res 853:68–73

37. Singhal AB, Benner T, Roccatagliata L et al (2005) A pilot study of normobaric oxygen therapy in acute ischemic stroke. Stroke 36:797–802

38. Moody RA, Mead CO, Ruamsuke S, Mullan S (1970) Therapeutic value of oxygen at normal and hyperbaric pressure in experimental head injury. J Neurosurg 32:51–54

39. Chen T, Qian YZ, Di X (2000) Lactate/glucose dynamics after rat fluid percussion brain injury. J Neurotrauma 17:135–142

40. Reinert M, Schaller B, Widmer HR, Seiler R, Bullock R (2004) Influence of oxygen therapy on glucose-lactate metabolism after diffuse brain injury. J Neurosurg 101:323–329

41. Menzel M, Doppenberg EM, Zauner A et al (1999) Cerebral oxygenation in patients after severe head injury: monitoring and effects of arterial hyperoxia on cerebral blood flow, metabolism and intracranial pressure. J Neurosurg Anesthesiol 11:240–251

42. Oddo M, Levine JM, Frangos S et al (2012) Brain lactate metabolism in humans with subarachnoid hemorrhage. Stroke 43:1418–1421

43. Magnoni S, Ghisoni L, Locatelli M et al (2003) Lack of improvement in cerebral metabolism after hyperoxia in severe head injury: a microdialysis study. J Neurosurg 98:952–958

44. Reinert MA, Barth HU, Rothen et al (2003) Effects of cerebral perfusion pressure and increased fraction of inspired oxygen on brain tissue oxygen, lactate and glucose in patients with severe head injury. Acta Neurochir 145:341–350

45. Tolias CM, Reinert M, Seiler R, Gilman C, Scharf A, Bullock MR (2004) Normobaric hyperoxia-induced improvement in cerebral metabolism and reduction in intracranial pressure in patients with severe head injury: a prospective historical cohort-matched study. J Neurosurg 101:435–444

46. Vilalta A, Sahuquillo J, Poca MA, Merino MA et al (2011) Normobaric hyperoxia in traumatic brain injury: does brain metabolic state influence the response to hyperoxic challenge? J Neurotrauma 28:1139–1148
47. Figaji AA, Zwane E, Graham Fieggen A, Argent AC, Le Roux PD, Peter JC (2010) The effect of increased inspired fraction of oxygen on brain tissue oxygen tension in children with severe traumatic brain injury. Neurocrit Care 12:430–437
48. Diringer MN, Aiyagari V, Zazulia AR, Videen TO, Powers WJ (2007) Effect of hyperoxia on cerebral metabolic rate for oxygen measured using positron emission tomography in patients with acute severe head injury. J Neurosurg 106:526–529
49. Maloney-Wilensky E, Le Roux P (2010) The physiology behind direct brain oxygen monitors and practical aspects of their use. Childs Nerv System 26:419–430
50. Le Roux P (2013) Physiological monitoring of the severe traumatic brain injury patient in the intensive care unit. Curr Neurol Neurosci Rep 13:331
51. Beynon C, Kiening KL, Orakcioglu B, Unterberg AW, Sakowitz OW (2012) Brain tissue oxygen monitoring and hyperoxic treatment in patients with traumatic brain injury. J Neurotrauma 29:2109–2123
52. Hlatky R, Valadka AB, Goodman JC et al (2004) Patterns of energy substrates during ischemia measured in the brain by microdialysis. J Neurotrauma 21:894–906
53. Dings J, Meixensberger J, Jager A et al (1998) Clinical experience with 118 brain tissue oxygen partial pressure catheter probes. Neurosurgery 43:1082–1095
54. Santbrink H, Maas AIR, Avezaat CJJ (1996) Continuous monitoring of partial pressure of brain tissue oxygen in patients with severe head injury. Neurosurgery 38:21–31
55. Kiening KL, Unterberg AW, Bardt TF et al (1996) Monitoring of cerebral oxygenation in patients with severe head injuries: brain tissue PO2 versus jugular vein oxygen saturation. J Neurosurg 85:751–757
56. van den Brink WA, van Santbrink H, Steyerberg EW et al (2000) Brain oxygen tension in severe head injury. Neurosurgery 46:868–878
57. Bardt TF, Unterberg AW, Hartl R et al (1998) Monitoring of brain tissue PO2 in traumatic brain injury: effect of cerebral hypoxia on outcome. Acta Neurochir Suppl 71:153–156
58. Maloney-Wilensky E, Gracias V, Itkin A et al (2009) Brain tissue oxygen and outcome after severe traumatic brain injury: a systematic review. Crit Care Med 37:2057–2063
59. Chang JJ, Youn TS, Benson D et al (2009) Physiologic and functional outcome correlates of brain tissue hypoxia in traumatic brain injury. Crit Care Med 37:283–290
60. Oddo M, Levine JM, Mackenzie L et al (2011) Brain hypoxia is associated with short-term outcome after severe traumatic brain injury independently of intracranial hypertension and low cerebral perfusion pressure. Neurosurgery 69:1037–1045
61. Longhi L, Valeriani V, Rossi S et al (2002) Effects of hyperoxia on brain tissue oxygen tension in cerebral focal lesions. Acta Neurochir Suppl 81:315–317
62. Ponce LL, Pillai S, Cruz J et al (2012) Position of probe determines prognostic information of brain tissue pO2 in severe traumatic brain injury. Neurosurgery 70:1492–1502
63. Ramakrishna R, Stiefel M, Udoteuk J et al (2008) Brain oxygen and outcome in patients with aneurysmal subarachnoid hemorrhage. J Neurosurg 109:1075–1082
64. Bohman LE, Sanborn M, Pisapia J, et al (2012) Long term outcome of patients with aneurysmal subarachnoid hemorrhage treated with brain oxygen-directed therapy. Neurocrit Care 17 (abst)
65. Johnston AJ, Steiner LA, Coles JP et al (2005) Effect of cerebral perfusion pressure augmentation on regional oxygenation and metabolism after head injury. Crit Care Med 33:189–195
66. Rose JC, Neill TA, Hemphill JC 3rd (2006) Continuous monitoring of the microcirculation in neurocritical care: an update on brain tissue oxygenation. Curr Opin Crit Care 12:97–102
67. Gracias VH, Guillamondegui OD, Stiefel MF et al (2004) Cerebral cortical oxygenation: a pilot study. J Trauma 56:469–447
68. Stiefel MF, Udoetek J, Spiotta A et al (2006) Conventional neurocritical care and cerebral oxygenation after traumatic brain injury. J Neurosurg 105:568–575

69. Le Roux P, Lam AM, Newell DW et al (1997) Cerebral arteriovenous difference of oxygen: a predictor of cerebral infarction and outcome in severe head injury. J Neurosurg 87:1–8
70. Gopinath SP, Valadka AB, Uzura M et al (1999) Comparison of jugular venous oxygen saturation and brain tissue PO2 as monitors of cerebral ischemia after head injury. Crit Care Med 27:2337–2345
71. Tolias CM, Reinert M, Seiler R et al (2004) Normobaric hyperoxia-induced improvement in cerebral metabolism and reduction in intracranial pressure in patients with severe head injury: a prospective historical cohort-matched study. J Neurosurg 101:435–444
72. Gupta AK, Hutchinson PJ, Fryer T et al (2002) Measurement of brain tissue oxygenation performed using positron emission tomography scanning to validate a novel monitoring method. J Neurosurg 96:263–268
73. Al-Rawi PG, Hutchinson PJ, Gupta AK et al (2000) Multiparameter brain tissue monitoring correlation between parameters and identification of CPP thresholds. Zentralbl Neurochir 61:74–79
74. Dohmen C, Bosche B, Graf R et al (2007) Identification and clinical impact of impaired cerebrovascular autoregulation in patients with malignant middle cerebral artery infarction. Stroke 3:56–61
75. Oddo M, Frangos S, Maloney-Wilensky E et al (2010) Effect of shivering on brain tissue oxygenation during induced normothermia in patients with severe brain injury. Neurocrit Care 2:10–16
76. Weiner GM, Lacey MR, Mackenzie L et al (2010) Decompressive craniectomy for elevated intracranial pressure and its effect on the cumulative ischemic burden and therapeutic intensity levels after sever traumatic brain injury. Neurosurgery 66:1111–1119
77. Figaji AA, Zwane E, Fieggen AG et al (2009) Pressure autoregulation, intracranial pressure and brain tissue oxygenation in children with severe traumatic brain injury. J Neurosurg Pediatr 4:420–428
78. Smith MJ, Maggee S, Stiefel M et al (2005) Packed red blood cell transfusion increases local cerebral oxygenation. Crit Care Med 33:1104–1108
79. Muench E, Horn P, Bauhuf C et al (2007) Effects of hypervolemia and hypertension on regional cerebral blood flow, intracranial pressure, and brain tissue oxygenation after subarachnoid hemorrhage. Crit Care Med 35:1844–1851
80. Spiotta AM, Stiefel MF, Gracias VH et al (2010) Brain tissue oxygen-directed management and outcome in patients with severe traumatic brain injury. J Neurosurg 113:571–580
81. Narotam PK, Morrison JF, Nathoo N (2009) Brain tissue oxygen monitoring in traumatic brain injury and major trauma: outcome analysis of a brain tissue oxygen-directed therapy. J Neurosurg 111:672–682
82. Martini RP, Deem S, Yanez ND et al (2009) Management guided by brain tissue oxygen monitoring and outcome following severe traumatic brain injury. J Neurosurg 111:644–649
83. Nangunoori R, Maloney-Wilensky E, Stiefel MD et al (2012) Brain tissue oxygen based therapy and outcome after severe traumatic brain injury: a systematic literature review. Neurocrit Care 17:131–138
84. Hazelton JL, Balan I, Elmer GI et al (2010) Hyperoxic reperfusion after global cerebral ischemia promotes inflammation and long-term hippocampal neuronal death. J Neurotrauma 27:753–762
85. Richards EM, Fiskum G, Rosenthal RE, Hopkins I, McKenna MC (2007) Hyperoxic reperfusion after global ischemia decreases hippocampal energy metabolism. Stroke 38:1578–1584
86. Deakin CD, Nolan JP, Soar J et al (2010) European Resuscitation Council Guidelines for Resuscitation 2010 Section 4. Adult advanced life support. Resuscitation 81:1305–1352
87. Kilgannon JH, Jones AE, Parrillo JE et al (2011) Relationship between supranormal oxygen tension and outcome after resuscitation from cardiac arrest. Circulation 123:2717–2722
88. Bellomo R, Bailey M, Eastwood GM et al (2011) Arterial hyperoxia and in-hospital mortality after resuscitation from cardiac arrest. Crit Care 15:R90

89. Brenner M, Stein D, Hu P, Kufera J, Wooford M, Scalea T (2012) Association between early hyperoxia and worse outcomes after traumatic brain injury. Arch Surg 147:1042–1046
90. Davis DP, Meade W, Sise MJ et al (2009) Both hypoxemia and extreme hyperoxemia may be detrimental in patients with severe traumatic brain injury. J Neurotrauma 26:2217–2223
91. Danilov CA, Fiskum G (2008) Hyperoxia promotes astrocyte cell death after oxygen and glucose deprivation. Glia 56:801–808
92. Blasiole B, Bayr H, Vagni VA et al (2013) Effect of Hyperoxia on Resuscitation of Experimental Combined Traumatic Brain Injury and Hemorrhagic Shock in Mice. Anesthesiology 118:649–663
93. Meier J, Kemming GI, Kisch-Wedel H, Blum J, Pape A, Habler OP (2004) Hyperoxic ventilation reduces six-hour mortality after partial fluid resuscitation from hemorrhagic shock. Shock 22:240–247
94. Balan IS, Fiskum G, Hazelton J, Cotto-Cumba C, Rosenthal RE (2006) Oximetry guided reoxygenation improves neurological outcome after experimental cardiac arrest. Stroke 37:3008–3013
95. Xu F, Liu P, Pascual JM, Xiao G, Lu H (2012) Effect of hypoxia and hyperoxia on cerebral blood flow, blood oxygenation, and oxidative metabolism. J Cereb Blood Flow Metab 32:1909–1918

Part III
Mechanical Ventilation

Intubation in the ICU: We Could Improve our Practice

A. De Jong, B. Jung, and S. Jaber

Introduction

Airway management is a commonly performed procedure in the intensive care unit (ICU). Hypoxemia and cardiovascular collapse represent the initial and most serious life-threatening complications associated with difficult airway access, both in emergency intubation in the critically ill [1–4] and in planned intubations (e. g., scheduled surgery or invasive procedures) [5]. To prevent and limit the incidence of life-threatening complications following intubation, several pre-oxygenation techniques and intubation algorithms have been entertained.

The objectives of the present chapter are to:
1) describe new tools (e. g., the MACOCHA Score) to better identify patients at high-risk of difficult intubation and related complications;
2) describe new strategies for improving pre-oxygenation before intubation (e. g., continuous positive airway pressure [CPAP] or non-invasive ventilation [NIV]);
3) propose an intubation bundle (the Montpellier-ICU intubation algorithm) to limit complications related to the intubation procedure;
4) report recent data on the role of videolaryngoscopes in the ICU; and, finally,
5) propose an algorithm for secure airway management in the ICU (The Montpellier-airway ICU algorithm).

Which Patients are 'At Risk' of Complications During Intubation?

All ICU patients could be considered at risk of complications during intubation. The main indication for intubation in the ICU is acute respiratory failure [1–4]. In

A. De Jong · B. Jung · S. Jaber ✉
Intensive Care Unit, Anesthesia and Critical Care Department, Saint Eloi Teaching Hospital,
University Montpellier 1, 34295 Montpellier, France
e-mail: s-jaber@chu-montpellier.fr

J.-L. Vincent (Ed.), *Annual Update in Intensive Care and Emergency Medicine 2014*, 107
DOI 10.1007/978-3-319-03746-2_9, © Springer International Publishing Switzerland
and BioMed Central Ltd. 2014

these cases, the risk of hypoxemia and cardiovascular collapse during the intubation process (often crucial) is particularly elevated (15 to 50 %) [3]. Respiratory muscle weakness ('ventilatory insufficiency') and gas exchange impairment ('respiratory insufficiency') are often present. It is thus worth anticipating that life-threatening complications may occur during intubation [6]. Obesity and pregnancy are the two main situations where functional residual capacity (FRC) is decreased and where the risk of atelectasis is increased leading to hypoxemia [6]. Other 'at risk' patients include those who cannot safely tolerate a mild degree of hypoxemia (epilepsy, cerebrovascular disease, coronary artery disease, sickle cell disease, etc. ...). Finally, patients considered to be 'difficult to intubate', in particular require adequate pre-oxygenation [7].

How to Identify Risk Factors for Difficult Intubation in the ICU?

Although several predictive risk factors and scores for difficult intubation have been identified in anesthesia practice, until recently no (*a priori*) clinical score had been developed for ICU patients. However, a recent study assessed risk factors for difficult intubation in the ICU [3] and developed a predictive score of difficult intubation, the MACOCHA score, which was then externally validated. The main predictors of difficult intubation were related to the patient (Mallampati score III or IV, obstructive sleep apnea syndrome, reduced mobility of cervical spine, limited mouth opening), the pathology (coma, severe hypoxia) and the operator (non-anesthesiologist) (Table 1). By optimizing the discrimination threshold, the discriminative ability of the score is high. In order to reject difficult intubation with certainty, a cut-off of 3 or greater seems appropriate, providing an optimal negative predictive value (97 % and 98 % in the original and validation cohorts, respectively) and sensitivity (76 % and 73 % in the original and validation cohorts, respectively). The MACOCHA score enables patients at risk of difficult intubation to be identified and further studies are needed to determine whether calculating this

Table 1 MACOCHA score calculation worksheet

	Points
– *Factors related to patient*	
Mallampati score III or IV	5
Obstructive sleep apnea syndrome	2
Reduced mobility of cervical spine	1
Limited mouth opening < 3 cm	1
– *Factors related to pathology*	
coma	1
Severe hypoxemia (< 80 %)	1
– *Factor related to operator*	1
Non-anesthesiologist	
Total	**12**

Coded from 0 to 12, 0 = easy, 12 = very difficult

score before each intubation could help reduce the incidence of difficult intubations and related complications.

Of note, the Intubation Difficulty Scale (IDS) is a quantitative scale of intubation difficulty, which can be useful for objectively comparing the complexity of endotracheal intubation, but *a posteriori* and not *a priori* [21].

How to Improve Pre-oxygenation Before Intubation?

Spontaneous Ventilation

Several maneuvers in spontaneous ventilation (e. g., 3–8 vital capacities vs 3 minutes tidal volume breathing) exist to improve pre-oxygenation before intubation and seem to be almost equally effective [8]. Some technical details, however, can make a significant difference. First, the clinician needs to make sure that the facemask properly fits the patient's facial morphology. Second, fresh gas flow needs to be set at a high range to homogenize ventilation through the lungs and to decrease the impact of leaks [9, 10]. Third, leaks should be avoided and diagnosed either by a flaccid reservoir bag or by the absence of a normal capnograph waveform, because leaks impair the efficacy of pre-oxygenation.

End-tidal oxygen concentration (EtO_2 in %) is available as a surrogate for oxygen alveolar pressure (PAO_2) which reflects, in part, the oxygen reserve in the lungs; the target commonly adopted is 90 % [11]. This target is reached more quickly when pure oxygen is administered. Although the clinician must be aware of the potential complication of de-nitrogenation-induced atelectasis, the benefit of reaching an end-inspiratory oxygen fraction of 90 % before attempting intubation outweighs the risk of developing atelectatic-related hypoxia in 'at risk' patients.

In critically ill patients, the advantage of a prolonged period of pre-oxygenation has not been clearly demonstrated. Most such patients present with acute respiratory failure with a certain amount of shunt, a reduced FRC, and do not respond to administration of oxygen as well as patients scheduled for surgery [12]. Mort et al. demonstrated a moderate increase in arterial oxygen pressure (PaO_2) after 4 min of oxygen therapy before intubation (from 62 to 88 mmHg before and after oxygen therapy) [12]; despite pre-oxygenation, half of the 34 patients included in the study experienced severe hypoxia during intubation.

Position

Patient position is an important factor and limits the decrease in FRC. Studies have reported that pre-oxygenation in the semi-sitting position or in the 25° head-up position can achieve higher PaO_2. It may also prolong the time to hypoxemia in obese patients scheduled for surgery [13, 14]. To our knowledge, thus far only one study, performed in non-obese patients scheduled for surgery, has reported a beneficial impact of semi-sitting (20° head up) during pre-oxygenation in terms of time to desaturation [15]. This position seems not to be beneficial in pregnant patients, probably because of the gravid uterus constraining the diaphragm in its upper position and because of the detrimental effect of the sitting position on vena caval back flow [16]. In the critically ill, there are so far no pre-oxygenation studies evaluating the semi-sitting versus the supine positions.

Non-invasive Ventilation with Positive Pressure

Positive end-expiratory pressure (PEEP) with high-flow oxygen has been evaluated as a pre-oxygenation method in the morbidly obese. The aim of positive pressure used as a pre-oxygenation method is to increase the proportion of aerated lung, thereby limiting the decrease in FRC. This limitation in FRC decrease will result in an increase in lung oxygen stores, and may also help keep the closing capacity below the FRC. The closing capacity is the volume of air at which airways begin to close during expiration. The volume of air between the closing capacity and the residual volume is called the closing volume.

The first study was performed in the early 2000s and found that applying 7 cmH$_2$O of CPAP for 3 minutes did not prolong time to desaturation in morbidly obese women [17]. Important limitations of this study were the absence of ventilation between the onset of apnea and intubation, and the relative brevity of the pre-oxygenation (only 3 minutes). Later studies, however, showed a benefit of applying CPAP with oxygen during pre-oxygenation in morbidly obese patients [18, 19]. Compared to O$_2$ alone, CPAP of 10 cmH$_2$O + O$_2$ for 5 min increased the time to desaturate and reduced the amount of atelectasis following intubation [18, 19]. Immediately after intubation, the amount of atelectasis measured by computed tomography (CT) was 10 % in the oxygen group compared to only 2 % in the 10 cmH$_2$O PEEP group [18].

In a landmark study of morbidly obese patients, our group showed that NIV using a pressure support ventilation (PSV) level of 8 cmH$_2$O and PEEP of 6 cmH$_2$O for 5 minutes was safe, feasible, and efficient [20]. We reported that 95 % of patients could reach the end-expiratory oxygen fraction target of 90 % with NIV compared to 50 % in the oxygen group [20]. The impact of the combination of both semi-sitting position and NIV in obese and non-obese surgical patients needs to be evaluated.

Pre-oxygenation with NIV in pregnant patients has never been formally evaluated, as it may be harmful because of the risk of aspiration in this patient population.

NIV as a pre-oxygenation maneuver has also been evaluated in critically ill patients; our group reported its benefits compared to administration of oxygen alone [21]. Indeed, in a randomized controlled trial including hypoxemic patients, the incidence of severe hypoxemia (SpO$_2$ < 80 %) within 30 min after intubation was 7 % in the NIV group (PSV 5–15 cmH$_2$O, PEEP 5–10 cmH$_2$O, FiO$_2$ = 100 %), compared to 42 % in the oxygen group. To perform NIV for 3 to 5 min in critically ill patients, the facial mask available in every ICU room is adequate. The patient should be in the semi-sitting position, FiO$_2$ set at 100 %, inspiratory pressure set to

Box 1 The Montpellier-ICU intubation algorithm, adapted from [2]

PRE-INTUBATION

1. Presence of two operators

2. Fluid loading (isotonic saline 500 ml or starch 250 ml) in absence of cardiogenic edema

3. Preparation of long-term sedation

4. Pre-oxygenate for 3 min with NIV in case of acute respiratory failure (FiO_2 100 %, pressure support ventilation level between 5 and 15 cmH_2O to obtain an expiratory tidal volume between 6 and 8 ml/kg and PEEP of 5 cmH_2O)

PER-INTUBATION

5. Rapid sequence induction:

– Etomidate 0.2–0.3 mg/kg or ketamine 1.5–3 mg/kg

– Succinylcholine 1–1.5 mg/kg (in absence of allergy, hyperkalemia, severe acidosis, acute or chronic neuromuscular disease, burn patient for more than 48 h and medullar trauma)

– Rocuronium: 0.6 mg/kg IVD in case of contraindication to succinylcholine or prolonged stay in the ICU or risk factor for neuromyopathy

6. Sellick maneuver

POST-INTUBATION

7. Immediate confirmation of tube placement by capnography

8. Norepinephrine if diastolic blood pressure remains < 35 mmHg

9. Initiate long-term sedation

10. Initial 'protective ventilation': tidal volume 6–8 ml/kg, PEEP < 5 cmH_2O and respiratory rate between 10 and 20 cycles/min, FiO_2 100 % for a plateau pressure < 30 cmH2O

11. Recruitment maneuver: CPAP 40 cmH_2O during 40 s, FiO_2 100 % (if no cardiovascular collapse)

12. Maintain intubation cuff pressure from 25–30 cmH_2O

NIV: non-invasive ventilation; CPAP: continuous positive airway pressure ; FiO_2: inspired fraction of oxygen

observe a tidal volume of 6 to 10 ml/kg and respiratory rate of 10 to 25 cycles/min. The duration of the procedure usually corresponds with the time needed to prepare the drugs and equipment for intubation. NIV was included in a bundle and was associated with a decrease in life-threatening hypoxemia following intubation in a multicenter study [1, 2] (Box 1).

Recruitment Maneuver

As discussed earlier, the rationale of use NIV during pre-oxygenation is to recruit lung tissue available for gas exchange: 'Open the lung' with the PSV and 'keep the lung open' with PEEP, which limits alveolar de-recruitment. Conversely, the combination of de-nitrogenation (with 100 % O_2) and the apneic period associated with the intubation procedure can dramatically decrease the aerated lung volume ratio, thereby causing atelectasis. In obese patients pre-oxygenated without positive pressure, the proportion of atelectasis following intubation can represent 10 % of the total lung volume [18]. One option to limit alveolar de-recruitment after intubation is to ventilate the patient using a bag-valve balloon. However, it is not possible to measure the pressure delivered when patients are ventilated using this method.

A recruitment maneuver (RM) consists of a transient increase in inspiratory pressure. Several maneuvers exist, but the one best described in this situation consists of applying a CPAP of $40\,cmH_2O$ for 30 to 40 s [22–24]. In the ICU, a randomized controlled trial was conducted by our group in 40 critically ill patients requiring intubation for acute hypoxemic respiratory failure [22]. Compared to no RM, an RM performed immediately after intubation was associated with a higher PaO_2 (under 100 % FiO_2) 5 min (93 ± 36 vs $236 \pm 117\,mmHg$) and 30 min (110 ± 39 and $180 \pm 79\,mmHg$) after intubation.

In the operating room, an initial study assessed the impact of applying several PEEP (0, 5, $10\,cmH_2O$) values following intubation in obese and non-obese patients scheduled for surgery [24]. At each step, end-expiratory lung volume, static elastance, gas exchange and dead space were measured. In both obese and non-obese patients, PEEP of $10\,cmH_2O$ compared with zero end-expiratory pressure (ZEEP) improved end-expiratory lung volume and elastance without effects on oxygenation. We then randomized 66 morbidly obese patients (body mass index $46 \pm 6\,kg/m^2$) scheduled for surgery into 3 groups: Conventional pre-oxygenation, pre-oxygenation with NIV and pre-oxygenation with NIV + post-intubation RM [23]. The study demonstrated that the combination of pre-oxygenation with NIV + post-intubation RM helped maintain lung volumes and oxygenation during anesthesia induction more so than pre-oxygenation with either pure oxygen alone or with NIV. One of the main take home messages of this study was that to improve PaO_2 5 min after intubation, an RM added to NIV could be performed. Both oxygenation (PaO_2, $234 \pm 73\,mmHg$ vs $128 \pm 54\,mmHg$) and capnia ($PaCO_2$ 42 ± 3 vs $40 \pm 3\,mmHg$) were improved in the RM + NIV group compared to NIV alone.

Bundle to Limit Complications Related to Intubation (The Montpellier-ICU Intubation Algorithm)

Pre-oxygenation and RMs are only two of the procedures that can improve airway safety. Managing the airway of 'at risk' patients presents some unique challenges for the anesthesiologist/intensivist. The combination of a limited physiologic reserve in these patients and the potential for difficult mask ventilation and intubation mandates careful planning with a good working knowledge of alternative tools and strategies, should conventional attempts at securing the airway fail. Pre-oxygenation techniques can be combined to limit the risk of hypoxia during intubation attempts. To limit the incidence of severe complications occurring after this potentially hazardous procedure, we believe that the whole process (pre-, per- and post-intubation) should be guided by protocols geared toward patient safety. We designed a multicenter study and described how implementation of such a bundle protocol could improve the safety of airway management in the ICU [1, 2]. This bundle, the Montpellier-ICU intubation algorithm, is summarized in Box 1.

Briefly, pre-intubation period interventions consisted of fluid loading if there was no cardiogenic edema, pre-oxygenation with NIV in the case of acute respiratory failure, preparation of sedation by the nursing team and the presence of two operators. NIV applied during the 3-min pre-oxygenation phase was performed with an ICU ventilator (most often those which served to provide invasive mechanical ventilation) and a standard face mask. The PSV level was set between 5 and 15 cmH$_2$O, adjusted to obtain an expired tidal volume of 6 to 8 ml/kg of ideal body weight. The FiO$_2$ was set at 100 % and we used a PEEP level of 5 cm H$_2$O.

During the intubation period, rapid sequence induction (RSI) was recommended using short-acting, well tolerated hypnotics (etomidate or ketamine), and a rapid onset muscle relaxant (succinylcholine), with application of cricoid pressure (Sellick maneuver). The Sellick maneuver was performed to prevent gastric contents from leaking into the pharynx, by external obstruction of the esophagus, and associated inhalation of substances into the lungs, as well as vomiting into an unprotected airway.

Just after the intubation (post-intubation period), we recommended verifying the tube's position by capnography (a technique which allows the endotracheal position of the tube to be confirmed and verifies the absence of esophageal placement), initiation of long-term sedation as soon as possible (to avoid agitation) and use of 'protective' mechanical ventilation settings, as defined by the ARDS network. At any time, vasopressors were mandatory in the event of severe hemodynamic collapse.

Intubation Devices: Role of Videolaryngoscopes in the ICU

Videolaryngosopes are indirect rigid fiberoptic laryngoscopes with a video camera mounted at the end of an angled blade. The blade is inserted into the mouth in the midline and guided down the back of the tongue until the glottis is visualized. The tip of the endotracheal tube can then be visualized on the video screen and is positioned to enter the glottic inlet. New videolaryngoscope devices are suggested to improve airway management both in anesthesia care and in critically ill patients [25]. In recent years, the role of videolaryngoscopes has been debated, particularly in the ICU where there has been a lack of scientific evidence and generally intubation conditions are more difficult than in the operating room [26]. Recently, however, videolaryngoscopes, such as C-Mac [27, 28] or Glide-scope [29, 30], have demonstrated their effectiveness in the ICU setting. Moreover, a recent study [31] assessed a new mixed videolaryngoscope that can be used as a direct or indirect view laryngoscope. This before-after prospective study showed that the systematic use of a mixed videolaryngoscope for intubation in a quality improvement process using an airway management algorithm significantly reduced the incidence of difficult laryngoscopy and/or difficult intubation. In multivariate analysis, standard laryngoscope use was an independent risk factor for difficult laryngoscopy and/or difficult intubation, as were Mallampati score III or IV and non-expert operator status. Moreover, in the subgroup of patients with difficult intubation predicted by the MACOCHA score [3], incidence of difficult intubation was much higher in the standard laryngoscope group (47 %) than in the mixed videolaryngoscope group (0 %).

In summary, videolaryngoscopes seem to be effective at reducing difficult intubation in ICU patients, but a large multicenter study is needed to assess whether complications of intubation are decreased using videolaryngoscopes.

Airway Management Algorithm

As previously recommended in the operating room [32], an airway management algorithm is advised in the ICU (Fig. 1). First, the difficulty of intubation is evaluated using the MACOCHA score. The availability of equipment for management of a difficult airway is checked. During the procedure, the patient should be ventilated in case of desaturation to < 80 %. In case of inadequate ventilation and unsuccessful intubation, emergency non-invasive airway ventilation (supraglottic airway) must be used. If a difficult intubation is predicted (MACOCHA score ≥ 3), the presence of two operators, use of a metal blade, and use of a malleable stylet are recommended. The videolaryngoscopy or combo videolaryngoscopy are also recommended in case of predicted difficult intubation. In other cases, choice of the device is at the discretion of the physician. In cases of abundant secretions even after aspiration, direct laryngoscopy is preferred rather than videolaryngoscopy. Finally, in cases of intubation failure, an intubating stylet (malleable stylet or long flexible angulated stylet) should be added first, followed successively by the use of videolaryngoscopy if not initially used, an intubation laryngeal mask airway, fiberoscopy and finally the use of rescue percutaneal or surgical airway.

Studies are needed to assess whether applying this protocol in the ICU enables reduction of difficult intubation and complications. In each ICU, this airway management algorithm could be adapted according to local ICU practice.

Conclusions

Pre-oxygenation is a standard of care before intubation in the operating room and in the ICU. The aim of pre-oxygenation is to increase the lungs' stores of oxygen. In the critically ill patient, the combination of pure oxygen, NIV, de-nitrogenation and post-intubation recruitment maneuvers outweighs the potential risk of post-intubation atelectasis. Moreover, potential risk factors for difficult intubation should be assessed in ICU patients, in order to identify patients at risk of difficult intubation using a simple score applicable at the bedside. An intubation bundle should then be applied in order to reduce complications of intubation. Finally, an airway management algorithm is strongly advised in the ICU, as in the operating room. In this setting, new intubation devices, such as videolaryngoscopes, should be used after an appropriate training program.

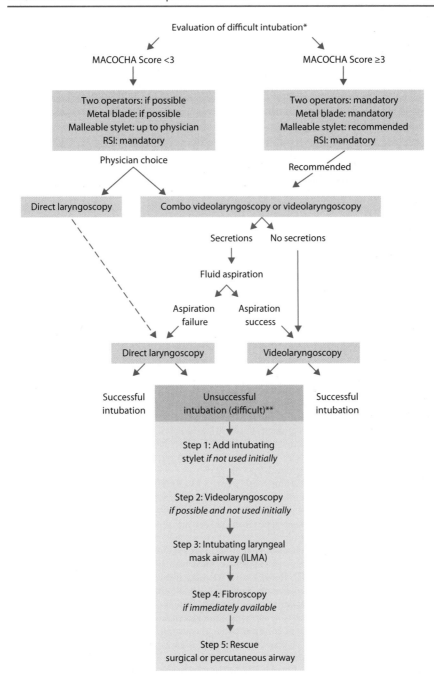

Fig. 1 Airway management algorithm in the intensive care unit.
* The availability of equipment for management of a difficult airway is checked;
** During the whole procedure, the patient should be ventilated in case of desaturation < 80 %. In case of inadequate ventilation and unsuccessful intubation, emergency non-invasive airway ventilation (supra-glottic airway) must be used. RSI: rapid sequence induction

References

1. Jaber S, Amraoui J, Lefrant J-Y et al (2006) Clinical practice and risk factors for immediate complications of endotracheal intubation in the intensive care unit: a prospective, multiple-center study. Crit Care Med 34:2355–2361
2. Jaber S, Jung B, Corne P et al (2010) An intervention to decrease complications related to endotracheal intubation in the intensive care unit: a prospective, multiple-center study. Intensive Care Med 36:248–255
3. De Jong A, Molinari N, Terzi N et al (2013) Early identification of patients at risk for difficult intubation in ICU: Development and validation of the MACOCHA score in a multicenter cohort study. Am J Respir Crit Care Med 187:832–839
4. Martin LD, Mhyre JM, Shanks AM, Tremper KK, Kheterpal S (2011) 3,423 emergency tracheal intubations at a university hospital: airway outcomes and complications. Anesthesiology 114:42–48
5. Peterson GN, Domino KB, Caplan RA, Posner KL, Lee LA, Cheney FW (2005) Management of the difficult airway: a closed claims analysis. Anesthesiology 103:33–39
6. Duggan M, Kavanagh BP (2007) Atelectasis in the perioperative patient. Curr Opin Anaesthesiol 20:37–42
7. Apfelbaum JL, Hagberg CA, Caplan RA et al (2013) Practice Guidelines for Management of the Difficult Airway: An Updated Report by the American Society of Anesthesiologists Task Force on Management of the Difficult Airway. Anesthesiology 118:251–270
8. Tanoubi I, Drolet P, Donati F (2009) Optimizing preoxygenation in adults. Can J Anaesth J Can Anaesthésie 56:449–466
9. Sum Ping SJT, Makary LF, Van Hal MD (2009) Factors influencing oxygen store during denitrogenation in the healthy patient. J Clin Anesth 21:183–189
10. Russell EC, Wrench I, Feast M, Mohammed F (2008) Pre-oxygenation in pregnancy: the effect of fresh gas flow rates within a circle breathing system. Anaesthesia 63:833–836
11. Hedenstierna G (2009) Respiratory physiology. In: Miller RD, Eriksson LI, Fleisher LA, Wiener-Kronish JP, Young WL (eds) Miller's anaesthesia. Elsevier, Philadelphia
12. Mort TC, Waberski BH, Clive J (2009) Extending the preoxygenation period from 4 to 8 mins in critically ill patients undergoing emergency intubation. Crit Care Med 37:68–71
13. Dixon BJ, Dixon JB, Carden JR et al (2005) Preoxygenation is more effective in the 25 degrees head-up position than in the supine position in severely obese patients: a randomized controlled study. Anesthesiology 102:1110–1115
14. Altermatt FR, Muñoz HR, Delfino AE, Cortínez LI (2005) Pre-oxygenation in the obese patient: effects of position on tolerance to apnoea. Br J Anaesth 95:706–709
15. Ramkumar V, Umesh G, Philip FA (2011) Preoxygenation with 20° head-up tilt provides longer duration of non-hypoxic apnea than conventional preoxygenation in non-obese healthy adults. J Anesth 25:189–194
16. Baraka AS, Hanna MT, Jabbour SI et al (1992) Preoxygenation of pregnant and nonpregnant women in the head-up versus supine position. Anesth Analg 75:757–759
17. Cressey DM, Berthoud MC, Reilly CS (2001) Effectiveness of continuous positive airway pressure to enhance pre-oxygenation in morbidly obese women. Anaesthesia 56:680–684
18. Coussa M, Proietti S, Schnyder P et al (2004) Prevention of atelectasis formation during the induction of general anesthesia in morbidly obese patients. Anesth Analg 98:1491–1495
19. Gander S, Frascarolo P, Suter M, Spahn DR, Magnusson L (2005) Positive end-expiratory pressure during induction of general anesthesia increases duration of nonhypoxic apnea in morbidly obese patients. Anesth Analg 100:580–584
20. Delay J-M, Sebbane M, Jung B et al (2008) The effectiveness of noninvasive positive pressure ventilation to enhance preoxygenation in morbidly obese patients: a randomized controlled study. Anesth Analg 107:1707–1713
21. Baillard C, Fosse J-P, Sebbane M et al (2006) Noninvasive ventilation improves preoxygenation before intubation of hypoxic patients. Am J Respir Crit Care Med 174:171–177

22. Constantin JM, Futier E, Cherprenet AL et al (2010) A recruitment maneuver increases oxygenation after intubation of hypoxemic intensive care unit patients: a randomized controlled study. Crit Care 14:R76

23. Futier E, Constantin JM, Pelosi P et al (2011) Noninvasive ventilation and alveolar recruitment maneuver improve respiratory function during and after intubation of morbidly obese patients: a randomized controlled study. Anesthesiology 114:1354–1363

24. Futier E, Constantin JM, Petit A et al (2010) Positive end-expiratory pressure improves end-expiratory lung volume but not oxygenation after induction of anaesthesia. Eur J Anaesthesiol 27:508–513

25. Asai T (2012) Videolaryngoscopes: do they truly have roles in difficult airways? Anesthesiology 116:515–517

26. Cook T, Behringer EC, Benger J (2012) Airway management outside the operating room: hazardous and incompletely studied. Curr Opin Anaesthesiol 25:461–469

27. Noppens RR, Geimer S, Eisel N, David M, Piepho T (2012) Endotracheal intubation using the C-MAC® video laryngoscope or the Macintosh laryngoscope: A prospective, comparative study in the ICU. Crit Care 16:R103

28. Ng I, Hill AL, Williams DL, Lee K, Segal R (2012) Randomized controlled trial comparing the McGrath videolaryngoscope with the C-MAC videolaryngoscope in intubating adult patients with potential difficult airways. Br J Anaesth 109:439–443

29. Kory P, Guevarra K, Mathew JP, Hegde A, Mayo PH (2013) The impact of video laryngoscopy use during urgent endotracheal intubation in the critically ill. Anesth Analg 117:144–149

30. Lakticova V, Koenig SJ, Narasimhan M, Mayo PH (2014) Video laryngoscopy is associated with increased first pass success and decreased rate of esophageal intubations during urgent endotracheal intubation in a medical intensive care unit when compared to direct laryngoscopy. J Intensive Care Med (in press)

31. De Jong A, Clavieras N, Conseil M et al (2013) Implementation of a Combo video laryngoscope for intubation in critically ill patients. A before-after comparative study. Intensive Care Med 39:2144–2152

32. Amathieu R, Combes X, Abdi W et al (2011) An algorithm for difficult airway management, modified for modern optical devices (Airtraq laryngoscope; LMA CTrach™): a 2-year prospective validation in patients for elective abdominal, gynecologic, and thyroid surgery. Anesthesiology 114:25–33

Oral Care in Intubated Patients: Necessities and Controversies

S. Labeau and S. Blot

Introduction

Healthcare professionals in both the community and hospital settings are responsible for maintaining good oral health of patients who are not able to perform this simple activity themselves. Cancer patients receiving chemotherapy or radiotherapy, institutionalized elderly, and patients in a critical care environment (intensive care unit [ICU]) are undeniably among the most vulnerable patients, in whom oral status deserves adequate attention because they may suffer from poor oral health [1, 2].

Oral health deteriorates following admission to hospital, and in the critical care setting in particular [3]. Patients who are tracheally intubated and mechanically ventilated are most prone to bad oral health, as a result of various physiological, pathological, mechanical and immunological factors [2, 4, 5]. In addition to issues relating to patient comfort, a lack of oral hygiene is associated with increased morbidity [6, 7]. Poor oral health may lead to the development of caries, thus causing permanent damage to teeth. Potentially lethal complications, such as ventilator-associated pneumonia (VAP), may also be the result of inadequate oral care. The added costs of complications are exponentially higher than the expenses associated with thorough prevention so that complications due to inadequate oral hygiene may carry a substantial health-economic burden [8].

Despite the ostensible advantages of providing adequate oral care to critically ill patients, oral care practices remain inconsistent, and mouth care is often still

S. Labeau
Faculty of Education, Health and Social Work, University College Ghent, Ghent, Belgium

S. Blot ✉
Faculty of Education, Health and Social Work, University College Ghent, Ghent, Belgium
Dept. of Internal Medicine, Faculty of Medicine and Health Sciences, Ghent University, Ghent, Belgium
e-mail: stijn.blot@ugent.be

J.-L. Vincent (Ed.), *Annual Update in Intensive Care and Emergency Medicine 2014*,   119
DOI 10.1007/978-3-319-03746-2_10, © Springer International Publishing Switzerland
2014

perceived as a comfort measure. There is, therefore, an urgent need for defined oral care procedures that are well supported by scientific evidence. This chapter provides a non-extensive overview of the growing interest in oral care, problem statement, impact of bad oral health, and oral care practice.

A Growing Interest in Oral Care

Interest in oral care by healthcare professionals and investigators has long been limited. Only in recent years has the number of studies related to this important topic begun to increase. As a consequence of this delay, evidence-based recommendations for oral care are not yet available, and several questions remain unanswered. The current lack of evidence pertains to various aspects of oral care, such as the best method, the best frequency, the best product and the best concentration of the best product [9].

The growing interest in oral care was well illustrated by Dale et al. who explored the evolution of nursing discourse in oral hygiene for tracheally intubated and mechanically ventilated patients by searching the online CINAHL and MEDLINE databases for nurse-authored English language articles published between 1960 and 2011 in peer-reviewed journals, and that discussed oral problems or related care for intubated adult patients [10]. Their review resulted in the identification of 84 publications that met the inclusion criteria. The early literature, defined as published between 1960 and 1985, revealed just six publications, three of these being descriptive evaluative studies and three with a narrative review design. Of the remaining 78 publications, 63 were published in or later than the year 2000. Among these, only six, however, were randomized controlled trials, with the earliest being published in 2006 [10].

This evolution in nursing interest for an efficient and effective means to deliver oral care to tracheally intubated patients clearly demonstrates growing awareness of their responsibility in a professional domain that still needs to be extensively charted.

Problem Statement

Several, often interrelated, mechanisms are involved in the deterioration of oral health in critically ill tracheally intubated patients.

Oral Flora

In healthy persons, the oropharynx is mainly colonized by Gram-positive streptococci and dental microorganisms. Within 48 hours of hospital admission, however, dramatic changes in this flora take place. Critical illness induces an increased vulnerability to colonization with exogenous microbes, leading to a shift in commensal oral flora towards a predominance of Gram-negative organisms and *Staphylococcus aureus* [1, 5]. Critically ill patients have increased levels of proteases in their oral secretions, which cause a depletion of fibronectin, a glycoprotein that interferes with binding of Gram-negative bacteria to epithelial cells and acts as a reticuloendothelial-mediated host defense system [11]. As a result, organisms such as *Pseudomonas aeruginosa* easily attach to the buccal and pharyngeal epithelial cell receptors [12]. Increased activity of proteolytic enzymes, such as elastases and proteases, and loss of fibronectin, followed by adherence of Gram-negative bacteria have been shown to be associated events [13–15]. The length of stay in the ICU is, moreover, an important contributing factor because the degree of colonization of the oral cavity with respiratory pathogens such as *S. aureus*, *Streptococcus pneumoniae*, *Hemophilus influenza*, and *Acinetobacter baumannii* increases to over 70 % with increasing severity of illness and length of stay in a critical care environment [16].

Dental Plaque

Dental plaque results from colonization and growth of aerobic, anaerobic and filamentous microorganisms on the surface of teeth and soft tissues [12]. It is a dynamic and complex system connecting microorganisms embedded in an extracellular matrix. Dental plaque starts to build up on teeth within 72 hours after cessation of an adequate oral hygiene regimen [17] and is not easily removed. Biofilm formation enhances bacterial replication and the ability of bacteria to overcome host defense mechanisms [18].

A recent systematic review demonstrated that hospitalization was associated with increased dental plaque accumulation leading to increased risk of inflammatory conditions in the mouth, such as periodontal disease [3]. A study comparing the colonization of dental plaque by respiratory pathogens in medical ICU patients with age-matched, untreated control subjects found higher dental plaque levels in the ICU patients [2]. More recently, a prospective, longitudinal observational study collected dental plaque samples of ICU patients from up to six sites per patient in order to determine microbiological change from baseline to seven days [19]. For patients who were still in the ICU on day 14, additional analysis was conducted. Of the 50 patients recruited, 36 were available for review at one week. A statistically significant ($p < 0.01$) increase in total viable microbe counts by a median of 2.26×10^6 cfu/ml from baseline to week one (95 % CI: 3.19×10^6, 1.24×10^7) was identified [19].

Dental plaque may be an important reservoir for pathogens, and dental plaque in ICU patients can be colonized by potential respiratory pathogens [2, 5, 19].

Drugs

Various drugs that are frequently used in the ICU negatively influence oral health. Exposure to antibiotics may promote colonization of the oral cavity by opportunistic pathogens [1, 2], and several medications cause xerostomia, which has a damaging impact on oral health [20]. The latter include antihypertensives, anticholinergics, antihistamines, antipsychotics, anorectics, anticonvulsants, antineoplastics, sympathicomimetics, antidepressants, and diuretics [20].

Endotracheal Tube

The presence of an oral endotracheal tube (ETT), in combination with the use of sedative drugs, inhibits or hampers swallowing. As a result, accumulated debris in the oral cavity creates a perfect environment for the multiplication of microorganisms. As the most important mechanism in the development of VAP is aspiration of oropharyngeal secretions into the lower respiratory tract, the presence of an ETT provides a direct pathway for translocation of microorganisms from the oropharynx to the lower respiratory tract, through an open glottis [21].

Evidence-based guidelines recommend the oral route of intubation with regard to the prevention of VAP [22]. However, oral intubation simultaneously causes the patient's mouth to be continuously open, resulting in xerostomia that induces drying of the mucous membranes, accumulation of dental plaque and reduction in the distribution of salivary immune factors [5]. Contrarily, ETTs may cause hypersalivation by inducing a hyperactive gag reflex [1, 23].

ETTs are also mechanical barriers that may hamper adequate examination and evaluation of the oral cavity and limit access for oral care [1, 24].

Finally, endotracheal intubation facilitates bacterial adherence to the mucosa by reducing mucosal immunoglobulin A, increasing protease production, damaging mucous membranes, increasing airway pH, and increasing the numbers of airway receptors for bacteria because of acute illness and antimicrobial use [2, 4, 16, 21].

Salivary Flow

Saliva contains natural antimicrobial proteins, including lysozyme, lactoferrin, lactoperoxidase, immunoglobulins, proline-rich proteins, cystatins, histatins, Von Ebner gland protein, secretory leukocyte proteinase inhibitor, and chromogranin A [25, 26]. Salivary flow, therefore, contributes considerably to maintaining oral health through its antimicrobial, lubricating and buffering properties [5, 27]. The buffering capacity plays an important role in limiting the deleterious effects of acid-producing bacteria on the teeth [11]. In critically ill patients, the production and distribution of saliva is threatened by several factors, including fever, diarrhea, extensive burn injury, and reduced or insufficient fluid intake [27]. As mentioned above, xerostomia can additionally result from drug administration [1, 2, 5, 20, 24,

27] and from orally inserted ETTs [1, 5, 20, 24]. Importantly, stress and anxiety may in turn induce xerostomia [5].

Xerostomia can facilitate oropharyngeal colonization with Gram-negative bacteria, the development of mucositis [27], and the accumulation of dental plaque. It also reduces the distribution of salivary immune factors, such as salivary immunoglobulin A, which protects against respiratory pathogens, and lactoferrin, which is bactericidal against several major pathogens, including *S. aureus, P. aeruginosa* and *H. influenzae* [5].

Impact of Poor Oral Health

Reduced salivary flow has been directly, positively related to development of caries [17]. Stomatitis increases the risk of bacterial translocation and may result in sepsis and subsequent multiple organ failure [28]. Bacterial plaque development may be followed by gingivitis, inducing a shift at the gingival surface from predominantly streptococcus and *Actinomyces spp.* to aerobic Gram-negative bacilli. In case of dental plaque accumulation, subgingival inflammation may progress to periodontitis, which, in turn, has been associated with systemic diseases such as bacteremia, rheumatoid arthritis or cardiovascular diseases [17, 28].

Substantial evidence supports the relationship between poor oral health, the oral microflora and VAP [2]. Nosocomial pneumonia is responsible for up to 50 % attributable mortality and considerable morbidity in the ICU [29]. Micro-aspiration of contaminated upper airway secretions along leaks and defects of the tracheal seal of the cuff is assumed to play a pivotal role in VAP development, with oropharyngeal colonization among the most critical risk factors [4, 5, 21, 30].

Oral Care Practice

Nurses' Attitudes Towards Oral Care

In the past decade, the attitude of ICU nurses towards oral care appears to have undergone some positive change. An American survey of 77 nursing care providers in 2003 reported that oral hygiene was generally directed towards patient comfort rather than towards preventing infection. Additionally, oral care priority was rated only 54 on a 100-point scale [31].

A 2004 survey among nurses in two ICUs in a London hospital found that 62 % of 103 participants had received some training in oral need assessment and 74 % in oral care methods; 58 % requested initial or further training in oral care. On a 10-point Lickert scale, 13.5 % of the nurses rated oral care as a low priority (grades 4–6) [24].

Also in 2004, a survey by Furr et al. aimed to determine the factors that affect quality of care. The survey was completed by 556 respondents in 102 American ICUs. The oral care education nurses had received, along with having sufficient time to provide care, prioritizing oral care, and not viewing oral care as unpleasant were found to have direct effects on the quality of the oral care provided [32].

In 2007, a survey in 59 European ICUs revealed that oral care was considered a high priority by most of the respondents (88 %) [33]. Although 77 % of participants indicated that they had received adequate training on this issue, the vast majority (93 %) stated that they would like additional oral care education. Importantly, 32 % of participants considered cleaning the oral cavity as a difficult and unpleasant task, and 68 % considered it difficult. Moreover, 37 % of respondents felt that, despite their efforts, oral hygiene worsens over time in tracheally intubated patients. The authors concluded that it is an important challenge to train and educate nurses in such a way that their attitude becomes more positive [33].

Education

The positive effect of oral care education on ICU nurses' knowledge and practice is well illustrated by a study using a quasi-experimental design to evaluate the effectiveness of an evidence-based practice education program, incorporating oral care with 0.12 % chlorhexidine oral rinse solution. In a convenience sample of 44 registered nurses, there was a statistically significant difference in the total oral care educational level (p = 0.009) as well as an increased frequency of providing oral care (p = 0.001) after a 30 min educational program [34].

Current Practice

A recent Turkish study found a wide variety in the type and frequency of oral care measures among 101 ICU nurses. Surprisingly, the most commonly used solution for oral care was sodium bicarbonate (79.2 %), and the most frequently used equipment was foam swabs (82.2 %). Oral care was carried out less than every 4 h per day by 44.5 % of the nurses. Oral care products and solutions were reported to be different in almost every unit [35].

In Swiss ICUs, also, a large variety of oral care practices was identified. A survey yielding completed questionnaires from 21 ICUs revealed that all performed mechanical tooth cleaning with toothbrushes, with 90 % of these also applying toothpaste; 75 % of the centers surveyed additionally used oral antiseptics with chlorhexidine as the preferred product in 67 % of the cases. Iodine use was not reported. Remarkably, 29 % reported using other mouth wash solutions, most of which do not possess any pronounced or proven antiseptic properties. Oral hygiene measures were performed 3 times per day by 75 % of the centers and twice a day by the remaining 25 %. Saliva substitute was additionally administered by 1/3 of the centers. Oral hygiene was exclusively administered by the nursing staff [36].

Oral care practices in Europe appear to differ from those in the United States. In European ICUs, the use of foam swabs and moisturizers is rather rare [33], whereas in the US these are used very frequently (at least every 12 hours in more than 90 %

of the respondents) [37]. The beneficial effect of foam swabs, however, remains unconfirmed [38, 39]. Electric toothbrushes are very rarely used in either European or American ICUs [37].

The accent of oral care practice in Europe is clearly on mouthwashes, mostly with chlorhexidine. Indeed, chlorhexidine mouthwashes have been associated with a decrease in dental plaque [40], incidence of respiratory infections [41], VAP [40, 42] and in nosocomial infections in general [41]. A systematic review and random effects meta-analysis of randomized trials assessing the effect of oral care with chlorhexidine or povidone-iodine on the prevalence of VAP versus oral care without these antiseptics in adult mechanically ventilated patients included 14 studies with 2,481 patients; 12 investigated the effect of chlorhexidine (2,341 patients) and two of povidone-iodine (140 patients). Overall, antiseptic use resulted in a significant risk reduction in rates of VAP (RR 0.67; 95 % CI 0.50–0.88; p = 0.004). Chlorhexidine application was shown to be effective (RR 0.72; 95 % CI 0.55–0.94; p = 0.02), whereas the effect of povidone-iodine remains unclear (RR 0.39; 95 % CI 0.11–1.36; p = 0.14). Favorable effects were more pronounced in subgroup analyses for 2 % chlorhexidine (RR 0.53, 95 % CI 0.31–0.91), and in cardiosurgical studies (RR 0.41, 95 % CI 0.17–-0.98) [9].

Chemical and/or Mechanical Cleaning

The oral cavity can be cleaned either mechanically, chemically, or by combining both methods. Chemical cleaning can be performed with mouthwashes, of which chlorhexidine appears to be the most effective product with respect to VAP prevention (cfr. supra) [9].

Mouthwashes alone will nevertheless not eliminate dental plaque, and the formation of a biofilm protects potentially deleterious bacteria against chemical agents. Foam swabs and toothettes are frequently used in the United States, but their value in removing plaque formation is unproven and highly questionable [1, 33, 37–39]. A toothbrush is a more adequate tool when it comes to thorough mechanical cleaning of the oral cavity [38, 39]. Although not always easy to perform in ICUs, this practice leads to improved oral health, decreased gingival inflammation, and cost savings through the elimination of toothettes [43]. Although the size of the toothbrush itself does not seem to influence its ability to remove dental plaque, a small-headed or pediatric toothbrush may be more useful in patients with oral ETTs [1].

Recently, there has been a growing interest in assessing the effect of oral care involving toothbrushing on the development of VAP. Alhazzani et al. [44] and Gu et al. [45] simultaneously conducted a systematic review and meta-analysis exploring this issue. Because of variations in inclusion criteria between the research groups, six [44] and four [45] randomized controlled trials were identified for analysis, respectively (Table 1). Both meta-analyses yielded identical results, namely that toothbrushing does not significantly reduce the incidence of VAP (risk ratio 0.77, 95 % CI 0.50–1.21). In addition to some methodological concerns related to

Table 1 Results of randomized controlled trials comparing an oral care protocol that includes toothbrushing with an oral care protocol without toothbrushing

Author	Setting	Ventilator-associated pneumonia occurrence rate		Risk ratio (95 % confidence interval)
		Toothbrush group	Control group	
Munro 2009 [46]	Medical, surgical and trauma ICU	48/97 (47.4 %)	45/95 (47.4 %)	1.04 (0.78–1.40)
Pobo 2009 [55]	Medical, surgical and trauma ICU	15/74 (20.3 %)	18/73 (24.7 %)	0.82 (0.45–1.50)
Yao 2011 [47]	Neurosurgical ICU	4/28 (14.3 %)	14/25 (56.0 %)	0.26 (0.10–0.67)
Lorente 2012 [56]	Medical, surgical and trauma ICU	21/217 (9.7 %)	24.219 (11.0 %)	0.88 (0.51–1.54)

the fact that VAP diagnosis was exclusively based on a Clinical Pulmonary Infection Score ≥ 6 in two studies [46, 47] in both meta-analyses, the results should not lead to the conclusion that there is no need for toothbrusing in oral care. Toothbrushing is essential to remove dental plaque and maintain oral health in any individual, and helps alleviate the oral discomfort that patients with oral ETTs are particularly prone to [48, 49]. Providing oral care that does not involve toothbrushing should be considered as bad practice and cannot be listed among current controversies in the prevention of VAP as its primary goal is not the avoidance of pneumonia [50, 51].

Oral tool kits are now available that contain all the materials needed to provide oral care for 24 hours. It has been demonstrated that the availability of such kits at the bedside increases the frequency and comprehensiveness of the oral care provided [52].

Frequency of Oral Care

The optimal frequency to administer oral care is another controversial issue for which evidence-based recommendations are still lacking. Grap et al. compared self-reported frequencies of oral care interventions by ICU nurses with the frequencies documented in the patients' medical records [31]. Although a majority of the 170 nurses surveyed reported providing oral care 2 or 3 times daily for non-intubated patients, and 5 times daily or even more for intubated patients, the authors identified a mean of only 1.2 times daily per patient based on the unit's flow sheets. In a replication study with a sample of 181 nurses, findings were generally comparable to those of the original study, with participants self-reporting more oral care than was actually documented in writing: the overall documented frequency of oral care for non-intubated patients was 1.8 for the previous 24 hours, whereas the self-reported frequency was 3; in intubated patients the main documented frequency was 3.3, whereas the self-reported frequency was 4.2 [53]. The results of the surveys by Grap et al. [31] and Hanneman and Gusick [53] support the statement by Cutler and Davis that "the disparity between what nurses think they do and what is actually documented raises questions about the reliability of documentation and the consistency of practice" [52].

It has been suggested that oral care be provided based upon an 'at risk' calculator score, or anywhere between every two and four hours, depending on the patient's condition [54]. Cutler and Davis propose swabbing every two hours or as needed while limiting deep endotracheal suctioning to every six hours [52]. Another protocol proposes toothbrushing every two hours combined with oral moistening every two hours while the ETT remains *in situ* [54]. It has also been advised to use oral assessment scores to determine mouth care regimes [12].

Assessment of the Oral Cavity

Oral care can only be effective if preceded by an adequate and thorough assessment of the oral cavity. Despite the fact that assessment tools are available, they do not seem to be used often in daily nursing practice [1, 24]. This observation may be due to a lack of time or knowledge, or because they do not assist the bedside nurses in identifying specific problems such as *Candida* or *Herpes simplex* [1]. Collaborative interactions with a dental hygienist have been proposed, but have not been routinely employed either in the care of the critically ill or to advise nursing staff in practical oral care [54].

In their survey on oral care practices, Jones et al. found that 98 % of respondents reported performing an oral needs assessment routinely, but only 26 % appeared to use a written assessment tool [24]. Binkley et al. consider the use of an oral health assessment tool to be a substantial advantage as it stimulates awareness and allows the practitioner to monitor the value of their interventions [37]. Jones et al. recommend that the use of an oral assessment tool be made a priority in ICUs [24]. Again, because nurses feel that, despite their efforts, oral hygiene worsens over time in patients who have an ETT *in situ* [33, 37], the use of an assessment tool might help counter this perception [37].

The BRUSHED Assessment Model was suggested by Hayes and Jones to encourage nurses to look for particular signs during oral care by means of a simple mnemonic [23]. Routine inspection of the elements in the model (Bleeding, Redness, Ulceration, Saliva, Halitosis, External factors, Debris) may sharpen awareness of the different problems that may arise, and may result in systematic and vigilant cleaning of the oral cavity.

Protocols

In a non-randomized trial with use of a historical control group, Mori and colleagues demonstrated a significant decrease in the relative risk of VAP (relative risk: 0.37, 95 % CI 0.277 to 0.62) after introduction of an oral care protocol in a medical-surgical ICU of a university hospital [42]. The VAP incidence decreased from 10.4

to 3.9 per 1,000 ventilator days [42]. Koeman et al. also found a significantly decreased risk of VAP when using either a chlorhexidine (hazard ratio: 0.35, 95 % CI 0.16 to 0.79; p = 0.012) or a chlorhexidine/colistin solution (hazard ratio: 0.45, 95 % CI 0.22 to 0.93; p = 0.030) in comparison with a placebo solution [30]. These studies indicate that investment in an oral care protocol may be beneficial.

While awaiting solid evidence, we recommend thorough mechanical cleaning with use of a toothbrush twice daily with additional chemical decontamination using a chlorhexidine 2 % oral care solution preferably every 6 hours. For patients with a tendency to develop mouth dryness, repeated administration of ice chips may help to enhance patient comfort. In such patients, application of moisturizers can be recommended as well. As micro-aspiration of subglottic secretions is the principal mechanism in the pathogenesis of VAP, we recommend performing deep oropharyngeal aspiration of subglottic secretions at least every two hours. We propose this approach as a 'best practice' model, acknowledging a lack of validation of this protocol and, therefore, we stress the need for well-designed randomized trials on this issue.

Conclusion

Although strong evidence-based recommendations are lacking, it is clear that preserving oral health is crucial to avoid the development of mouth and respiratory infections in intubated patients. Good oral health can be achieved by combining mechanical and chemical cleaning/decontamination of the oral cavity several times per day, along with an adequate oral assessment. Based on the literature currently available, we have proposed a non-validated best practice protocol.

Oral care in the critically ill patient with an ETT *in situ* is often perceived as a difficult and unpleasant task. Moreover, efforts to preserve adequate hygiene are often not perceived as beneficial. Thus, implementation of a protocol with the aim of improving oral care should be accompanied by substantial efforts to increase awareness of the problem, investment in a more positive attitude, and adequate in-service training.

References

1. McNeill HE (2000) Biting back at poor oral hygiene. Intensive Crit Care Nurs 16:367–372
2. Scannapieco FA (2006) Pneumonia in nonambulatory patients: The role of oral bacteria and oral hygiene. J Am Dent Assoc 137:21S–25S
3. Terezakis E, Needleman I, Kumar N, Moles D, Agudo E (2011) The impact of hospitalization on oral health: a systematic review. J Clin Periodontol 38:628–636
4. Grap MJ, Munro CL, Elswick RK, Sessler CN, Ward KR (2004) Duration of action of a single, early oral application of chlorhexidine on oral microbial flora in mechanically ventilated patients: A pilot study. Heart Lung 33:83–91
5. Munro CL, Grap MJ (2004) Oral health and care in the intensive care unit: State of the science. Am J Crit Care 13:25–33

6. Janssens JP (2005) Pneumonia in the elderly (geriatric) population. Curr Opin Pulm Med 11:226–230
7. Terpenning M, Shay K (2002) Oral health is cost-effective to maintain but costly to ignore. J Am Geriatr Soc 50:584–585
8. Vandijck DM, Decruyenaere JM, Blot SI (2006) The value of sepsis definitions in daily ICU-practice. Acta Clin Belg 61:220–226
9. Labeau SO, Van de Vyver K, Brusselaers N, Vogelaers D, Blot SI (2011) Prevention of ventilator-associated pneumonia with oral antiseptics: a systematic review and meta-analysis. Lancet Infect Dis 11:845–854
10. Dale C, Angus JE, Sinuff T, Mykhalovskiy E (2013) Mouth care for orally intubated patients: A critical ethnographic review of the nursing literature. Intensive Crit Care Nurs 29:266–274
11. Brennan MT, Bahrani-Mougeot F, Fox PC et al (2004) The role of oral microbial colonization in ventilator-associated pneumonia. Oral Surg Oral Med Oral Pathol Oral Radiol Endod 98:665–672
12. Berry AM, Davidson PM (2006) Beyond comfort: oral hygiene as a critical nursing activity in the intensive care unit. Intensive Crit Care Nurs 22:318–328
13. Woods DE, Straus DC, Johanson WG Jr, Bass JA (1981) Role of salivary protease activity in adherence of gram-negative bacilli to mammalian buccal epithelial cells in vivo. J Clin Invest 68:1435–1440
14. Dal Nogare AR, Toews GB, Pierce AK (1987) Increased salivary elastase precedes gram-negative bacillary colonization in postoperative patients. Am Rev Respir Dis 135:671–675
15. Wang PL, Azuma Y, Shinohara M, Ohura K (2001) Effect of Actinobacillus actinomycetem-comitans protease on the proliferation of gingival epithelial cells. Oral Dis 7:233–237
16. Pesola G (2004) Ventilator-associated pneumonia in institutionalized elders: Are teeth a reservoir for respiratory pathogens? Chest 126:1401–1403
17. Estes RJ, Meduri GU (1995) The pathogenesis of ventilator-associated pneumonia: I. Mechanisms of bacterial transcolonization and airway inoculation. Intensive Care Med 21:365–383
18. Costerton JW, Lewandowski Z, Caldwell DE, Korber DR, Lappin-Scott HM (1995) Microbial biofilms. Annu Rev Microbiol 49:711–745
19. Sachdev M, Ready D, Brealey D et al (2013) Changes in dental plaque following hospitalisation in a critical care unit: an observational study. Crit Care 17:R189
20. Barnett J (1991) A reassessment of oral healthcare. Prof Nurse 6:703–704 (706–708)
21. Safdar N, Crnich CJ, Maki DG (2005) The pathogenesis of ventilator-associated pneumonia: Its relevance to developing effective strategies for prevention. Respir Care 50:725–739
22. Dodek PM, Keenan S, Cook DJ et al (2004) Evidence-Based Clinical Practice Guideline for the Prevention of Ventilator-Associated Pneumonia. Annals of Internal Medicine 141:305–313
23. Hayes J, Jones C (1995) A collaborative approach to oral care during critical illness. Dent Health (London) 34:6–10
24. Jones H, Newton JT, Bower EJ (2004) A survey of the oral care practices of intensive care nurses. Intensive Crit Care Nurs 20:69–76
25. Amerongen AV, Veerman EC (2002) Saliva-the defender of the oral cavity. Oral Dis 8:12–22
26. Edgerton M, Koshlukova SE (2000) Salivary histatin 5 and its similarities to the other antimicrobial proteins in human saliva. Adv Dent Res 14:16–21
27. Dennesen P, van der Ven A, Vlasveld M et al (2003) Inadequate salivary flow and poor oral mucosal status in intubated intensive care unit patients. Crit Care Med 31:781–786
28. Holmstrup P, Poulsen AH, Andersen L, Skuldbol T, Fiehn NE (2003) Oral infections and systemic diseases. Dent Clin North Am 47:575–598
29. Rello J, Sole-Violan J, Sa-Borges M et al (2005) Pneumonia caused by oxacillin-resistant Staphylococcus aureus treated with glycopeptides. Crit Care Med 33:1983–1987
30. Koeman M, van der Ven AJ, Hak E et al (2006) Oral decontamination with chlorhexidine reduces the incidence of ventilator-associated pneumonia. Am J Respir Crit Care Med 173:1348–1355

31. Grap MJ, Munro CL, Ashtiani B, Bryant S (2003) Oral care interventions in critical care: Frequency and documentation. Am J Crit Care 12:113–118
32. Furr LA, Binkley CJ, McCurren C, Carrico R (2004) Factors affecting quality of oral care in intensive care units. J Adv Nurs 48:454–462
33. Rello J, Koulenti D, Blot S et al (2007) Oral care practices in intensive care units: a survey of 59 European ICUs. Intensive Care Med 33:1066–1070
34. Zurmehly J (2013) Oral care education in the prevention of ventilator-associated pneumonia: quality patient outcomes in the intensive care unit. J Contin Educ Nurs 44:67–75
35. Turk G, Kocacal Guler E, Eser I, Khorshid L (2012) Oral care practices of intensive care nurses: a descriptive study. International journal of nursing practice 18:347–353
36. Gmur C, Irani S, Attin T, Menghini G, Schmidlin PR (2013) Survey on oral hygiene measures for intubated patients in Swiss intensive care units. Schweizer Monatsschr Zahnmed 123:394–409
37. Binkley C, Furr LA, Carrico R, McCurren C (2004) Survey of oral care practices in US intensive care units. Am J Infect Control 32:161–169
38. Pearson LS (1996) A comparison of the ability of foam swabs and toothbrushes to remove dental plaque: implications for nursing practice. J Adv Nurs 23:62–69
39. Pearson LS, Hutton JL (2002) A controlled trial to compare the ability of foam swabs and toothbrushes to remove dental plaque. J Adv Nurs 39:480–489
40. Fourrier F, Cau-Pottier E, Boutigny H, Roussel-Delvallez M, Jourdain M, Chopin C (2000) Effects of dental plaque antiseptic decontamination on bacterial colonization and nosocomial infections in critically ill patients. Intensive Care Med 26:1239–1247
41. DeRiso AJ 2nd, Ladowski JS, Dillon TA, Justice JW, Peterson AC (1996) Chlorhexidine gluconate 0.12 % oral rinse reduces the incidence of total nosocomial respiratory infection and nonprophylactic systemic antibiotic use in patients undergoing heart surgery. Chest 109:1556–1561
42. Mori H, Hirasawa H, Oda S, Shiga H, Matsuda K, Nakamura M (2006) Oral care reduces incidence of ventilator-associated pneumonia in ICU populations. Intensive Care Med 32:230–236
43. Stiefel KA, Damron S, Sowers NJ, Velez L (2000) Improving oral hygiene for the seriously ill patient: implementing research-based practice. Medsurg Nurs 9:40–43
44. Alhazzani W, Smith O, Muscedere J, Medd J, Cook D (2013) Toothbrushing for critically ill mechanically ventilated patients: A systematic review and meta-analysis of randomized trials evaluating ventilator-associated pneumonia. Crit Care Med 41
45. Gu WJ, Gong YZ, Pan L, Ni YX, Liu JC (2012) Impact of oral care with versus without toothbrushing on the prevention of ventilator-associated pneumonia: a systematic review and meta-analysis of randomized controlled trials. Crit Care 16:R190
46. Munro CL, Grap MJ, Jones DJ, McClish DK, Sessler CN (2009) Chlorhexidine, toothbrushing, and preventing ventilator-associated pneumonia in critically ill adults. Am J Crit Care 18:428–437 (quiz 438)
47. Yao LY, Chang CK, Maa SH, Wang C, Chen CC (2011) Brushing teeth with purified water to reduce ventilator-associated pneumonia. J Nurs Res 19:289–297
48. Labeau SO, Blot SI (2013) Oral care for mechanically ventilated patients involving toothbrushing. Crit Care Med 41:e136–e137
49. Labeau SO, Blot SI (2013) Toothbrushing for preventing ventilator-associated pneumonia. Crit Care 17:417
50. Labeau SO, Blot SI (2012) Toothbrushing does not need to reduce the risk of VAP to be indispensable. Eur J Clin Microbiol Infect Dis 31:3257–3258
51. Lorente L, Blot S, Rello J (2010) New issues and controversies in the prevention of ventilator-associated pneumonia. Am J Respir Crit Care Med 182:870–876
52. Cutler CJ, Davis N (2005) Improving oral care in patients receiving mechanical ventilation. Am J Crit Care 14:389–394

53. Hanneman SK, Gusick GM (2005) Frequency of oral care and positioning of patients in critical care: a replication study. Am J Crit Care 14:378–386 (quiz 387)
54. Abidia RF (2007) Oral care in the intensive care unit: a review. J Contemp Dent Pract 8:76–82
55. Pobo A, Lisboa T, Rodriguez A et al (2009) A randomized trial of dental brushing for preventing ventilator-associated pneumonia. Chest 136:433–439
56. Lorente L, Lecuona M, Jimenez A et al (2012) Ventilator-associated pneumonia with or without toothbrushing: a randomized controlled trial. Eur J Clin Microbiol Infect Dis 31:2621–2629

Sleep and Mechanical Ventilation in Critically Ill Patients

C. Psarologakis, S. Kokkini, and D. Georgopoulos

Introduction

Sleep in critically ill patients has been recently recognized as an important concept of modern intensive care. Impaired sleep in intensive care unit (ICU) patients may have serious cardiorespiratory, neurological, immunological, and metabolic consequences [1]. Several factors, such as pre-existing medical or chronic sleep disorders, severity of illness, the acute illness that precipitated the ICU admission, the ICU environment, alterations in circadian rhythm, various medications and mechanical ventilation, may place critically ill patients at risk of poor sleep quality [1]. Among these factors, mechanical ventilation has attracted considerable interest in recent years. Mechanical ventilation may affect sleep by several direct and indirect mechanisms, mainly involving aspects of control of breathing and patient-ventilator interaction, and the use of medications to facilitate care. Studies indicate that carefully chosen ventilator modes and titration of ventilator settings may have an impact on sleep quality in these patients. In this chapter, we will summarize the current knowledge about this important but largely ignored issue.

Basic Principles of Control of Breathing During Sleep

Although extensive discussion of control of breathing during sleep is beyond the scope of this chapter, some important issues relevant to mechanical ventilation may help the reader to understand the relationship between mechanical ventilation and sleep patterns.

C. Psarologakis · S. Kokkini · D. Georgopoulos ✉
Department of Intensive Care Medicine, University Hospital of Heraklion, Medical School,
University of Crete, Heraklion, Crete, Greece
e-mail: georgop@med.uoc.gr

J.-L. Vincent (Ed.), *Annual Update in Intensive Care and Emergency Medicine 2014*,
DOI 10.1007/978-3-319-03746-2_11, © Springer International Publishing Switzerland
2014

Data from experimental studies in animals and healthy subjects have shown that control of breathing differs markedly between wakefulness and sleep [2–4]. In contrast to wakefulness, during non-rapid eye movement (NREM) sleep, respiration is dominated mainly by chemical feedback. This feedback refers to the response of respiratory muscle pressure (Pmus) to PaO_2, $PaCO_2$ and pH. It has been shown that NREM sleep unmasks a highly sensitive $PaCO_2$ apneic threshold, such that apnea is induced by small transient reductions in $PaCO_2$ below eupnea [2, 4, 5]. This effect does not occur during wakefulness, in which it has been shown that manipulation of chemical stimuli over a wide range has no appreciable effect on respiratory rate (Fig. 1) [6, 7]. Unlike in NREM sleep, in both phasic and tonic rapid eye movement (REM) sleep, ventilatory control was believed to be largely independent of chemoreceptor drive but dominated by behavioral factors [8]. Earlier studies suggested that during REM sleep the sensitivity to CO_2 is significantly reduced, whereas on the other hand there is a non-chemoreceptor activation of respiratory neurons and absence of apnoeic threshold [8,9]. However, Meza et al. showed no significant difference between REM and NREM sleep in terms of the response of Pmus to chemical stimuli [5]. During both REM and NREM sleep, even a small change in tidal volume (V_T) that was inevitably associated with chemical stimuli alteration resulted in a corresponding response of Pmus [5]. This finding indicates that chemical feedback dominates respiration during all stages of sleep.

Not only is chemical feedback a major determinant of breathing during sleep, its magnitude is influenced by the wakefulness/sleep stage. Compared to wakefulness, several studies have shown that the sensitivity to chemical stimuli is reduced during sleep. This reduction applies to all stages of sleep, although data in REM sleep are scanty. Some of this reduction in chemosensitivity may be secondary to an increase in upper airway resistance but this is unlikely to be the sole explanation because $PaCO_2$ increases during sleep even when the upper airways are by-passed [10].

The fact that control of breathing differs between wakefulness and sleep (and possible sedation) is relevant to mechanical ventilation. Ventilatory settings and/or ventilator modes which are appropriate during wakefulness may not be so during sleep and *vice versa*.

Sleep in Mechanically Ventilated Patients

Surveys of ICU survivors have shown that sleep deprivation and the inability to sleep rank among the top three major sources of anxiety and stress during the ICU stay (along with pain and intubation) [11]. Moreover, sleep abnormalities, as detected by polysomnograpy, are extremely common in mechanically ventilated critically ill patients [12, 13]. Notwithstanding that sleep scoring using conventional rules may not be feasible in some patients because of the absence of stage-2 markers and abnormal electroencephalogram (EEG) features during wakefulness [14], critically ill patients exhibit considerable reduction (or absence) in REM and NREM slow-wave sleep (SWS, deep sleep), increased duration of stage 1 (light sleep) and more frequent arousals and awakenings than normal [1, 12, 13]. Thus, although to-

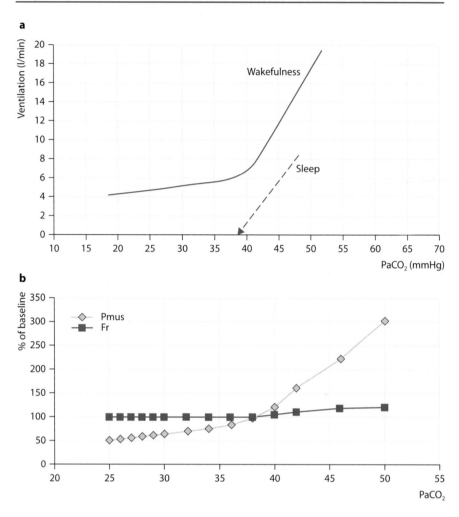

Fig. 1 **a** Schematic representation of ventilatory response to CO_2 in normal subjects. Note that in awake patients, the response is linear in the hypercapnic range. In the hypocapnic range the slope progressively decreases with decreasing $PaCO_2$. Apnea is not observed. During sleep, apnea develops when $PaCO_2$ is reduced 2–3 mmHg below the eupneic level. Data for awake subjects are based on refs. [6] and [7]. Data for asleep subjects are based on refs. [2–5]. **b** Intensity of inspiratory effort (Pmus) and breathing frequency (Fr) (expressed as % of the values at eupnea) as a function of $PaCO_2$ during wakefulness. Data based on [6]

tal sleep time in mechanically ventilated patients may be normal or even increased, the quality of sleep is poor and these patients are considered to be qualitatively sleep deprived [1, 12, 13]. As was stated earlier, this may cause serious consequences leading to more days on mechanical ventilation, longer ICU stays and increased morbidity [1].

It is of interest to note that REM and SWS sleep are considered to have the most restorative effects. Animal studies have shown that both REM sleep deprivation and sleep fragmentation contribute to reduction in neurogenesis in the hippocampal dentate gyrus [15, 16]. Furthermore, reductions in both NREM (SWS and stage 2) and REM sleep decrease the number of brain cells that subsequently develop into adult neurons [17]. These effects of REM and SWS reduction may be linked to cognitive dysfunction [17], frequently observed in ICU survivors. In addition to these effects, human studies have shown that REM and SWS stages are crucial for memory formation and learning process [18]. It follows that critically ill patients, in whom reduction (or even absence) of REM and SWS is the rule, may exhibit both memory and learning problems. Since defects in memory formation and learning process abnormalities have been linked to delirium and post-traumatic stress disorder [17], poor sleep quality during the ICU stay may partly explain the high incidence of these disorders in critically ill patients.

Why Might Mechanical Ventilation Affect Sleep?

During mechanical ventilation, the pressure provided by the ventilator (Paw) is incorporated into the system that controls breathing [19]. In mechanically ventilated patients, the total pressure applied to the respiratory system at time t $[P_{TOT}(t)]$ is the sum of Pmus(t) and Paw(t). $P_{TOT}(t)$ is dissipated to overcome the elastic and resistive pressures of the respiratory system according to the equation of motion:

$$P_{TOT}(t) = Pmus(t) + Paw(t) = V'(t) \times Rrs + \Delta V(t) \times Ers \qquad (1)$$

where V' and ΔV are instantaneous flow and volume (in relation to passive FRC), respectively, Rrs is respiratory system resistance and Ers is respiratory system elastance. The relationships of Eq. 1 determine the volume-time profile during mechanical ventilation, which, via neuro-mechanical, chemical and behavioral feedback systems, affects the Pmus waveform. The ventilator pressure, by changing flow and volume, may influence these feedback systems, and thus alter either the patient's control of breathing itself or its expression. In addition, Pmus, depending on several factors, alters the Paw waveform. Thus, during mechanical ventilation, ventilatory output is not under the exclusive influence of a patient's control of breathing; instead, it represents the final expression of an interaction between ventilator-delivered pressure and patient respiratory effort [19, 20].

During sleep, respiration is mainly under the influence of chemical feedback and to a lesser extent of neuro-mechanical feedback systems [5]. Thus, to the extent that mechanical ventilation interferes with these feedback systems, it might be an important determinant of sleep in ventilated patients.

How Does Mechanical Ventilation Affect Sleep?

Theoretically, mechanical ventilation may affect sleep by:
1) promoting unstable breathing;
2) inducing dyssynchrony between patient effort and ventilator delivered pressure;
3) altering the Pmus (patient's respiratory effort); and
4) the use of sedatives and analgesic agents to facilitate its process.

Unstable Breathing and Mechanical Ventilation

Unstable breathing and central apneas are well recognized causes of sleep fragmentation [21]. Although the mechanism(s) by which these events may disrupt sleep is not well established, fluctuation of sympathetic tone during the cycles of unstable breathing may be involved [21].

The pathophysiologic mechanisms by which mechanical ventilation causes unstable breathing may be best explained using the engineering concept of loop gain, as proposed by Khoo and colleagues [22]. Theoretically, in a closed system governed mainly by chemical control (as occurs during sleep or sedation, see earlier), a transient change in ventilation at a given metabolic rate ($\Delta V'_{initial}$) will result in a transient change in alveolar gas tensions. This change is sensed by peripheral and central chemoreceptors, which, after a variable delay, exert a corrective ventilatory response ($\Delta V'_{corrective}$). This corrective response is in the opposite direction to the initial perturbation. The ratio of $\Delta V'_{corrective}$ to $\Delta V'_{initial}$ defines the loop gain, a dimensionless index that is the mathematical product of three types of gain: Plant gain (the relationship between the change in gas tensions in mixed pulmonary capillary blood and $\Delta V'_{initial}$), feedback gain (the relationship between gas tensions at the chemoreceptor level and those at the mixed pulmonary capillary level), and controller gain (the relationship between $\Delta V'_{corrective}$ and the change in gas tensions at the chemoreceptor level) (Fig. 2). Loop gain has both a magnitude and a dynamic component [22, 23]. In this system, instability occurs when the corrective response is $180°$ out of phase with the initial disturbance (dynamic component) and the loop gain is ≥ 1 (magnitude component). This instability leads to fluctuation in chemical stimuli, namely $PaCO_2$. If $PaCO_2$ reaches the apneic threshold, apnea occurs.

Positive-pressure ventilation exerts multiple effects on loop gain by influencing almost all the factors that determine plant, feedback and controller gains. These effects are complex and, at times, opposing and variable. Nevertheless, the effect of mechanical ventilation on controller gain exerts the most powerful influence on the propensity to develop breathing instability [23]. The magnitude and direction of the change in controller gain depends on the ventilator mode, the level of assistance, the mechanics of the respiratory system, and the Pmus waveform. Disease states may also interfere with the effects of mechanical ventilation on loop gain [23, 24].

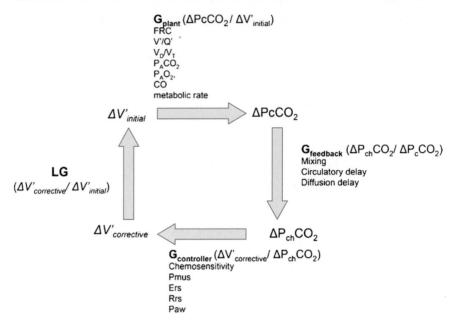

Fig. 2 Schematic representation of the "Loop Gain" model of respiratory chemical control system. Total loop gain is the product of the three component gains: G_{plant}, $G_{feedback}$, and $G_{controller}$. Below each component are depicted physiologic parameters that influence the component gain, and consequently the total loop gain and the propensity for an individual to develop periodic breathing. Mechanical ventilation or medication (e. g., sedative agents) may modify some of these parameters and thus alter an individual's intrinsic propensity to develop periodic breathing. FRC: functional residual capacity; V'/Q': ventilation-perfusion ratio; V_D/V_T: dead space fraction; P_ACO_2 and P_AO_2: alveolar partial pressure of CO_2 and O_2, respectively, CO: cardiac output; Pmus: pressure developed by respiratory muscles; Paw: airway (ventilator) pressure; Ers and Rrs: elastance and resistance of respiratory system respectively

In addition to CO_2, O_2 and pH can play a key role in destabilizing breathing in ventilated patients during sleep. It is well known that hypoxia, acting via peripheral chemoreceptor stimulation, decreases $PaCO_2$ and, as a result, it reduces the plant gain (stabilizing influence); for a given change in alveolar ventilation, $PaCO_2$ will change less when baseline $PaCO_2$ is low [3, 25]. Hypoxia, however, increases the controller gain to a much greater extent, because the slope of the ventilatory response to CO_2 below eupnea increases and becomes a highly destabilizing influence [3, 25]. Similar principles apply if pH is considered a chemical stimulus. Acidemia decreases the plant gain (lowers $PaCO_2$) and increases, to a much lesser extent, the controller gain [3, 25]. During mechanical ventilation, the propensity towards unstable breathing in the face of changing O_2 and pH depends on a complex interaction between the effects of these stimuli and mechanical ventilation on plant, feedback and controller gains.

Patient-ventilator Dyssynchrony

Patient-ventilator dyssynchrony is a common phenomenon during mechanical ventilation [26]. Dyssynchrony occurs either when cycling of the ventilator is not in phase with patient effort or when the instantaneous ventilatory demands of the patients are not met by the gas delivered by the ventilator. Several types of asynchrony exist, but it is not known whether a particular type of asynchrony affects sleep more than another [26]. Nevertheless, ineffective efforts, which are considered the most extreme form of asynchrony, might cause sleep disruption, since this type of asynchrony is a form of airway obstruction, a well-known cause of arousals and sleep fragmentation [27]. However, studies that examined the effects of dyssynchrony on sleep showed contradictory results (see below).

Sleep and Respiratory Effort

Indirect data from recent studies indicate that sleep in critically ill patients may be influenced by the magnitude of a patient's inspiratory effort. It has been shown that, compared to low pressure support, controlled mechanical ventilation (passive mechanical ventilation) is associated with better sleep both in terms of quantity and quality [28]. It seems that there is a negative relationship between patient effort and sleep quality and quantity. Thus, to the extent that the mode of mechanical ventilation as well as the ventilator settings are major determinants of Pmus [20], mechanical ventilation may affect sleep by simply altering the respiratory effort.

Sleep and Medications that Facilitate the Process of Mechanical Ventilation

Sedative agents (e. g., gamma aminobutyric acid A [$GABA_A$] agonists) and analgesics (e. g., opioids) are commonly used in critically ill patients in order to facilitate the process of mechanical ventilation. A widely held belief is that sedation in critically ill patients promotes sleep and thus reduces the detrimental effects of sleep deprivation or poor sleep quality. It has been shown that in ~50 % of mechanically ventilated pa tients, the dose of sedatives (benzodiazepine, propofol) is increased during the night (11 pm–7 am) [29]. However, data from recent studies do not support this practice. Kondili et al. have shown that propofol administration to achieve the recommended level of sedation in critically ill patients (Ramsay 3) does not increase sleep efficiency and by suppressing REM sleep further worsens the already impaired sleep quality of these patients [30]. These effects of $GABA_A$ agonists on sleep may explain the link between the use of these agents and the incidence of delirium and post-traumatic stress disorders [29]. Similar to sedative agents, reduction of REM sleep has also been observed when opioids are used for analgesia [31].

Sleep Patterns and Mechanical Ventilation

As stated earlier, mechanical ventilation affects sleep through several mechanisms. Modes of mechanical ventilator and/or ventilator settings may affect sleep by influencing these mechanisms. The effects on sleep may, however, be unpredictable because these influences may be opposing.

In order to understand the interaction between sleep and mechanical ventilation, we should realize that the ventilator mode and settings are major determinants of driving pressure for flow and thus of arterial blood gases and chemical feedback. Assume that in a ventilated patient $PaCO_2$ decreases because of an increase in the set level of assistance or a decrease in metabolic rate and/or dead space $(V_D)/V_T$ ratio. During sleep, as the sensitivity to CO_2 dictates (i.e., chemical feedback), the intensity of inspiratory effort will decrease, whereas the breathing frequency will change minimally [20]. This operation of chemical feedback (down-regulation of inspiratory effort) serves to minimize or even to prevent the decrease in $PaCO_2$. Thus, it is obvious that the proper operation of chemical feedback depends almost exclusively on the relationship between the intensity of patient inspiratory effort (expressed by the pressure time product of Pmus, PTP-Pmus) and the volume delivered by the ventilator (V_T) [7]. Similarly, if $PaCO_2$ increases (by a decrease in assistance level, increase in metabolic rate and/or V_D/V_T ratio), the patient will increase the intensity of inspiratory effort and, to a much lesser extent, the respiratory frequency. Thus, V_T/PTP-Pmus per breath is critical for the effectiveness of chemical feedback to compensate for changes in chemical stimuli $(PaCO_2)$ [20].

During sleep, conventional modes of assisted mechanical ventilation, such as pressure support and volume assist-control without back-up rate, may promote unstable breathing [32]. Indeed, it has been shown that with these modes, high assist results in high V_T/PTP-Pmus, leading to impaired neuroventilatory coupling [7]. This effect may have serious consequences, because in the presence of high V_T/PTP-Pmus (i.e., high assist) the system becomes unstable [20]. Under this circumstance, there is a possibility for fluctuation in chemical stimuli (mainly $PaCO_2$) which may result in periodic breathing and sleep disruption [5, 33]. Patients with pre-existing diseases that predispose to periodic breathing (e.g., patients with congestive heart failure or brain damage) are at high risk of unstable breathing with conventional modes of assisted mechanical ventilation [24, 32]. Parthasarathy and Tobin studied the effect of pressure support and assist control ventilation with back-up rate on sleep fragmentation in 11 mechanically ventilated critical ill patients [32]. Total sleep fragmentation, measured as the sum of arousals and awakenings, was approximately 50 % greater during pressure support than during assist-control ventilation (79 vs. 54 events/hour). During pressure support, one third of these events were due to central apneas as contrasted with rates of zero during assist-control ventilation (Fig. 3). The most important determinant of central apneas was the difference between the basic level of end-tidal CO_2 and the patient's apneic threshold: A small difference was associated with a higher probability of central apneas. An experimental increase in dead space resulted in a significant decrease in sleep fragmentation by increasing basic end-tidal CO_2 in those patients

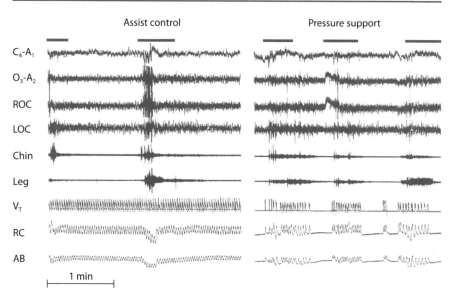

Fig. 3 Polysomnographic tracings during assist-control and pressure support ventilation in a representative patient. Electroencephalogram (C4-A1, O3-A2), electrooculogram (ROC, LOC), electromyograms (Chin and Leg), integrated tidal volume (V_T), rib-cage (RC), and abdominal (AB) excursions on respiratory inductive plethysmography are shown. Notice: 1) the periodic breathing during pressure support; and 2) that arousals and awakenings, indicated by horizontal bars, were more numerous during pressure support than during assist-control ventilation. From [32] with permission

with central apneas on pressure support (83 and 44 events per hour, respectively, for the two experimental conditions). The relationship between sleep fragmentation and central apneas is also highlighted by a study by Alexopoulou et al. which showed that the presence of unstable breathing in mechanically ventilated critically ill patients was associated with a fourfold increase in sleep fragmentation index [34].

Theoretically, unstable breathing during sleep in mechanically ventilated patients may be prevented or attenuated with modes that decrease the volume delivered by a ventilator in response to any reduction in the intensity of patient effort. Proportional-assist ventilation (PAV) and neurally-adjusted ventilator assist (NAVA) are such modes of support, because with these modalities there is a tight link between effort and ventilator [35]. Nevertheless, if the assist setting during both modes is such that controller gain increases considerably and the inherent loop gain of the patient is relatively high, then the patient will be at risk of developing unstable breathing [33]. During conventional modes, decreasing assist may improve breathing stability by decreasing V_T/PTP-Pmus ratio [20]. However, the effects of this strategy on sleep are unpredictable; lowering the assist improves breathing stability (beneficial effect on sleep), but increases respiratory effort (harmful effect on sleep). Similar reasoning should apply with PAV and NAVA.

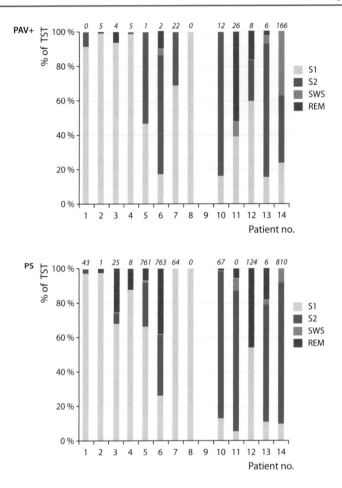

Fig. 4 Sleep architecture in each patient with proportional assist ventilation with load adjustable gain factors (PAV+, upper panel) and with pressure support ventilation (PS, lower panel). Patient no. 9 did not achieve sleep during the entire recording period. Asynchrony events (events per hour of sleep) are shown in each patient and for both modes of mechanical ventilation (*italics*). Notice that compared to pressure support, PAV+ significantly decreased the asynchrony events per hour of sleep, but did not improve sleep architecture. REM: rapid eye movement; S1, S2: sleep stages 1 and 2, respectively; SWS: slow-wave sleep; TST: total sleep time. From [38] with permission

It has been proposed that patient-ventilator dyssynchrony may be another important mechanism of sleep disruption. If this is true, assisted modes of mechanical ventilation that are associated with improvement in patient-ventilator synchrony (such as PAV and NAVA) should result in improved sleep quality in critically ill patients but data so far are controversial. Two studies have shown that reducing patient-ventilator asynchrony using PAV [36] or NAVA [37] results in sleep improvement. Other studies, however, do not support the hypothesis that patient-ventilator synchrony plays a central role in determining sleep quality in mechan-

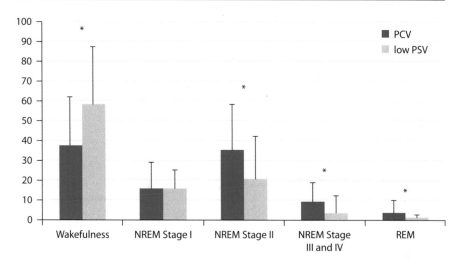

Fig. 5 Comparison of quantity of sleep stages expressed as a percentage of total recording time during the entire night between pressure-controlled ventilation (PCV, passive mechanical ventilation) and low-level pressure-support ventilation (low-PSV). *p < 0.01. From [28] with permission

ically ventilated patients. Alexopoulou et al. examined patient-ventilator asynchrony in 14 non-sedated critically ill patients ventilated with PAV+ (i. e., PAV with automatic measurement of respiratory system mechanics) and pressure support. Interestingly, although PAV+ was associated with considerably better synchrony between the patient and the ventilator, this mode failed to improve sleep (Fig. 4) [38]. Fanfulla et al. demonstrated, in patients admitted to a step-down unit after ICU discharge, that the role of patient-ventilator asynchronies in sleep fragmentation was negligible [39]. Cabello et al. [40] studied the effects of common ventilator modes (assist-control and pressure support) on sleep and observed that patient-ventilator asynchrony explained a small percentage (less than 10%) of sleep fragmentation. However, the interpretation of all these studies is complicated by the fact that patients' respiratory efforts were not controlled.

The effects of assist-control and pressure support on sleep architecture were investigated by Toublanc et al. in a report on 20 mechanically ventilated patients at the end of the weaning period [41]. In this randomized crossover study, patients were assigned to receive either assist-control or low pressure support ventilation for 4 hours. With assist-control, the V_T and ventilator frequency were set so as to provide the patient's minute ventilation. The authors showed that ventilation on assist-control, unlike pressure support, was associated with a significant increase in the time that a patient spent in sleep stages 1 and 2, a reduction in wakefulness during the first part of the night, and a significant increase in sleep stages 3 and 4 during the second part of the night. These results indicate better sleep with assist-control than with pressure support. It is likely that the difference in sleep quality is the result of the different assistance provided by the two modes and not of the mode itself. This hypothesis is supported by a study by Andrejak et al. which demonstrated that mechanically ventilated patients with acute-on-chronic respiratory failure had significantly improved sleep quality and quantity when respiratory muscles were rested at night using pressure-controlled ventilation (passive mechanical ventilation) compared to using low-level pressure support ventilation (Fig. 5) [28]. Collectively, these findings indicate that sleep may be improved if the ventilator settings (or mode) meet or even exceed the ventilatory demands of the patient. However under this circumstance, the ratio of V_T/PTP-Pmus might be high, making the system unstable, and thus the use of sufficient back-up rate is mandatory for sleep improvement.

Because of discrepancies in the control of breathing between wakefulness and sleep, it is possible to have excessive or inadequate control during sleep at settings determined during wakefulness. Fanfulla et al. investigated the effect of different ventilator settings on sleep quality in nine patients with neuromuscular disease receiving long term non-invasive mechanical ventilation (NIV) [42]. The authors evaluated breathing patterns and sleep architecture during ventilation with two non-invasive pressure support ventilation settings titrated: 1) on simple clinical parameters, and 2) to the patient's respiratory effort. The authors showed that during wakefulness, both strategies were effective in improving arterial blood gases. However, during sleep, NIV settings based on clinical parameters did not predict ventilatory synchrony, but settings based on respiratory effort did improve synchrony and resulted in better sleep. This study highlights the importance of wakefulness/sleep state in ventilator setting titration, a difficult task because the caregiver usually cannot tell what state (sleep/wakefulness) a patient is in.

Conclusions

Sleep in mechanically ventilated patients is characterized by poor quality. Mechanical ventilation may contribute to this through several direct and indirect mechanisms, such as the promotion of unstable breathing, patient-ventilator dyssynchrony, increased respiratory effort and the use of sedatives and opioids to facilitate care. Taking into account that a particular ventilatory strategy may have both beneficial and harmful effects on sleep, carefully chosen ventilator settings and/or mode of mechanical ventilation specifically targeting these mechanisms may have a great impact on sleep quality.

References

1. Parthasarathy S, Tobin MJ (2004) Sleep in the intensive care unit. Intensive Care Med 30:197–206
2. Dempsey JA, Skatrud JB (1986) A sleep-induced apneic threshold and its consequences. Am Rev Respir Dis 133:1163–1170
3. Dempsey JA, Smith CA, Przybylowski T et al (2004) The ventilatory responsiveness to CO(2) below eupnoea as a determinant of ventilatory stability in sleep. J Physiol 560:1–11

4. Skatrud JB, Dempsey JA (1983) Interaction of sleep state and chemical stimuli in sustaining rhythmic ventilation. J Appl Physiol 55:813–822
5. Meza S, Giannouli E, Younes M (1998) Control of breathing during sleep assessed by proportional assist ventilation. J Appl Physiol 84:3–12
6. Georgopoulos D, Mitrouska I, Bshouty Z et al (1997) Respiratory response to CO2 during pressure-support ventilation in conscious normal humans. Am J Respir Crit Care Med 156:146–154
7. Mitrouska J, Xirouchaki N, Patakas D, Siafakas N, Georgopoulos D (1999) Effects of chemical feedback on respiratory motor and ventilatory output during different modes of assisted mechanical ventilation. Eur Respir J 13:873–882
8. Douglas NJ (1984) Control of breathing during sleep. Clin Sci (Lond) 67:465–471
9. Douglas NJ, White DP, Weil JV, Pickett CK, Zwillich CW (1982) Hypercapnic ventilatory response in sleeping adults. Am Rev Respir Dis 126:758–762
10. Onal E, Lopata M (1982) Periodic breathing and the pathogenesis of occlusive sleep apneas. Am Rev Respir Dis 126:676–680
11. Rotondi AJ, Chelluri L, Sirio C et al (2002) Patients' recollections of stressful experiences while receiving prolonged mechanical ventilation in an intensive care unit. Crit Care Med 30:746–752
12. Freedman NS, Gazendam J, Levan L, Pack AI, Schwab RJ (2001) Abnormal sleep/wake cycles and the effect of environmental noise on sleep disruption in the intensive care unit. Am J Respir Crit Care Med 163:451–457
13. Cooper AB, Thornley KS, Young GB et al (2000) Sleep in critically ill patients requiring mechanical ventilation. Chest 117:809–818
14. Drouot X, Roche-Campo F, Thille AW et al (2012) A new classification for sleep analysis in critically ill patients. Sleep Med 13:7–14
15. Guzman-Marin R, Bashir T, Suntsova N, Szymusiak R, McGinty D (2007) Hippocampal neurogenesis is reduced by sleep fragmentation in the adult rat. Neuroscience 148:325–333
16. Guzman-Marin R, Suntsova N, Bashir T et al (2008) Rapid eye movement sleep deprivation contributes to reduction of neurogenesis in the hippocampal dentate gyrus of the adult rat. Sleep 31:167–175
17. Meerlo P, Mistlberger RE, Jacobs BL, Heller HC, McGinty D (2009) New neurons in the adult brain: the role of sleep and consequences of sleep loss. Sleep Med Rev 13:187–194
18. McCoy JG, Strecker RE (2011) The cognitive cost of sleep lost. Neurobiol Learn Mem 96:564–582
19. Georgopoulos D, Roussos C (1996) Control of breathing in mechanically ventilated patients. Eur Respir J 9:2151–2160
20. Kondili E, Prinianakis G, Georgopoulos D (2003) Patient-ventilator interaction. Br J Anaesth 91:106–119
21. Bradley TD, Floras JS (2003) Sleep apnea and heart failure: Part II: central sleep apnea. Circulation 107:1822–1826
22. Khoo MC, Kronauer RE, Strohl KP, Slutsky AS (1982) Factors inducing periodic breathing in humans: a general model. J Appl Physiol 53:644–659
23. Younes M, Ostrowski M, Thompson W, Leslie C, Shewchuk W (2001) Chemical control stability in patients with obstructive sleep apnea. Am J Respir Crit Care Med 163:1181–1190
24. Klimathianaki M, Kondili E, Alexopoulou C, Prinianakis G, Georgopoulos D (2010) Effect of propofol on breathing stability in adult ICU patients with brain damage. Respir Physiol Neurobiol 171:232–238
25. Nakayama H, Smith CA, Rodman JR, Skatrud JB, Dempsey JA (2002) Effect of ventilatory drive on carbon dioxide sensitivity below eupnea during sleep. Am J Respir Crit Care Med 165:1251–1260
26. Kondili E, Xirouchaki N, Georgopoulos D (2007) Modulation and treatment of patient-ventilator dyssynchrony. Curr Opin Crit Care 13:84–89

27. Issa FG, McNamara SG, Sullivan CE (1987) Arousal responses to airway occlusion in sleeping dogs: comparison of nasal and tracheal occlusions. J Appl Physiol 62:1832–1836
28. Andrejak C, Monconduit J, Rose D et al (2013) Does using pressure-controlled ventilation to rest respiratory muscles improve sleep in ICU patients? Respir Med 107:534–541
29. Seymour CW, Pandharipande PP, Koestner T et al (2012) Diurnal sedative changes during intensive care: impact on liberation from mechanical ventilation and delirium. Crit Care Med 40:2788–2796
30. Kondili E, Alexopoulou C, Xirouchaki N, Georgopoulos D (2012) Effects of propofol on sleep quality in mechanically ventilated critically ill patients: a physiological study. Intensive Care Med 38:1640–1646
31. Wang D, Teichtahl H (2007) Opioids, sleep architecture and sleep-disordered breathing. Sleep Med Rev 11:35–46
32. Parthasarathy S, Tobin MJ (2002) Effect of ventilator mode on sleep quality in critically ill patients. Am J Respir Crit Care Med 166:1423–1429
33. Meza S, Mendez M, Ostrowski M, Younes M (1998) Susceptibility to periodic breathing with assisted ventilation during sleep in normal subjects. J Appl Physiol 85:1929–1940
34. Alexopoulou C, Kondili E, Vakouti E et al (2007) Sleep during proportional-assist ventilation with load-adjustable gain factors in critically ill patients. Intensive Care Med 33:1139–1147
35. Kacmarek RM (2011) Proportional assist ventilation and neurally adjusted ventilatory assist. Respir Care 56:140–148
36. Bosma K, Ferreyra G, Ambrogio C et al (2007) Patient-ventilator interaction and sleep in mechanically ventilated patients: pressure support versus proportional assist ventilation. Crit Care Med 35:1048–1054
37. Delisle S, Ouellet P, Bellemare P, Tetrault JP, Arsenault P (2011) Sleep quality in mechanically ventilated patients: comparison between NAVA and PSV modes. Ann Intensive Care 1:42–50
38. Alexopoulou C, Kondili E, Plataki M, Georgopoulos D (2013) Patient-ventilator synchrony and sleep quality with proportional assist and pressure support ventilation. Intensive Care Med 39:1040–1047
39. Fanfulla F, Ceriana P, D'Artavilla Lupo N et al (2011) Sleep disturbances in patients admitted to a step-down unit after ICU discharge: the role of mechanical ventilation. Sleep 34:355–362
40. Cabello B, Thille AW, Drouot X et al (2008) Sleep quality in mechanically ventilated patients: comparison of three ventilatory modes. Crit Care Med 36:1749–1755
41. Toublanc B, Rose D, Glerant JC et al (2007) Assist-control ventilation vs. low levels of pressure support ventilation on sleep quality in intubated ICU patients. Intensive Care Med 33:1148–1154
42. Fanfulla F, Delmastro M, Berardinelli A, Lupo ND, Nava S (2005) Effects of different ventilator settings on sleep and inspiratory effort in patients with neuromuscular disease. Am J Respir Crit Care Med 172:619–624

The Importance of Weaning for Successful Treatment of Respiratory Failure

J. Bickenbach, C. Brülls, and G. Marx

Introduction

Identification of acute respiratory failure and treatment of the underlying cause(s) are crucial but also difficult challenges in ICU management. Weaning from mechanical ventilation must be conducted in a timely manner because invasive, prolonged mechanical ventilation can be a significant hazard with a negative influence on the weaning process. Interestingly, the process of weaning from mechanical ventilation represents approximately 40–50 % of the duration of mechanical ventilation [1–3] and is directly associated with patient prognosis [4].

Our knowledge of the pathophysiological aspects of mechanical ventilation have increased in recent years. Here we review recent aspects of ventilator-induced complications, their impact on weaning from mechanical ventilation and the role of weaning protocols as well as the potential role of specialized weaning units.

Ventilator-associated Complications

Ventilator-induced Lung Injury

Despite the necessity and the vital role of mechanical ventilation, it exposes the lung to mechanical stress. This effect can have an important impact on the pathophysiology especially when high inspiratory pressures are used. During one of the most distinctive forms of acute respiratory failure, the acute respiratory distress syndrome (ARDS), in particular, considerable heterogeneous damage to the lung occurs and coexistence of normally aerated, consolidated and collapsed lung regions can be

J. Bickenbach ✉ · C. Brülls · G. Marx
Department of Surgical Intensive Care, University Hospital RWTH Aachen,
52074 Aachen, Germany
e-mail: jbickenbach@ukaachen.de

J.-L. Vincent (Ed.), *Annual Update in Intensive Care and Emergency Medicine 2014*,
DOI 10.1007/978-3-319-03746-2_12, © Springer International Publishing Switzerland
2014

found [5], thus promoting different regional alveolar stresses and strains, which are the main determinants of ventilator-induced lung injury (VILI) [6, 7]. VILI describes the phenomenon of further damage to alveoli because of mechanical stress and progressive overdistension of lung tissue, resulting in mechanotransduction and an inflammatory response. In other areas, especially atelectatic lung regions, enormous sheer stress due to cyclic opening and closing of alveoli can be found (atelectrauma) [8].

New imaging technologies can support the analysis of regional ventilation and related alveolar morphologies in the heterogeneously damaged lung. For example, electrical impedance tomography (EIT) is a non-invasive imaging modality which can be used at the bedside, and offers information about regional ventilation of the lung. The method is based on visualization and quantification of tissue impedance determined by applying non-hazardous electrical currents and measuring the resulting voltages at the surface of the thorax. EIT-based measurements are able to identify lung heterogeneity, as is typical in ARDS [9], and to guide modification of positive end-expiratory pressure (PEEP) and tidal volumes for prevention of further VILI [10].

Regarding the effects of mechanical ventilation on the alveolar network, intravital microscopy enables direct visualization of alveolar dynamics. Early studies showed that alveoli could be identified according to their different mechanical behavior when changing ventilatory settings [11–13]. Advancements in intravital microscopy led to a technique that offers imaging of alveolar mechanics with a flexible miniprobe applicable not only *in vivo*, but also in real time and without surgical opening of the thorax. The fibered confocal laser scanning microscopy (CLSM) provides images of alveolar structure giving depth information that is advantageous over conventional microscopy. Use in a porcine model of acute lung injury (ALI) showed regional effects of recruitment after incremental PEEP (Fig. 1) [14, 15]. Based on these findings, translation into clinical use would be of enormous interest. Thus, clinical studies need to be conducted, particularly in intensive care settings where patients need to be treated with mechanical ventilation because of respiratory insufficiency. The technique of CLSM may help to better understand the mechanical behavior of alveolar structure during mechanical ventilation and their effects on pulmonary function. CLSM may be an interesting technique for endoscopic use in patients, for example in association with diagnostic bronchoscopies.

For prevention of VILI, the most evident therapeutic measure we have at the moment is lung-protective ventilation with reduction of tidal volume to 6 ml/kg body weight and limitation of plateau pressures to 30 cmH$_2$O [16]. However, the discussion about lung-protective strategies has not ended yet. Remarkably, a recent study demonstrated that in patients with severe ARDS (PaO$_2$/FiO$_2$ $\leq$ 150), even smaller tidal volumes ($\approx$ 3 ml/kg), combined with extracorporeal CO$_2$-elimination were associated with a significantly higher number of ventilator-free days than higher tidal volumes ($\approx$ 6 ml/kg) without extracorporeal CO$_2$-elimination [17].

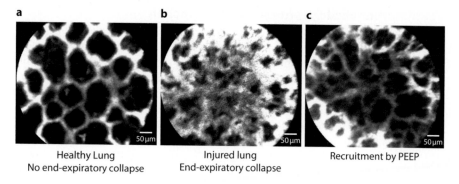

Healthy Lung   Injured lung   Recruitment by PEEP
No end-expiratory collapse   End-expiratory collapse

Fig. 1 Confocal laser scanning microscopy (CLSM) for imaging of alveolar structure in a porcine model of acute lung injury. Images show **a** alveoli of a healthy lung, **b** after experimental lung injury by lavage and **c** after alveolar recruitment by positive end-expiratory pressure (PEEP)

Ventilator-associated Pneumonia

Intensive care unit (ICU) patients receiving mechanical ventilation are at high risk of developing ventilator-associated pneumonia (VAP), with an incidence of 8 %–28 % in patients who are mechanically ventilated for > 24 hours [18]. The pathophysiological mechanisms of VAP are well known and, in particular, aspiration of colonized pharyngeal secretions along the cuff of the endotracheal tube (ETT) plays an important role in the development of VAP, gaining access to the airway via folds in the wall of the cuff. A bacterial biofilm gradually forms on the inner surface of the ETT and acts as a hatchery for microbes. Other crucial mechanisms for VAP development are the absence of effective coughing as well as a relevant reduction in mucociliary clearance in analgosedated patients [19].

The incidence of VAP can be reduced by shortening invasive mechanical ventilation, but preventive measures have also been shown to reduce the rate of VAP, especially those that reduce colonization of the airway (e. g., oral care with chlorhexidine, closed tracheal suction systems, patient positioning for reduction of aspiration) [18, 20, 21]. Ricard et al. conducted a study in which European ICU staff were interviewed about adherence to current prevention strategies. Interestingly, overall median adherence to VAP prevention measures was 72 % (34.5–83.0); however, data revealed a large discrepancy between countries [22].

These studies emphasize the impact of a bundle approach, because no single preventive measure may preclude VAP. Thus it is of importance to a) identify patients at risk of VAP early, and b) treat them with a bundle of preventive measures. Implementation and educational processes are challenging and need broader permeation.

Ventilator-induced Diaphragmatic Dysfunction

Mechanical ventilation harms the diaphragm. There has been evidence for more than a decade that ventilator-induced diaphragmatic dysfunction (VIDD), as a collective term for diaphragm muscle atrophy and contractile dysfunction, is a clinical reality [23] and it is accepted that it endangers the weaning process. There has been growing evidence about the pathophysiology of this condition, pointing at inactivity as a major contributor to VIDD leading to generation of reactive oxygen species (ROS), mainly from mitochondria [24]. ROS damage contractile proteins and activate the proteolytic and apoptotic cascade resulting in contractile deficit and muscle atrophy [25]. This process is rapid and occurs in less than one day of mechanical ventilation [26].

Mitochondrial ROS production originating from an uncoupling of the respiratory chain is one major contributor to VIDD and scavenging of mitochondrial ROS can ameliorate contractile dysfunction and prevent muscle atrophy [27]. Picard and colleagues investigated specimens from organ donors ventilated for 15 h–176 h and compared them to diaphragm biopsies from short-term ventilated (6 h) lung surgery patients [28]. These authors hypothesized that nutritive imbalance, comparable to the metabolic syndrome, might be responsible for the uncoupling in the respiratory chain. They revealed lipid accumulation, concomitant down-regulation of mitochondrial biogenesis and damage of mitochondrial DNA. Although it cannot be simply concluded that nutritive oversupply triggers ROS production (or that the opposite occurs), their findings are a further landmark in our understanding of VIDD [29]. Compared to these findings of oversupply, the results of Davis and colleagues [30] may seem contradictory. After 6 hours of mechanical ventilation in rats, blood flow and oxygen delivery to the diaphragm decreased significantly compared to after 30 minutes of mechanical ventilation. This finding was found solely in the diaphragm but not in other investigated respiratory or hindlimb muscles, raising the question as to whether hypoxia-induced generation of ROS contributes to VIDD. This reduction in blood flow during mechanical ventilation may be one factor leading to alterations in angio-neogenetic factors that may induce further vessel sprouting in the diaphragm [31].

All these studies underline the crucial changes in diaphragm muscle physiology during mechanical ventilation and point to the need for early spontaneous breathing in ICU patients to avoid prolonged/difficult weaning. Importantly, spontaneous breathing in a sedated state seems to quickly restore diaphragm function, resulting in an increase in force of 59 % 4–7 hours after stopping mechanical ventilation [32] and supporting the relevance of spontaneous breathing trials (SBT). However, these data can only be interpreted for healthy individuals, in whom VIDD is the sole cause of diaphragm dysfunction. After infection and sepsis, in particular, diaphragm function is reduced further [33], and the danger of overloading is more likely.

Another interesting and clinical important novelty was the finding by Jung and colleagues [34], in a porcine model of VIDD, that prolonged hypercapnia for 72 h could prevent diaphragm atrophy. This observation is in contradiction to earlier findings of contractile impairment after acute hypercapnia [35]. Both findings are important in respect to weaning patients: Acute hypercapnia prior to extubation or SBTs should be avoided, whereas permissive hypercapnia during mechanical ventilation, if necessary to prevent further VILI, does not further reduce contractile force. Importantly, there is no evidence that different levels of VILI further aggravate contractile dysfunction [36].

Finally it should be emphasized that VIDD is only one aspect of respiratory weakness. Although not directly induced by mechanical ventilation, other acquired muscle weaknesses can occur in critical care patients. As is often the case in severe sepsis, critical illness myopathy may develop, thus weakening respiratory muscles and lead to prolonged weaning from mechanical ventilation [37].

The Weaning Process

Typical ventilator-induced complications thus have a marked influence on the length of mechanical ventilation and can lead to a prolonged weaning process. To minimize or to avert these mechanisms, invasive mechanical ventilation should be terminated as soon as possible (Fig. 2).

Inspection for Spontaneous Breathing Capacity

The essential condition for successful weaning is a balance between necessary and potential work of breathing at the best possible rate [38]. It is indispensable to achieve the necessary work of breathing without any mechanical support, so adequate respiratory muscle function must be seen as a basic prerequisite for successful weaning [39] .

Fig. 2 Impact of ventilator-induced complications on weaning

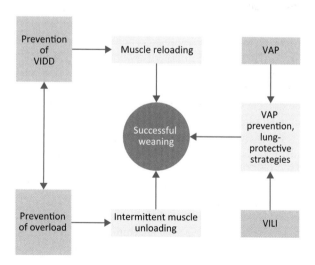

Hence, crucial aspects of weaning from mechanical ventilation are:
1. Evaluation of spontaneous breathing capacity
2. Performance of defined SBTs with regard to breathing capacity
3. Avoidance of extubation failure and high re-intubation rates

To standardize these clinical procedures, weaning protocols may be useful, especially for logistic reasons and for helping personnel to identify a preferably early time point for the weaning process. Several studies have demonstrated that protocol-based weaning can reduce both duration of mechanical ventilation and ventilator-associated complications (e. g., VAP) [40].

Regarding spontaneous breathing capacity, a 'traditional' procedure is complete liberation from the respirator with use of a T-piece trial. Trials over 30–120 min are sufficient for evaluation of spontaneous breathing capacity in patients [41]. However, to avoid early fatigue, a small amount of ventilator support to compensate for the work of breathing is recommended. Pressure support levels of 6–12 cmH$_2$O compensate respirator and tube-dependent work of breathing with a higher number of successful SBTs [42, 43]. However, large controlled studies demonstrating a clear benefit or advantage for one of the possible strategies are still lacking.

Patient-controlled Ventilation

Proportional-assist ventilation (PAV), as a modification of pressure support, allows individual pressure support, dependent on the patient's possible work of breathing. A defined amount of pressure support, with consideration of changes in compliance and resistance, may contribute to more effective ventilator support [44]. Other approaches with regard to patient-ventilator interaction are based on the reduction in asynchrony between respirator and patient, and on mechanical support that is individual for every breathing rate. These approaches may result in a reduction in stress and work of breathing. In neurally-adjusted ventilatory assist (NAVA), the respirator gives support in proportion to the electrical activity of the diaphragm, which needs to be measured with an esophageal captured electromyographic signal. Pressure support is then directly proportional to the intensity of the signal and will be continuously adapted to the signal intensity. This procedure, as demonstrated by Roze et al., seems promising as muscular fatigue can be rapidly identified and muscular recovery can be seen in patients with prolonged weaning [45]. However, large clinical trials need to be conducted to support the effect of NAVA on weaning.

Other closed-loop controlled strategies are targeted at patient-related, physiological feedback to drive ventilation and oxygenation (e. g., Intellivent with control of FiO$_2$ and PEEP). Arnal et al. studied the effects of Intellivent on patients with respiratory failure and demonstrated that in passive patients the system was effective. Intellivent provided a lower tidal volume and higher PEEP without any difference in oxygenation when compared to adaptive support ventilation (ASV), a ventilator mode for regulating airway pressure [46].

All these procedures considering patient-ventilator interactions seem promising and they may contribute to a shortened duration of mechanical ventilation. However, large clinical trials need to focus on patients undergoing prolonged weaning.

Identification of Difficult-to-Wean-Patients: Importance of Specialized Treatment

An unnecessary delay in liberation from the ventilator could, because of ventilator-associated complications, increase mortality rates [41, 47]. Thus, it is essential to begin the weaning process immediately after the underlying cause of respiratory failure has been addressed. Using recent classification of weaning [4], most patients (around 60 %) can be successfully extubated after one SBT (simple weaning), suggesting that only a short period of ventilator assistance was given or the underlying cause could be removed quickly. Roughly 30–40 % of patients present as 'difficult weaning', requiring up to three SBTs (or as long as 7 days) to be successfully extubated, and 6–15 % of patients need prolonged weaning, characterized as >3 SBTs (or longer than 7 days). This classification, although quite simple, seems relevant because different patients may need different management strategies during weaning. For example, in patients with prolonged weaning, a higher number of co-morbidities (chronic heart failure, severe chronic respiratory insufficiency) may influence treatment. Patients with prolonged weaning have worse outcomes [48] and this may be one reason why such patients should be managed in specialized units.

Remarkably, a multicenter study demonstrated that a significant proportion of postoperative patients as well as patients with pneumonia or acute respiratory insufficiency for other reasons exhibited prolonged weaning, resulting in worse outcomes [49]. This important study underlines the clinical relevance of weaning in a broad group of postoperative patients. In summary, prolonged weaning is time- and resource-consuming, demands multidisciplinary treatment and is probably best performed in specialized units with a high demand for quality. The German Society of Anesthesiology and Intensive Care Medicine has implemented a certification procedure for prolonged weaning, which demands different modules of quality management and a specific number of patients within the three weaning classification groups.

Conclusion

The process of weaning from mechanical ventilation can take considerable time. It is essential to identify the best time point to start weaning, because mechanical ventilation is associated with several complications that influence outcomes. The development of mechanical ventilation in recent years has been targeted on optimizing patient-ventilator interaction and synchrony; however, large clinical trials need to prove the relevance of these closed-loop systems. Patients undergoing prolonged weaning are increasingly present in postoperative care. Only a multi-professional, approach in specialized units can sufficiently counter this clinical challenge.

References

1. Esteban A, Anzueto A, Frutos F et al (2002) Characteristics and outcomes in adult patients receiving mechanical ventilation: a 28-day international study. JAMA 287:345–355
2. Goligher E, Ferguson ND (2009) Mechanical ventilation: epidemiological insights into current practices. Curr Opin Crit Care 15:44–51
3. Marelich GP, Murin S, Battistella F, Inciardi J, Vierra T, Roby M (2000) Protocol weaning of mechanical ventilation in medical and surgical patients by respiratory care practitioners and nurses: effect on weaning time and incidence of ventilator-associated pneumonia. Chest 118:459–467
4. Boles JM, Bion J, Connors A et al (2007) Weaning from mechanical ventilation. Eur Respir J 29:1033–1056
5. Steinberg J, Schiller HJ, Halter JM et al (2002) Tidal volume increases do not affect alveolar mechanics in normal lung but cause alveolar overdistension and exacerbate alveolar instability after surfactant deactivation. Crit Care Med 30:2675–2683
6. Chiumello D, Carlesso E, Cadringher P et al (2008) Lung stress and strain during mechanical ventilation for acute respiratory distress syndrome. Am J Respir Crit Care Med 78:346–355
7. Gattinoni L, Carlesso E, Caironi P (2012) Stress and strain within the lung. Curr Opin Crit Care 18:42–47
8. Halbertsma FJ, Vaneker M, Scheffer GJ, van der Hoeven JG (2005) Cytokines and biotrauma in ventilator-induced lung injury: a critical review of the literature. Neth J Med 63:382–392
9. Pulletz S, Kott M, Elke G et al (2012) Dynamics of regional lung aeration determined by electrical impedance tomography in patients with acute respiratory distress syndrome. Multidiscip Respir Med 7:44
10. Zick G, Elke G, Becher T et al (2013) Effect of PEEP and tidal volume on ventilation distribution and end-expiratory lung volume: A prospective experimental animal and pilot clinical study. PLoS One 8:e72675
11. Halter J, Steinberg JM, Schiller HJ et al (2003) Positive end-expiratory pressure after a recruitment maneuver prevents both alveolar collapse and recruitment/derecruitment. Am J Respir Crit Care Med 167:1620–1626
12. Schiller HJ, McCann UG, Carney DE, Gatto LA, Steinberg JM, Nieman GF (2001) Altered alveolar mechanics in the acutely injured lung. Crit Care Med 29:1049–1055
13. Schiller HJ, Steinberg J, Halter J et al (2003) Alveolar inflation during generation of a quasi-static pressure/volume curve in the acutely injured lung. Crit Care Med 31:1126–1133
14. Bickenbach J, Czaplik M, Dembinski R et al (2010) In vivo microscopy in a porcine model of acute lung injury. Respir Physiol Neurobiol 172:192–200
15. Czaplik M, Rossaint R, Koch E et al (2011) Methods for quantitative evaluation of alveolar structure during in vivo microscopy. Respir Physiol Neurobiol 176:123–129
16. The Acute Respiratory Distress Syndrome Network (2000) Ventilation with lower tidal volumes as compared with traditional tidal volumes for acute lung injury and the acute respiratory distress syndrome. N Engl J Med 342:1301–1308
17. Bein T, Weber-Carstens S, Goldmann A et al (2013) Lower tidal volume strategy ($\approx$ 3 ml/kg) combined with extracorporeal CO2 removal versus 'conventional' protective ventilation (6 ml/kg) in severe ARDS: the prospective randomized Xtravent-study. Intensive Care Med 39:847–856
18. Ramirez P, Bassi GL, Torres A (2012) Measures to prevent nosocomial infections during mechanical ventilation. Curr Opin Crit Care 18:86–92

19. Bickenbach J, Marx G (2013) Diagnosis of pneumonia in mechanically ventilated patients: What is the meaning of the CPIS? Minerva Anestesiol 79:1406–1414
20. Hunter JD (2006) Ventilator associated pneumonia. Postgrad Med J 82:172–178
21. Mietto C, Pinciroli R, Patel N, Berra L (2013) Ventilator associated pneumonia: evolving definitions and preventive strategies. Respir Care 58:990–1007
22. Ricard J, Conti G, Boucherie M et al (2012) A European survey of nosocomial infection control and hospital-acquired pneumonia prevention strategies. J Infect 65:285–291
23. Jaber S, Jung B, Matecki S, Petrof BJ (2011) Clinical review: ventilator-induced diaphragmatic dysfunction – human studies confirm animal model findings! Crit Care 15:206
24. Powers SK, Hudson MB, Nelson WB et al (2011) Mitochondria-targeted antioxidants protect against mechanical ventilation-induced diaphragm weakness. Crit Care Med 39:1749–1759
25. Whidden MA, Smuder AJ, Wu M, Hudson MB, Nelson WB, Powers SK (2010) Oxidative stress is required for mechanical ventilation-induced protease activation in the diaphragm. J Appl Physiol 108:1376–1382
26. Powers SK, Shanely RA, Coombes JS et al (2002) Mechanical ventilation results in progressive contractile dysfunction in the diaphragm. J Appl Physiol 92:1851–1858
27. Powers SK, Hudson MB, Nelson WB et al (2011) Mitochondria-targeted antioxidants protect against mechanical ventilation-induced diaphragm weakness. Crit Care Med 39:1749–1759
28. Picard M, Jung B, Liang F et al (2012) Mitochondrial dysfunction and lipid accumulation in the human diaphragm during mechanical ventilation. Am J Respir Crit Care Med 186:1140–1149
29. Lecuona E, Sassoon CS, Barreiro E (2012) Lipid overload: trigger or consequence of mitochondrial oxidative stress in ventilator-induced diaphragmatic dysfunction? Am J Respir Crit Care Med 186:1074–1076
30. Davis RT 3rd, Bruells CS, Stabley JN, McCullough DJ, Powers SK, Behnke BJ (2012) Mechanical ventilation reduces rat diaphragm blood flow and impairs oxygen delivery and uptake. Crit Care Med 40:2858–2866
31. Bruells CS, Maes K, Rossaint R et al (2013) Prolonged Mechanical Ventilation Alters the Expression Pattern of Angio-neogenetic Factors in a Pre-Clinical Rat Model. PloS one 8:e70524
32. Thomas D, Maes K, Agten A et al (2013) Time course of diaphragm function recovery after controlled mechanical ventilation in rats. J Appl Physiol 115:775–784
33. Callahan LA, Supinski GS (2009) Sepsis-induced myopathy. Crit Care Med 37:354–367
34. Jung B, Sebbane M, Le Goff C et al (2013) Moderate and prolonged hypercapnic acidosis may protect against ventilator-induced diaphragmatic dysfunction in healthy piglet: an in vivo study. Crit Care 17:R15
35. Jaber S, Jung B, Sebbane M et al (2008) Alteration of the piglet diaphragm contractility in vivo and its recovery after acute hypercapnia. Anesthesiology 108:651–658
36. Bruells CS, Smuder AJ, Reiss LK et al (2013) Negative pressure ventilation and positive pressure ventilation promote comparable levels of ventilator-induced diaphragmatic dysfunction in rats. Anesthesiology 119:652–662
37. Judemann K, Lunz D, Zausig YA, Graf BM, Zink W (2011) Intensive care unit-acquired weakness in the critically ill: critical illness polyneuropathy and critical illness myopathy. Anaesthesist 60:887–901
38. Lellouche F, Mancebo J, Jolliet P et al (2006) A multicenter randomized trial of computer-driven protocolized weaning from mechanical ventilation. Am J Respir Crit Care Med 174:894–900
39. Goldstone J (2002) The pulmonary physician in critical care. 10: difficult weaning. Thorax 57:986–991
40. Gupta P, Giehler K, Walters RW, Meyerink K, Modrykamien AM (2014) The effect of a mechanical ventilation discontinuation protocol in patients with simple and difficult weaning: impact on clinical outcomes. Respir Care (in press)

41. Esteban A, Alia I, Tobin MJ et al (1999) Effect of spontaneous breathing trial duration on outcome of attempts to discontinue mechanical ventilation. Spanish Lung Failure Collaborative Group. Am J Respir Crit Care Med 159:512–518
42. Brochard L, Rua F, Lorino H, Lemaire F, Harf A (1991) Inspiratory pressure support compensates for the additional work of breathing caused by the endotracheal tube. Anesthesiology 75:739–745
43. Ezingeard E, Diconne E, Guyomarc'h S et al (2006) Weaning from mechanical ventilation with pressure support in patients failing a T-tube trial of spontaneous breathing. Intens Care Med 32:165–169
44. Grasso S, Puntillo F, Mascia L et al (2000) Compensation for increase in respiratory workload during mechanical ventilation. Pressure-support versus proportional-assist ventilation. Am J Respir Crit Care Med 161:819–826
45. Rozé H, Repusseau B, Perrier V, et al (2013) Neuro-ventilatory efficiency during weaning from mechanical ventilation using neurally adjusted ventilatory assist. Br J Anaesth 111:955–960
46. Arnal JM, Wysocki M, Novotni D et al (2012) Safety and efficacy of a fully closed-loop control ventilation (IntelliVent-ASV®) in sedated ICU patients with acute respiratory failure: a prospective randomized crossover study. Intensive Care Med 38:781–787
47. Coplin WM, Pierson DJ, Cooley KD et al (2000) Implications of extubation delay in brain-injured patients meeting standard weaning criteria. Am J Respir Crit Care Med 161:1530–1536
48. Funk GC, Anders S, Breyer MK et al (2010) Incidence and outcome of weaning from mechanical ventilation according to new categories. Eur Respir J 35:88–94
49. Peñuelas O, Frutos-Vivar F, Fernández C et al (2011) Characteristics and outcomes of ventilated patients according to time to liberation from mechanical ventilation. Am J Respir Crit Care Med 184:430–437

Part IV
Lung Protective Strategies

Protective Lung Ventilation During General Anesthesia: Is There Any Evidence?

S. Coppola, S. Froio, and D. Chiumello

Introduction

In acute respiratory distress syndrome (ARDS) several studies have shown that mechanical ventilation with high tidal volume (V_T) and low levels of positive end-expiratory pressure (PEEP) can promote ventilator-induced lung injury (VILI), thus increasing morbidity and mortality [1]. An open lung strategy, combining the use of low V_T with adequate PEEP levels and recruitment maneuvers, has thus been recommended in ARDS patients [2–4]. In patients without ARDS admitted to intensive care units (ICUs), who required mechanical ventilation for at least 12 hours, the use of a high V_T significantly increased the inflammatory response [5, 6]. In contrast to critically ill patients, during general anesthesia, mechanical ventilation is required only for a few hours, thus the beneficial effects of lung-protective ventilation remain questionable. Moreover, there are limited data from few randomized controlled trials with only small cohorts of enrolled patients.

Two recent meta-analyses that enrolled patients from ICUs and the operating room (OR) showed that lung-protective ventilation was associated with lower mortality and postoperative complications [2, 7]. However, there are no recommendations regarding optimal ventilatory strategies in patients without lung injury during general anesthesia.

In the present article, we provide a comprehensive picture of the current literature on lung-protective ventilation during general anesthesia in patients without ARDS, focusing on the applications of this strategy in patients undergoing abdominal, thoracic and cardiac surgery.

S. Coppola · S. Froio · D. Chiumello ✉
Dipartimento di Anestesia, Rianimazione (Intensiva e Subintensiva) e Terapia del Dolore
Fondazione IRCCS Ca' Granda Ospedale Maggiore Policlinico, Milan University, Milan, Italy
e-mail: chiumello@libero.it

J.-L. Vincent (Ed.), *Annual Update in Intensive Care and Emergency Medicine 2014*,   159
DOI 10.1007/978-3-319-03746-2_13, © Springer International Publishing Switzerland
and BioMed Central Ltd. 2014

How Mechanical Ventilation is Applied in the Operating Room

Although the protective ventilation approach may be beneficial in a broader population with and without ARDS, the use of high V_T without PEEP is still common
during general anesthesia. A large French multicenter observational study, in which
more than 2,900 patients undergoing general anesthesia were enrolled, showed that
18 % of patients were ventilated with a V_T greater than 10 ml/kg body weight and
81 % without PEEP [8]. Moreover, a recruitment maneuver was applied in only 7 %
of patients.

Similarly a 5-year observational study, in which 45,575 patients were enrolled,
reported that although use of a V_T less than 10 ml/kg and PEEP levels greater than
5 cmH$_2$O increased progressively over time, 16–18 % of patients continued to receive a V_T greater than 10 ml/kg without application of PEEP [9]. The presence of
obesity and a short height were the main risk factors for receiving a large V_T during
prolonged anesthesia [10].

Rationale for Lung-protective Ventilation
During General Anesthesia

General anesthesia affects lung function primarily because of the loss of muscle
tone, which promotes a reduction in lung volume, an alteration in ventilation-
perfusion ratio and the onset of lung atelectasis. The development of atelectasis
is very common and occurs in more than 90 % of subjects undergoing general anesthesia [11, 12]. Atelectasis is mainly due to three basic mechanisms [13, 14]:

- compression atelectasis
- absorption atelectasis
- loss of surfactant atelectasis.

Compression atelectasis is caused by the alterations in chest wall mechanics induced by general anesthesia *per se* and by several other mechanisms, such as the
patient's position (head-down), the body mass index, the age of patient and the
type of surgery (abdominal surgery or laparoscopy), which increase intra-abdominal
pressure (IAP), thus decreasing chest compliance and functional residual capacity (FRC), with the consequent development of intraoperative atelectasis, intrapulmonary shunting and hypoxemia. Other factors related to surgery can contribute to
the reduction in pulmonary inflation and to the development of atelectasis, such as
a prolonged recumbent position intraoperatively, residual pain that reduces cough
effectiveness, and postoperative diaphragmatic dysfunction that can persist for up to
one week [15, 16]. If the FRC is reduced below closing capacity, airway closure will
occur; consequently the lung bases will be well perfused, but underventilated due
to airway closure and alveolar collapse. This phenomenon increases ventilation-
perfusion mismatch and promotes further atelectasis generation and hypoxemia.

Absorption atelectasis can be caused by exposure to high inspired fraction of
oxygen (FiO$_2$) levels. When oxygen is absorbed from the alveolar gas into the
capillary in distal occluded alveolar areas or where the ventilation-perfusion ratio is

low or high FiO_2 levels are delivered, reabsorption of gas is promoted and generates atelectasis [11].

Loss of surfactant atelectasis arises from alterations in surfactant induced by effects of general anesthesia on healthy lungs [17].

The presence of atelectasis is an important factor in the pathogenesis of postoperative pulmonary complications, such as hypoxemia, pulmonary infections and local inflammatory response [18]. Postoperative pulmonary complications in the first hours after surgery are mainly due to atelectasis in the dependent regions of the lungs. Lung atelectasis may also promote the development of VILI by lung overdistension and by cyclic opening and closing of lung units at the boundary between the normally inflated and collapsed lung units. On the basis of several studies of mechanical ventilation in ARDS patients, the same mechanisms of injury could be applied to mechanically ventilated patients during general anesthesia with healthy lungs. The use of recruitment maneuvers associated with adequate levels of PEEP could open and keep open previously collapsed lung regions. In addition, the use of a low-moderate V_T could avoid overstress-overdistension of lung units.

Protective versus Conventional Lung Ventilation Strategies during General Anesthesia

In Table 1, we provide a synopsis of randomized controlled trials (RCT) comparing protective *versus* conventional lung ventilation strategies during general anesthesia over time, in specific surgical settings showing the main outcomes explored in these studies. In Fig. 1, we show the numbers of RCTs that we considered, divided according to the type of surgery.

Abdominal Surgery

Postoperative pulmonary complications remain a significant problem after surgery. They occur in 5–10 % of all surgical patients and 9–40 % of those undergoing abdominal surgery experience postoperative pulmonary complications [19], which increase morbidity and mortality [19, 20]. Among the postoperative pulmonary complications, lung atelectasis is one of the principle mechanisms for the development of VILI, pneumonia and postoperative respiratory failure.

Table 1 Synopsis of randomized controlled trials comparing protective *versus* conventional lung ventilation strategy during general anesthesia. Studies are grouped according to specific surgical settings: abdominal, thoracic and cardiac surgery

	First author [ref]	Year	N° pts	V_T (ml/kg) Case	V_T (ml/kg) Control	PEEP (cmH$_2$O) Case	PEEP (cmH$_2$O) Control	Recruitment maneuver (Yes/No) Case	Recruitment maneuver (Yes/No) Control	Outcomes
Abdominal	Wrigge [21]	2000	39	6 / 6	15	0 / 10	0	No	No	Systemic IL-6, IL-10, TNF-α: similar
	Wrigge [22]	2004	30	6	12–15	10	0	No	No	Systemic/pulmonary IL-8-1-6-10-12, TNF-α: similar
	Determann [23]	2008	40	6	12	10	0	No	No	Lung epithelial injury biomarkers: similar
	Weingarten [25]	2010	40	6	10	12	0	Yes	No	Intraoperative PaO$_2$, Lung mechanics: better; Systemic IL-8, IL-6: similar
	Treschan [24]	2012	101	6	12	5	5	No	No	Postoperative dynamic spirometry: similar
	Severgnini [26]	2013	56	7	9	10	0	Yes	No	Clinical Pulmonary Infection Score: lower; Postoperative respiratory function: better
	Futier [27]	2013	400	6-8	10–12	6–8	0	Yes	No	Pulmonary/extrapulmonary complications: lower; Hospital stay: shorter
	PROVHILO [28]	–	900	<8	<8	12	≤2	Yes	No	Postoperative pulmonary complications
Thoracic	Schilling [33]	2005	32	5	10	0	0	No	No	Pulmonary TNF-α, IL-8, IL-10: lower TNF-α
	Michelet [36]	2006	52	5	9	5	0	No	No	Systemic IL-1β, IL-6, IL-8: lower; Oxygenation: better; Postoperative MV length: shorter
	Yang [35]	2011	100	6	10	5	0	No	No	Oxygenation: better; Postoperative pulmonary complications: lower

Continuation see next page

Table 1 *Continued*

	First author [ref]	Year	N° pts	Ventilatory strategy						Outcomes
				V_T (ml/kg)		PEEP (cmH$_2$O)		Recruitment maneuver (Yes/No)		
				Case	Control	Case	Control	Case	Control	
Cardiac	Chaney [49]	2000	25	6	12	5	5	No	No	Postoperative lung mechanics: better
	Koner [42]	2004	44	6	10 / 10	5	0 / 5	No	No	Systemic IL-6, TNF-α: similar; Hospital LOS: similar; Postoperative pulmonary function: similar
	Zupancich [44]	2005	40	8	10–12	10	2–3	No	No	Pulmonary and systemic Il-6, IL-8: lower
	Reis [47]	2005	62	4–6	6–8	10	5	Yes	No	Systemic Il-8, IL-10: lower
	Reis [48]	2005	69	4–6	6–8	10	5	Yes	No	Systemic IL-6, TNF-α, IFN-γ: similar; Postoperative hypoxemia: lower; Postoperative FRC: better
	Wrigge [41]	2005	44	6	12	9*	7*	No	No	Systemic TNF-α, IL-6-8-2-4-10: similar; Pulmonary TNF-α, IL-6-8-2-4-10: lower TNF-α
	Sundar [43]	2011	149	6	10	5*	4.9*	No	No	Time to extubation: similar; Extubation at 6–8 h after surgery: better; Reintubation: lower

Case: lung-protective ventilation group; Control: conventional ventilation group. Outcome results always refer to the case group. In the Thoracic surgery section, ventilatory parameters refer to one-lung ventilation. *PEEP levels set according to ARDSnetwork strategy. V_T: tidal volume; PEEP: positive end-expiratory pressure; MV: mechanical ventilation; FRC: functional residual capacity; IL: interleukin; TNF: tumor necrosis factor; IFN: interferon; pts: patients; PaO$_2$: partial pressure of oxygen in arterial blood; LOS: length of stay.

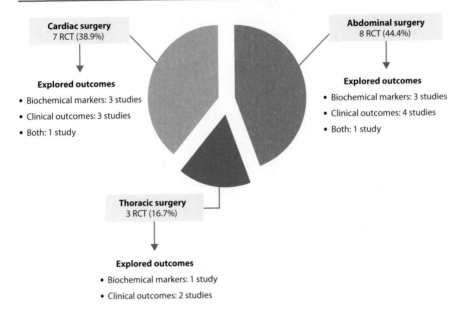

Cardiac surgery
7 RCT (38.9%)

Explored outcomes
• Biochemical markers: 3 studies
• Clinical outcomes: 3 studies
• Both: 1 study

Abdominal surgery
8 RCT (44.4%)

Explored outcomes
• Biochemical markers: 3 studies
• Clinical outcomes: 4 studies
• Both: 1 study

Thoracic surgery
3 RCT (16.7%)

Explored outcomes
• Biochemical markers: 1 study
• Clinical outcomes: 2 studies

Fig. 1 The number and percentage of randomized controlled trials (RCTs) included in Table 1, divided by type of surgery

In this context, Wrigge and colleagues investigated in two studies the effect of different ventilatory strategies on the release of inflammatory mediators in patients undergoing elective surgery [21, 22]. In the first study, 39 patients scheduled for extra-thoracic surgery (abdominal, vascular, bone and other) were randomized to one of three mechanical ventilation strategies: 1) V_T of 15 ml/kg ideal body weight without PEEP; 2) V_T of 6 ml/kg without PEEP; and 3) V_T of 6 ml/kg with PEEP 10 cmH$_2$O. Plasma levels of interleukin (IL)-6, IL-10 and tumor necrosis factor (TNF)-α were measured after one hour of mechanical ventilation [21]. In the second study, 64 patients undergoing general anesthesia were randomized to receive mechanical ventilation with a V_T of 12–15 ml/kg ideal body weight without PEEP, or with V_T of 6 ml/kg and PEEP levels of 10 cmH$_2$O. Local and systemic inflammatory biomarkers, including IL-8, IL-1, IL-6, IL-10, TNF-α and IL-12, were determined after 3 hours of mechanical ventilation [22]. Both studies were unable to find any significant differences in terms of inflammatory mediators and the authors concluded that, in contrast to patients with acute lung injury in whom there is a systemic inflammatory reaction during major surgery, in uninjured normal lungs short term mechanical ventilation alone with high V_T levels did not increase pulmonary or systemic inflammation related to surgery [21, 22]. No differences in biomarkers of lung epithelial injury were observed after 5 hours in a later study, which compared ventilation with V_T 12 ml/kg ideal body weight without PEEP versus V_T 6 ml/kg and PEEP 10 cmH$_2$O [23].

To explore the effect of a high compared to a low V_T for similar PEEP levels, Treschan et al. randomized patients to receive a V_T of 12 ml/kg body weight versus 6 ml/kg with a PEEP of 5 cmH$_2$O [24]. Except for the intraoperative oxygenation, which was higher in the high V_T group, there was no significant difference in forced vital capacity and forced expiratory volume in one second between groups, for up to five days after the surgery.

Different from the previous studies, Weingarten et al. evaluated an open lung strategy in which low V_T ventilation was associated with PEEP plus a recruitment maneuver in order to minimize atelectasis and shear stress in the lung parenchyma [25]. This open lung strategy, consisting of a V_T of 6 ml/kg predicted body weight with PEEP 12 cmH$_2$O and recruitment maneuvers, significantly improved only intraoperative oxygenation with no difference in the inflammatory response or length of hospital stay compared to a V_T of 10 ml/kg without PEEP [25]. These first studies seem to suggest that a protective ventilator strategy does not have any role in patients without lung injury [21–25]. However, these studies demonstrated that this mode of ventilation is feasible in open abdominal surgery with no adverse effects [23, 25]. In contrast to the previous studies, Severgnini et al., comparing a lung protective mechanical ventilation consisting of a V_T of 7 ml/kg ideal body weight with PEEP levels of 10 cmH$_2$O and recruitment maneuvers *versus* a V_T of 9 ml/kg without PEEP, showed beneficial effects of the lung-protective strategy during general anesthesia lasting more than 2 hours [26]. The lung-protective strategy improved postoperative respiratory function in terms of dynamic spirometry, oxygenation, and pulmonary complications for up to 5 days after surgery, without increasing the incidence of intraoperative complications. Although there was no significant difference in the hospital length of stay between groups, 20 % of the patients in the lung-protective group, compared with 40 % in the control group, were still in hospital on postoperative day 14 [26].

A recent multicenter randomized clinical trial in which lung-protective ventilation with a V_T of 6–8 ml/kg predicted body weight, PEEP 6–8 cmH$_2$O and recruitment maneuvers repeated every 30 minutes was compared with non-protective ventilation with V_T 10–12 ml/kg without PEEP, found that the lung-protective ventilation significantly reduced major pulmonary and extrapulmonary complications from 27.5 % to 10.5 % [27]. The lung-protective strategy also significantly reduced the proportion of patients who required postoperative ventilator assistance from 17 % to 5 % and the hospital length of stay.

Compared to the earlier studies [22–25], these two recent trials found a beneficial effect of a lung-protective strategy probably because of the large number of enrolled patients, the homogeneity of the selected population of patients undergoing open abdominal surgery with an expected duration of at least 2 hours, the standardization of fluid management, and the clinically relevant outcomes explored (not only lung inflammatory mediators) in the postoperative period.

These results demonstrate that in patients undergoing abdominal surgery a multifaceted open lung protective strategy can prevent the intraoperative alveolar opening and closing and overdistension of lung areas that lead to VILI and pulmonary complications. Currently, we are waiting for the results of the PROVHILO study, a worldwide multicenter RCT in which patients scheduled for abdominal surgery are being enrolled. In this study, all patients are ventilated with protective tidal volumes (in both groups, $V_T < 8$ ml/kg predicted body weight) and randomly assigned to a lung-protective strategy with use of recruitment maneuvers and PEEP levels of 12 cmH$_2$O or a conventional strategy without recruitment maneuvers and PEEP between 0 and 2 cmH$_2$O [28]. If the results of this study confirm those of the last two trials [27, 26], lung-protective strategies will be more widely applied in patients undergoing abdominal surgery [28].

Thoracic Surgery

During thoracic surgery, one-lung ventilation is an established procedure that could increase the risk of promoting VILI compared to double lung ventilation, because of greater reduction in lung volume and greater degree of alveolar collapse in dependent lung regions. Two retrospective studies of patients who had undergone elective pneumonectomy found that larger intraoperative V_T and higher inspiratory airway pressure were associated with the development of pulmonary edema and respiratory failure [29, 30]. Despite this, conventional mechanical ventilation in these patients consists of V_T between 8–12 ml/kg to prevent lung atelectasis with zero or low levels of PEEP to avoid shunt aggravation by redistribution of blood flow to non-ventilated regions [31, 32]. However this approach is not an evidence-based guideline.

Schilling et al., in a randomized study in patients scheduled for open thoracic surgery undergoing one-lung ventilation, showed that mechanical ventilation with V_T of 5 ml/kg ideal body weight compared to 10 ml/kg significantly decreased the pulmonary inflammatory response up to 2 hours postoperatively [33]. Subsequently, Licker et al. retrospectively evaluated the implementation of a lung-protective ventilation strategy in lung cancer resection combining a low V_T (< 8 ml/kg) with PEEP 4–10 cmH$_2$O and recruitment maneuvers *versus* a conventional V_T target ventilation of 9–12 ml/kg during two-lung ventilation and 8–10 ml/kg during one-lung ventilation without recruitment maneuvers and PEEP applied at the discretion of the anesthetist [34]. The lung-protective strategy significantly reduced the incidence of atelectasis (from 8.8 % to 5 %), postoperative acute lung injury (from 3.7 % to 0.9 %), ICU admission (from 9.4 % to 2.5 %) and length of hospital stay (from 14.5 ± 3.3 to 11.8 ± 4.1 days). These data were confirmed in a randomized study during elective lobectomy in which patients were ventilated with a high V_T of 10 ml/kg without PEEP compared to a low V_T of 6 ml/kg with 5 cmH$_2$O of PEEP and pressure controlled ventilation [35]. The lung-protective ventilation was associated with a lower incidence of lung infiltration or atelectasis (2 versus 10) and of cases of hypoxemia (1 versus 8).

During esophagectomy, a procedure requiring a prolonged period of one-lung ventilation, Michelet et al. demonstrated in an RCT that lung-protective ventilation (V_T 9 ml/kg during two-lung ventilation, reduced to 5 ml/kg during one-lung ventilation and PEEP 5 cmH$_2$O throughout the operative time) could prevent alterations in lung function and reduce the inflammatory response in patients without previous lung disease compared to conventional ventilation strategy (V_T 9 ml/kg during two- and one-lung ventilation without PEEP) [36].

The majority of studies so far have demonstrated that, during thoracic surgery, traditional intraoperative ventilatory settings seem to be harmful. An intraoperative open lung approach based on small V_T, moderate-high PEEP and recruitment maneuvers may be beneficial but further randomized clinical trials are necessary to generate clinical evidence.

Cardiac Surgery

In cardiac surgery, use of cardiopulmonary bypass (CPB), contact of the blood with artificial surfaces and ischemia/reperfusion of the heart and lungs are associated with a pulmonary and systemic inflammatory response, with activation of elements of the complement cascade, neutrophils and pro-inflammatory cytokines [37–39]. This systemic inflammatory response syndrome can be mild to severe in 10 to 35 % of cases and may induce an acute lung injury, which generally resolves within 24 hours. This clinical event contributes to increased morbidity and mortality [40]. In this context, injurious mechanical ventilation could aggravate the primary inflammatory response described above (first hit), representing a second hit. Moreover, during CPB, the lungs are not ventilated and either rest at low values of continuous positive pressure [41] or are completely disconnected from the ventilator [42–44]. Traditionally, ventilator settings in cardiac surgery patients included large V_T (10–15 ml/kg) in order to minimize atelectasis and minimal levels of PEEP to reduce hemodynamic consequences. Following the results of clinical trials in ARDS patients [45, 46], there has been increased interest in protective lung ventilatory strategies during cardiac anesthesia and several trials have tried to demonstrate the role of protective lung ventilation in this context.

Koner et al. found no differences in plasma levels of IL-6 and TNF-α 2 hours after the end of CBP among patients randomized to receive protective ventilation (V_T 6 ml/kg ideal body weight, PEEP 5 cmH$_2$O) or conventional V_T ventilation (V_T 10 ml/kg) with and without PEEP levels at 5 cmH$_2$O [42]. There were no differences among groups in the explored clinical outcomes, including total intraoperative fluid balance, intubation time and hospital length of stay [42].

Wrigge et al. measured pulmonary and plasma levels of different cytokines and chemokines (IL-2, IL-4, IL-6, IL-8, IL-10, TNF-α and interferon-γ) in patients ventilated with high or with low tidal volumes (V_T 12 ml/kg *versus* V_T 6 ml/kg ideal body weight). They observed higher values of TNF-α after 6 hours of ventilation with high V_T, with no differences in other inflammatory mediators [41].

However, a significantly reduced inflammatory response, in terms of pulmonary and systemic mediator levels (IL-6 and IL-8) was observed when applying a moderate PEEP level strategy (V_T 8 ml/kg with PEEP 10 cmH$_2$O) compared to a low PEEP and high V_T strategy (10–12 ml/kg with PEEP 2–3 cmH$_2$O) [44]. In comparison to previous studies [41, 42], this study evaluated a greater difference in PEEP levels and a longer duration of mechanical ventilation [44].

Reis et al. investigated the effect of open lung ventilation, consisting of low V_T (4–6 ml/kg) with moderate-high PEEP levels (10 cmH$_2$O) and recruitment maneuvers, on inflammatory mediators. In this study, they compared an early (immediately after intubation) and a late (at the end of CPB) application of the same open lung strategy, with conventional ventilation (V_T 6–8 ml/kg, PEEP 5 cmH$_2$O). Both the open lung approaches significantly decreased IL-8 and IL-10 levels after CPB [47]. Subsequently, the same authors showed that the early open lung approach significantly attenuated the reduction in postoperative FRC, for up to 5 days after surgery, and reduced the incidence of hypoxemic events during the first 3 days after extubation [48]. Ventilation and weaning times were similar among groups. This positive effect on postoperative FRC could be related to the prevention of additional lung injury caused by mechanical ventilation. Chaney et al. similarly reported better dynamic and static lung compliance and less shunt in patients ventilated with low compared to high V_T (6 *versus* 12 ml/kg) [49].

Recently Sundar and colleagues observed that a larger number of patients were extubated after 8 hours (53 % *versus* 31 %) when ventilated with a low V_T of 6 ml/kg ideal body weight compared to V_T 10 ml/kg with similar PEEP levels. Furthermore, a lower postoperative reintubation rate was observed. However, global time to extubation was similar between groups, as were ICU length of stay and 28-day mortality [43].

There is, therefore, a small amount of evidence from small studies in support of lung-protective ventilation in cardiac surgery patients [50]. However, the presence of several confounding factors, not related to mechanical ventilation, which could contribute to the development of a systemic inflammatory response and postoperative pulmonary complications, may have influenced the main outcome results. Hence, further studies with larger cohorts of patients are needed to confirm the still weak evidence in favor of lung-protective ventilation in cardiac anesthesia.

Conclusions

Mechanical ventilation is necessary for patients during general anesthesia. Although mechanical ventilation is considered a safe procedure, it can generate pulmonary stress and strain, promoting lung injury. There is increasing evidence that lung-protective ventilation may be beneficial in abdominal surgery (lower inflammatory response and better outcome). During thoracic and cardiac surgery, lung protective ventilation has only been associated with a reduced inflammatory response.

Lung-protective ventilation should be considered in the presence of pulmonary disease, prolonged anesthesia, in high-risk patients or for high-risk surgery. Although lung-protective ventilation may be beneficial for the lung, it may impair the cardiovascular system, reducing venous return and cardiac output and requiring the use of fluids and vasopressors. Thus, the risks and benefits of lung-protective ventilation need to be balanced in each individual patient.

References

1. Plotz FB, Slutsky AS, van Vught AJ, Heijnen CJ (2004) Ventilator-induced lung injury and multiple system organ failure: a critical review of facts and hypotheses. Intensive Care Med 30:1865–1872
2. Serpa NA, Cardoso SO, Manetta JA et al (2012) Association between use of lung-protective ventilation with lower tidal volumes and clinical outcomes among patients without acute respiratory distress syndrome: a meta-analysis. JAMA 308:1651–1659
3. De Prost N, Dreyfuss D (2012) How to prevent ventilator-induced lung injury? Minerva Anestesiol 78:1054–1066
4. Bernard GR, Artigas A, Brigham KL et al (1994) The American-European Consensus Conference on ARDS. Definitions, mechanisms, relevant outcomes, and clinical trial coordination. Am J Respir Crit Care Med 149:818–824
5. Pinheiro DO, Hetzel MP, dos Anjos SM, Dallegrave D, Friedman G (2010) Mechanical ventilation with high tidal volume induces inflammation in patients without lung disease. Crit Care 14:R39
6. Determann RM, Royakkers A, Wolthuis EK et al (2010) Ventilation with lower tidal volumes as compared with conventional tidal volumes for patients without acute lung injury: a preventive randomized controlled trial. Crit Care 14:R1
7. Hemmes SN, Serpa NA, Schultz MJ (2013) Intraoperative ventilatory strategies to prevent postoperative pulmonary complications: a meta-analysis. Curr Opin Anaesthesiol 26:126–133
8. Jaber S, Coisel Y, Chanques G et al (2012) A multicentre observational study of intra-operative ventilatory management during general anaesthesia: tidal volumes and relation to body weight. Anaesthesia 67:999–1008
9. Hess DR, Kondili D, Burns E, Bittner EA, Schmidt UH (2013) A 5-year observational study of lung-protective ventilation in the operating room: A single-center experience. J Crit Care 28:533–533
10. Fernandez-Bustamante A, Wood CL, Tran ZV, Moine P (2011) Intraoperative ventilation: incidence and risk factors for receiving large tidal volumes during general anesthesia. BMC Anesthesiol 11:22
11. Duggan M, Kavanagh BP (2005) Pulmonary atelectasis: a pathogenic perioperative entity. Anesthesiology 102:838–854
12. Cai H, Gong H, Zhang L, Wang Y, Tian Y (2007) Effect of low tidal volume ventilation on atelectasis in patients during general anesthesia: a computed tomographic scan. J Clin Anesth 19:125–129
13. Joyce CJ, Williams AB (1999) Kinetics of absorption atelectasis during anesthesia: a mathematical model. J Appl Physiol 86:1116–1125
14. Hedenstierna G, Rothen HU (2000) Atelectasis formation during anesthesia: causes and measures to prevent it. J Clin Monit Comput 16:329–335
15. Simonneau G, Vivien A, Sartene R et al (1983) Diaphragm dysfunction induced by upper abdominal surgery. Role of postoperative pain. Am Rev Respir Dis 128:899–903
16. Aubrun F, Gazon M, Schoeffler M, Benyoub K (2012) Evaluation of perioperative risk in elderly patients. Minerva Anestesiol 78:605–618
17. Otis DR Jr., Johnson M, Pedley TJ, Kamm RD (1993) Role of pulmonary surfactant in airway closure: a computational study. J Appl Physiol 75:1323–1333
18. Tusman G, Bohm SH, Warner DO, Sprung J (2012) Atelectasis and perioperative pulmonary complications in high-risk patients. Curr Opin Anaesthesiol 25:1–10

19. Arozullah AM, Daley J, Henderson WG, Khuri SF (2000) Multifactorial risk index for predicting postoperative respiratory failure in men after major noncardiac surgery. The National Veterans Administration Surgical Quality Improvement Program. Ann Surg 232:242–253

20. Smetana GW, Lawrence VA, Cornell JE (2006) Preoperative pulmonary risk stratification for noncardiothoracic surgery: systematic review for the American College of Physicians. Ann Intern Med 144:581–595

21. Wrigge H, Zinserling J, Stuber F et al (2000) Effects of mechanical ventilation on release of cytokines into systemic circulation in patients with normal pulmonary function. Anesthesiology 93:1413–1417

22. Wrigge H, Uhlig U, Zinserling J et al (2004) The effects of different ventilatory settings on pulmonary and systemic inflammatory responses during major surgery. Anesth Analg 98:775–781

23. Determann RM, Wolthuis EK, Choi G et al (2008) Lung epithelial injury markers are not influenced by use of lower tidal volumes during elective surgery in patients without preexisting lung injury. Am J Physiol Lung Cell Mol Physiol 294:L344–L350

24. Treschan TA, Kaisers W, Schaefer MS et al (2012) Ventilation with low tidal volumes during upper abdominal surgery does not improve postoperative lung function. Br J Anaesth 109:263–271

25. Weingarten TN, Whalen FX, Warner DO et al (2010) Comparison of two ventilatory strategies in elderly patients undergoing major abdominal surgery. Br J Anaesth 104:16–22

26. Severgnini P, Selmo G, Lanza C et al (2013) Protective mechanical ventilation during general anesthesia for open abdominal surgery improves postoperative pulmonary function. Anesthesiology 118:1307–1321

27. Futier E, Constantin JM, Paugam-Burtz C et al (2013) A trial of intraoperative low-tidal-volume ventilation in abdominal surgery. N Engl J Med 369:428–437

28. Hemmes SN, Severgnini P, Jaber S et al (2011) Rationale and study design of PROVHILO – a worldwide multicenter randomized controlled trial on protective ventilation during general anesthesia for open abdominal surgery. Trials 12:111

29. Fernandez-Perez ER, Keegan MT, Brown DR, Hubmayr RD, Gajic O (2006) Intraoperative tidal volume as a risk factor for respiratory failure after pneumonectomy. Anesthesiology 105:14–18

30. van der Werff YD, van der Houwen HK, Heijmans PJ et al (1997) Postpneumonectomy pulmonary edema. A retrospective analysis of incidence and possible risk factors. Chest 111:1278–1284

31. Cohen E (2001) Management of one-lung ventilation. Anesthesiol Clin North America 19:475–495

32. Wilson WCBJ (2005) Anesthesia for thoracic surgery. In: Miller RD (ed) Miller's Anesthesia, 6th edn. Elsevier Churchill Livingstone, Philadelphia, pp 1894–1895

33. Schilling T, Kozian A, Huth C et al (2005) The pulmonary immune effects of mechanical ventilation in patients undergoing thoracic surgery. Anesth Analg 101:957–965

34. Licker M, Diaper J, Villiger Y et al (2009) Impact of intraoperative lung-protective interventions in patients undergoing lung cancer surgery. Crit Care 13:R41

35. Yang M, Ahn HJ, Kim K et al (2011) Does a protective ventilation strategy reduce the risk of pulmonary complications after lung cancer surgery?: a randomized controlled trial. Chest 139:530–537

36. Michelet P, D'Journo XB, Roch A et al (2006) Protective ventilation influences systemic inflammation after esophagectomy: a randomized controlled study. Anesthesiology 105:911–919

37. De Somer F (2013) End-organ protection in cardiac surgery. Minerva Anestesiol 79:285–293

38. Butler J, Rocker GM, Westaby S (1993) Inflammatory response to cardiopulmonary bypass. Ann Thorac Surg 55:552–559

39. Wan S, LeClerc JL, Vincent JL (1997) Inflammatory response to cardiopulmonary bypass: mechanisms involved and possible therapeutic strategies. Chest 112:676–692

40. Cremer J, Martin M, Redl H et al (1996) Systemic inflammatory response syndrome after cardiac operations. Ann Thorac Surg 61:1714–1720
41. Wrigge H, Uhlig U, Baumgarten G et al (2005) Mechanical ventilation strategies and inflammatory responses to cardiac surgery: a prospective randomized clinical trial. Intensive Care Med 31:1379–1387
42. Koner O, Celebi S, Balci H, Cetin G, Karaoglu K, Cakar N (2004) Effects of protective and conventional mechanical ventilation on pulmonary function and systemic cytokine release after cardiopulmonary bypass. Intensive Care Med 30:620–626
43. Sundar S, Novack V, Jervis K et al (2011) Influence of low tidal volume ventilation on time to extubation in cardiac surgical patients. Anesthesiology 114:1102–1110
44. Zupancich E, Paparella D, Turani F et al (2005) Mechanical ventilation affects inflammatory mediators in patients undergoing cardiopulmonary bypass for cardiac surgery: a randomized clinical trial. J Thorac Cardiovasc Surg 130:378–383
45. The Acute Respiratory Distress Syndrome Network (2000) Ventilation with lower tidal volumes as compared with traditional tidal volumes for acute lung injury and the acute respiratory distress syndrome. N Engl J Med 342:1301–1308
46. Amato MB, Barbas CS, Medeiros DM et al (1998) Effect of a protective-ventilation strategy on mortality in the acute respiratory distress syndrome. N Engl J Med 338:347–354
47. Reis MD, Gommers D, Struijs A et al (2005) Ventilation according to the open lung concept attenuates pulmonary inflammatory response in cardiac surgery. Eur J Cardiothorac Surg 28:889–895
48. Reis MD, Struijs A, Koetsier P et al (2005) Open lung ventilation improves functional residual capacity after extubation in cardiac surgery. Crit Care Med 33:2253–2258
49. Chaney MA, Nikolov MP, Blakeman BP, Bakhos M (2000) Protective ventilation attenuates postoperative pulmonary dysfunction in patients undergoing cardiopulmonary bypass. J Cardiothorac Vasc Anesth 14:514–518
50. Wrigge H, Pelosi P (2011) Tidal volume in patients with normal lungs during general anesthesia: lower the better? Anesthesiology 114:1011–1013

Protective Mechanical Ventilation in the Non-injured Lung: Review and Meta-analysis

Y. Sutherasan, M. Vargas, and P. Pelosi

Introduction

Acute respiratory distress syndrome (ARDS) is one of the main causes of mortality in critically ill patients. Injured lungs can be protected by optimum mechanical ventilator settings, using low tidal volume (V_T) values and higher positive-end expiratory pressure (PEEP); the benefits of this protective strategy on outcomes have been confirmed in several prospective randomized controlled trials (RCTs). The question is whether healthy lungs need specific protective ventilatory settings when they are at risk of injury. We performed a systematic review of the scientific literature and a meta-analysis regarding the rationale of applying protective ventilatory strategies in patients at risk of ARDS in the perioperative period and in the intensive care unit (ICU).

Mechanism of Ventilator-Induced Lung Injury in Healthy Lungs

Several studies have reported the multiple hit theory as the main cause of ARDS in previously healthy lungs (transfusion, cardiopulmonary bypass [CPB], sepsis etc.). Recently, many investigators have reported that, in healthy lungs, mechanical venti-

Y. Sutherasan
Division of Pulmonary and Critical Care Unit, Department of Medicine, Ramathibodi Hospital, Mahidol University, Bangkok, Thailand

M. Vargas
Department of Neuroscience and Reproductive and Odontostomatological Sciences, University of Naples "Federico II", Naples, Italy

P. Pelosi ✉
AOU IRCCS San Martino-IST, Department of Surgical Sciences and Integrated Diagnostics, University of Genoa, Genoa, Italy
e-mail: ppelosi@hotmail.com

J.-L. Vincent (Ed.), *Annual Update in Intensive Care and Emergency Medicine 2014*, DOI 10.1007/978-3-319-03746-2_14, © Springer International Publishing Switzerland and BioMed Central Ltd. 2014

lation can aggravate the 'one hit' ventilator-induced lung injury (VILI), even when using the least injurious settings.

The pathophysiologic principles of VILI are complex and characterized by different overlapping interactions. These interactions include: (a) high V_T causing over distension; (b) cyclic closing and opening of peripheral airways during tidal breath resulting in damage of both the bronchiolar epithelium and the parenchyma (lung strain), mainly at the alveolar-bronchiolar junctions; (c) lung stress by increased transpulmonary pressure (the difference between alveolar and pleural pressure); (d) low lung volume associated with recruitment and de-recruitment of unstable lung units (atelectrauma); (e) inactivation of surfactant by large alveolar surface area oscillations associated with surfactant aggregate conversion, which increases surface tension [1]; (f) local and systemic release of lung-borne inflammatory mediators, namely biotrauma [2].

Recent experimental and clinical studies have demonstrated two main mechanisms leading to VILI: First, direct trauma to the cell promoting releasing of cytokines to the alveolar space and the circulation; second, the so-called 'mechanotransduction' mechanism. Cyclic stretch during mechanical ventilation stimulates alveolar epithelial and vascular endothelial cells through mechano-sensitive membrane-associated protein and ion channels [3]. High V_T ventilation led to an increase in expression of intrapulmonary tumor necrosis factor (TNF)-α and macrophage inflammatory protein-2 in mice without previous lung injury [4] and recruited leukocytes to endothelial cells [3]. Tissue deformation activates nuclear factor-kappa B (NF-κB) signaling consequent to the production of interleukin (IL)-6, IL-8, IL-1ß and TNF-α [3]. The cellular necrosis is associated with an inflammatory response in surrounding lung tissue [3].

Mechanotransduction is the conversion of mechanical stimuli to a biochemical response when alveolar epithelium or vascular endothelium is stretched during mechanical ventilation. The stimulus causes expansion of the plasma membrane and triggers cellular signaling via various inflammatory mediators influencing pulmonary and systemic cell dysfunction [3]. A high level of mechanical stretch is associated with increased epithelial cell necrosis, decreased apoptosis and increased IL-8 level [3]. Extracellular matrix (ECM), a three-dimensional fiber mesh, is composed of collagen, elastin, glycosaminoglycans (GAGs) and proteoglycans. The ECM represents the biomechanical behavior of the lung and plays a role in stabilizing lung matrix and fluid content. Mechanotransduction causes the mechanical force on ECM that causes the lung strain (the ratio between V_T and functional residual capacity [FRC]). High V_T ventilation causes ECM remodeling, influenced by the airway pressure gradient and the pleural pressure gradient [2, 5].

In animal models, VILI, defined by lung edema formation, develops when lung strain is greater than 1.5–2 [6]. Cyclic mechanical stress causes release and activation of matrix metalloproteinase (MMP). MMP plays an important role in regulating ECM remodeling and VILI. Lung strain also leads to modification of proteoglycan and GAGs. The fragmentation of GAGs may affect the development of the inflammatory response by interacting with various types of chemokine and acting as ligands for Toll-like receptors [5, 7]. In addition, the ECM has been demonstrated

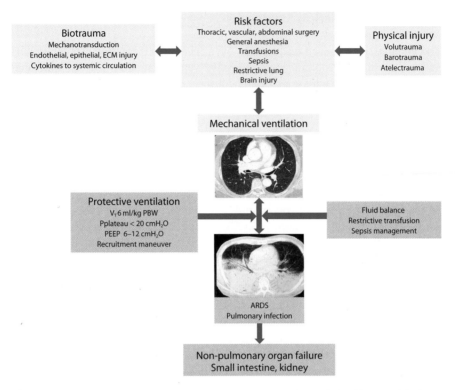

Fig. 1 Pathophysiology of ventilator-induced lung injury (VILI) in non-injured lungs and the lung-protective ventilatory approach. V_T: tidal volume; PBW: predicted body weight; PEEP: positive end-expiratory pressure; ARDS: acute respiratory distress syndrome; ECM: extracellular matrix

to be the signal of matrikines requiring proteolytic breakdown. Mechanical strain induces ECM breakdown [5].

During the perioperative period, general anesthesia and deep sedation with or without muscle paralysis markedly affect lung structure by reducing the tone of respiratory muscles and altering diaphragmatic position [8]. A direct effect of anesthetics on pulmonary surfactant, as well as the weight of the heart and greater intra-abdominal pressure in the supine position, promotes collapse of dependent lung regions and partial collapse of mid-pulmonary regions as a consequence of the reduction in end-expiratory lung volume. These alterations promote: (a) increase in lung elastance; (b) increase in lung resistance; and (c) impairment in gas exchange. The morphological alterations of the lungs are sustained at least for the first 24–72 hours postoperatively, particularly in patients undergoing high-risk surgery. In addition these alterations facilitate rapid shallow breathing and increased work of breathing as well as impaired gas-exchange [9] (Fig. 1).

Protective Ventilation Strategies

The previously mentioned mechanisms have encouraged intensive care physicians and anesthesiologists to consider 'protective ventilation strategies' in vulnerable non-injured lungs, which use physiologic low V_T values, moderate to high levels of PEEP and/or recruitment maneuvers.

Tidal Volume, Positive End-Expiratory Pressure and Recruitment Maneuvers

In Surgery

A recent large prospective cohort study conducted in different types of surgery demonstrated that the incidence of in-hospital mortality was about as high as the incidence of postoperative pulmonary complications which were associated with prolonged hospital stays [10]. Historically, use of large V_T (10–15 ml/kg) was advocated during the perioperative period to prevent impaired oxygenation and re-open collapsed lung units [11]. Nowadays, lung protective ventilation has become the standard of care in patients with ARDS. Secondary analysis of the ARDS network trial database revealed that the reduction in V_T from 12 to 6 ml/kg predicted body weight (PBW) yielded benefit, regardless of the level of plateau pressure [12]. Over the last few decades, clinicians have tended to decrease V_T from 8.8 ml/kg actual body weight (ABW) to 6.9 ml/kg ABW in critically ill patients [13].

Applying a PEEP ≥ 8 cm H_2O and using recruitment maneuvers may increase end-expiratory lung volume (EELV) beyond airway closure, certainly preventing atelectasis. However, the adverse effect of PEEP and recruitment maneuvers is a possible reduction in right ventricular (RV) preload and an increase in RV afterload. These consequences may lead to lower stroke volume and potentially became problematic during surgery. Therefore, the role of low V_T ventilation and moderate to high PEEP levels with recruitment maneuvers in previously non-injured lungs is still controversial during surgery.

In terms of lung mechanics and gas exchange, during cardiac surgery protective ventilation with a V_T of 6 ml/kg and PEEP 5 cm H_2O can improve lung mechanics and prevent postoperative shunting compared to conventional or standard ventilation with V_T of 12 ml/kg and PEEP 5 cm H_2O [14].

In patients undergoing CPB surgery, Koner et al. found no differences in plasma levels of TNF-α or IL-6 in patients ventilated with V_T of 6 ml/kg plus PEEP 5 cm H_2O, with V_T 10 ml/kg plus PEEP 5 cm H_2O or with V_T 10 ml/kg but zero end-expiratory pressure (ZEEP) [15]. Wrigge et al. also reported that ventilation with V_T of 6 ml/kg or with 12 ml/kg for 6 hours did not affect serum TNF-α, IL-6, or IL-8 concentrations in CPB surgery; only bronchoalveolar lavage (BAL) fluid TNF-α levels were significantly higher in the higher V_T group [16]. In contrast, Zupancich et al. showed that serum and BAL fluid IL-6 and IL-8 levels were elevated in a conventional ventilation group compared to a protective ventilation group after 6 hours of ventilation [17].

During major thoracic and abdominal surgery, there was no difference in the time course of tracheal aspirate and plasma TNF-α, IL-1, IL-6, IL-8, IL-12, or IL-10 in patients receiving conventional ventilation (V_T 12–15 ml/kg ideal body weight [IBW] and PEEP 0 cm H_2O) and those receiving protective ventilation (V_T 6 ml/kg IBW and PEEP 10 cm H_2O) [18]. In abdominal surgery, Wolthuis et al. demonstrated attenuation of pulmonary IL-8, myeloperoxidase and elastase in a protective ventilation group [19]. In terms of clinical outcomes, elderly patients undergoing major abdominal surgery ventilated with 6 ml/kg PBW, 12 cm H_2O PEEP and receiving a recruitment maneuver by sequentially increasing PEEP in 3 steps to 20 cm H_2O had no hemodynamic effects and achieved better intraoperative PaO_2 and dynamic lung compliance compared with patients receiving conventional ventilation with V_T 10 ml/kg without PEEP and recruitment maneuvers. However, this study showed no differences in IL-6 and IL-8 levels [20].

In a prospective study of 3434 cardiac surgery patients, only 21 % of patients received V_T < 10 ml/kg PBW; V_T values of more than 10 ml/kg PBW were an independent risk factor for multiple organ failure [21]. Obesity, female gender and short height are risk factors for receiving V_T of more than 10 ml/kg [22].

Treschan et al. demonstrated that applying V_T of 6 ml/kg PBW during major abdominal surgery did not attenuate postoperative lung function impairment compared to V_T values of 12 ml/kg PBW with the same PEEP level of 5 cm H_2O [23]. However, Severgnini et al. showed that compared to conventional ventilation (V_T 9 ml/kg IBW without PEEP), application of protective ventilation during abdominal surgery lasting more than 2 hours (V_T 7 ml/kg IBW, PEEP 10 cm H_2O, and recruitment maneuver) improved pulmonary function tests for up to 5 days, with reduced modified Clinical Pulmonary Infection Scores (mCPIS), lower rates of postoperative pulmonary complications, and better oxygenation [24]. A study conducted by Futier et al. (IMPROVE study) emphasizes the benefits of low V_T with PEEP and recruitment maneuver. This large RCT demonstrated that major pulmonary and extrapulmonary complications within 7 days after major abdominal surgery occurred in 21 patients (10.5 %) in the protective ventilation group (V_T 6–8 ml/kg PBW, PEEP 6–8 cm H_2O and recruitment maneuver) compared with 55 patients (27.5 %) in the conventional ventilation group (V_T 10–12 ml/kg PBW without PEEP); furthermore, patients in the protective ventilation group had shorter lengths of hospital stay than those in the conventional group [25].

Higher V_T ventilation seems to be an inflammatory stimulus for the lungs. However, as shown in the studies mentioned earlier, in terms of resultant local and systemic inflammatory responses processes, results are still debated [15, 16, 18, 26]. Application of lower V_T is challenging because it can possibly increase the risk of atelectasis. Nevertheless, Cai et al. showed that applying ventilation with V_T of 6 ml/kg alone was associated with no difference in the amount of atelectasis compared to ventilation with V_T of 10 ml/kg [27] and application of PEEP may additionally counteract this effect [24]. Several studies have shown that protective ventilation can improve lung mechanics, gas exchange and decrease the incidence of postoperative pulmonary complications [24, 25, 28] (Table 1).

Table 1 Characteristics and impact of protective ventilation in surgical patients

First author, Year [Ref]	No	Design	Patient population	Protective ventilation		Standard ventilation		Main outcome of protective ventilation
				Tidal volume	PEEP (cmH$_2$O)	Tidal volume	PEEP (cmH$_2$O)	
Chaney 2000 [14]	25	RCT	CABG	6 ml/kg	≥ 5	12 ml/kg	≥ 5	Better lung mechanics and less shunt
Wrigge 2004 [18]	62	RCT	Major thoracic or abdominal surgery	6 ml/kg IBW	10	12 or 15 ml/kg IBW	0	No difference in BAL or plasma cytokines
Koner 2004 [15]	44	RCT	CABG	6 ml/kg	5	10 ml/kg 10 ml/kg	5 0	No difference in plasma cytokines, Better oxygenation in PEEP groups
Wrigge 2005 [16]	44	RCT	CABG	6 ml/kg IBW	9[a]	12 ml/kg IBW	7[a]	No difference in BAL and plasma cytokines
Zupancich 2005 [17]	40	RCT	CABG	8 ml/kg	10	10 ml/kg	2–3	Decrease in BAL and plasma cytokines
Cai 2006 [27]	16	RCT	Neurosurgery	6 ml/kg	0	10 ml/kg	0	No difference in amount of atelectasis or gas exchange
Determann 2008 [26]	40	RCT	Abdominal surgery	6 ml/kg IBW	10	12 ml/kg IBW	0	No difference in BAL and plasma of Clara cell protein, advanced glycation end products and surfactant proteins
Wolthuis 2008 [19]	40	RCT	Abdominal surgery	6 ml/kg IBW	10	12 ml/kg IBW	0	Attenuated the increase in BAL myeloperoxidase
Weingarten 2010 [20]	40	RCT	Abdominal surgery Age >65 years	6 ml/kg PBW[b]	12	10 ml/kg PBW	0	Better intraoperative oxygenation, no difference in biomarkers
Fernandez-Bustamante 2011 [22]	429	Cross-sectional	Abdominal surgery	< 8 ml/kg PBW 8–10 ml/kg PBW	– –	> 10 mL/kg PBW	–	Obesity, female gender or short height risk factors for receiving large V_T

Continuation see next page

Table 1 *Continued*

First author, Year [Ref]	No	Design	Patient population	Protective ventilation		Standard ventilation		Main outcome of protective ventilation
				Tidal volume	PEEP (cmH$_2$O)	Tidal volume	PEEP (cmH$_2$O)	
Sundar 2011 [28]	149	RCT	Cardiac surgery	6 ml/kg PBW	$\geq 5^a$	10 ml/kg PBW	$\geq 5^a$	Less postoperative reintubation and intubated patients at 6–8 hours after surgery.
Lellouche 2012 [21]	3434	Observational	Cardiac surgery	<10 ml/kg PBW	–	10–12 ml/kg PBW >12 ml/kg PBW	– –	V$_T$ ≥ 10 ml/kg independent risk factor for organ failure and prolonged ICU stay
Treschan 2012 [23]	101	RCT	Upper abdominal surgery	6 ml/kg PBW	5	12 ml/kg PBW	5	Did not improve lung function
Severgnini 2013 [24]	56	RCT	Open abdominal surgery	7 ml/kg IBW^b	10	9 ml/kg IBW	0	Better pulmonary function test and mCPIS score, fewer chest X-ray findings.
Futier 2013 [25]	400	RCT	Major abdominal surgery	6–8 ml/kg PBW^b	6–8	10–12 ml/kg PBW	0	Less postoperative pulmonary and extra pulmonary complications.

No: number of patients; CABG: coronary artery bypass surgery; BAL: bronchoalveolar lavage; IBW: ideal body weight; PBW: predicted body weight; RCT: randomized control trial; ICU: intensive care unit; MV: mechanical ventilation; V$_T$: tidal volume; mCPIS: modified Clinical Pulmonary Infection Score.
^{a} Level of PEEP set according to the sliding scale based on PaO$_2$/FiO$_2$ ladder.
^{b} With recruitment maneuver.

To better investigate the impact of protective ventilation itself involving low V_T or PEEP and recruitment maneuvers, a large RCT including 900 patients and investigating the effect on postoperative pulmonary complications of an open lung strategy with high PEEP and recruitment maneuvers in short term mechanical ventilation has recently been completed (PROVHILO) [29]. Finally, the impact of current mechanical ventilatory practice during general anesthesia on postoperative pulmonary complications will be revealed by another large prospective observational study (LAS VEGAS) [30].

In the Intensive Care Unit

In a study comparing mechanical ventilation with V_T of 6 ml/kg and 12 ml/kg but with the same level of PEEP (5 cm H_2O) in a surgical ICU, the low V_T group had a lower, but not significantly, incidence of pulmonary infections, duration of intubation, and duration of ICU stay [31]. Pinheiro de Oliveira et al. demonstrated in trauma and general ICU patients that protective ventilation (V_T 5–7 ml/kg PBW and PEEP 5 cm H_2O) attenuated pulmonary IL-8 and TNF-α compared with high V_T ventilation (10–12 ml/kg PBW and PEEP 5 cm H_2O) after 12 hours of mechanical ventilation. Nevertheless, there were no differences in number of days on mechanical ventilation, length of ICU stay or mortality between the 2 groups [32]. Determann et al. also reported that conventional ventilation with V_T 10 ml/kg was associated with a significantly lower clearance rate of plasma IL-6 compared to protective ventilation with a V_T 6 ml/kg PBW [33]. This trial was stopped early because more patients in the conventional ventilation group developed acute lung injury (ALI, 10 patients [13.5 %] vs. 2 patients [2.6 %], p = 0.01) [33].

Not only a high V_T but also the time of exposure can lead to the release of pro-inflammatory mediators and an increase in the wet-to-dry ratio in the lung [34]. In a large retrospective cohort study in ICU patients who received mechanical ventilation for > 48 hours, 24 % of 332 patients developed acute lung injury (ALI) within 5 days. A V_T > 6 ml/kg PBW (OR 1.3 for each ml above 6 ml/kg PBW, p < 0.001), history of blood transfusion, acidemia, and history of restrictive lung disease were independent risk factors for development of ALI [35]. The incidence of ARDS decreased from 28 % to 10 % when applying a quality improvement intervention, namely setting V_T at 6–8 ml/kg PBW in patients at risk of ARDS plus using a restrictive protocol for red blood cell (RBC) transfusion [36]. Lower V_T ventilation was also not associated with differences in sedative drug dosage [37].

Recent Meta-analyses

Serpa Neto et al. [38] performed a meta-analysis of 20 trials that compared higher and lower V_T ventilation in critically ill patients and surgical patients who did not meet the consensus criteria for ARDS. Patients who received lower V_T ventilation showed a decrease in the development of ALI (risk ratio [RR] 0.33, 95 % CI 0.23–0.47, number needed to treat [NNT] 11), pulmonary infection (RR 0.45, 95 % CI 0.22–0.92, NNT 26), atelectasis (RR 0.62, 95 % CI 0.41–0.95) and mortality (RR

0.64, 95 % CI 0.46–0.86, NNT 23) [38]. However, there are some limitations that need to be addressed in the design of this meta-analysis. Some of the included studies were small, five studies were observational and studies included various types of clinical settings, such as sepsis in the ICU and one-lung ventilation in the operating room [36, 39]. Therefore, the results of this study cannot be considered as definitive.

To better specify the effect of protective ventilation in cardiac and abdominal surgical patients, excluding ICU patients, Hemmes et al. [40] performed a meta-analysis focusing on the effects of protective ventilation on the incidence of postoperative pulmonary complications and included eight articles. These authors demonstrated that applying protective ventilation decreased the incidence of lung injury (RR 0.40, 95 % CI 0.22–0.70, NNT 37), pulmonary infection (RR 0.64, 95 % CI 0.43–0.97, NNT 27) and atelectasis (RR 0.67, 95 % CI 0.47–0.96, NNT 31). When comparing lower PEEP and higher PEEP, higher PEEP also attenuated postoperative lung injury (RR 0.29, 95 % CI 0.14–0.60, NNT 29), pulmonary infection (RR 0.62, 95 % CI 0.40–0.96, NNT 33) and atelectasis (RR 0.61, 95 % CI 0.41–0.91, NNT 29).

The most recent systematic review was performed by Fuller et al. [41]. These authors hypothesized that low V_T is associated with a decreased incidence in the progression to ARDS in patients without ARDS at the time of initiation of mechanical ventilation. Thirteen studies were included and only one was a RCT. The majority of these studies showed that low V_T could decrease the progression of ARDS. However, a formal meta-analysis was not conducted because of the marked heterogeneity and variability of baseline ARDS among included patients [41].

Meta-analysis Including the Most Recent Trials

From the results of two additional recently published RCTs, which included overall more than 400 patients [24, 25], we hypothesized that the use of a protective ventilator strategy, defined as physiologically low V_T with moderately high PEEP with or without recruitment maneuvers, could lead to a substantial decrease in pulmonary complications in non-injured lungs and may affect mortality. Therefore, we conducted a new meta-analysis restricted to RCTs in patients undergoing surgery and critically ill patients, and excluding one-lung ventilation. Studies were identified by two authors through a computerized blind search of Pubmed using a sensitive search strategy. Articles were selected for inclusion in the systematic review if they evaluated two types of ventilation in patients without ARDS or ALI at the onset of mechanical ventilation in the operating room or ICU. Protective ventilation was defined as low V_T with or without high PEEP, and standard ventilation was defined as high V_T with or without low PEEP. Articles not reporting outcomes of interest were excluded. Data were independently extracted from each report by two investigators using a data recording form developed for this purpose. We extracted data regarding study design, patient characteristics, type of ventilation, and mean change in arterial blood gases, lung injury development, and ICU and hospital length of stay, overall survival, and incidence of atelectasis. The longest follow-up period in each trial up to hospital discharge was used in the analysis. After extraction, the data were reviewed and compared by a third investigator. Whenever needed, we obtained additional information about a specific study by directly questioning the principal investigator. We assessed allocation concealment, the baseline similarity of groups (with regard to age, severity of illness, and severity of lung injury), and early treatment cessation.

The primary endpoint was the development of lung injury in each study group. Secondary endpoints included incidence of lung infection, atelectasis, length of ICU stay, length of hospital stay and mortality. Continuous outcome data were evaluated with a meta-analysis of risk ratio performed with a fixed-effects model according to Mantel and Haenszel. When heterogeneity was $>25\,\%$, we performed a meta-analysis with mixed random effect using the DerSimonian and Laird method. Results were graphically represented using Forest plot graphs. The homogeneity assumption was measured by the I^2, which describes the percentage of total variation across studies that is due to heterogeneity rather than to chance; a value of $0\,\%$ indicates no observed heterogeneity, and larger values show increasing heterogeneity. Parametric variables are presented as mean and standard deviation, and nonparametric variables as median and interquartile range (IQR). All analyses were conducted with OpenMetaAnalyst (version 6), Prism 6 (GraphPad software) and SPSS version 20 (IBM SPSS). For all analyses, 2-sided p values less than 0.05 were considered significant. To evaluate potential publication bias, a weighted linear regression was used, with the natural log of the OR as the dependent variable and the inverse of the total sample size as the independent variable. This is a modified Macaskill's test, which gives more balanced type I error rates in the tail probability areas in comparison to other publication bias tests [42].

Seventeen articles were included in the meta-analysis [14–20, 23–28, 31–33, 43]. Three studies were conducted in critically ill patients and the others in surgical patients. Six of the studies were in cardiac surgery, 6 in major abdominal surgery, 1 in neurosurgery, and 1 in thoracic surgery. A total of 1362 patients, comprising 682 patients with protective ventilation and 680 patients with conventional ventilation, were analyzed. Characteristics of the included RCTs are shown in Table 2. Nine studies evaluated inflammatory mediators as their primary outcome. The development of pulmonary complications was the primary outcome in three studies. The average V_T values in the protective ventilation and conventional ventilation groups were 6.1 ml/kg IBW and 10.7 ml/kg, respectively. The average plateau pressures were $<20\,cm\,H_2O$ in both groups, significantly lower in the protective ventilation group than in the conventional ventilation group. The protective ventilation groups had higher levels of $PaCO_2$ and more acidemia, although within the normal ranges (Table 3).

The protective ventilation group had a lower incidence of ALI (RR 0.27, 95 % CI 0.12–0.59) and lung infection (RR 0.35, 95 % CI 0.25–0.63); however, application of protective ventilation did not affect atelectasis (RR 0.76, 95 % CI 0.33–1.37) or mortality (RR 1.03; 95 % CI 0.67–1.58) compared with conventional ventilation (Figs. 2 and 3). There were no differences in length of ICU stay (weighted mean

Table 2 Characteristics of the studies included in the meta-analysis

First author, Year [Ref]	Number of patients	Protective ventilation		Standard ventilation		Setting	Design	Primary outcome
		V_T (ml/kg)	N	V_T (ml/kg)	N			
Lee 1990 [31]	103	6	47	12	56	ICU	RCT	Duration of MV
Chaney 2000 [14]	25	6	12	12	16	Surg	RCT	Lung mechanics
Wrigge 2004 [18]	62	6	30	12	32	Surg	RCT	Cytokines in BAL
Koner 2004 [15]	44	6	15	10	29	Surg	RCT	Cytokines in blood
Wrigge 2005 [16]	44	6	22	12	22	Surg	RCT	Cytokines in BAL
Zupancich 2005 [17]	40	8	20	10	20	Surg	RCT	Cytokines in BAL
Michelet 2006 [43]	52	5	26	9	26	Surg	RCT	Cytokines in blood
Cai 2007 [27]	16	6	8	10	8	Surg	RCT	Atelectasis
Wolthius 2008 [19]	40	6	21	12	19	Surg	RCT	Pulmonary Inflammation
Determan 2008 [26]	40	6	21	12	19	Surg	RCT	Cytokines in BAL
Weingarten 2010 [20]	40	6	20	10	20	Surg	RCT	Oxygenation
Determann 2010 [33]	150	6	76	10	74	ICU	RCT	Cytokines in BAL
Pinheiro de Oliveira 2010 [32]	20	6	10	12	10	ICU	RCT	Cytokines in BAL
Sundar 2011 [28]	149	6	75	10	74	Surg	RCT	Duration of MV
Treschan 2012 [23]	101	6	50	12	51	Surg	RCT	Spirometry
Severgnini 2013 [24]	55	7	27	9	28	Surg	RCT	Change in mCPIS
Futier 2013 [25]	400	6–8	200	10–12	200	Surg	RCT	Pulmonary and extrapulmonary complications

BAL: bronchoalveolar lavage; ICU: intensive care unit; MV: mechanical ventilation; Surg: surgical; V_T: tidal volume; mCPIS: modified Clinical Pulmonary Infection Score.

difference [WMD] –0.40, 95 % CI –1.02; 0.22) or length of hospital stay (WMD 0.13, 95 %CI –0.73; 0.08) (Fig. 4) between the protective ventilation and conventional ventilation groups. The I^2 test revealed no heterogeneity in the analysis of lung injury and mortality, but there was heterogeneity in the analysis of atelectasis and length of stay.

Table 3 Demographic, ventilation and laboratory characteristics of the patients included in the different studies

	Protective ventilation ($n = 682$)	Standard ventilation ($n = 680$)	p
Age, years	61 (8.4)	61 (7.7)	0.96
Weight, kg	77.5 (10.1)	77.2 (9.5)	0.82
Tidal volume, ml/kg	6.1 (0.63)	10.7 (1.2)	0.00
PEEP, cm H_2O	7.6 (2.4)	2.5 (2.6)	0.00
Plateau pressure, cm H_2O	17.2 (2.2)	19.9 (3.9)	0.03
Respiratory rate, breaths/min	16.7 (3.2)	10.1 (3.5)	0.00
PaO_2/FiO_2	331.6 (62.3)	332.5 (64.3)	0.94
$PaCO_2$, mmHg	42.6 (5.5)	38.4 (4.8)	0.01
pH	7.37 (0.3)	7.40 (0)	0.01

Results are shown as mean ($\pm$SD). FiO_2: fraction of inspired oxygen; PEEP: positive end-expiratory pressure.

Our meta-analysis including the most recent trials suggests that among surgical and critically ill patients without lung injury, protective mechanical ventilation with use of lower V_T, with or without PEEP, is associated with better clinical pulmonary outcomes in term of ARDS incidence and pulmonary infection but does not decrease atelectasis, mortality or length of stay. The plateau pressure in the conventional group was less than 20 cm H_2O, indicating that ARDS can occur even below the previously-believed safe plateau pressure level. The meta-analysis by Serpa Neto et al. [38] demonstrated that mortality was significantly lower with protective ventilation than in our study. This finding can be explained by the fact that we included only RCTs in our meta-analysis and the two most recent RCTs were not analyzed in the previous study. We summarize the characteristics of each recent meta-analysis Table 4.

In Specific Populations

Donors

A prospective multicenter study in brain death patients reported that 45 % of potential lung donors have a $PaO_2/FiO_2 < 300$, making them ineligible for lung donation. The authors suggest that mechanical ventilation management should be changed to protective ventilation settings to improve the supply of donor lungs [44]. Mascia et al. compared a protective mechanical ventilation strategy, including V_T of 6–8 ml/kg PBW, PEEP of 8–10 cm H_2O, apnea tests performed by using continuous positive airway pressure (CPAP), closed circuit for airway suction and recruitment maneuver performed after each ventilator disconnection, with conventional ventilation, namely V_T of 10–12 ml/kg PBW, PEEP 3–5 cm H_2O, apnea test performed by disconnecting the ventilator and open circuit airway suctioning, in potential donors. The authors clearly demonstrated that the number of lungs that met lung donor eligibility criteria after the 6-hour observation period and the number of lungs eligible to

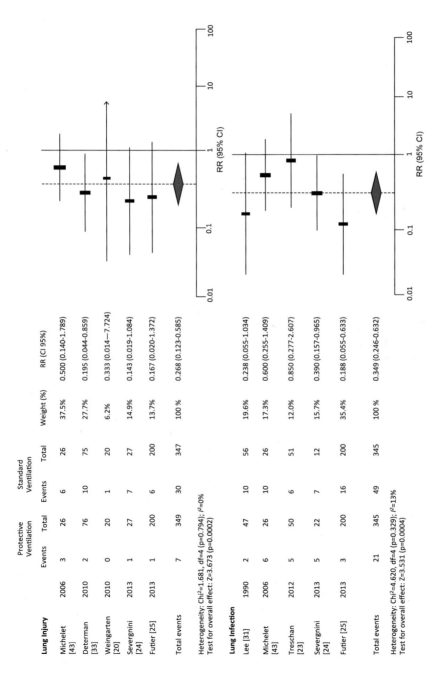

Lung Injury		Protective Ventilation		Standard Ventilation			
		Events	Total	Events	Total	Weight (%)	RR (CI 95%)
Michelet [43]	2006	3	26	6	26	37.5%	0.500 (0.140-1.789)
Determan [33]	2010	2	76	10	75	27.7%	0.195 (0.044-0.859)
Weingarten [20]	2010	0	20	1	20	6.2%	0.333 (0.014—7.724)
Severgnini [24]	2013	1	27	7	27	14.9%	0.143 (0.019-1.084)
Futier [25]	2013	1	200	6	200	13.7%	0.167 (0.020-1.372)
Total events		7	349	30	347	100 %	0.268 (0.123-0.585)

Heterogeneity: Chi²=1.681, df=4 (p=0.794); I²=0%
Test for overall effect: Z=3.673 (p=0.0002)

Lung Infection							
Lee [31]	1990	2	47	10	56	19.6%	0.238 (0.055-1.034)
Michelet [43]	2006	6	26	10	26	17.3%	0.600 (0.255-1.409)
Treschan [23]	2012	5	50	6	51	12.0%	0.850 (0.277-2.607)
Severgnini [24]	2013	5	22	7	12	15.7%	0.390 (0.157-0.965)
Futier [25]	2013	3	200	16	200	35.4%	0.188 (0.055-0.633)
Total events		21	345	49	345	100 %	0.349 (0.246-0.632)

Heterogeneity: Chi²=4.620, df=4 (p=0.329); I²=13%
Test for overall effect: Z=3.531 (p=0.0004)

Fig. 2 Effect of protective ventilation on lung injury and infection in surgical and ICU patients

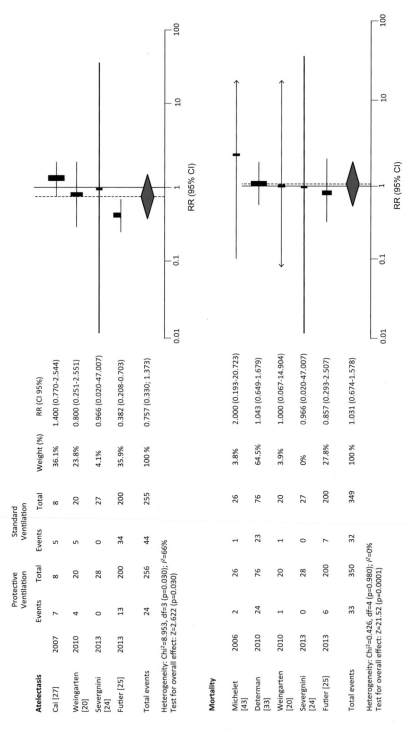

Fig. 3 Effect of protective ventilation on atelectasis and mortality in surgical and ICU patients

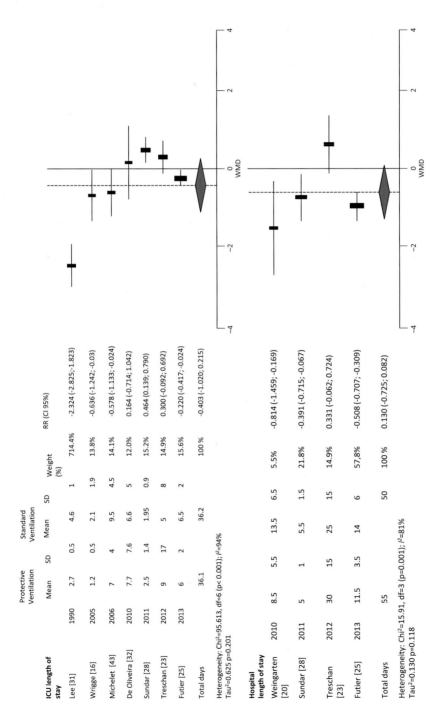

ICU length of stay		Protective Ventilation		Standard Ventilation		Weight (%)	RR (CI 95%)
		Mean	SD	Mean	SD		
Lee [31]	1990	2.7	0.5	4.6	1	714.4%	-2.324 (-2.825;-1.823)
Wrigge [16]	2005	1.2	0.5	2.1	1.9	13.8%	-0.636 (-1.242; -0.03)
Michelet [43]	2006	7	4	9.5	4.5	14.1%	-0.578 (-1.133; -0.024)
De Oliveira [32]	2010	7.7	7.6	6.6	5	12.0%	0.164 (-0.714; 1.042)
Sundar [28]	2011	2.5	1.4	1.95	0.9	15.2%	0.464 (0.139; 0.790)
Treschan [23]	2012	9	17	5	8	14.9%	0.300 (-0.092; 0.692)
Futier [25]	2013	6	2	6.5	2	15.6%	-0.220 (-0.417; -0.024)
Total days		36.1		36.2		100 %	-0.403 (-1.020; 0.215)

Heterogeneity: Chi²=95.613, df=6 (p< 0.001); I²=94%
Tau²=0.625 p=0.201

Hospital length of stay							
Weingarten [20]	2010	8.5	5.5	13.5	6.5	5.5%	-0.814 (-1.459; -0.169)
Sundar [28]	2011	5	1	5.5	1.5	21.8%	-0.391 (-0.715; -0.067)
Treschan [23]	2012	30	15	25	15	14.9%	0.331 (-0.062; 0.724)
Futier [25]	2013	11.5	3.5	14	6	57,8%	-0.508 (-0.707; -0.309)
Total days		55		50		100 %	0.130 (-0.725; 0.082)

Heterogeneity: Chi²=15.91, df=3 (p=0.001); I²=81%
Tau²=0.130 p=0.118

Fig. 4 Effect of protective ventilation on ICU and hospital lengths of stay in surgical and ICU patients

Table 4 Characteristics and outcomes of three recent meta-analyses

Author, year [ref]	Serpa Neto et al. 2012 [38]		Hemmes et al. 2013 [40]		Our meta-analysis	
Number of studies	20 articles		8 articles		17 articles	
Number of RCTs	15 articles		6 articles		17 articles	
Populations	ICU and surgical patients		Only surgical patients		ICU and surgical patients	
Search strategy until (year)	2012		2012		2013	
Statistical analysis	Fixed effect + Mantel and Haenszel		Fixed effect + Mantel and Haenszel		Fixed effect + Mantel and Haenszel, when $I^2 > 25\%$ random effect plus DerSimonian and Laird	
Number of patients	2833		1669		1362	
	PV group	CV group	PV group	CV group	PV group	CV group
V_T (ml/kg)	6.5	10.6	6.1	10.4	6.1	10.7
PEEP (cm H_2O)	6.4	3.4	6.6	2.7	7.6	2.5
Plateau pressure (cmH$_2$O)	16.6	21.4	16.6	20.5	17.2	19.9
Main outcome						
ALI	RR 0.33; 95 %CI 0.23–0.47		RR 0.40; 95 % CI 0.22–0.70		RR 0.27; 95 % CI 0.12–0.59	
Pulmonary infection	RR 0.52; 95 %CI 0.33–0.82		RR 0.64; 95 % CI 0.43–0.97		RR 0.35; 95 % CI 0.25–0.63	
Atelectasis	RR 0.62; 95 %CI 0.41–0.95		RR 0.67; 95 % CI 0.47–0.96		RR 0.76; 95 % CI 0.33–1.37	
Mortality	RR 0.64; 95 %CI 0.46–0.86		No data		RR 1.03; 95 % CI 0.67–1.58	
ICU length of stay	No data		No data		WMD –0.40; 95 %CI –1.02; 0.22	
Hospital length of stay	No data		No data		WMD 0.13; 95 %CI –0.73; 0.08	
Homogeneity test	Found heterogeneity in pulmonary infection outcome		Found heterogeneity in atelectasis outcome		Found heterogeneity in atelectasis, ICU length of stay and hospital length of stay outcome	

RCT: randomized control trial; V_T: tidal volume; PEEP: positive end-expiratory pressure; PV: protective ventilation; CV: conventional ventilation; ICU: intensive care unit; RR: risk ratio; 95 % CI: 95 % confidence interval. WMD: weighted mean difference.

be harvested were nearly two times higher with protective ventilation compared to traditional mechanical ventilation [45]. The authors concluded that these strategies can prevent the lungs from ARDS caused by brain injury and can recruit atelectasis.

One-Lung Ventilation

Michelet et al. demonstrated that during one-lung ventilation, protective ventilation resulted in higher PaO_2/FiO_2 ratios and shortened duration of postoperative mechanical ventilation in patients undergoing esophagectomy compared to conventional ventilation [43]. In patients undergoing esophagectomy, protective ventilation during one-lung ventilation causes lower serum levels of IL-1, IL-6, and IL-8 [43, 46]. In lobectomy patients, during one lung ventilation, Yang et al. reported that applying V_T of 6 ml/kg PBW, PEEP 5 cm H_2O and FiO_2 0.5 decreased the incidence of pulmonary complications and improved oxygenation indices compared to conventional ventilation [47].

Obesity

Obesity can aggravate atelectasis formation and is one of the risk factors for receiving high V_T values [21]. In morbid obesity, the forced vital capacity, maximal voluntary ventilation and expiratory reserve volume are markedly reduced. During anesthesia, an increase in body mass index correlates well with decreasing lung volume, lung compliance and oxygenation [48] but increasing lung resistance. The decrease of FRC is linked with atelectasis formation consequent to hypoxemia [49]. Ventilator management during anesthesia in obesity should be set as follows: (a) low V_T; (b) open lung approach with PEEP and recruitment maneuvers; (c) low FiO_2, less than 0.8 [49]. Because of the effects of chest wall and intra-abdominal pressure, we recommend careful monitoring of airway plateau pressure, intrinsic PEEP and transpulmonary pressure. Further studies are warranted to define protective ventilation settings in this group and particularly during the perioperative period.

Conclusions

Although, mechanical ventilation is a supportive tool in patients with respiratory failure and during the perioperative period, it has proved to be a double-edged sword. Mechanisms of VILI are now better understood. Implementation of protective ventilator strategies, consisting of V_T of 6 ml/kg, PEEP of 6–12 cm H_2O and recruitment maneuvers can decrease the development of ARDS, pulmonary infection and atelectasis but not mortality in previously non-injured lungs in the perioperative period and the ICU.

References

1. De Prost N, Dreyfuss D (2012) How to prevent ventilator-induced lung injury? Minerva Anestesiol 78:1054–1066
2. Pelosi P, Negrini D (2008) Extracellular matrix and mechanical ventilation in healthy lungs: back to baro/volotrauma? Curr Opin Crit Care 14:16–21
3. Lionetti V, Recchia FA, Ranieri VM (2005) Overview of ventilator-induced lung injury mechanisms. Curr Opin Crit Care 11:82–86

4. Wilson MR, Choudhury S, Goddard ME, O'Dea KP, Nicholson AG, Takata M (2003) High tidal volume upregulates intrapulmonary cytokines in an in vivo mouse model of ventilator-induced lung injury. J Appl Physiol 95:1385–1393

5. Pelosi P, Rocco PR (2008) Effects of mechanical ventilation on the extracellular matrix. Intensive Care Med 34:631–639

6. Protti A, Cressoni M, Santini A et al (2011) Lung stress and strain during mechanical ventilation: any safe threshold? Am J Respir Crit Care Med 183:1354–1362

7. Souza-Fernandes AB, Pelosi P, Rocco PR (2006) Bench-to-bedside review: the role of glycosaminoglycans in respiratory disease. Crit Care 10:237

8. Duggan M, Kavanagh BP (2005) Pulmonary atelectasis: a pathogenic perioperative entity. Anesthesiology 102:838–854

9. Tusman G, Bohm SH, Warner DO, Sprung J (2012) Atelectasis and perioperative pulmonary complications in high-risk patients. Curr Opin Anaesthesiol 25:1–10

10. Pearse RM, Moreno RP, Bauer P et al (2012) Mortality after surgery in Europe: a 7 day cohort study. Lancet 380:1059–1065

11. Bendixen HH, Hedley-Whyte J, Laver MB (1963) Impaired oxygenation in surgical patients during general anesthesia with controlled ventilation. A concept of atelectasis. N Engl J Med 269:991–996

12. Hager DN, Krishnan JA, Hayden DL, Brower RG, Network ACT (2005) Tidal volume reduction in patients with acute lung injury when plateau pressures are not high. Am J Respir Crit Care Med 172:1241–1245

13. Esteban A, Frutos-Vivar F, Muriel A et al (2013) Evolution of mortality over time in patients receiving mechanical ventilation. Am J Respir Crit Care Med 188:220–230

14. Chaney MA, Nikolov MP, Blakeman BP, Bakhos M (2000) Protective ventilation attenuates postoperative pulmonary dysfunction in patients undergoing cardiopulmonary bypass. J Cardiothorac Vasc Anesth 14:514–518

15. Koner O, Celebi S, Balci H, Cetin G, Karaoglu K, Cakar N (2004) Effects of protective and conventional mechanical ventilation on pulmonary function and systemic cytokine release after cardiopulmonary bypass. Intensive Care Med 30:620–626

16. Wrigge H, Uhlig U, Baumgarten G et al (2005) Mechanical ventilation strategies and inflammatory responses to cardiac surgery: a prospective randomized clinical trial. Intensive Care Med 31:1379–1387

17. Zupancich E, Paparella D, Turani F et al (2005) Mechanical ventilation affects inflammatory mediators in patients undergoing cardiopulmonary bypass for cardiac surgery: a randomized clinical trial. J Thorac Cardiovasc Surg 130:378–383

18. Wrigge H, Uhlig U, Zinserling J et al (2004) The effects of different ventilatory settings on pulmonary and systemic inflammatory responses during major surgery. Anesth Analg 98:775–781

19. Wolthuis EK, Choi G, Dessing MC et al (2008) Mechanical ventilation with lower tidal volumes and positive end-expiratory pressure prevents pulmonary inflammation in patients without preexisting lung injury. Anesthesiology 108:46–54

20. Weingarten TN, Whalen FX, Warner DO et al (2010) Comparison of two ventilatory strategies in elderly patients undergoing major abdominal surgery. Br J Anaesth 104:16–22

21. Lellouche F, Dionne S, Simard S, Bussieres J, Dagenais F (2012) High tidal volumes in mechanically ventilated patients increase organ dysfunction after cardiac surgery. Anesthesiology 116:1072–1082

22. Fernandez-Bustamante A, Wood CL, Tran ZV, Moine P (2011) Intraoperative ventilation: incidence and risk factors for receiving large tidal volumes during general anesthesia. BMC Anesthesiol 11:22

23. Treschan TA, Kaisers W, Schaefer MS et al (2012) Ventilation with low tidal volumes during upper abdominal surgery does not improve postoperative lung function. Br J Anaesth 109:263–271

24. Severgnini P, Selmo G, Lanza C et al (2013) Protective mechanical ventilation during general anesthesia for open abdominal surgery improves postoperative pulmonary function. Anesthesiology 118:1307–1321
25. Futier E, Constantin JM, Paugam-Burtz C et al (2013) A trial of intraoperative low-tidal-volume ventilation in abdominal surgery. N Engl J Med 369:428–437
26. Determann RM, Wolthuis EK, Choi G et al (2008) Lung epithelial injury markers are not influenced by use of lower tidal volumes during elective surgery in patients without preexisting lung injury. Am J Physiol Lung Cell Mol Physiol 294:L344–350
27. Cai H, Gong H, Zhang L, Wang Y, Tian Y (2007) Effect of low tidal volume ventilation on atelectasis in patients during general anesthesia: a computed tomographic scan. J Clin Anesth 19:125–129
28. Sundar S, Novack V, Jervis K et al (2011) Influence of low tidal volume ventilation on time to extubation in cardiac surgical patients. Anesthesiology 114:1102–1110
29. Hemmes SN, Severgnini P, Jaber S et al (2011) Rationale and study design of PROVHILO – a worldwide multicenter randomized controlled trial on protective ventilation during general anesthesia for open abdominal surgery. Trials 12:111
30. Hemmes SN, de Abreu MG, Pelosi P, Schultz MJ (2013) ESA Clinical Trials Network 2012: LAS VEGAS – Local assessment of ventilatory management during general anaesthesia for surgery and its effects on postoperative pulmonary complications: a prospective, observational, international, multicentre cohort study. Eur J Anaesthesiol 30:205–207
31. Lee PC, Helsmoortel CM, Cohn SM, Fink MP (1990) Are low tidal volumes safe? Chest 97:430–434
32. de Pinheiro Oliveira R, Hetzel MP, dos Anjos Silva M, Dallegrave D, Friedman G (2010) Mechanical ventilation with high tidal volume induces inflammation in patients without lung disease. Crit Care 14:R39
33. Determann RM, Royakkers A, Wolthuis EK et al (2010) Ventilation with lower tidal volumes as compared with conventional tidal volumes for patients without acute lung injury: a preventive randomized controlled trial. Crit Care 14:R1
34. Bregeon F, Roch A, Delpierre S et al (2002) Conventional mechanical ventilation of healthy lungs induced pro-inflammatory cytokine gene transcription. Respir Physiol Neurobiol 132:191–203
35. Gajic O, Dara SI, Mendez JL et al (2004) Ventilator-associated lung injury in patients without acute lung injury at the onset of mechanical ventilation. Crit Care Med 32:1817–1824
36. Yilmaz M, Keegan MT, Iscimen R et al (2007) Toward the prevention of acute lung injury: protocol-guided limitation of large tidal volume ventilation and inappropriate transfusion. Crit Care Med 35:1660–1666
37. Wolthuis EK, Veelo DP, Choi G et al (2007) Mechanical ventilation with lower tidal volumes does not influence the prescription of opioids or sedatives. Crit Care 11:R77
38. Serpa Neto A, Cardoso SO, Manetta JA et al (2012) Association between use of lung-protective ventilation with lower tidal volumes and clinical outcomes among patients without acute respiratory distress syndrome: a meta-analysis. JAMA 308:1651–1659
39. Licker M, Diaper J, Villiger Y et al (2009) Impact of intraoperative lung-protective interventions in patients undergoing lung cancer surgery. Crit Care 13:R41
40. Hemmes SN, Serpa Neto A, Schultz MJ (2013) Intraoperative ventilatory strategies to prevent postoperative pulmonary complications: a meta-analysis. Curr Opin Anaesthesiol 26:126–133
41. Fuller BM, Mohr NM, Drewry AM, Carpenter CR (2013) Lower tidal volume at initiation of mechanical ventilation may reduce progression to acute respiratory distress syndrome: a systematic review. Crit Care 17:R11
42. Peters JL, Sutton AJ, Jones DR, Abrams KR, Rushton L (2006) Comparison of two methods to detect publication bias in meta-analysis. JAMA 295:676–680
43. Michelet P, D'Journo XB, Roch A et al (2006) Protective ventilation influences systemic inflammation after esophagectomy: a randomized controlled study. Anesthesiology 105:911–919

44. Mascia L, Bosma K, Pasero D et al (2006) Ventilatory and hemodynamic management of potential organ donors: an observational survey. Crit Care Med 34:321–327
45. Mascia L, Pasero D, Slutsky AS et al (2010) Effect of a lung protective strategy for organ donors on eligibility and availability of lungs for transplantation: a randomized controlled trial. JAMA 304:2620–2627
46. Lin WQ, Lu XY, Cao LH, Wen LL, Bai XH, Zhong ZJ (2008) Effects of the lung protective ventilatory strategy on proinflammatory cytokine release during one-lung ventilation. Ai Zheng 27:870–873
47. Yang M, Ahn HJ, Kim K et al (2011) Does a protective ventilation strategy reduce the risk of pulmonary complications after lung cancer surgery?: a randomized controlled trial. Chest 139:530–537
48. Pelosi P, Croci M, Ravagnan I et al (1998) The effects of body mass on lung volumes, respiratory mechanics, and gas exchange during general anesthesia. Anesth Analg 87:654–660
49. Pelosi P, Gregoretti C (2010) Perioperative management of obese patients. Best Pract Res Clin Anaesthesiol 24:211–225

Dynamics of Regional Lung Inflammation: New Questions and Answers Using PET

J. Batista Borges, G. Hedenstierna, and F. Suarez-Sipmann

Introduction

> When the image is new, the world is new (Gaston Bachelard).

> The work of the eyes is done. Go now and do the heart-work on the images imprisoned within you (Rainer Maria Rilke).

The meaning of the term 'inflammation' has undergone considerable evolution. It was originally defined around the year 25 A.D. by Aulus Cornelius Celsus [1] and described the body's acute reaction following a traumatic event, such as a microscopic tear of a ligament or muscle. His original wording: "*Notae vero inflammationis sunt quatour: rubor et tumor cum calore et dolore*" (true signs of inflammation are four: redness and swelling with heat and pain) still holds. Disturbance of function (*functio laesa*) is the legendary fifth cardinal sign of inflammation and was added by Galen in the second century A.D. [2]. Recent articles [3] highlight the complicated role that inflammation plays in chronic illnesses, including metabolic, cardiovascular and neurodegenerative diseases. In addition to these difficult-to-treat diseases, more research and research tools are needed to illuminate therapeutic

J. Batista Borges
Hedenstierna laboratory, Department of Surgical Sciences, Section of Anesthesiology & Critical Care, Uppsala University, Uppsala, Sweden
Pulmonary Divison, Heart Institute (Incor) Hospital das Clínicas da Faculdade de Medicina da Universidade de São Paulo, São Paulo, Brazil

G. Hedenstierna
Hedenstierna laboratory, Department of Medical Sciences, Clinical Physiology, Uppsala University, Uppsala, Sweden

F. Suarez-Sipmann ✉
Hedenstierna laboratory, Department of Surgical Sciences, Section of Anesthesiology & Critical Care, Uppsala University, Uppsala, Sweden
CIBERES, Madrid, Spain
e-mail: fsuarez.sipmann@surgsci.uu.se

J.-L. Vincent (Ed.), *Annual Update in Intensive Care and Emergency Medicine 2014*, DOI 10.1007/978-3-319-03746-2_15, © Springer International Publishing Switzerland 2014

strategies in another difficulty-to-treat inflammatory malady, the acute respiratory distress syndrome (ARDS).

In more than 40 years of extensive research on ARDS, little advance has been made in terms of outcome improvement [4] and much debate remains over pivotal concepts regarding the pathophysiology and almost every aspect of its treatment [5]. ARDS is a frequent and important cause of morbidity and mortality in critically ill patients [4, 6]. Some 74,500 persons die of acute lung injury (ALI) in the United States each year, a figure that is comparable to the number of adult deaths attributed to breast cancer or human immunodeficiency virus (HIV) disease in 1999 [6]. More importantly, ARDS occurs with a higher incidence than previously reported, currently estimated to be about 190,600 cases per year in the United States with a mortality rate of 38.5 %, and therefore has a substantial impact on public health [6].

The Inflammatory Component of ARDS and Ventilator-induced Lung Injury

Dysregulated inflammation, inappropriate accumulation and activity of leukocytes and platelets, uncontrolled activation of coagulation pathways, and altered permeability of alveolar endothelial and epithelial barriers are central pathophysiologic concepts in ARDS [7–9]. Activation of the innate immune response by binding of microbial products or cell injury-associated endogenous molecules (danger-associated molecular patterns [DAMPs]) to pattern recognition receptors, such as the Toll-like receptors (TLRs) on the lung epithelium and alveolar macrophages, is now recognized as a potent driving force for acute lung inflammation. Newly reported innate immune effector mechanisms, such as formation of neutrophil extracellular traps – lattices of chromatin and antimicrobial factors that capture pathogens but can also cause endothelial injury – and histone release by neutrophils may contribute to alveolar injury. Signaling between inflammatory and hemostatic effector cells, such as platelet-neutrophil interaction, is also important. The delicate balance between protective and injurious innate and adaptive immune responses and hemostatic pathways may determine whether alveolar injury continues or is repaired and resolved.

Mechanical ventilation strategies designed to protect from the so-called ventilator-induced lung injury (VILI) reduce accumulation of pulmonary edema by preserving barrier properties of the alveolar endothelium and alveolar epithelium. Reductions in markers of lung epithelial injury have also been observed in clinical studies. These mechanical ventilation approaches aimed to attenuate VILI downregulate mechanosensitive pro-inflammatory pathways, resulting in reduced neutrophil accumulation in the alveoli and lower plasma levels of interleukin (IL)-6, IL-8, and soluble tumor necrosis factor (TNF) receptor 1.

VILI can induce or aggravate ARDS [10]. Mechanical cell deformation can be converted to biochemical changes, including production of pro-inflammatory cytokines. The proposed mechanism of VILI involves direct tissue damage due to mechanical stretch and activation of specific intracellular pathways involved in 'mechanotransduction' [11]. Of note, the development of hyaline membranes and increased permeability require the presence of polymorphonuclear leukocytes (PMN), suggesting that in addition to mechanical damage, inflammation is also necessary for mechanical ventilation to induce injury.

Much controversy remains about the precise contribution, kinetics, and primary role of each one of the putative VILI mechanisms and how best to design a full-bodied mechanical ventilation strategy capable of minimizing the majority of them [12]. A pressing unanswered question remains over the relative role of lung cyclic stretch, in even moderate degrees, vs. low-volume injury. Low-volume injury promotes local concentration of stresses in the vicinity of collapsed regions in heterogeneously aerated lungs together with cyclical recruitment of airways and alveoli. This mechanism tends to predominate in more dependent regions of the lungs and to occur in previously damaged lungs prone to collapse [13, 14]. Tremblay et al. showed increased production of inflammatory cytokines in lungs ventilated without positive end-expiratory pressure (PEEP) [15]. Conversely, stretch tends to occur in non-dependent regions and results from increased regional lung volume. Overstretching of alveolar walls causes endothelial and epithelial breaks and interstitial edema. Detachment of endothelial cells from the basement membrane and death of epithelial cells with denuding of the epithelial basement membrane become obvious after 20 min of mechanical ventilation with very high tidal volumes (V_T) [16]. The excessive deformation of epithelial and endothelial cells, as well as of the extracellular matrix, leads to an increased pro-inflammatory response. In some studies, low-volume injury was shown to predominate [13, 14, 17], whereas in others, including laboratory [18] and clinical studies [19], overdistension was the prevailing VILI mechanism.

Lung Inflammation Assessed by Positron Emission Tomography

Since inflammation in the lung seems to be a mediator in all causes of VILI [15, 20] and neutrophils play an important role in the inflammatory response to injurious mechanical ventilation [21], a research tool suitable for tracking regional inflammatory responses in the course of VILI and during lung protective ventilation strategies is of great interest.

Positron emission tomography (PET) is an advanced nuclear medicine technique used for non-invasive and quantitative measurements of radioactivity concentration within living tissues. It is based on the physical properties of certain isotopes that, when decaying, emit a positron, a particle with a mass equal to an electron but with a positive charge. The positron almost immediately collides with an electron and both are annihilated. In this process, two high-energy photons are created and leave the site of annihilation in opposite directions. The PET scanner is equipped with a large number of scintillation detectors arranged in a ring surrounding the object of interest. When two photons with equal energies are detected in coincidence, the event is stored in a dedicated data array called a sinogram. Typically, many millions of coincidences are stored during a PET scan. Coincidences are collected for a finite amount of time, called a time-frame. With modern PET scanners, a time-frame can range from a few seconds up to several minutes. Dynamic PET is a term used when several time-frames are collected from the same area of the body to track the changes in radioactivity concentration over time. The complete sinogram is then converted into a three-dimensional data array in a process called image reconstruction. Each data entry in this new data array contains the actual radioactivity concentration of a certain portion of the body within the specified time-frame. The three-dimensional image array can be viewed as a stack of tomographic slices on a computer display with color codes for the actual radioactivity concentration. When kinetic information is wanted, the dynamic PET data are processed further with dedicated computer software. Regions of interest are placed at will within the tissue and data resembling the changes in concentration over time are extracted. In advanced kinetic analysis, the time-activity curves of both the blood and the tissue of interest are needed. Advanced kinetic analysis typically involves the use of computer-aided mathematical modeling.

In ALI, the non-barrier functions of the pulmonary endothelium have been emphasized. But the barrier function *per se* is essential in preserving the most important purpose of the lungs: the adequate exchange of respiratory gases. PET studies have shown that measures of barrier function are a non-specific index of lung injury, indicating functional not structural lung injury [22, 23]. For example, PET imaging methods allow the rate at which proteins move across the endothelial barrier from vascular to extravascular compartments to be measured, the so called pulmonary transcapillary escape rate (PTCER). Palazzo et al. [24] used PET imaging to measure PTCER in an *in vivo* canine model of unilateral pulmonary ischemia-reperfusion injury and found that it was increased in the ischemic lung. Interestingly, both lungs had an increased PTCER compared with control non-ischemic lungs, suggesting that injury in one lung can lead to similar injury in the contralateral lung, a finding that has been observed in an analogous clinical setting, such as acute unilateral pneumonia. Calandrino et al. [22] described that, while PTCER and extravascular density, a close correlate to extravascular lung water (EVLW), were both elevated in ARDS patients they correlated poorly with one another on a regional basis. Moreover, as extravascular density returned to normal, PTCER remained elevated suggesting that lung tissue injury might be 'subclinical' but still present, even after pulmonary edema has actually resolved. This observation was further confirmed by Sandiford et al. [25] who examined the regional distribution of PTCER and extravascular density more closely in ARDS patients and found ventral-dorsal gradients only for extravascular density but not for PTCER. Once more, functional injury was detected even in lung regions that appeared to be free of structural injury. The finding that the lungs of ARDS patients are more diffusely involved than what might otherwise be assumed from just structural radiological imaging, such as computed tomography (CT), helps explain why ARDS lungs are so vulnerable to VILI: radiographically 'normal' lung, i.e., lung with a normal EVLW content in non-dependent lung regions may still be abnormal and vulnerable to mechanical stresses caused by mechanical ventilation. These data tell us that non-dependent regions of ARDS lung are 'at risk' because they demonstrate subclinical evidence of injury, which can be made manifest by inappropriate ventilator use. Jones et al. [26] showed a surprisingly high pulmonary uptake of [18F]-fluorodeoxyglucose (18F-FDG) in patients with head injury at risk of developing ARDS but without lung symptoms at the time of the scan. This signal may reflect sequestration of primed neutrophils in lung capillaries. *In vitro* studies in isolated human neutrophils have demonstrated that the uptake of deoxyglucose is increased to the same extent in cells that are only primed or primed and stimulated [27]. This finding indicates the vulnerability of these patients while on ventilatory support, because, even though neutrophils remain in a primed state, any additional stimulus precipitates actual tissue damage.

PET with 18F-FDG, a glucose-analog tracer, offers the opportunity to study regional lung inflammation *in vivo* with the advantage over conventional histological methods of preserving the integrity of the lung. 18F-FDG is taken up predominantly by metabolically active cells and has been recognized as a key marker of neutrophilic inflammation in the inflamed non-tumoral lung [14, 21, 28–33].

The type of lung cells responsible for 18F-FDG uptake (K_i) has been the matter of extensive investigation in models of ALI. 18F-FDG is a non-specific tracer, because it labels any cell with intense glucose uptake. However, several studies performed in humans [34] and animal models [29] have shown that, during pulmonary inflammation, most of the 18F-FDG uptake as measured by K_i can be attributed to activated neutrophils [35], even when macrophages are more abundant [30]. Although not usually characterized by an intense 18F-FDG uptake [36], macrophages may play a role in the generation of VILI [37]. The latest evidence [38] suggests that macrophages, as well as type 2 epithelial cells, might contribute to the 18F-FDG uptake signal during VILI. Therefore, although the overall 18F-FDG uptake signal is a complex mixture of the metabolic activity of many cell types, prior [29, 34–36] and very recent studies [17] have established that the major influence on the regional signal is the high metabolic activity of recruited neutrophils. In the acutely injured lung, images can therefore be interpreted, with a good approximation, as the regional distribution of neutrophilic inflammation.

There is a theoretical concern that in ALI, 18F-FDG may leak to the alveolar spaces becoming a major and non-specific determinant of the 18F-FDG signal, potentially causing a false, non-inflammation related increase in the measured uptake (K_i). The presence of edema, however, does not seem to affect the measurement of K_i, as suggested by Chen and Schuster [29], who measured glucose uptake with 18F-FDG in anesthetized dogs after intravenous oleic acid-induced ALI or after low-dose intravenous endotoxin followed by oleic acid. The rate of 18F-FDG uptake was significantly elevated in both endotoxin-treated groups, but not in the group treated only with oleic acid, leading the authors to conclude that pulmonary vascular leak, and consequently edema, does not significantly contribute to the K_i in ARDS lungs.

Higher Uptake in Normally and Poorly Aerated Lung

This *in vivo* non-invasive molecular imaging method has brought new insights into the role of low-volume vs. high-volume injury mechanisms [14, 32, 39]. Increased inflammation was found in normally aerated lung regions in a mixed population of patients with ARDS [39], an interesting finding differing from the classically assumed VILI targets in either overstretched or collapsed lung regions. Although thought-provoking, the study could not locate the regional onset of lung inflammation or determine the relative importance of the different mechanisms of VILI, as studied patients ranged in severity and duration of their ARDS.

We proceeded one step further by studying the location and magnitude of early inflammatory changes using PET imaging of ^{18}F-FDG in a porcine experimental model of ARDS. We evaluated the individual contributions of regional injurious mechanisms during early stages of VILI. To accomplish this aim, we created an experimental VILI model and designed a study that produced lungs heterogeneously aerated with significant amounts of non-aerated, poorly and normally aerated, and hyperinflated lung tissue (shown by CT). Within the same lung, we simultaneously found tidal hyperinflation, predominantly located in the non-dependent lung region, and collapse with tidal recruitment, mostly located in the dependent region. Remarkably, these two regions, classically comprising the major mechanisms of VILI, had ^{18}F-FDG uptakes similar to the healthy control group. On the other hand, the remaining regions situated in the intermediate portions of the lung presented a significantly higher uptake. Similarly, in the normal and poorly aerated regions we found the highest differences in ^{18}F-FDG uptake as compared to healthy controls, whereas the hyperinflated and non-aerated regions were similar to the control group (Fig. 1). We believe these findings challenge the current notion that hyperinflation and/or repeated collapse and re-expansion of alveolar units play the major role in early VILI. Instead, our data suggest that tidal stretch was highest in the poorly and normally aerated regions and this mechanism is the most important trigger of inflammation in these conditions. They also support the concept that the smaller the ventilated lung, the higher the VILI-triggering forces will be, as a larger fraction of V_T is delivered to a smaller lung volume.

An intriguing yet unanswered question raised by our data is whether the increased susceptibility to VILI was related to small length-scale heterogeneities of the lung parenchyma or of the airways [40], below the resolution limit of the CT, occurring in the poorly or even in the normally aerated regions. These heterogeneities would tend to produce an uneven distribution of V_T within lung regions and might have contributed to VILI. Perlman and Bhattacharya used real-time confocal microscopy to determine the micromechanics of alveolar perimeter distension in perfused rat lungs [41]. These investigators were able to image a 2-μm thick optical section under the pleura. Five to eight segments were identified within each alveolus. The average length of these segments was compared during normal inflation and hyperinflation. They found segmental distension to be heterogeneous within a single alveolus. Similarly, by using synchrotron-based X-ray tomographic

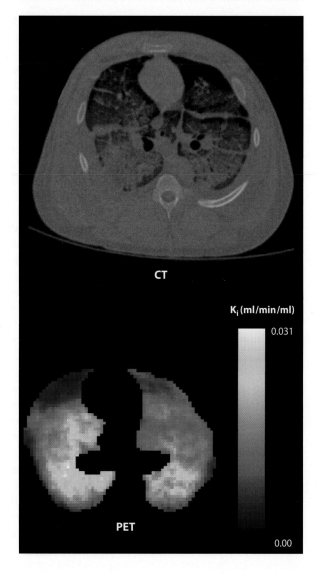

Fig. 1 Representative positron emission tomography (PET) image of net [^{18}F]fluoro-2-deoxy-D-glucose (^{18}F-FDG) uptake rate (K_i) in an experimental model of ventilator-induced lung injury. Note the predominance of activity in the normal and poorly aerated regions as seen in the corresponding computed tomography (CT) image

CT

K_i (ml/min/ml)

0.031

PET

0.00

microscopy on isolated rat lungs, Rausch et al. [42] estimated that local strains developing in alveolar walls were as much as four times higher than the global, with 'strain hotspots' occurring within the thinnest parts of the alveolar walls. When studying 3D microscopic distribution of lung parenchyma, using it as an input to their finite element modeling of alveolar expansion, they observed that thin regions may become overstretched, whereas regions with tissue accumulation remain unchallenged. These data fit with our own results and strongly suggest that a tidal stretch of the 'healthy' aerated parts of the heterogeneous aerated ARDS lungs can play a primary role in the activation of the inflammatory signaling cascade.

Furthermore, our finding of increased inflammation in normally aerated regions is in agreement with those of Bellani and colleagues [39] who, in their study of ARDS patients, determined that the metabolic activity of aerated regions was associated with both plateau pressure and regional V_T normalized by end-expiratory lung gas. Interestingly, neither they nor we found an association between cyclic alveolar recruitment-derecruitment and increased metabolic activity. Some key differences between this clinical study and our experimental observations highlight their complementary nature in terms of understanding VILI: 1) the time on mechanical ventilation before the clinical PET study averaged nine days and ranged from two to sixteen days, likely mixing distinct phases of ARDS and VILI pathophysiology, whereas our experimental study focused on early (hours) ARDS; 2) patients had limited tidal recruitment (2.9 % of the total lung weight) due to the lung-protective mechanical ventilation strategy applied, raising the question whether conditions with higher tidal recruitment would have produced more inflammation in those or in other regions, which our experimental data ruled out; 3) likewise, the amount of tissue undergoing hyperinflation was much smaller in the clinical study compared to our experimental study, because of the relatively low plateau pressures and V_T used in the patients. We observed that, even in more extreme ventilatory conditions with significant amounts of collapse, tidal recruitment, and hyperinflation, lung inflammation still predominates in the poorly and normally aerated regions.

At least three mechanisms could explain the increased K_i in poorly aerated regions: 1) alveolar cyclic recruitment at the subvoxel level; 2) cyclic opening and closing of small airways; or 3) increased tidal stretch. Measurements based on fluorescent microspheres confirmed the existence of ventilation heterogeneity down to length scales of $2 \, cm^3$ [43], and findings from synchrotron CT suggested that heterogeneity of specific ventilation (defined as ventilation per unit gas volume) can occur at lung volumes as low as $1 \, mm^3$ [44]. Recently, Wellman et al. have elegantly developed methods using PET to assess heterogeneity of specific ventilation at length scales below and above the effective image resolution of 12 mm [40]. Sub-resolution specific ventilation heterogeneity was reflected by multi-compartment voxel-level tracer kinetics during washout of $[^{13}N]$nitrogen (^{13}NN) from alveolar air space. These authors modeled the washout kinetics of ^{13}NN with PET to examine how specific ventilation heterogeneity at different length scales was influenced by lung aeration. They showed that airway narrowing or alveolar derecruitment can occur in poorly aerated lung regions especially at low length scales with a significant component derived from sub-resolution ($< 12 \, mm$) length scales. Components of specific ventilation heterogeneity at all studied length scales (< 12 to 60 mm) were highest in poorly aerated regions. Rylander et al., when studying the size and distribution of a "poorly aerated" compartment in ARDS patients, observed an uneven distribution of ventilation due to the presence of small-airway closure and/or obstruction [45]. Of note, airway dysfunction has been increasingly recognized as an important contributor to pulmonary impairment in patients with ARDS [46]. Animal models of ARDS have shown that, in addition to damage to the parenchyma, small airway injuries are characterized by bronchiolar epithelial necrosis and sloughing and by rupture of alveolar-bronchiolar attachments [47]. In humans who died with ARDS, small airway changes were characterized by wall thickening with inflammation, extracellular matrix remodeling, and epithelial denudation [46, 48].

Putting together all these aspects, it seems that, during VILI, the collapsed dependent and hyperinflated non-dependent regions may indirectly damage the normally and poorly aerated lung regions, by diverting the V_T to those regions submitting them to higher tidal stretch. We believe that the local consequences of the stretch in non-dependent regions and the local consequences of the mechanisms related to collapse in dependent regions are less important than the remote consequent stretches inflicted to the remainder intermediately located "baby lung" in terms of regional inflammation. Our findings highlight that we cannot determine which mechanism of VILI is more critical to oppose, but rather they emphasize the importance of strategies capable of minimizing both, collapse and hyperinflation, thereby unloading the small-aerated lung.

The effects of a protective ventilation strategy on topographic lung inflammatory cell activity have been recently described [17]: In a model of endotoxemic ALI, de Prost et al. found that mechanical ventilation had an important effect in determining the regional distribution and degree of early neutrophilic inflammation. When comparing protective ventilation (V_T 8 mL/kg and PEEP titrated to obtain a plateau pressure (Pplat) of $30\,cmH_2O$) with injurious ventilation (zero PEEP and V_T titrated to obtain a Pplat of $30\,cmH_2O$), the former resulted in a more homogeneously distributed uptake. Their findings are compatible with the concept that ventilation strategy plays an early pathogenic role in determining the profile of inflammatory cell distribution before lung injury is established and emphasize that the prevention of VILI should be a key aspect of patient management, even when mechanical ventilation periods and the underlying level of injury are limited [49]. Such results support former suggestion that heterogeneous inflammation may be an important element in the pathogenesis of ARDS [13]. Of note, these results indicate that in early endotoxemia during mechanical ventilation with no PEEP, inflammation predominates in the dependent regions.

Perspectives

As we have discussed, PET provides unique and unprecedented information to shed light on the inflammatory component of ARDS and VILI. The development of new and more selective/specific tracers to detect early inflammation has the potential to further enhance PET's capabilities and contributions. TNF-α is a well-known pro-inflammatory cytokine produced by monocytes and macrophages. It mediates the immune response by recruiting white blood cells to sites of inflammation and is involved in acute responses to injury. TNF-α appears in the circulation during the onset of sepsis-induced lung injury and is suggested to be an important early mediator of ALI. Interestingly, neutrophil recruitment induced by pure mechanical lung stretch has a significant TNF-α component [50].

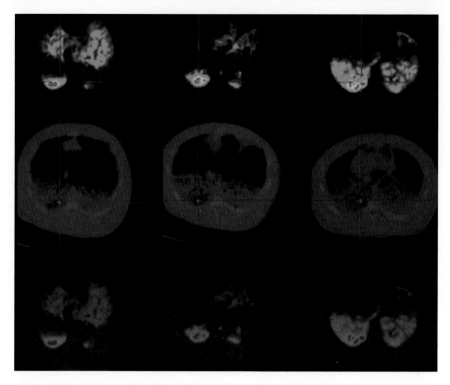

Fig. 2 Animals submitted to an experimental model of VILI were studied with positron emission tomography/computed tomography (PET/CT). PET images of the lung were obtained dynamically after injection of a tracer based on TNF-α. The images were generated with a novel approach with the pre-normalization of data before application of principal component analysis (PCA). PCA is a multivariate technique that has become an attractive tool in analyzing dynamic PET images because is a data-driven technique that emphasizes the regions with different kinetics without modeling assumptions. Three different slices at three different levels from the same animal are shown. Coloring is according to a relative scale for each image with black representing minimal and red maximal activity. Note the predominance of the activity in the poorly aerated regions

We have explored a new meaningful PET tracer based on TNF-α using a fusion protein of two affibody molecules fused genetically. Affibody molecules are a class of small protein domains that compete with receptor binding and have been shown to function as good imaging agents in the clinical setting. In preliminary tests *in vivo*, using an experimental model of ARDS, we tested a novel positron-emitting ligand of gallium, ^{68}Ga-TNFα. In the same way as with ^{18}F-FDG, PET images were obtained dynamically and at the end of the experiment tissue samples were taken from the lung and the abdomen. Significant activity inside the lung tissue was evidenced on the PET/CT images (Fig. 2). Tissue samples showed TNF-α (as analyzed with enzyme-linked immunosorbent assay [ELISA]) in the lung parenchyma and in small intestine tissue 4 hours after establishing the lung injury model. We confirmed that the used ligand of TNF-α bound to inflamed lung tissue and thus may become a future useful marker of inflammation especially when repeated studies are desirable.

Conclusions

Dynamic PET/CT imaging of ^{18}F-FDG has provided new relevant information on the location and distribution of inflammation in early VILI. The findings suggest that normally and poorly aerated regions – corresponding to intermediate gravitational zones – are the primary targets of the inflammatory process accompanying early VILI. This may be attributed to the small aerated lung volume that receives most of the ventilation and has potential implications in the way we approach lung protective ventilation.

References

1. Celsus AC (1478) Cornelii Celsi De medicina liber incipit. A Nicolao [Laurentii] impressvs, Florentiae
2. Rather LJ (1971) Disturbance of function (functio laesa): the legendary fifth cardinal sign of inflammation, added by Galen to the four cardinal signs of Celsus. Bull N Y Acad Med 47:303–322
3. Mueller K (2013) Inflammation. Inflammation's yin-yang. Introduction. Science 339:155
4. Phua J, Badia JR, Adhikari NKJ et al (2009) Has mortality from acute respiratory distress syndrome decreased over time?: A systematic review. Am J Respir Crit Care Med 179:220–227
5. Malhotra A, Drazen JM (2013) High-Frequency Oscillatory Ventilation on Shaky Ground. N Engl J Med 368:863–865
6. Rubenfeld GD, Caldwell E, Peabody E et al (2005) Incidence and outcomes of acute lung injury. N Engl J Med 353:1685–1693
7. Ware LB, Matthay MA (2000) The acute respiratory distress syndrome. N Engl J Med 342:1334–1349
8. Matthay MA, Zimmerman GA (2005) Acute lung injury and the acute respiratory distress syndrome: four decades of inquiry into pathogenesis and rational management. Am J Respir Cell Mol Biol 33:319–327
9. Matthay MA, Ware LB, Zimmerman GA (2012) The acute respiratory distress syndrome. J Clin Invest 122:2731–2740
10. Santos Dos CC, Slutsky AS (2000) Invited review: mechanisms of ventilator-induced lung injury: a perspective. J Appl Physiol 89:1645–1655
11. Vlahakis NE, Hubmayr RD (2005) Cellular stress failure in ventilator-injured lungs. Am J Respir Crit Care Med 171:1328–1342
12. Malhotra A (2007) Low-tidal-volume ventilation in the acute respiratory distress syndrome. N Engl J Med 357:1113–1120
13. Otto CM, Markstaller K, Kajikawa O et al (2008) Spatial and temporal heterogeneity of ventilator-associated lung injury after surfactant depletion. J Appl Physiol 104:1485–1494
14. de Prost N, Costa EL, Wellman T et al (2011) Effects of surfactant depletion on regional pulmonary metabolic activity during mechanical ventilation. J Appl Physiol 111:1249–1258
15. Tremblay L, Valenza F, Ribeiro SP et al (1997) Injurious ventilatory strategies increase cytokines and c-fos m-RNA expression in an isolated rat lung model. J Clin Invest 99:944–952

16. Dreyfuss D, Saumon G (1998) Ventilator-induced lung injury: lessons from experimental studies. Am J Respir Crit Care Med 157:294–323
17. de Prost N, Costa EL, Wellman T et al (2013) Effects of ventilation strategy on distribution of lung inflammatory cell activity. Crit Care 17:R175
18. Tsuchida S, Engelberts D, Peltekova V et al (2006) Atelectasis causes alveolar injury in nonatelectatic lung regions. Am J Respir Crit Care Med 174:279–289
19. Terragni PP, Rosboch G, Tealdi A et al (2007) Tidal hyperinflation during low tidal volume ventilation in acute respiratory distress syndrome. Am J Respir Crit Care Med 175:160–166
20. Ranieri VM, Suter PM, Tortorella C et al (1999) Effect of mechanical ventilation on inflammatory mediators in patients with acute respiratory distress syndrome: a randomized controlled trial. JAMA 282:54–61
21. Musch G, Venegas JG, Bellani G et al (2007) Regional gas exchange and cellular metabolic activity in ventilator-induced lung injury. Anesthesiology 106:723–735
22. Calandrino FSJ, Anderson DJ, Mintun MA, Schuster DP (1988) Pulmonary vascular permeability during the adult respiratory distress syndrome: a positron emission tomographic study. Am Rev Respir Dis 138:421–428
23. Schuster DP (1995) What is acute lung injury? What is ARDS? Chest 107:1721–1726
24. Palazzo R, Hamvas A, Shuman T et al (1992) Injury in nonischemic lung after unilateral pulmonary ischemia with reperfusion. J Appl Physiol 72:612–620
25. Sandiford P, Province MA, Schuster DP (1995) Distribution of regional density and vascular permeability in the adult respiratory distress syndrome. Am J Respir Crit Care Med 151:737–742
26. Jones HA, Clark JC, Minhas PS et al (1998) Pulmonary neutrophil activation following head trauma. Am J Respir Crit Care Med 157:A349 (abst)
27. Jones HA, Cadwallader KA, White JF et al (2002) Dissociation between respiratory burst activity and deoxyglucose uptake in human neutrophil granulocytes: implications for interpretation of (18)F-FDG PET images. J Nucl Med 43:652–657
28. Bellani G, Messa C, Guerra L et al (2009) Lungs of patients with acute respiratory distress syndrome show diffuse inflammation in normally aerated regions: a [18F]-fluoro-2-deoxy-D-glucose PET/CT study. Crit Care Med 37:2216–2222
29. Chen DL, Schuster DP (2004) Positron emission tomography with [18F]fluorodeoxyglucose to evaluate neutrophil kinetics during acute lung injury. Am J Physiol Lung Cell Mol Physiol 286:L834–L840
30. Jones HA, Clark RJ, Rhodes CG et al (1994) In vivo measurement of neutrophil activity in experimental lung inflammation. Am J Respir Crit Care Med 149:1635–1639
31. Jones HA, Sriskandan S, Peters AM et al (1997) Dissociation of neutrophil emigration and metabolic activity in lobar pneumonia and bronchiectasis. Eur Respir J 10:795–803
32. Costa ELV, Musch G, Winkler T et al (2010) Mild endotoxemia during mechanical ventilation produces spatially heterogeneous pulmonary neutrophilic inflammation in sheep. Anesthesiology 112:658–669
33. de Prost N, Tucci MR, Melo MFV (2010) Assessment of lung inflammation with 18F-FDG PET during acute lung injury. AJR Am J Roentgenol 195:292–300
34. Chen DL, Rosenbluth DB, Mintun MA, Schuster DP (2006) FDG-PET imaging of pulmonary inflammation in healthy volunteers after airway instillation of endotoxin. J Appl Physiol 100:1602–1609
35. Oehler R, Weingartmann G, Manhart N et al (2000) Polytrauma induces increased expression of pyruvate kinase in neutrophils. Blood 95:1086–1092
36. Jones HA, Schofield JB, Krausz T et al (1998) Pulmonary fibrosis correlates with duration of tissue neutrophil activation. Am J Respir Crit Care Med 158:620–628
37. Wilson MR, O'Dea KP, Zhang D et al (2009) Role of lung-marginated monocytes in an in vivo mouse model of ventilator-induced lung injury. Am J Respir Crit Care Med 179:914–922

38. Saha D, Takahashi K, de Prost N et al (2013) Micro-autoradiographic assessment of cell types contributing to 2-deoxy-2-[(18)F]fluoro-D-glucose uptake during ventilator-induced and endotoxemic lung injury. Mol Imaging Biol 15:19–27
39. Bellani G, Guerra L, Musch G et al (2011) Lung regional metabolic activity and gas volume changes induced by tidal ventilation in patients with acute lung injury. Am J Respir Crit Care Med 183:1193–1199
40. Wellman TJ, Winkler T, Costa ELV et al (2012) Effect of regional lung inflation on ventilation heterogeneity at different length scales during mechanical ventilation of normal sheep lungs. J Appl Physiol 113:947–957
41. Perlman CE, Bhattacharya J (2007) Alveolar expansion imaged by optical sectioning microscopy. J Appl Physiol 103:1037–1044
42. Rausch SMK, Haberthur D, Stampanoni M et al (2011) Local Strain Distribution in Real Three-Dimensional Alveolar Geometries. Ann Biomed Eng 39:2835–2843
43. Robertson HT, Altemeier WA, Glenny RW (2000) Physiological implications of the fractal distribution of ventilation and perfusion in the lung. Ann Biomed Eng 28:1028–1031
44. Porra L, Monfraix S, Berruyer G et al (2004) Effect of tidal volume on distribution of ventilation assessed by synchrotron radiation CT in rabbit. J Appl Physiol 96:1899–1908
45. Rylander C, Tylén U, Rossi-Norrlund R et al (2005) Uneven distribution of ventilation in acute respiratory distress syndrome. Crit Care 9:R165–R171
46. Pires-Neto RC, Morales MMB, Lancas T et al (2013) Expression of acute-phase cytokines, surfactant proteins, and epithelial apoptosis in small airways of human acute respiratory distress syndrome. J Crit Care 28:111.e9–111.e15
47. D'Angelo E, Koutsoukou A, Della Valle P et al (2008) Cytokine release, small airway injury, and parenchymal damage during mechanical ventilation in normal open-chest rats. J Appl Physiol 104:41–49
48. Morales MMB, Pires-Neto RC, Inforsato N et al (2011) Small airway remodeling in acute respiratory distress syndrome: a study in autopsy lung tissue. Crit Care 15:R4
49. Fernandez-Perez ER, Keegan MT, Brown DR et al (2006) Intraoperative tidal volume as a risk factor for respiratory failure after pneumonectomy. Anesthesiology 105:14–18
50. Wilson MR, Choudhury S, Takata M (2005) Pulmonary inflammation induced by high-stretch ventilation is mediated by tumor necrosis factor signaling in mice. Am J Physiol Lung Cell Mol Physiol 288:L599–L607

Non-conventional Modes of Ventilation in Patients with ARDS

L. Morales Quinteros and N. D. Ferguson

Introduction

Acute respiratory distress syndrome (ARDS) is a life-threatening form of acute respiratory failure characterized by acute hypoxemia and by diffuse pulmonary infiltrates on chest radiography. ARDS represents a common pathway of lung injury that arises in a variety of clinical settings, most often associated with pneumonia, sepsis, and trauma. Many treatments have been explored in ARDS, but most success has come through avoidance of iatrogenic ventilator-associated lung injury by manipulation of the mechanical ventilator. Using conventional ventilation, we now know that strategies that limit tidal volumes and inspiratory pressures, and which employ higher levels of positive end-expiratory pressure (PEEP) lead to significant reductions in mortality [1, 2]. In recent years there has been an increasing interest in non-conventional modes of ventilation. In this chapter, we review several of these 'new' modes and discuss their applicability to the patient with ARDS.

Non-conventional Ventilatory Modes in ARDS

The majority of intensive care units (ICUs) use conventional ventilator strategies, such as volume assist-control, pressure control, or pressure support to ventilate patients with mild-moderate ARDS. However, in patients with severe and refractory hypoxic respiratory failure, units differ between using high PEEP and so called 'non-conventional' modes to maintain oxygenation. Newer ventilators can be set to modes other than the pressure-control and volume-control modes of older machines. Technological advances and computerized control of mechanical ventilators have made it possible to deliver ventilatory assistance in new modes. In fact,

L. Morales Quinteros · N. D. Ferguson ✉
Interdepartmental Division of Critical Care, University of Toronto, Toronto, Canada
e-mail: n.ferguson@utoronto.ca

J.-L. Vincent (Ed.), *Annual Update in Intensive Care and Emergency Medicine 2014*,
DOI 10.1007/978-3-319-03746-2_16, © Springer International Publishing Switzerland
2014

there has been a growing interest in the use of alternative modes of mechanical ventilation that fulfill the principles of lung-protective ventilation, preventing lung injury and asynchony, promoting better oxygenation and faster weaning. We call these innovations non-conventional modes to differentiate them from the traditional volume-control and pressure-control modes. Here we will examine the physiological rationale, and give an overview on how four of these these non-conventional ventilatory modes work, as well as the clinical evidence for their use in adult patients who have ARDS.

Pressure-regulated Volume Control

Overview and physiology

Pressure-regulated volume control (PRVC), is a mode of mechanical ventilation that automatically adjusts inspiratory pressure in response to dynamic changes in patient mechanics and efforts. On a breath-to-breath basis, the ventilator in PRVC mode will adjust the delivered inspiratory pressure to achieve the goal tidal volume (Fig. 1). One can think of PRVC as a traditional pressure control mode that automatically adjusts itself to deliver a target tidal volume. Thus the clinician sets an inspiratory time and a goal tidal volume. Once these settings are entered, the ventilator will deliver a series of test breaths to establish the inspiratory pressure required to deliver the goal tidal volume with the chosen inspiratory time. The ventilator subsequently measures tidal volume on a breath-to-breath basis. If a change in respiratory system mechanics or patient effort causes the delivered tidal volume to be below goal, the ventilator will increase the inspiratory pressure on the next breath and *vice versa*.

Advantages
- Ensures safe tidal volumes over time in a patient with improving respiratory system compliance.
- Patient has very little work of breathing requirement.
- Variable minute ventilation to meet patient demand.
- Decelerating flow waveform for improved gas distribution.
- Breath by breath analysis.

Disadvantages and risks
- Varying mean airway pressures.
- When patient demand is increased, pressure level may diminish when support is needed.
- May be tolerated poorly in awake non-sedated patients.

Evidence in ARDS
There are two studies that have compared volume-controlled ventilation with this mode in patients with ARDS: PRVC did not improve clinical outcomes but it may achieve lower pressure airways [3, 4].

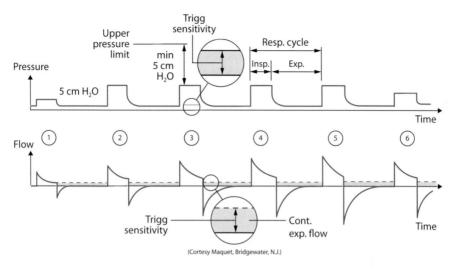

(Cortesy Maquet, Bridgewater, N.J.)

Fig. 1 Pressure-regulated volume control. (*1*) Test breath (5 cm H_2O); (*2*) pressure is increased to deliver set volume; (*3*) maximum available pressure; (*4*) breath delivered at preset VE, at preset respiratory frequency, and during preset inspiratory time; (*5*) when tidal volume corresponds to set value, pressure remains constant; (*6*) if preset volume increases, pressure decreases; the ventilator continually monitors and adapts to the patient's needs

High-frequency Oscillatory Ventilation

Overview and physiology

High-frequency oscillatory ventilation (HFOV) is an alternative mode of ventilation that uses a relatively constant and higher mean airway pressure along with very small tidal volumes to achieve many of the goals of lung protection (Fig. 2). Although HFOV is a recent arrival in the adult critical care unit, it has been used and studied extensively in neonatal and pediatric ICUs over the past 30 years. In the early 1970s, Lunkenheimer and colleagues [5] published their findings with the surprising observation that they could achieve adequate CO_2 clearance using an electromagnetic vibrator at high respiratory frequencies of up to 40 Hz. Around the same time, Bryan in Toronto [6], noted similar phenomena while measuring lung impedance during anesthesia. Over the next decade, a series of experiments on animals and humans helped develop HFOV into a viable treatment option for neonates with respiratory distress syndrome.

A feature of HFOV is the relative ability to decouple oxygenation and ventilation. Oxygenation is dependent on the mean airway pressure (with the overall objective of reducing the intrapulmonary shunting of blood) and the fraction of inspired oxygen (FiO_2), whereas ventilation (and tidal volume) is inversely related to the frequency and is directly related to the excursion of the diaphragm of the oscillator (pressure amplitude, ΔP).

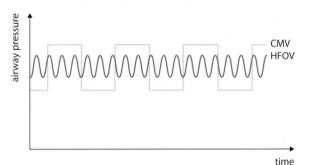

Fig. 2 Pressure-time curve contrasting conventional pressure control ventilation (CMV) with large tidal swings in pressure (*light blue line*) versus high-frequency oscillatory ventilation (HFOV, *dark blue line*)

Advantages

- The main benefit of HFOV in ALI/ARDS may be its ability to fulfill the doctrine of lung protective ventilation optimally and to attenuate ventilator-induced lung injury (VILI).
- Limiting excess distension of alveoli by delivering small tidal volumes, one should expect avoidance of barotrauma and volutrauma.
- The high mean airway pressures used in HFOV allow maintenance of high end-expiratory lung volume (an 'open lung'), greater alveolar recruitment and the prevention of end-expiratory alveoloar collapse and hence avoidance of atelectrauma.
- HFOV consistently leads to improved oxygenation.

Disadvantages

- High mean airway pressure delivered by HFOV may increase intrathoracic pressure, causing a decrease in venous return, cardiac output and cerebral perfusion.
- Higher mean airway pressure during HFOV may result in barotrauma.
- Heavy sedation and frequently paralysis are needed during HFOV.

Clinical evidence in ARDS

Supported by this strong physiologic rationale for lung protection, positive animal data, and successful clinical use of HFOV in the setting of neonatal/pediatric respiratory failure, there has been a growing interest in the use of HFOV in adults who have ARDS. Until recently, clinical studies on the application of HFOV in adults have mainly been case series in 'rescue' situations in which conventional ventilation arguably has failed. In addition, a number of small clinical trials suggested a mortality benefit in adults with ARDS treated with HFOV, but these trials were confounded by small sample sizes and outdated control ventilation strategies [7, 8]

To address this issue, two larger randomized controlled trials were conducted to compare HFOV with lung-protective conventional mechanical ventilation in terms of mortality in adult ARDS. In the OSCAR study, Young et al. [9] randomized 795 people with ARDS in 13 UK centers to receive HFOV or usual care conventional ventilation. There was no difference in the primary outcome of 30-day

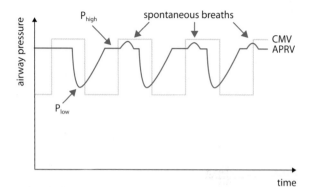

Fig. 3 Pressure-time curve schematic showing spontaneous breathing during airway pressure release ventilation (APRV). CMV: conventional mechancial ventilation

mortality between the two groups (HFOV 42 % vs. conventional ventilation 41 %). Meanwhile, in the OSCILLATE study, Ferguson et al. [10] randomized 548 people at 39 centers in 5 countries (including the U.S. and Canada) with ARDS to either HFOV or protocolized conventional ventilation using low tidal volumes, recruitment maneuvers and high PEEP. This study was stopped early because of an excess mortality in the HFOV arm. In-hospital mortality was 47 % in the HFOV group compared to 35 % in the control group (relative risk of death with HFO, 1.33; 95 % confidence interval, 1.09 to 1.64; p = 0.005). Possible factors that might explain this excess mortality in the HFOV arm were a greater use of sedation, neuromuscular blocker use, and longer and higher rates of vasoactive drugs, as well as chance alone. In light of these considerations, the results of these two studies preclude the routine use of this mode in patients with ARDS. There may still be a place for HFOV in the setting of rescue therapy.

Airway Pressure Release Ventilation

Overview and physiology

Airway pressure release ventilation (APRV) was described by Downs and Stock in 1987 [11] as a modified form of continuous positive airway pressure (CPAP) to enhance oxygenation by augmenting alveolar recruitment and allowing spontaneous breathing throughout the ventilation cycle. APRV functions essentially as two levels of CPAP, where patients spend most of the time at the higher level (Phigh), with intermittent, brief releases to the lower CPAP level (Plow) to facilitate ventilation. Throughout this ventilatory CPAP cycle, patients are also able to breath spontaneously, adding to ventilation and potentially contributing to many of the purported benefits of APRV (Fig. 3).

Advantages

- Allows spontaneous breathing (with potentially less need for sedation or paralysis) and potentially reduced atrophy of the diaphragm during critical illness.
- Can provide a relatively high mean airway pressure to improve oxygenation.

- Allows patients to breath spontaneously while continuing lung recruitment.
- May improve venous return and cardiac output with subsequent increase in oxygen delivery, compared with equivalent modes of ventilation.

Disadvantages
- Potential for high (unmeasured) transpulmonary pressures during spontaneous breaths.
- Potential for decruitment during release breaths.
- Potential for volutrauma with large release volumes.

Clinical evidence in ARDS

The clinical evidence evaluating the use of APRV in ARDS patients is currently limited to observational studies [12] and small randomized trials. Small studies have demonstrated that compared with conventional ventilation, patients ventilated with APRV have lower peak airway pressures but higher mean airway pressures with comparable oxygenation and ventilation parameters. Despite considerable enthusiasm among some groups, to date no studies have demonstrated convincing improvements in clinical outcomes with APRV.

Putensen et al [13], randomized 30 patients with multiple trauma to either APRV with spontaneous breathing ($n = 15$) or pressure-control ventilation ($n = 15$) for 72 hours. Weaning was performed with APRV in both groups. APRV was associated with increases in lung compliance and oxygenation and reduction of shunting. Interestingly, the use of APRV was associated with shorter duration of ventilatory support (15 vs 21 days), shorter length of ICU stay (23 vs 30 days), and shorter duration of sedation and use of vasopressors. An important confounder in this trial, however, was that all patients on pressure-control ventilation were initially paralyzed, favoring the APRV group. In 2004, a study randomized 58 patients with acute lung injury (ALI) after stabilization to either APRV or pressure-controlled synchronized intermittent mandatory ventilation [14]. There were no significant differences in the clinically important outcomes, such as ventilator-free days, sedation days, need of hemodialysis, or ICU-free days.

Neurally-adjusted Ventilatory Assist

Overview and physiology

Diaphragmatic electromyography (EMG) as a tool to study respiration was first described in 1959. In the 1990s, however, work was done by Sinderby et al. [15] who developed electrodes lodged in a nasogastric tube that permitted reliable diaphragm EMG signal acquisition, reflecting the patient's neural respiratory drive in real time, and minimizing artifacts and noise. The mode of ventilation that converts this electrical activity into a proportionally assisted and synchronized breath is known as neutrally-adjusted ventilatory assist (NAVA).

The purpose of mechanical ventilation is to provide appropriate unloading of the respiratory muscles and to maintain adequate gas exchange until the respiratory disease that is responsible for the patient's respiratory failure has improved. Short-term mechanical ventilation itself is associated with rapid diaphragmatic dysfunction and atrophy [16–18]. Partial support modes that permit diaphragmatic effort or allow for periods of spontaneous breathing may alleviate some of the ventilator-induced diaphragmatic dysfunction (VIDD). On the other hand, patient-ventilator asynchrony is present in 25 % of patients receiving mechanical ventilation in the ICU [19] and may contribute to patient discomfort, sleep fragmentation, higher use of sedation, development of delirium, VILI, prolonged mechanical ventilation, and ultimately death.

How does it work?

During spontaneous breathing, the respiratory signal originates in the brainstem and is transmitted down the phrenic nerve to the diaphragm, causing electrical excitation. The diaphragm then contracts, creating negative pressure in the chest. This negative pressure results in air being drawn into the lung, producing lung expansion and changes in pulmonary pressures, flow, and volume. Neural feedback from various sensors regulates the respiratory drive during spontaneous breathing on a breath-by-breath basis. This regulation system involves responses to stretch receptors in the lung, the Hering-Breuer reflex, and changes in lung compliance, upper airway receptors, peripheral chemoreceptors in the carotid body, and central chemoreceptors localized in the brainstem.

The NAVA approach to mechanical ventilation is based on the patient's neural respiratory output. By using a nasogastric tube with embedded electrodes, the electrical activity of the diaphragm (Edi) is detected and is transmitted to the ventilator. The ventilator assists the spontaneous breath by delivering pressure directly and linearly proportional to the Edi. Therefore, the peak inspiratory pressure (PIP) delivered is proportional to the neural respiratory drive. Inspiration (pressure delivery) is maintained until the electrical activity decreases by 30 % of the peak pressure generated, and then the breath is terminated. NAVA works on the principle that there is nothing wrong with the patient's respiratory neural center, just an imbalance between the amount of work of breathing they need to do and their ability to do that work. NAVA, like other forms of proportional assist ventilation allows the patient to drive the ventilator, rather than the ventilator driving the patient.

Advantages

- Optimal ventilation based on the patient's ongoing needs, providing them the ability to use physiologic feedback to control ventilation and comfort for each breath.
- Reduced work of breathing, fewer missed patient trigger efforts. Intrinsic PEEP will not affect triggering in NAVA.
- Improved synchrony – the patient's diaphragmatic electrical activity controls onset, breath delivery and cycling off of the breath.
- Reduced need for sedation and/or paralysis.

Disadvantages

- Cannot be used if the respiratory center, phrenic nerve and neuromuscular junction are not intact.
- The Edi signal may not be present if patient is over ventilated. This may be a result of too high a pressure support level or NAVA level if in NAVA mode.
- Contraindications to insertion of a nasogastric tube (malformations, bleeding, varices, tumors, infections, stenosis or rupture).

Clinical evidence in ARDS

The evidence base for NAVA in ARDS is limited to small studies showing feasibility and focused on physiological endpoints. Colombo et al. [20] compared varying levels of pressure support with matched NAVA levels in 14 patients with acute respiratory failure of varied etiologies. Gas exchange was not affected by the mode or assist level. The differences in breathing pattern, ventilator assistance, and respiratory drive and timing between PSV and NAVA were small, overall, at the two lower assist levels. At the highest assist, however, tidal volumes were greater, breathing frequency lower, and electrical activity of the diaphragm smaller in PSV than in NAVA. There was mismatch between neural and flow-based timing in PSV but not in NAVA and the rate of asynchronous events exceeded 10 % in five (36 %) patients on PSV, but none on NAVA. In summary, compared to PSV, NAVA averted the risk of over-assistance, avoided patient-ventilator asynchronies, and improved the overall patient-ventilator interaction.

In 15 ICU patients, Lecomte et al. [21] progressively increased the NAVA level, hypothesizing that the corresponding increase in airway pressure and tidal volume would be limited at a NAVA level where adequate unloading of the respiratory muscles was achieved. Indeed, tidal volume reached a plateau at around 6 ml/kg, while diaphragm electrical activity progressively decreased in response to increases in NAVA support. Meanwhile, Patroniti and colleagues [22] compared different assistance levels of NAVA versus PSV examining the effects on respiratory pattern, breathing variability, and the incidence of tidal volumes above 8 and 10 ml/kg. These authors found that NAVA improved synchrony, while maintaining oxygenation and protective tidal volumes.

Conclusions

ARDS remains a life-threatening form of respiratory failure with long term consequences in survivors. Mechanical ventilation represents the mainstay supportive treatment of ARDS and several of the non-conventional modes may have a role in future management. Of the four modes we reviewed here, PRVC is closest to conventional ventilation and is already in common use because much of the evidence about conventional lung protective ventilation can reasonably be applied to this mode. There are new data available about HFOV that suggest it should be used cautiously in adults with ARDS and likely reserved as rescue therapy for refractory hypoxemia. APRV has potential pros – the ability to recruit the lung while simultaneously preserving spontaneous breathing – and cons – the potential for cyclic overdistention and atelectrauma – the balance of which has not yet been adequately described. Large trials are needed in this area. Finally, NAVA represents a paradigm shift in how patients interact with ventilators, resulting in excellent synchrony and essentially putting the patient back in charge of their respiratory pattern. How this will translate into effects on clinical outcomes in ARDS has not yet been assessed.

New modes of conventional ventilation are appearing all the time, often with very limited data about their clinical implications. As an ICU community we should take it upon ourselves to adequately study these innovations. Until such time as data on outcomes become available, one must weigh the potential benefits of choosing a novel mode of ventilation against the existing data for conventional modes. Whatever mode is ultimately chosen for a patient, clinicians should always keep in mind that simply selecting a given mode is not enough – how we use it may be even more important.

References

1. The Acute Respiratory Distress Syndrome Network (2000) Ventilation with lower tidal volumes as compared with traditional tidal volumes for acute lung injury and the acute respiratory distress syndrome. N Engl J Med 342:1301–1308
2. Briel M, Meade M, Mercat A et al (2010) Higher vs lower positive end-expiratory pressure in patients with acute lung injury and acute respiratory distress syndrome: systematic review and meta-analysis. JAMA 303:865–873
3. Guldager H, Nielsen SL, Carl P et al (1997) A comparison of volume control and pressure-regulated volume control ventilation in acute respiratory failure. Crit Care 1:75–77
4. Riverso P, Bernardi PL, Corsa D et al (1998) A comparison of ventilation techniques in ARDS. Volume controlled vs pressure regulated volume control. Minerva Anestesiol 64:339–343
5. Lunkenheimer PP, Rafflenbeul W, Keller H et al (1972) Application of transtracheal pressure oscillations as a modification of "diffusion respiration". Br J Anaesth 44:627
6. Bryan AC (2001) The oscillations of HFO. Am J Respir Crit Care Med 163:816–817
7. Derdak S, Mehta S, Stewart TE et al (2002) High-frequency oscillatory ventilation for acute respiratory distress syndrome in adults: a randomized, controlled trial. Am J Respir Crit Care Med 166:801–808
8. Sud S, Sud M, al Friedrichet JO (2010) High frequency oscillation in patients with acute lung injury and acute respiratory distress syndrome (ARDS): systematic review and meta-analysis. BMJ 340:1–11
9. Young D, Lamb SE, Shah S et al (2013) High-frequency oscillation for acute respiratory distress syndrome. N Engl J Med 368:806–813
10. Ferguson ND, Cook DJ, Guyatt GH et al (2013) High-frequency oscillation in early acute respiratory distress syndrome. N Engl J Med 10:795–805
11. Downs JB, Stock MC (1987) Airway pressure release ventilation: a new concept in ventilatory support. Crit Care Med 15:459–461
12. Gonzalez M, Arroliga A, Frutos-Vivar F et al (2010) Airway pressure release ventilation versus assist-control ventilation: a comparative propensity score and international cohort study. Intensive Care Med 36:817–827
13. Putensen C, Zech S, Wrigge H et al (2001) Long term effects of spontaneous breathing during ventilatory support during ventilatory support in patients with acute lung injury. Am J Respir Crit Care Med 164:43–49

14. Varpula T, Valta P, Niemi R et al (2004) Airway pressure release ventilation as a primary ventilatory mode in acute respiratory distress syndrome. Acta Anaesthesiol Scand 48:722–731
15. Sinderby C, Navalesi P, Beck J et al (1999) Neural control of mechanical ventilation in respiratory failure. Nature Med 5:1433–1436
16. Levine S, Nguyen T, Taylor N et al (2008) Rapid disuse atrophy of diaphragmatic fibers in mechanically ventilated humans. N Engl J Med 358:1327–1335
17. Froese AB, Bryan C (1974) Effects of anesthesia and paralysis on diaphragmatic mechanics in man. Anesthesiology 41:242–255
18. Knisely AS, Leal SM, Singer DB (1988) Abnormalities of diaphragmatic muscle in neonates with ventilated lungs. J Pediatr 113:1074–1077
19. Thille AW, Cabello B, Galia F, Lyazidi A, Brochard L (2008) Reduction of patient-ventilator asynchrony by reducing tidal volume during pressure-support ventilation. Intensive Care Med 34:1477–1486
20. Colombo D, Cammarota G, Bergamaschi V, De Lucia M, Corte FD, Navalesi P (2008) Physiological response to varying levels of pressure support and neurally adjusted ventilatory assist in patients with acute respiratory failure. Intensive Care Med 34:2010–2018
21. Lecomte F, Brander L, Jalde F et al (2009) Physiological response to increasing levels of neurally adjusted ventilatory assist (NAVA). Respir Physiol Neurobiol 166:117–124
22. Patroniti N, Bellani G, Saccavino E et al (2012) Respiratory pattern during neurally adjusted ventilatory assist in acute respiratory failure patients. Intensive Care Med 38:230–239

Part V
Acute Respiratory Distress Syndrome

ARDS: A Clinical Syndrome or a Pathological Entity?

P. Cardinal-Fernández, A. Ballén Barragán, and J. A. Lorente

Introduction

Despite substantial advances in the understanding of the pathogenesis of the acute respiratory distress syndrome (ARDS), no specific pharmacologic treatment has been shown to affect outcome [1]. This failure has been attributed in part to a lack of a reliable definition for ARDS [2, 3]. Indeed, how the target population is defined for a clinical trial affects the results and their generalizability. Studies including patients with a low probability of responding to the treatment under study (because they are unlikely to have the diagnosis or because of other reasons) are likely to yield false-negative results [4, 5]. Thus a reliable definition of ARDS is essential for research (clinical trials, epidemiologic studies, and studies on pathogenesis) and for clinical practice (to reliably make a diagnosis of ARDS and provide appropriate treatment). In this context several relevant questions arise: What are the different diagnostic criteria for the definition of ARDS? What are the diagnostic test characteristics of these different criteria considering diffuse alveolar damage (DAD) as the histological reference for the diagnosis of ARDS? Does the clinical phenotype of ARDS correlate with one or with more histological entities? Is DAD the sole histological manifestation of ARDS?

P. Cardinal-Fernández
Department of Critical Care, Hospital Universitario de Getafe, Madrid, Spain
CIBER de Enfermedades Respiratorias, Madrid, Spain

A. Ballén Barragán
Department of Pathology, Hospital Universitario de Getafe, Madrid, Spain

J. A. Lorente ✉
Department of Critical Care, Hospital Universitario de Getafe, Madrid, Spain
CIBER de Enfermedades Respiratorias, Madrid, Spain
Universidad Europea de Madrid, Madrid, Spain
e-mail: joseangel.lorente@salud.madrid.org

J.-L. Vincent (Ed.), *Annual Update in Intensive Care and Emergency Medicine 2014*,
DOI 10.1007/978-3-319-03746-2_17, © Springer International Publishing Switzerland
2014

Original Definition

Although much has been written on ARDS, it is of interest to review how patients with ARDS were identified in the first description of the syndrome [6]. The first description of ARDS appeared in 1967, when Ashbaugh and colleagues described 12 patients with acute respiratory distress (4 with multiple trauma, 1 with chest trauma, 1 with gunshot wound to the chest, 1 with gunshot wound to the abdomen, 1 with pancreatitis, and 4 with probable viral pneumonia) characterized by "dyspnea, tachypnea, cyanosis that is refractory to oxygen therapy, decreased lung compliance, and diffuse alveolar infiltrates evident on the chest radiograph" [6]. X-ray findings included patchy, bilateral alveolar infiltrates, frequently confused with acute heart failure and mild pulmonary edema, evolving before death to consolidation. The theoretical relationship of this syndrome to an alveolar surface agent was postulated. Similar cases of respiratory failure in combination with prolonged cardiopulmonary bypass (CPB), congestive atelectasis, viral pneumonia and with fat-embolism had been reported (cited in [6]) at the time of this initial report [6].

The microscopic appearance of lung tissue in five patients who died early in their course was described as "hyperemia, dilated engorged capillaries, and areas of alveolar atelectasis". Interstitial and intra-alveolar hemorrhage and edema were also common [6]. Alveolar macrophages were numerous. A striking finding was the presence of hyaline membranes in all but one patient. Diffuse interstitial fibrosis without notable hyperemia was present in two patients who died after a protracted course. Both patients had hyaline membranes.

The Concept of ARDS

In classical thought, a definition was taken to be a statement of the essence of a thing. A definition of the object must include the essential attributes that form its "essential nature". What then is ARDS? A recently convened international expert panel conference agreed that "ARDS is a type of acute diffuse, inflammatory lung injury, leading to increased pulmonary vascular permeability, increased lung weight, and loss of aerated lung tissue" [3]. Very similar definitions have been provided in other consensus conferences and review articles, all of which include acute inflammation and increased endothelial and epithelial permeability to protein as elements of the ARDS conceptual model [7, 8].

The clinical hallmark of this syndrome includes:
(i)   a risk factor for the development of ARDS;
(ii) severe hypoxemia;
(iii) bilateral pulmonary infiltrates;
(iv) no clinical evidence of cardiogenic pulmonary edema (although ARDS can also occur in the setting of left ventricular [LV] failure);
(v)   the presence of physiological abnormalities, such as increased venous admixture, increased physiological dead space, and decreased lung compliance [3, 9].

The corresponding pathologic findings are lung edema, inflammation and hemorrhage, hyaline membranes, and alveolar epithelial cell injury (i. e., DAD) [3, 10].

ARDS Definitions

ARDS is caused by an inflammatory insult to the alveolocapillary membrane that results in increased permeability and subsequent interstitial and alveolar edema [9]. However, it is not yet possible to measure capillary and alveolar permeability at the bedside. Thus, diagnosis has to rely on a combination of clinical, gas exchange and X-ray findings that reflect the presence of pulmonary inflammation and hyperpermeability pulmonary edema. These criteria lack sufficient specificity (see below), as they often identify patients that do not fit the conceptual model of ARDS.

In the case of ARDS, four clinical definitions are commonly used to define this population for studies: the American-European consensus conference (AECC) definition [7], the lung injury score (LIS) [11], the Delphi definition [12] and the Berlin definition [3].

The 1994 AECC considered as diagnostic criteria gas exchange (PaO_2/FiO_2 ratio ≤ 200), X-ray findings (bilateral infiltrates), clinical presentation (acute onset) and evidence for absence of hydrostatic pulmonary edema (pulmonary artery occlusion pressure [PAOP] ≤ 18 mmHg or no clinical suspicion of left atrial hypertension) [7]. This definition also recognized different degrees of severity, defining acute lung injury (ALI) as a less severe form of respiratory dysfunction characterized by a $PaO_2/FiO_2 \leq 300$, and ARDS if gas exchange is more severely affected with a PaO_2/FiO_2 ratio ≤ 200.

The LIS definition included a score from 0 to 4 in four domains (PaO_2/FiO_2 ratio, presence of consolidation in 0 to 4 quadrants on chest X-ray, positive end-expiratory pressure (PEEP) level, and compliance) [11]. The total score is divided by the number of domains. ARDS is diagnosed if LIS > 2.5.

The Delphi definition also assessed four domains: Hypoxemia (PaO_2/FiO_2 ratio ≤ 200 with PEEP ≥ 10 cmH$_2$O); chest X-ray (bilateral airspace disease); onset (within 72 h of the insult); and non-cardiogenic origin of the edema (subjective assessment on the absence of clinical evidence of congestive heart failure) [12]. All four criteria have to be present for a diagnosis of ARDS, in addition to at least one of two additional criteria: Objective evidence of non-cardiogenicon-cardiogenic edema (PAOP ≤ 8 mmHg or LV ejection fraction $\geq 40\%$) or presence of a recognized risk factor for ARDS.

The Berlin Definition

The Berlin definition proposed three mutually exclusive categories of ARDS based on the degree of hypoxemia: Mild (200 mmHg $< PaO_2/FiO_2 \leq 300$ mmHg with PEEP or continuous positive airway pressure [CPAP] ≥ 5 cmH$_2$O), moderate $(100\,\text{mmHg} < \text{PaO}_2/\text{FIO}_2 \leq 200\,\text{mmHg}$ with PEEP $\geq 5\,\text{cmH}_2\text{O})$, and severe $(\text{PaO}_2/\text{FiO}_2 \leq 100\,\text{mmHg}$ with PEEP $\geq 5\,\text{cmH}_2\text{O})$ [3].

Using the Berlin definition, stages of mild, moderate, and severe ARDS were associated with increased mortality (27 %, 95 % confidence interval [CI] 24–30 %; 32 %, 95 % CI 29–34 %; and 45 %, 95 % CI 42–48 %, respectively) and increased median duration of mechanical ventilation in survivors (5 days, interquartile range [IQR] 2–11; 7 days, IQR 4–14; and 9 days, IQR 5–17, respectively). Although not part of the definition, a subgroup of particular severity was identified, characterized by a $\text{PaO}_2/\text{FiO}_2 \leq 100\,\text{mmHg}$ and either a respiratory system compliance $\leq 20\,\text{ml/cmH}_2\text{O}$ or a corrected minute ventilation $\geq 13\,\text{l/min}$ (corrected minute ventilation is a surrogate of dead space ventilation and is calculated as the measured minute ventilation multiplied by the arterial partial pressure of carbon dioxide [PaCO_2] divided by 40 mmHg). This higher-risk subgroup among patients with severe ARDS included 15 % of the entire ARDS population and had a mortality of 52 % (95 % CI 48–56 %). Patients with severe ARDS who did not meet the higher-risk subset criteria included 13 % of the entire ARDS population and had a mortality rate of 37 % (95 % CI 33–41) [3].

This updated and revised Berlin Definition for ARDS addressed a number of the limitations of the AECC definition:

(i)   the timing from insult to onset of disease was stated as "acute onset" in the AECC definition, and within a specified timeframe (1 week since the insult) in the Berlin definition;

(ii) the ALI category ($\text{PaO}_2/\text{FiO}_2$ ratio ≤ 300 in the AECC) becomes a subgroup of ARDS patients with less severity;

(iii) the gas exchange criterion ($\text{PaO}_2/\text{FiO}_2$ ratio ≤ 300 for ALI and ≤ 200 for ARDS, regardless of PEEP) has to be met with a minimal PEEP $\geq 5\,\text{cmH}_2\text{O}$ in the Berlin definition;

(iv) the chest radiograph criterion is clarified (bilateral opacities not fully explained by effusions, lobar/lung collapse, or nodules; findings could be demonstrated on CT scan instead of chest radiograph);

(v)   the cardiogenic cause of the pulmonary edema criterion is modified (it is only required that hydrostatic edema is not the primary cause of respiratory failure);

(vi) the presence of a risk factor, not considered in the AECC, is required in the Berlin definition (the diagnosis can be made in the absence of a risk factor, but in this case hydrostatic edema has to be objectively ruled out).

One of the main advantages of the Berlin definition is the proposal of diagnostic criteria sensitive to disease severity, because there is evidence of differential effects of interventions depending on ARDS severity. For example, an individual patient meta-analysis of three large randomized clinical trials of high PEEP suggested harm in patients with mild ARDS, a group unlikely to have DAD [13]. Another meta-analysis suggested benefit from prone ventilation only for the most severe ARDS cases [14].

Specificity of the Definitions According to the Histological Findings

Although the pathologic correlate of ARDS is DAD, studies have demonstrated only moderate agreement between the clinical diagnosis of ARDS and DAD at autopsy [2, 15–19]. In a series of autopsy cases, Pinheiro et al. found that DAD was present in 5 of 10 patients with the clinical diagnosis of ARDS (50%) and in 2 of 12 without a clinical diagnosis of ARDS [16]. Sarmiento et al. studied 17 cases with extrapulmonary ARDS and found that DAD was present in 15 (88%) [17]. In another series of 49 autopsy cases with the clinical diagnosis of pneumonia and ARDS, the same group found that DAD was present in 31 (63%) [18]. In a series of 64 patients with a clinical diagnosis of ARDS who died and had a clinical autopsy, de Hemptinne et al. found typical DAD lesions on histological examination in only 32 (50%) [19].

Studies on the specificity of the diagnosis of ARDS using lung biopsy specimens show similar results. Kao et al. studied 41 patients with ARDS of < 1 week duration who underwent open lung biopsy for diagnostic purposes, and found that DAD was present in only 12 (29%) [20]. In a series of 57 patients with ARDS undergoing open-lung biopsy, DAD was found in only 23 (40%) [21].

The diagnostic test properties of the different definitions have been formally studied. Esteban et al., using a modified AECC definition (requiring four-quadrant air-space disease to make the diagnosis of ARDS instead of bilateral chest X-ray infiltrates as stated in the AECC definition), studied 382 patients who died in the intensive care unit (ICU) and had an autopsy examination. Among 127 patients with a diagnosis of ARDS, only 84 (66%) had DAD [15]. Sensitivity was 75% and specificity 84%. Specificity decreased to 75% among patients with a risk factor for ARDS, and was greater in cases with extrapulmonary ARDS than in cases with pulmonary ARDS (78% versus 69%).

Ferguson et al. compared the diagnostic test properties of three different ARDS definitions [2] in a study of 138 cases receiving mechanical ventilation for more than 12 h that died in the ICU and were autopsied (excluding those that died > 14 days after the last intubation). DAD was present in 42 patients and clinical ARDS was diagnosed in 82, 53 and 46 patients, using AECC, LIS, and Delphi definitions, respectively. In patients with a clinical diagnosis of ARDS, DAD was present at autopsy in 35/82 (43%), 31/53 (58%), and 29/46 (63%) patients, using AECC, LIS, and Delphi definitions, respectively. Sensitivities and specificities (95% confidence intervals) were, respectively, 0.83 (0.72–0.95) and 0.51 (0.41–0.61) (AECC); 0.74 (0.61–0.87) and 0.77 (0.69–0.86) (LIS); and 0.69 (0.55–0.83) and 0.82 (0.75–0.90) (Delphi definition).

In a more recent study in a large series of 712 autopsy cases, among the 356 patients who met the Berlin definition of ARDS, only 159 (45%) had DAD [22]. The Berlin definition had sensitivity and specificity for identification of DAD of 89% and 63%, respectively, among all autopsies studied, and 98% and 31% among patients with at least one risk factor for ARDS. The presence of DAD varied with the severity of ARDS according to the Berlin definition: DAD was found in 12%, 40%

and 58 % of patients with mild, moderate and severe ARDS, respectively, according to the Berlin definition. In this study, 14 % of patients meeting the clinical diagnostic criteria for ARDS had normal lungs at autopsy examination [22]. This finding may represent atelectasis that resolved during the fixation process or false positive X-ray interpretation because of the presence of pleural effusion or soft tissue opacities [23, 24].

A number of conditions can be diagnosed in patients with the clinical syndrome of ARDS that do not show DAD on histological examination, including pneumonia, edema, malignancy and other conditions [16–22] (Box 1).

Box 1:
Pathological entities diagnosed in patients with the clinical syndrome of ARDS and who do not have diffuse alveolar damage (DAD) on histological examination [16–22]
- Pneumonia
- Diffuse alveolar hemorrhage
- Edema
- Pulmonary embolism
- Pulmonary infarction
- Metastatic disease
- Pulmonary lymphoma
- Lymphangitic tumor
- Emphysema
- Specific bacterial or fungal infections
    - Tuberculosis
    - *Pneumocystis jiroveci* pneumonia
    - Allergic bronchopulmonary aspergillosis
    - Cytomegalovirus pneumonitis
- Eosinophilic pneumonia
- Fibrosis
- Organizing pneumonia
- Wegener´s granulomatosis
- Usual interstitial pneumonia (UIP)
- Desquamative interstitial pneumonia (DIP)
- Bronchiolitis obliterans organizing pneumonia (BOOP)
- Non-specific interstitial pneumonitis
- Organizing pneumonia
- Interstitial pneumonitis
- Bronchiolitis
- Drug reaction
- Hypersensitivity pneumonia
- Metastatic calcification

What are the Clinical Correlates of DAD?

DAD is the histological manifestation of ALI due to a variety of insults that damage the alveolar epithelium and the capillary endothelium. Epithelial and endothelial injury result in the formation of cell debris that form, in combination with coagulation and other plasma proteins, intraalveolar eosinophilic linear structures termed hyaline membranes. The acute phase is followed by a reparative organizing, proliferative, or fibroproliferative stage, characterized by rapid proliferation of fibroblasts within the interstitium. The presence of histologically diffuse fibroblast proliferation differentiates DAD in the organizing phase from usual interstitial pneumonia (UIP), in which fibrosis is manifested by collagen deposition rather than by massive fibroblast proliferation [25].

DAD is the defining characteristic of acute interstitial pneumonia (AIP) [26]. The term AIP was introduced in 1986 by Katzenstein et al. to designate the cases previously known as the Hamman-Rich syndrome, in order to distinguish these cases clinically and histologically from chronic forms of idiopathic interstitial lung disease, such as UIP (the histological correlate of idiopathic pulmonary fibrosis) [27,28]. AIP is an idiopathic pulmonary disease that is characterized by rapid onset of respiratory failure. The clinical manifestations of AIP fit into what is clinically defined as ARDS. Radiologically, AIP is characterized by the presence of bilateral lung infiltrates, patchy or diffuse, often described as alveolar. CT shows bilateral ground-glass opacities and/or bilateral airspace consolidation [25]. Histological findings in AIP are those of DAD: Formation of hyaline membranes (acute phase), followed by fibroblast migration into the alveolar septa and finally interstitial thickening by fibroblasts. Other findings are alveolar collapse/atelectasis, hyperplasia of type 2 pneumocytes, edema within the alveolar septa, thrombi within small pulmonary arteries, squamous metaplasia, and mild interstitial chronic inflammation. AIP differs clinicopathologically from the other types of interstitial pneumonia in that it shows diffuse interstitial fibrosis [25].

The term AIP is applied to cases of DAD of unknown cause. The lack of an identifiable etiology defines the entity, in analogy to UIP, which is a term used when there is a known etiology, and idiopathic pulmonary fibrosis, a term used when the etiology is unknown [25]. As AIP is an idiopathic entity, other causes of DAD should be excluded before making the diagnosis. Causes of DAD include sepsis, drug toxicity (most commonly chemotherapeutic agents, such as bleomycin and busulfan, amiodarone and nitrofurantoin), connective tissue disease, complications of lung transplantation, oxygen toxicity, and aspiration. Indeed, any risk factor for ARDS (as the clinical syndrome designating cases with DAD of known cause) can be included in the list, such as sepsis, trauma, blood transfusion, or pancreatitis.

The differential diagnosis of AIP (i. e., idiopathic DAD) should include causes of acute respiratory failure and alveolar infiltrates on the chest X-ray (e. g., hydrostatic pulmonary edema), and known causes of DAD (e. g., ARDS). In addition, some patients with known UIP/idiopathic pulmonary fibrosis develop superimposed DAD, often of unknown cause, and also present clinically as ARDS [29]. Whether DAD presents different histological characteristics according to the cause was examined by Kang et al. [30] who studied 26 autopsy cases of DAD. Clinicians were asked to classify the cases into those due to infection ($n = 7$), tumor chemotherapy or drug toxicity ($n = 16$) or AIP ($n = 3$). Unfortunately, cases of DAD due to other causes were excluded. All cases with DAD had clinical criteria for a diagnosis of ARDS. Intraalveolar fibrosis was observed in most cases. All 7 cases of DAD due to severe infection showed multiple organ dysfunction syndrome, only 2 of 7 patients showed interstitial myofibroblast proliferation, and thrombi were identified in 4 of 7. When DAD was attributed to tumor chemotherapy or drug toxicity, only 3 of 16 patients showed multiple organ dysfunction syndrome, 15 showed interstitial myofibroblast proliferation, and 6 showed thrombi formation. Of the 3 cases diagnosed as AIP, none showed multiple organ dysfunction syndrome, 3 showed marked interstitial myofibroblast proliferation, and thrombi were identified in 1. The cases in the severe infection group showed a predominance of intra-alveolar myofibroblasts, whereas myofibroblasts were markedly present not only in the intra-alveolar spaces but also within the swollen alveolar interstitia in most cases of DAD due to tumor chemotherapy and drug toxicity and AIP [30]. These results suggest that the pathophysiologic mechanism of DAD caused by severe infection involves a systemic insult, and the mechanism underlying DAD due to tumor chemotherapy or drug toxicity appears to involve interstitial pneumonia-like lesions, similar to AIP.

Is DAD the Sole Histological Correlate of ARDS?

Many experts agree that the most common histological finding in ARDS is DAD [19, 21, 30–33]. ARDS shows the same rapid evolution from diffuse pulmonary edema to fibrosis through the proliferation of myofibroblasts and collagen deposition in the alveoli. The injury/repair process includes microvascular thrombosis, endothelial and epithelial injury, inflammation, apoptosis, and fibrosis [34, 35]. The question is whether DAD is the sole histological manifestation of ARDS? The definitions alluded to above define merely a clinical entity and do not require particular histological findings. On the other hand, without reference to any histological pattern, ARDS is a term that does not define a specific clinicopathological entity and encompasses a heterogeneous list of conditions rather than a well-defined clinicopathological entity [19, 21,32,36].

The answer depends on the conceptual model of ARDS. One may consider ARDS as a primary clinical phenotype with a variety of pathologic findings or as a pathologically defined entity with variable clinical presentations [2, 3, 15, 22, 23, 37]. As stated, members of the recently convened Berlin definition panel were not in complete agreement that DAD is the sole pathologic correlate of ARDS [37], and some considered pneumonia and non-cardiogenic edema as compatible with ARDS when clinical criteria are met [23]. It is interesting to note that, in the study by Thille et al., if the pathological findings of pneumonia without DAD were added to the cases of DAD, then DAD or pneumonia, or both, was identified in 88 % of the ARDS cases by the Berlin definition [22, 23]. Thus the Berlin definition is quite specific for identifying cases of DAD and pneumonia, which is the most common clinical cause of ARDS, and it has been proposed that pneumonia in the histological examination be added to the pathological correlate of ARDS, which would be important for clinical-pathological studies of ARDS [23]. The Berlin definition identifies a group of patients having respiratory failure due to acute lung inflammation (DAD and pneumonia without DAD). The finding of a higher frequency of DAD in patients with greater ARDS severity [22] suggests that patients with pneumonia but still without hyaline membranes could represent a less severe form of lung injury. Further, it is reasonable to think that these patients with the clinical syndrome of ARDS and pneumonia (albeit without hyaline membranes) at autopsy examination have lung inflammation and increased alveolocapillary permeability, as the defining characteristics of ARDS. Indeed, that patients with clinical ARDS and pneumonia without DAD on histological examination have a different clinical course and different response to therapies than patients with DAD has not been proven.

The diagnostic criteria of the Berlin definition identify a clinical phenotype of ARDS that includes DAD, pneumonia and other findings such as alveolar hemorrhage and edema [23]. Indeed, transient hydrostatic edema coexists with increased permeability to protein in approximately 30 % of patients with a clinical diagnosis of ARDS [38]. In addition, mortality was reduced with low tidal volume ventilation in all patients with ALI associated with various conditions, which likely included patients who did not have DAD [39, 40].

Conclusions

Current clinical definitions of ARDS identify patients with DAD with a low specificity. Only around 50–60 % of patients with the clinical syndrome are found at autopsy or lung biopsy to show the characteristic histological findings of DAD. This lack of specificity represents a challenge for appropriate patient selection for clinical trials to test new therapies, and makes it harder for clinicians to make the diagnosis in a specific manner and, therefore, be able to implement effective preventive or therapeutic measures in patients with ARDS. The lack of correlation between the clinical manifestations and the histological findings emphasizes the need for a more complete biological characterization of the syndrome, including research on diagnostic biomarkers (e. g., gene expression patterns, proteomics, metabolomics) for the identification of cases according to their clinicopathological phenotype.

References

1. Fanelli V, Vlachou A, Ghannadian S, Simonetti U, Slutsky AS, Zhang H (2013) Acute respiratory distress syndrome: new definition, current and future therapeutic options. J Thorac Dis 5:326–334
2. Ferguson ND, Frutos-Vivar F, Esteban A et al (2005) Acute respiratory distress syndrome: under recognition by clinicians and diagnostic accuracy of three clinical definitions. Crit Care Med 33:2228–2234

3. The ARDS Definition Task Force (2012) Acute respiratory distress syndrome: the Berlin definition. JAMA 307:2526–2533
4. Sackett DL (2001) Why randomized controlled trials fail but needn't: 2. Failure to employ physiological statistics, or the only formula a clinician-trialist is ever likely to need (or understand!). CMAJ 165:1226–1237
5. Wood KA, Huang D, Angus DC (2003) Improving clinical trial design in acute lung injury. Crit Care Med 31:S305–S311
6. Ashbaugh DG, Bigelow DB, Petty TL, Levine BE (1967) Acute respiratory distress in adults. Lancet 2:319–323
7. Bernard GR, Artigas A, Brigham KL et al (1994) The American-European Consensus Conference on ARDS: definitions, mechanisms, relevant outcomes, and clinical trial coordination. Am J Respir Crit Care Med 149:818–824
8. Matthay MA, Ware LB, Zimmerman GA (2012) The acute respiratory distress syndrome. J Clin Invest 122:2731–2740
9. Villar J (2001) What is the acute respiratory distress syndrome? Respiratory Care 56:1539–1545
10. Katzenstein AL, Bloor CM, Leibow AA (1976) Diffuse alveolar damage – the role of oxygen, shock, and related factors: a review. Am J Pathol 85:209–228
11. Murray JF, Matthay MA, Luce JM et al (1988) An expanded definition of the adult respiratory distress syndrome. Am Rev Respir Dis 138:720–723
12. Ferguson ND, Davis AM, Slutsky AS et al (2005) Development of a clinical definition for acute respiratory distress syndrome using the Delphi technique. J Crit Care 20:147–154
13. Briel M, Meade M, Mercat A et al (2010) Higher vs lower positive end-expiratory pressure in patients with acute lung injury and acute respiratory distress syndrome: systematic review and meta-analysis. JAMA 303:865–873
14. Cesana BM, Antonelli P, Chiumello D, Gattinoni L (2010) Positive end-expiratory pressure, prone positioning, and activated protein C: a critical review of meta-analyses. Minerva Anestesiol 76:929–936
15. Esteban A, Fernández-Segoviano P, Frutos-Vivar F et al (2004) Comparison of clinical criteria for the acute respiratory distress syndrome with autopsy findings. Ann Intern Med 141:440–445
16. Pinheiro BV, Muraoka FS, Assis RV et al (2007) Accuracy of clinical diagnosis of acute respiratory distress syndrome in comparison with autopsy findings. J Bras Pneumol 33:423–428
17. Sarmiento X, Almirall J, Guardiola JJ et al (2011) Estudio sobre la correlación clínico-patológica en el síndrome de distrés respiratorio agudo secundario. Med Intensiva 35:22–27
18. Sarmiento X, Guardiola JJ, Almirall J et al (2011) Discrepancy between clinical criteria for diagnosing acute respiratory distress syndrome secondary to community acquired pneumonia with autopsy findings of diffuse alveolar damage. Respir Med 105:1170–1175
19. de Hemptinne Q, Remmelink M, Brimioulle S, Salmon I, Vincent JL (2009) ARDS: a clinico-pathological confrontation. Chest 135:944–949
20. Kao KC, Tsai YH, Wu YK et al (2006) Open lung biopsy in early-stage acute respiratory distress syndrome. Critical Care 10:R106
21. Patel SR, Karmpaliotis D, Ayas NT et al (2004) The role of open-lung biopsy in ARDS. Chest 125:197–202
22. Thille AW, Esteban A, Fernández-Segoviano P et al (2013) Comparison of the Berlin definition for the acute respiratory distress syndrome with autopsy. Am J Respir Crit Care Med 187:761–767
23. Thompson BT, Matthay MA (2013) The Berlin Definition of ARDS versus pathological evidence of diffuse alveolar damage. Am J Respir Crit Care Med 187:675–677
24. Rubenfeld GD, Caldwell E, Granton JT, Hudson LD, Matthay MA (1999) Interobserver variability in applying a radiographic definition for ARDS. Chest 116:1347–1353

25. Mukhopadhyay S, Parambil JG (2012) Acute interstitial pneumonia (AIP): Relationship to Hamman-Rich syndrome, DAD (DAD), and acute respiratory distress syndrome (ARDS). Semin Respir Crit Care Med 33:476–485
26. American Thoracic Society, European Respiratory Society American Thoracic Society (2002) European Respiratory Society International Multidisciplinary Consensus Classification of the Idiopathic Interstitial Pneumonias. This joint statement of the American Thoracic Society (ATS), and the European Respiratory Society (ERS) was adopted by the ATS board of directors, June 2001 and by the ERS Executive Committee, June 2001. Am J Respir Crit Care Med 165:277–304
27. Katzenstein AL, Myers JL, Mazur MT (1986) Acute interstitial pneumonia: a clinicopathologic, ultrastructural, and cell kinetic study. Am J Surg Pathol 10:256–267
28. Katzenstein A-LA, Mukhopadhyay S, Myers JL (2008) Diagnosis of usual interstitial pneumonia and distinction from other fibrosing interstitial lung diseases. Hum Pathol 39:1275–1294
29. Collard HR, Moore BB, Flaherty KR et al (2007) Idiopathic Pulmonary Fibrosis Clinical Research Network Investigators. Acute exacerbations of idiopathic pulmonary fibrosis. Am J Respir Crit Care Med 176:636–643
30. Kang D, Nakayama T, Togashi M et al (2009) Two forms of diffuse alveolar damage in the lungs of patients with acute respiratory distress syndrome. Hum Pathol 40:1618–1627
31. Kaarteenaho R, Kinnula VL (2011) DAD: a common phenomenon in progressive interstitial lung disorders. Pulm Med 2011:531302.
32. Ware LB, Matthay MA (2000) The acute respiratory distress syndrome. N Engl J Med 342:1334–1349
33. Matthay MA, Zimmerman GA, Esmon C et al (2003) Future research directions in acute lung injury: Summary of a National Heart, Lung, and Blood Institute working group. Am J Respir Crit Care Med 167:1027–1035
34. Tomashefski JF Jr, Davies P, Boggis C, Greene R, Zapol WM, Reid LM (1983) The pulmonary vascular lesions of the adult respiratory distress syndrome. Am J Pathol 112:112–126
35. Moloney ED, Evans TW (2003) Pathophysiology and pharmacological treatment of pulmonary hypertension in acute respiratory distress syndrome. Eur Respir J 21:720–727
36. Schwarz MI, Albert RK (2004) "Imitators" of the ARDS: implications for diagnosis and treatment. Chest 125:1530–1535
37. Ferguson ND, Fan E, Camporota L et al (2012) The Berlin definition of ARDS: an expanded rationale, justification, and supplementary material. Intensive Care Med 38:1573–1582
38. Wheeler AP, Bernard GR, Thompson BT et al (2006) Pulmonary-artery versus central venous catheter to guide treatment of acute lung injury. N Engl J Med 354:2213–2224
39. Eisner MD, Thompson BT, Hudson LD et al (2001) Efficacy of low tidal volume ventilation in patients with different clinical risk factors for acute lung injury and the acute respiratory distress syndrome. Am J Respir Crit Care Med 164:231–236
40. The Acute Distress Syndrome Network (2000) Ventilation with lower tidal volumes as compared with traditional tidal volumes for acute lung injury and the acute respiratory distress syndrome. N Engl J Med 342:1301–1308

Novel Pharmacologic Approaches for the Treatment of ARDS

R. Herrero, Y. Rojas, and A. Esteban

Introduction

Acute respiratory distress syndrome (ARDS) is a heterogeneous disease, which is defined by the acute onset of hypoxemic respiratory failure with bilateral infiltrates on chest radiography due primarily to non-cardiogenic pulmonary edema [1]. Only two supportive strategies have shown to improve survival in patients with acute lung injury (ALI)/ARDS, namely lung protective ventilation that reduces the stretch of the lungs and a conservative fluid strategy [2, 3]. The mortality of ARDS, however, remains high and no pharmacological therapies have effectively improved the outcome of these patients so far.

Studies of the pharmacologic management of ARDS, such as trials of anti-inflammatory agents, anticoagulants, surfactant, vasodilators, and β_2 agonists, have shown conflicting results [4]. Potential reasons for such conflicting results may be:
 1) the heterogeneity of the pathophysiologic processes leading to lung injury;
 2) failure to apply therapies to subgroups of patients with an homogeneous disease process; and
 3) inappropriate dosing and route of administration of the drugs.
In the last decade, there has been extensive research into potential therapeutic targets and methods of drug administration that could help in the development of specific pharmacological drugs to prevent or mitigate the development of ARDS.

R. Herrero ✉ · Y. Rojas · A. Esteban
Unidad De Cuidados Intensivos, Fundacion Para La Investigacion Biomedica, Hospital
Universitario De Getafe, Ciber De Enfermedades Respiratorias, Universidad Europea De Madrid,
Getafe, Madrid, Spain
e-mail: raquelher@hotmail.com

J.-L. Vincent (Ed.), *Annual Update in Intensive Care and Emergency Medicine 2014*,   231
DOI 10.1007/978-3-319-03746-2_18, © Springer International Publishing Switzerland
2014

Pathophysiology

Early in ARDS, there is widespread neutrophilic alveolitis with disruption of the alveolar epithelial and endothelial barriers, which leads to the formation of protein-rich edema in the interstitium and alveolar spaces [5]. There is activation of alveolar macrophages and neutrophil recruitment, cell death in the alveolar epithelium and vascular endothelium, deposition of hyaline membranes on the denudated basement membrane, deficient surfactant production that contributes to alveolar collapse, and formation of microthrombi. This scenario evolves to a fibro-proliferative process that fills the airspaces with granulation tissue containing proliferating alveolar type II cells, as well as new blood vessels and extracellular matrix rich in collagen and fibrin. In some patients, this process progresses to irreversible lung fibrosis [6].

Modulation of Neutrophil Migration and Activation

A considerable quantity of neutrophils is present in the bronchoalveolar lavage (BAL) fluid from patients with ARDS. Persistence of elevated numbers of neutrophils correlates with worsening gas exchange and with poor prognosis [7]. The regulation of neutrophil lifespan is known to be critical for maintaining an effective host response and preventing excessive inflammation. One of the mechanisms that controls the number of neutrophils in the lung is the induction of apoptosis. Interestingly, neutrophils are less susceptible to undergo apoptosis under hypoxic conditions, as occurs in the alveoli in ARDS. In this line, the hypoxia-inducible factor (HIF) oxygen-sensing pathway has been shown to play a role in prolonging neutrophil survival during hypoxia. The expression and transcriptional activity of HIF are regulated by the oxygen-sensitive prolyl hydroxylases (PHD1-3) [8]. This suggests that modulation of HIF and PHD1-3 expression aimed at enhancing neutrophil apoptosis may be a potential approach to downregulate inflammation in the early phase of ARDS.

Active neutrophils release a series of enzymes that contribute to lung damage. Neutrophil elastase is a serine protease stored in the azurophilic granules of leukocytes that has been implicated in the pathology of ARDS. Neutrophil elastase seems to promote inflammation, endothelial and epithelial cell injury, extracellular matrix damage and collagen deposition that leads pulmonary fibrosis [9–11]. Sivelestat was the first neutrophil elastase inhibitor tested in humans and it suppressed the production of neutrophil elastase and interleukin (IL)-8, resulting in improved respiratory function in patients with ARDS secondary to cardiopulmonary bypass [12]. In animal models of lung fibrosis, sivelestat not only decreased inflammatory cell recruitment in the acute phase, but also reduced collagen deposition in lung parenchyma in the fibroproliferative phase of ARDS resulting in less fibrosis and better static compliance of the lung. This beneficial effect was also associated with a decrease in transforming growth factor (TGF)-β1 activation and expression of phospho-SMAD2/3, which are mechanisms involved in lung fibrosis [9, 11]. AZD9668 (N-{[5-(methanesulfonyl)pyridin-2-yl]methyl}

-6-methyl-5-(1-methyl-1H-pyrazol-5-yl)-2-oxo-1-[3-(trifluoromethyl)phenyl]-1,2-dihydropyridine-3-carboxamide) is another novel neutrophil elastase inhibitor that can be administered orally. It exerts selective and rapid inhibition of neutrophil elastase that is also reversible. Oral administration of AZD9668 to mice or rats prevented human neutrophil elastase-induced lung tissue injury as assessed by decreased matrix protein degradation products in BAL fluid and reduced inflammatory responses in the lung in acute and chronic lung injury models. Therefore, neutrophil elastase inhibitors may be drugs that could potentially reduce lung inflammation and diminish structural and functional pulmonary changes in human ARDS [13].

Endothelial Protection

Because the cardinal feature of ALI/ARDS is an increase in lung vascular permeability, often precipitated by an exuberant inflammatory response with subsequent endothelial barrier disruption, strategies aimed at promoting endothelial barrier function could serve as novel therapies in this setting. In this regard, several promising agonists have been identified, including lipid mediators (sphingosine 1-phosphate, resolvins), statins, ang-1/2-Tie2 system and activated protein C (APC). All these agonists have in common the ability to directly mediate endothelial cell signaling and induce characteristic actin cytoskeletal rearrangement leading to endothelial cell barrier protection [14].

Sphingosine 1-phosphate

There is increasing evidence that sphingolipids contribute to different pulmonary disorders, including ALI. Sphingolipids are essential constituents of plasma membranes and regulate many pathophysiological cellular responses inducing apoptosis and cell survival, vascular permeability, mast cell activation, and airway smooth muscle functions [15].

Sphingosine-1-phosphate (S1P) exerts a protective effect against ALI. S1P is a potent angiogenic factor that preserves human lung endothelial cell integrity and barrier function [16] preventing the alveolar flooding demonstrated in animal models of ARDS. S1P is a naturally occurring bioactive sphingolipid that acts extracellularly (via its G protein-coupled receptors, S1P1-5) and intracellularly on various targets. The synthesis of S1P is catalyzed by sphingosine kinases 1 and 2, and the degradation of S1P is mediated by lipid S1P phosphatases and S1P lyase, contributing to the control of the S1P cellular responses [15, 16] (Fig. 1). S1P enhances vascular barrier function through a series of cellular events initiated by activation of its G-protein coupled receptor, S1P1, and the subsequent downstream activation of Rho and Rac1. Activation of these intracellular signals results in endothelial cytoskeletal reorganization to form strong cortical actin rings in the cell periphery, and reinforcement of focal adhesions and paracellular junctional complexes

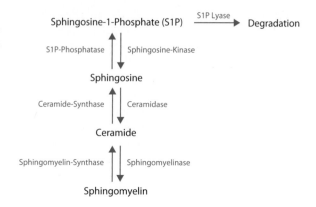

Fig. 1 Overview of sphingolipid metabolism. *Arrows* indicate regulatory enzymes

(cadherin, paxillin, catenins, zona occludens), that prevent excessive vascular permeability [16, 17].

Recent studies show that stimulating the S1P-SIP1 axis reduces vascular permeability, which can be of great value to treat ARDS. S1Ps and S1P analogs, such as FTY720 and ftysiponate, serve as protective agents limiting the disruption of the pulmonary microvascular endothelial barrier and lung edema formation, as well as attenuating parenchymal accumulation of inflammatory cells, which limit the development of ARDS [16, 18]. Another strategy is the prevention of degradation of S1P via inhibition of S1P lyase (S1PL). All these results can be particularly relevant as lung injury was associated with an enhanced S1PL expression and decreased S1P levels in lung tissue in some models of lipopolysaccharide (LPS)-induced ARDS. 2-acetyl-4(5)-[1(R),2(S),3(R),4-tetrahydroxybutyl]-imidazole inhibited S1PL in lung tissue and BAL fluid and reduced lung injury and inflammation in animal models [19].

Resolvins

Resolvins are docosahexaenoic acid (DHA)-derived lipid mediators that constitute novel endogenous pathways of local-acting mediators that possess both anti-inflammatory and pro-resolvin properties [19]. A novel resolvin D1 (RvD1) suppressed production of pro-inflammatory mediators by primary human cells, such as small airway epithelial cells and monocytes, in a dose-dependent manner *in vitro* [20] and attenuated inflammation in LPS-induced ALI *in vivo* [21]. This attenuated lung inflammation was mediated by the suppression of nuclear factor-kappa B (NF-κB) activation through a mechanism partly dependent on peroxisome proliferator-activated receptor gamma (PPARγ) activation. Also, RvD1 significantly reduced macrophages and neutrophil exocytosis and upregulated the expression of the anti-inflammatory cytokine, IL-10, which accelerated the resolution of lung inflammation [20]. In addition, these endogenous mediators seem to have anti-fibrotic and host-directed antimicrobial actions [19]. Thus, resolvins constitute a novel genus of chemical mediators that could be useful for the design of new therapies for ARDS.

Statins

Statins are a class of 3-hydroxy-3-methylglutaryl-coenzyme A-reductase inhibitors that have pleiotropic properties. Statins not only lower cholesterol, but also have other non-lipid-lowering effects that can be beneficial for the management of sepsis and sepsis-induced ARDS, particularly associated with pneumonia [22]. In this context, statins confer lung protection by preserving endothelial function and integrity, reducing vascular leak, and exerting anti-inflammatory and anti-thrombotic effects. In experimental studies of endotoxin-induced lung injury, simvastatin preserved protein permeability preventing lung edema formation, attenuated neutrophil migration to the lung, and reduced endothelial cell-derived cytokine expression (IL-6, IL-8, monocyte chemotactic protein [MCP]-1, regulated upon activation normal T cell expressed and presumably secreted [RANTES]). These protective effects of statins are mediated through the upregulation of the activity of integrin-β4 in endothelial cells. These findings support statins as useful drugs and integrin-β4 as a novel therapeutic target in patients with ALI [23].

Angiopoietin-1/2 System

The angiopoietin (Ang)-1/2 system has been recognized to play a major role in various features of human sepsis and ALI. Ang-1 and Ang-2 bind to the endothelial and the soluble form of the Tie2 receptor (sTie2). Ang-1 induces activation of the endothelial Tie2 receptor, and reduces pulmonary inflammation and endothelial cell permeability. Ang-2 prevents Ang-1 from binding to the endothelial Tie2 receptor, and consequently leads to pulmonary inflammation and increased endothelial cell permeability [24, 25]. This suggests that the Ang-1/2-Tie2 system should be further investigated as it constitutes a potential target for treating patients with ARDS.

Activated Protein C

APC, an endogenous protein that promotes fibrinolysis and inhibits thrombosis, can modulate the coagulation and inflammation associated with ALI. Restoring normal alveolar levels of APC was expected to prevent the progression of pulmonary coagulopathy and to mitigate the intensity of lung damage. However, a recent clinical trial demonstrated that APC did not improve outcomes in patients with ALI, suggesting that the method of APC administration may be important. It has been speculated that APC inhalation, instead of intravenous administration, might provide the expected benefit to patients with ARDS [26, 27]. Furthermore, combination of APC with other anticoagulant agents (including anti-thrombin and

Fig. 2 Schematic of the renin-angiotensin system. ACE: angiotensin-converting enzyme; ACE2: angiotensin-converting enzyme 2; AT$_1$: angiotensin II type 1 receptor; AT$_2$: angiotensin II type 2 receptor

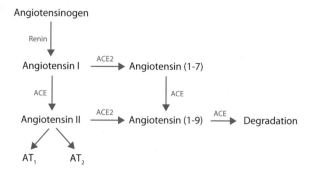

heparin) and pro-fibrinolytic agents (such as plasminogen activators) could be more effective in attenuating pulmonary coagulopathy and inflammation, but this has not been tested yet.

Regulation of the Renin-angiotensin System

Recent studies indicate that the renin-angiotensin system plays a critical role in acute lung diseases. Angiotensin II, a key effector peptide of the system, causes vasoconstriction and exerts multiple biological functions. Angiotensin-converting enzyme (ACE) and ACE2 are homologs with different key functions in the renin-angiotensin system. ACE cleaves angiotensin I to generate angiotensin II, whereas ACE2 reduces angiotensin II levels and thereby functions as a negative regulator of the angiotensin system (Fig. 2). Capillary blood vessels in the lung are a major site of ACE expression and angiotensin II production in the human body [28]. ACE, angiotensin II and the angiotensin II type 1 receptor (AT1) induce apoptosis in the alveolar wall, alter alveolar capillary barrier integrity leading to lung edema, and promote collagen deposition, which can result in lung fibrosis with the consequent impairment of lung function. In contrast, ACE2 and the angiotensin II type 2 receptor (AT2) protect against all these effects (Fig. 2). Indeed, inhibiting ACE and AT1 as well as increasing ACE2 and AT2 activity attenuated lung injury in several animal models of ARDS, and may represent novel approaches for the treatment of ARDS [29–32].

Endotoxin Signaling

Many drugs targeting endotoxin or the endotoxin-induced cytokine storm have been developed with therapeutic purposes in sepsis and sepsis-induced ARDS. Toll-like receptor 4 (TLR4) is activated by LPS or endotoxin, the major component of the outer membrane of Gram-negative bacteria, and constitutes a potent inflammatory stimulus implicated in septic shock and septic-induced ARDS. Activation of TLR4 by LPS depends on LPS binding protein (LBP)-catalyzed extraction and transfer of individual LPS molecules from aggregated LPS to CD14 and then from CD14 to MD2, followed by engagement and dimerization of TLR4. TLR4 signaling may also be activated by stimuli other than LPS. Chemical (acid aspiration) or virus (influenza) insults may cause ALI via the generation of host-derived, oxidized phospholipids that potently stimulate TLR-4 [33]. Eritoran is a potent, well-tolerated, synthetic TLR4 antagonist that protects against influenza-induced ARDS in mice, improving the survival of these animals even when administered as late as 6 days post-infection. Eritoran binds to CD14, which inhibits ligand binding to MD2:TLR4 complexes preventing TLR4 dimerization and activation [34]. In viral infection, eritoran blocks oxidized phospholipid-induced TLR4 signaling, mitigates the subsequent cytokine storm, and also helps to control viral titer. Despite the lack of benefit in severe septic patients (ACCESS trial) [38], eritoran could still be effective in influenza infection and, perhaps, in ALI mediated by non-infectious agents, but its most effective timing and dosing remain unknown. Based on endotoxin challenge studies in animals, the prophylactic or very early administration of eritoran in patients at-risk or with ARDS could be more effective in controlling the 'sepsis cascade'. Antagonism of TLR4 signaling could therefore become a useful therapy for ARDS [35, 36].

Cell Adhesion Molecules

The cell adhesion molecules, integrins and selectins, are transmembrane cell surface receptors that regulate leukocyte migration and activation, endothelial/epithelial cytokine expression and alveolar-capillary protein permeability in the lung [37]. The $\alpha v\beta 5$ and $\alpha v\beta 6$ integrins have an important role on pulmonary endothelial and epithelial cells, respectively. Dysfunction of these molecules alters alveolar endothelial- and epithelial-cell functions and barrier integrity, leading to alveolar flooding. In addition, $\alpha v\beta 6$ integrin, which is upregulated in injured epithelial cells, plays a robust role in the development of lung fibrosis via activation of the TGF-β (a pro-fibrotic cytokine). Prevention of leukocyte-epithelial adhesion by using antagonists of integrins, such as XVA143 (antagonist of α-L/β-2 integrin) or BIO1211 (antagonist of α-4/β-1 integrin), protects alveolar epithelial cells from injury in inflammatory lung diseases [38].

These results identify integrins and selectins as promising therapeutic targets for ALI, in particular in sepsis-induced ARDS [39]. Inhibition of these integrins by specific antibodies has shown therapeutic effects in models of septic shock [40, 41]. In fact, these families of adhesion molecules have been under intense investigation by the pharmaceutical industry. In this regard, antagonists of integrin $\alpha v\beta 3$ (e. g., abciximab), integrin $\alpha L\beta 2$ (efalizumab), and integrin $\alpha 4\beta 1$ (natalizumab) are currently US FDA-approved for acute coronary syndromes, psoriasis and multiple sclerosis, respectively. However, none has been approved for indications related to ARDS. Recently, positive results in phase II clinical trials with a small-molecule selectin antagonist (bimosiamose) and a small-molecule integrin $\alpha 4\beta 1$ antagonist (valategrast, R411) for the management of asthma and chronic obstructive pulmonary disease (COPD) have generated great enthusiasm [37]. The efficacy of these molecules against the development of ARDS may therefore warrant further investigation.

MicroRNA

ARDS is a disease affected by various genetic and non-genetic factors. MicroRNAs (miRNAs) have emerged as a novel class of gene regulators which play critical roles in complex diseases including ARDS. From animal models of ALI, including LPS- and ventilator-induced lung injury (VILI), several miRNAs (e. g., miR-146a, miR-155, miR-16) have been identified as important regulators of inflammatory responses in the lung. For example, upregulation of miR-16 significantly down-regulates IL-6 and TNF-α expression in LPS-induced lung injury [42]. In addition, some miRNAs (hsa-miR-374a, hsa-miR-374b, hsa-miR-520c-3p, and hsa-miR-1290) have been involved in endothelial cell barrier dysfunction and in the increased vascular permeability and formation of lung edema in injured lungs. These miRNAs seem to control endothelial cell barrier via regulation of non-muscle myosin light chain kinase (nmMLCK) expression in human lung endothelium *in vitro*. Thereby, modulation of miRNAs could have important beneficial effects on controlling the development and progression of ARDS [43].

Antihistamines

Endogenous histamine is widely distributed in the lungs and is an important mediator of early and late inflammatory responses. Histamine promotes neutrophil migration, increases cytokine expression, and enhances capillary permeability leading to protein leak. In animal models of ALI, inhaled endotoxin causes an increase in histamine concentration in BAL fluid. Administration of mepyramine (H1-receptor antagonist) or ranitidine (H_2-receptor antagonist) attenuates the increased histamine concentration, but only the administration of ranitidine was associated with a significant reduction in neutrophil numbers and in protein permeability. This study suggests that endogenous histamine may be involved in the recruitment of neutrophils and protein leaks in endotoxin-induced ALI via the H_2 receptors [44]. Also, scavenging of endogenous histamine by the arthropod-derived histamine binding protein, EV131, mitigates endotoxin-induced lung injury, supporting the notion that histamine-mediated signaling could be a potential target in ARDS [45].

Stimulators of Lung Repair

Growth Factors

A series of growth factors, such as keratinocyte-, epithelial-, basic fibroblast-, hepatocyte- and vascular endothelial-growth factor, are emerging as important candidates to repair the damaged pulmonary alveolar capillary membrane. To this end, the synergistic interaction of these growth factors, which directly or indirectly affect pulmonary endothelial and epithelial cells, appears to promote the repair process of lung damage. As an example, the combined effect of trefoil factor family peptides and growth factors, such as epithelial growth factor (EGF), stimulated epithelial proliferation and repair [46].

Erythropoietin

A number of preclinical studies have revealed beneficial effects of exogenous erythropoietin (EPO) administration in various experimental models of ARDS. EPO provides protection by modulating multiple early signaling pathways involved in apoptosis, inflammation and peroxidation. Furthermore, EPO appears to confer vascular protection by promoting angiogenesis. However, only preliminary studies exist and more experimental and clinical data are necessary to clarify the efficacy and cytoprotective mechanisms of EPO [47].

Hyaluronan

Hyaluronan constitutes the major glycosaminoglycan in lung tissue and has diverse functions in normal lung homeostasis and pulmonary disease. Hyaluronan and its degradation products, produced by hyaluronidase enzymes and reactive oxygen species (ROS), are implicated in different aspects of the ALI process. The different activities of hyaluronan and its degradation products are regulated by multiple hyaluronan-binding proteins, including CD44, TLR4, hyaluronan-binding protein 2 (HABP2), and receptor for hyaluronan-mediated motility (RHAMM). Recent research indicates that exogenous administration of high molecular weight hyaluronan can serve as a novel therapeutic intervention for lung diseases, including LPS-induced ALI, sepsis/VILI, and airway hyperactivity [48].

Nanomedicine

Novel long-acting biocompatible and biodegradable phospholipid micelles have been developed to inhibit different targets implicated in ALI. For example, nano-sized micelles have been developed to trigger receptor expressed on myeloid cells 1 (TREM-1), ROS and heat shock protein (Hsp)90, all effectors thought to be involved in ALI. The main limitations of some peptide drugs for clinical use are the short half-life (minutes) and their water-insolubility. To overcome these limitations, some groups have developed micellar-targeted peptides in which the peptide drug remains in its active form for longer (hours) and increases its stability and bioavailability [49]. These long-acting micellar nanomedicines have provided significant advancement in the treatment of ARDS in experimental models, which could be extended to the clinical setting. Another advance is the novel nanovesicle aerosols composed of non-lamellar phospholipids that were developed as pulmonary surfactant aerosols and have been successfully used as therapy in mice with acid-induced lung injury. Currently existing intratracheal surfactants are ineffective because they are inactivated by albumin leakage and other mechanisms. The nanovesicle aerosols of non-lamellar lipids improve the resistance of pulmonary surfactants to inhibition, and may therefore be promising as a non-invasive aerosol therapy in ALI [50].

Conclusions

Despite decades of clinical trials and experimental research, there is no effective pharmacologic therapy for the treatment of all patients with ARDS. Multiple biochemical and biological targets, however, have been identified that could give rise to future drug discovery and development. Several aspects should be taken into account in order to guarantee the efficacy of those potential new drugs. Better stratification may help to identify subgroups of patients with ARDS that benefit from targeted interventions, given the heterogeneity of patients with ARDS and the multiple etiologies of this disease (direct versus indirect ARDS). Combinations of different therapeutic strategies could also improve outcomes for these patients compared with therapies based on single agents. Finally, we also need to optimize the dose, timing and route of administration as well as to determine the potential toxicity of the novel pharmacologic agents for their future use in the management of patients with ARDS.

Acknowledgements

This work was funded by the Centro de Investigación Biomédica en Red de Enfermedades Respiratorias (CIBERES) and the Instituto de Salud Carlos III (Fondo de Investigación Sanitaria, FIS PI12/0245, PI0902624, PI0902644, PI1102791).

References

1. Ranieri VM, Rubenfeld GD, Thompson BT et al (2012) Acute respiratory distress syndrome: the Berlin Definition. JAMA 307:2526–2533
2. Wiedemann HP, Wheeler AP, Bernard GR et al (2006) Comparison of two fluid-management strategies in acute lung injury. N Engl J Med 354:2564–2575

3. Petrucci N, Iacovelli W (2004) Ventilation with lower tidal volumes versus traditional tidal volumes in adults for acute lung injury and acute respiratory distress syndrome. Cochrane Database Syst Rev CD003844
4. Frank AJ, Thompson BT (2010) Pharmacological treatments for acute respiratory distress syndrome. Curr Opin Crit Care 16:62–68
5. Ware LB, Matthay MA (2000) The acute respiratory distress syndrome. N Engl J Med 342:1334–1349
6. Thille AW, Esteban A, Fernandez-Segoviano P et al (2013) Comparison of the Berlin definition for acute respiratory distress syndrome with autopsy. Am J Respir Crit Care Med 187:761–767
7. Steinberg KP, Milberg JA, Martin TR, Maunder RJ, Cockrill BA, Hudson LD (1994) Evolution of bronchoalveolar cell populations in the adult respiratory distress syndrome. Am J Respir Crit Care Med 150:113–122
8. Walmsley SR, Chilvers ER, Thompson AA et al (2011) Prolyl hydroxylase 3 (PHD3) is essential for hypoxic regulation of neutrophilic inflammation in humans and mice. J Clin Invest 121:1053–1063
9. Fujino N, Kubo H, Suzuki T et al (2012) Administration of a specific inhibitor of neutrophil elastase attenuates pulmonary fibrosis after acute lung injury in mice. Exp Lung Res 38:28–36
10. Chua F, Dunsmore SE, Clingen PH et al (2007) Mice lacking neutrophil elastase are resistant to bleomycin-induced pulmonary fibrosis. Am J Pathol 170:65–74
11. Takemasa A, Ishii Y, Fukuda T (2012) A neutrophil elastase inhibitor prevents bleomycin-induced pulmonary fibrosis in mice. Eur Respir J 40:1475–1482
12. Ryugo M, Sawa Y, Takano H et al (2006) Effect of a polymorphonuclear elastase inhibitor (sivelestat sodium) on acute lung injury after cardiopulmonary bypass: findings of a double-blind randomized study. Surg Today 36:321–326
13. Stevens T, Ekholm K, Granse M et al (2011) AZD9668: pharmacological characterization of a novel oral inhibitor of neutrophil elastase. J Pharmacol Exp Ther 339:313–320
14. Jacobson JR (2009) Pharmacologic therapies on the horizon for acute lung injury/acute respiratory distress syndrome. J Investig Med 57:870–873
15. Uhlig S, Gulbins E (2008) Sphingolipids in the lungs. Am J Respir Crit Care Med 178:1100–1114
16. Abbasi T, Garcia JG (2013) Sphingolipids in lung endothelial biology and regulation of vascular integrity. Handb Exp Pharmacol 201:201–226
17. Wang L, Dudek SM (2009) Regulation of vascular permeability by sphingosine 1-phosphate. Microvasc Res 77:39–45
18. Natarajan V, Dudek SM, Jacobson JR et al (2013) Sphingosine-1-phosphate, FTY720, and sphingosine-1-phosphate receptors in the pathobiology of acute lung injury. Am J Respir Cell Mol Biol 49:6–17
19. Serhan CN, Chiang N (2008) Endogenous pro-resolving and anti-inflammatory lipid mediators: a new pharmacologic genus. Br J Pharmacol 153:200–215
20. Hsiao HM, Sapinoro RE, Thatcher TH et al (2013) A novel anti-inflammatory and pro-resolving role for resolvin D1 in acute cigarette smoke-induced lung inflammation. PLoS One 8:e58258
21. Liao Z, Dong J, Wu W et al (2012) Resolvin D1 attenuates inflammation in lipopolysaccharide-induced acute lung injury through a process involving the PPARgamma/NF-kappaB pathway. Respir Res 13:110
22. Chalmers JD, Short PM, Mandal P, Akram AR, Hill AT (2010) Statins in community acquired pneumonia: Evidence from experimental and clinical studies. Respir Med 104:1081–1091
23. Chen W, Sammani S, Mitra S, Ma SF, Garcia JG, Jacobson JR (2012) Critical role for integrin-beta4 in the attenuation of murine acute lung injury by simvastatin. Am J Physiol Lung Cell Mol Physiol 303:L279–L285
24. van der Heijden M, van Nieuw Amerongen GP, Koolwijk P, van Hinsbergh VW, Groeneveld AB (2008) Angiopoietin-2, permeability oedema, occurrence and severity of ALI/ARDS in septic and non-septic critically ill patients. Thorax 63:903–909

25. van der Heijden M, van Nieuw Amerongen GP, van Hinsbergh VW, Groeneveld AB (2010) The interaction of soluble Tie2 with angiopoietins and pulmonary vascular permeability in septic and nonseptic critically ill patients. Shock 33:263–268
26. Glas GJ, Van Der Sluijs KF, Schultz MJ, Hofstra JJ, Van Der Poll T, Levi M (2013) Bronchoalveolar hemostasis in lung injury and acute respiratory distress syndrome. J Thromb Haemost 11:17–25
27. Bo L, Bian J, Li J, Wan X, Zhu K, Deng X (2011) Activated protein C inhalation: a novel therapeutic strategy for acute lung injury. Med Sci Monit 17:HY11–HY13
28. Imai Y, Kuba K, Penninger JM (2007) Angiotensin-converting enzyme 2 in acute respiratory distress syndrome. Cell Mol Life Sci 64:2006–2012
29. Imai Y, Kuba K, Rao S et al (2005) Angiotensin-converting enzyme 2 protects from severe acute lung failure. Nature 436:112–116
30. Wang R, Ibarra-Sunga O, Verlinski L, Pick R, Uhal BD (2000) Abrogation of bleomycin-induced epithelial apoptosis and lung fibrosis by captopril or by a caspase inhibitor. Am J Physiol Lung Cell Mol Physiol 279:L143–L151
31. Bechara RI, Pelaez A, Palacio A et al (2005) Angiotensin II mediates glutathione depletion, transforming growth factor-beta1 expression, and epithelial barrier dysfunction in the alcoholic rat lung. Am J Physiol Lung Cell Mol Physiol 289:L363–L370
32. Marshall RP, Gohlke P, Chambers RC et al (2004) Angiotensin II and the fibroproliferative response to acute lung injury. Am J Physiol Lung Cell Mol Physiol 286:L156–L164
33. Imai Y, Kuba K, Neely GG et al (2008) Identification of oxidative stress and Toll-like receptor 4 signaling as a key pathway of acute lung injury. Cell 133:235–249
34. Kim HM, Park BS, Kim JI et al (2007) Crystal structure of the TLR4-MD-2 complex with bound endotoxin antagonist Eritoran. Cell 130:906–917
35. Wong YN, Rossignol D, Rose JR, Kao R, Carter A, Lynn M (2003) Safety, pharmacokinetics, and pharmacodynamics of E5564, a lipid A antagonist, during an ascending single-dose clinical study. J Clin Pharmacol 43:735–742
36. Mullarkey M, Rose JR, Bristol J et al (2003) Inhibition of endotoxin response by e5564, a novel Toll-like receptor 4-directed endotoxin antagonist. J Pharmacol Exp Ther 304:1093–1102
37. Woodside DG, Vanderslice P (2008) Cell adhesion antagonists: therapeutic potential in asthma and chronic obstructive pulmonary disease. BioDrugs 22:85–100
38. Sheppard D (2012) Modulation of acute lung injury by integrins. Proc Am Thorac Soc 9:126–129
39. Su G, Hodnett M, Wu N et al (2007) Integrin alphavbeta5 regulates lung vascular permeability and pulmonary endothelial barrier function. Am J Respir Cell Mol Biol 36:377–386
40. Puthawala K, Hadjiangelis N, Jacoby SC et al (2008) Inhibition of integrin alpha(v)beta6, an activator of latent transforming growth factor-beta, prevents radiation-induced lung fibrosis. Am J Respir Crit Care Med 177:82–90
41. Kyriakides C, Austen W Jr, Wang Y, Favuzza J, Moore FD Jr, Hechtman HB (2000) Endothelial selectin blockade attenuates lung permeability of experimental acid aspiration. Surgery 128:327–331
42. Cai ZG, Zhang SM, Zhang Y, Zhou YY, Wu HB, Xu XP (2012) MicroRNAs are dynamically regulated and play an important role in LPS-induced lung injury. Can J Physiol Pharmacol 90:37–43
43. Adyshev DM, Moldobaeva N, Mapes B, Elangovan V, Garcia JG (2013) MicroRNA regulation of nonmuscle myosin light chain kinase expression in human lung endothelium. Am J Respir Cell Mol Biol 49:58–66
44. Kim TH, Yoon HJ, Lim CM, Kim EK, Kim MJ, Koh Y (2005) The role of endogenous histamine on the pathogenesis of the lipopolysaccharide (LPS)-induced, acute lung injury: a pilot study. Inflammation 29:72–80
45. Ryffel B, Couillin I, Maillet I et al (2005) Histamine scavenging attenuates endotoxin-induced acute lung injury. Ann NY Acad Sci 1056:197–205

46. Lindsay CD (2011) Novel therapeutic strategies for acute lung injury induced by lung damaging agents: the potential role of growth factors as treatment options. Hum Exp Toxicol 30:701–724
47. Kakavas S, Demestiha T, Vasileiou P, Xanthos T (2011) Erythropoetin as a novel agent with pleiotropic effects against acute lung injury. Eur J Clin Pharmacol 67:1–9
48. Lennon FE, Singleton PA (2011) Role of hyaluronan and hyaluronan-binding proteins in lung pathobiology. Am J Physiol Lung Cell Mol Physiol 301:L137–L147
49. Sadikot RT, Rubinstein I (2009) Long-acting, multi-targeted nanomedicine: addressing unmet medical need in acute lung injury. J Biomed Nanotechnol 5:614–619
50. Kaviratna AS, Banerjee R (2012) Nanovesicle aerosols as surfactant therapy in lung injury. Nanomedicine 8:665–672

Outcome of Patients with Acute Respiratory Distress Syndrome: Causes of Death, Survival Rates and Long-term Implications

M. Zambon, G. Monti, and G. Landoni

Introduction

Several treatments for patients with acute respiratory distress syndrome (ARDS) have been proposed since its first description in 1967 [1], and a large amount of research has been conducted. Despite many negative experimental and clinical trials, in the last 15 years some treatments have received general consensus and application. Above all, there are protective ventilation strategies, but also prone positioning, neuromuscular blockers, conservative fluid balance, and extracorporeal membrane oxygenation (ECMO). Nevertheless, ARDS remains a major problem in intensive care units (ICU) patients. In this review, we first discuss the reasons why patients still die from ARDS; then, we review mortality rates and long-term outcomes of ARDS patients.

Causes of Mortality

ARDS is often part of a systemic condition that can include other entities, such as sepsis of pulmonary or non-pulmonary origin, trauma, acute kidney injury, etc. Although several predictors of mortality have been reported, it is a difficult and sometimes impossible challenge to understand the causes that lead to multiple organ dysfunction syndrome (MODS) and to fatal outcomes in patients with ARDS. Interestingly, predictors of mortality for ARDS were found to be the same markers of severity of illness, and models using variables selected from ARDS patients predicted mortality as well as non-specific severity scores, such as APACHE III [2]. In fact, the most frequent cause of death described in ARDS patients is MODS [3]. Causes that lead to MODS in ARDS patients are summarized in Fig. 1.

M. Zambon · G. Monti · G. Landoni ✉
Department of Anesthesia and Intensive Care, San Raffaele Scientific Institute, Milan, Italy
e-mail: landoni.giovanni@hsr.it

J.-L. Vincent (Ed.), *Annual Update in Intensive Care and Emergency Medicine 2014*,
DOI 10.1007/978-3-319-03746-2_19, © Springer International Publishing Switzerland
2014

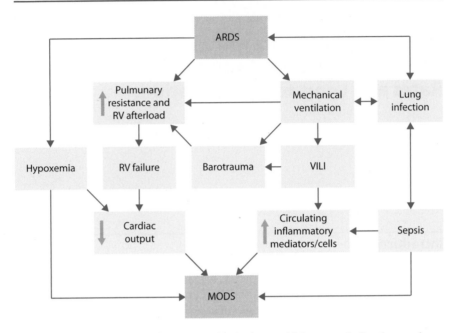

Fig. 1 Schematic representation of causes that lead to multiple organ dysfunction syndrome (MODS) in patients with acute respiratory distress syndrome (ARDS). VILI: ventilator-induced lung injury; RV: right ventricular

Refractory Hypoxemia

The main clinical characteristic of ARDS is, by definition, a severe form of hypoxemia; therefore, one might be led to believe that refractory hypoxemia is the main cause of death in these patients. The recent Berlin definition of ARDS [4] created three categories (mild, moderate, severe) based on the degrees of hypoxemia, and these were associated with increased mortality (27 %, 32 % and 45 % respectively). However, death from refractory hypoxemia is relatively uncommon. A key article published in 1986 by Montgomery and colleagues reported that, in a series of 47 patients who had ARDS, refractory hypoxemia was responsible for only 16 % of the deaths. Sepsis/MODS was the leading cause of death in these patients [5]. Bersten and colleagues [6] found that in their 168 ARDS patients, respiratory failure contributed to death in 24 % and was the only cause of death in just 9 % of patients. Other investigators have reported similar findings [7–9].

Ventilator-induced Lung Injury

A large number of investigations in the last 20 years have focused on the harmful effects of mechanical ventilation. It is now clear that efforts to improve gas exchange with aggressive ventilation have deleterious effects on the lungs: Ventilator-induced lunch injury (VILI) is a well-recognized cause of increased mortality. Damage is caused either by mechanical or biological mechanisms.

Barotrauma (and its consequence, pneumothorax) was a frequent complication of mechanically ventilated patients with ARDS before the implementation of low tidal volume ventilation; in a study by Boussarsar and colleagues, the incidence of barotrauma increased dramatically when patients were ventilated with plateau pressures higher than $35\,cmH_2O$ [10]. However, in a retrospective analysis of a large cohort of mechanically ventilated patients where tidal volumes and airway pressure were limited, barotrauma still occurred in 6.5 % of patients with ARDS and was associated with a significant increase in mortality [11].

Another important mechanism of injury is the release of inflammatory mediators from the lungs, which increases when patients are ventilated with higher tidal volumes. These mediators (including interleukin [IL]-6, tumor necrosis factor [TNF], IL-1 and IL-8) may have systemic effects, impairing the functions of other organs. There is correlation between changes in a multiple organ failure score over 72 hours and changes in plasma concentration of a number of inflammatory mediators [12]. Imay and colleagues found that mechanical ventilation led to epithelial cell apoptosis in the kidney and small intestine [13].

Mechanical ventilation can activate polymorphonuclear leukocytes; the consequent release of elastase is correlated with the degree of systemic inflammatory response and multiple organ failure [14]. All these data may explain the high rate of MODS observed in patients with ARDS and the decrease in morbidity and mortality in patients treated with a lung protective strategy.

Sepsis

Sepsis is the condition most often associated with ARDS. In a study assessing consecutive cohorts of patients who had ARDS from 1982, 1990, 1994 and 1998, Stapleton and co-workers identified sepsis as the leading cause of death [9]. In the recent PROSEVA trial, more than 80 % of patients with severe ARDS had sepsis [15]. Although sepsis is a well-recognized risk factor for mortality in ARDS patients, the direct cause-effect relationship of infection on ARDS mortality is still unclear. Several studies have reported no significant effects of pulmonary infection on mortality rates [16–18].

Right Ventricular Failure

Increased pulmonary vascular resistance and pulmonary hypertension in severe forms of acute respiratory failure were described more than 35 years ago [19]. In ARDS patients, microvascular obstruction, high respiratory pressures (namely high positive end-expiratory pressure [PEEP]) and hypercapnia, through the raise in pulmonary arterial pressure and the increased right ventricular (RV) afterload,

may cause RV failure. Acute cor pulmonale in ARDS patients has been associated
with high mortality rates [20, 21]. In 1985, Jardin and co-workers found that when
patients were ventilated with large tidal volumes and excessive airway pressures,
the combination of acute cor pulmonale and lung parenchimal destruction led to
death in 100 % of cases [21]. However, in an observational study by the same group
after the implementation of protective ventilatory strategies and prone positioning,
the effect of RV dysfunction on mortality was not significant. It has to be noted
that in the group of patients with acute cor pulmonale, more patients were ventilated in the prone position; this markedly improved PaO_2/FiO_2 ratio and allowed an
immediate reduction in PEEP, implementing a sort of "RV protective" ventilatory
strategy [22].

Has Mortality From ARDS Decreased?

In large epidemiologic studies conducted in the past decade, mortality rates for
ARDS patients were as high as 40–60 % [23, 24]. A systematic analysis by Krafft
et al. [25] concluded that the mortality rate of ARDS patients remained constant
from 1967, year of the first description by Ashbaugh [1], to 1994, at the time of the
American-European Consensus Conference (AECC) definition criteria [26]. Despite quite a large amount of research in the field, no great advances seem to have
been made in the treatment of critically ill patients with severe respiratory failure.
In the last decade, however, several single center studies have described improved
survival of ARDS patients [27, 28]. More recently, two French multicenter randomized controlled trials evaluating neuromuscular blocking agents and prone position
in severe ARDS patients obtained 28-days mortalities in the treatment groups as
low as 23 % and 16 % respectively [15, 29].

A systematic analysis of studies on ARDS published using the AECC definitions
included 72 papers published from 1994 to 2006 and 11,426 patients. Studies about
specific subgroups of ARDS patients (such as trauma, transfusion-related acute lung
injury [TRALI], sepsis-related ARDS) were excluded, because of the known differences in outcomes of different subgroups of ARDS patients. The authors found
a significant trend towards a reduction in mortality over the years [30]. As expected,
mortality rates in randomized controlled trials was lower than that of observational
studies, because of the selected populations enrolled in controlled studies, the better
care provided in high quality centers and the Hawthorne effect. However, the trend
in mortality reduction is present both in epidemiologic studies and in interventional
trials. A possible limitation of these kinds of analyses is the heterogeneity in patient
populations among studies, and the different time of the outcome measurement (28-
day vs. ICU vs. hospital mortality). Nevertheless, aggregated data should minimize
these biases.

Interestingly, the same analysis conducted by another group concluded that there
had been no change in outcomes from ARDS over the years [31]. This opposite result can be explained by methodological issues [32]. The decline in mortality rates
is even stronger if we consider that severity of illness has generally increased over

time [33, 34]. The main reason for the decline in mortality rates is commonly believed to be the implementation of protective ventilatory strategies. After the landmark ARDS network trial on low tidal volume ventilation versus high tidal volume ventilation [35], protective ventilatory strategies have been progressively implemented, even though translating this evidence-based therapy into practice has presented some difficulties [36]. Ventilating patients with lower tidal volumes, mainly reducing the incidence of VILI, could be the keystone in the ventilatory management of severely hypoxemic patients. Erickson and co-workers, in a large retrospective cohort study of patients enrolled in ARDS network trials in the same time period as the two systematic analyses, suggested a reduction in mortality over time. Interestingly, after adjusting for clinical covariates including lower tidal volume ventilation, the temporal trend persisted, indicating that factors other than lower tidal volume ventilation were responsible for this survival improvement [37].

Another factor influencing the decrease in mortality could be the change in the case mix of ARDS patients. Some authors suggest that there has been a decline in hospital-acquired ARDS, perhaps secondary to a lower rate of nosocomial infections and a more conservative use of blood products [33]. ARDS in patients with severe sepsis and septic shock is typically associated with higher mortality rates. Better care of septic patients with implementation of sepsis bundles may have participated in the decrease in ARDS mortality.

Long-term Outcome and Quality of Life

The long-term clinical outcomes of patients who survive ARDS has received great interest in the last decade; with higher survival rates and increased patient disease severity, more patients are exposed to morbidity that may persist for years. Quality of life (QOL) measures, in addition to long-term mortality evaluation, should therefore be encouraged.

The most widely used instruments to evaluate long term QOL can be divided into questionnaires and physiological tests. Included in the first group is the widely used Medical Outcome Study Short Form 36-Item Health Survey (or SF-36), which measures QOL in eight different domains (physical functioning and role, bodily pain, general health, vitality, social functioning, emotional role and mental health), each scored from 0 (worst) to 100 (best). Every domain can be compared with those of an age and sex matched control population. Another questionnaire is the St. George's Respiratory Questionnaire (SGRQ), a 76-item pulmonary specific questionnaire, with results grouped in 3 domains (symptoms, activity and impacts) and an overall score; in SGRQ the lower the score, the better the QOL.

The second group of tests includes spirometry and pulmonary functioning testing and the functional 6-minute walking test, in which the larger the number of meters walked in 6 minutes, the better the result. A very comprehensive way to evaluate QOL is the return of the patient to his/her previous job, but this measure is rarely reported.

Important issues related to QOL after ARDS can be extrapolated from a meta-analysis published in 2006 by Dowdy et al. [38], which evaluated QOL in 557 ARDS survivors. First, QOL after ARDS is decreased, similar in different population studies and more dependent on factors related to ARDS (e. g., impact of critical illness, ARDS specific effect) than population factors. This finding is shown consistently both by a reduction of performance in QOL questionnaires and by a universally reported reduction of meters in the 6-minute walking tests [39]. Second, QOL recovery is both domain and time-specific. For example, considering the SF-36 domains, Cheung et al. [40] reported an increasing value in the physical role domain from the 1st to the 2nd year (from 30 % to 60 % of predicted, although not statistically significant). Similar results were reported by Heyland and colleagues [41] in a 1-year follow up study.

More recently Herridge et al. [42] reported the 5 year results from the same cohort of patients, showing a further increase in the physical domain performance, especially in the younger group of patients, but none had a score as high as the predicted score at 5 years for the general population. In other domains of SF-36, conflicting results are reported: in the series by Herridge et al. [42], emotional role and mental health were constantly high throughout the years (more than 75); in the series by Heyland and colleagues [41], however, they were constantly depressed (less than 65).

Interestingly, in a cohort of 18 patients with ARDS who were treated with ECMO for refractory hypoxemia, SF-36 assessed at 8 months was significantly lower across all domains compared to sex- and age-matched healthy individuals, and was lower than other ARDS survivors in the domains of general health, mental health, vitality and social function [43].

Apart from SF-36 evaluation, an interesting psychiatric study with a very long follow up (up to 8 years) showed that about half of the ARDS survivors reached DSM-IV diagnostic criteria for post-traumatic stress disorder (PTSD) or sub-PTSD. At follow up, 40 % of patients were still suffering from PTSD or sub-PTSD [44].

Variability in cognitive functions could be related also to an important finding, highlighted by Mikkelsen et al. in 2012: Being exposed to lower partial pressure of arterial oxygen (PaO$_2$) during ARDS is associated with cognitive and psychiatric impairment, as previously hypothesized by the researchers [45]. The degree of hypoxemia in different series of patients could be one of the intrinsic ARDS factors that may alter subsequent QOL evolution in the mental health domains. Moreover, the impact of ARDS could also spread to the QOL of the patient's family. Tansey et al. reported a reduction of about 1.5 standard deviations in the mental component score of the SF-36 in the patient's informal caregiver [46].

Trying to understand which survivors of ARDS are at greater risk of reduced QOL is very important to improve early QOL and, perhaps, to develop prophylactic interventions for high-risk patients. Kim et al. [47] evaluated whether there was a relationship between the causes of ARDS (pulmonary versus extrapulmonary) and subsequent QOL. These authors showed more serious sequelae in primary ARDS but these were not associated with a worse QOL. However, this study had few patients enrolled ($n = 29$), probably too few to detect a significant difference. In contrast, Parker et al. [48] demonstrated that patients with secondary lung injuries had worse scores in all SF-36 domains in a 1-year follow-up study. Similar results were reported in a study by Masclans et al. [49], who failed to show a correlation between the cause of ARDS, a sepsis origin, the extent of compromise in pulmonary function testing and the results of computed tomography (CT) scans. The only association identified was the robust positive correlation observed between 1-month and 6-month QOL, indicating that it is possible to identify patients with poor long-term QOL at an early stage.

Conclusions

Mortality rates for ARDS seem to have decreased over time. Nevertheless, the most severe forms of ARDS are still associated with mortality rates of around 40 %. The main cause of death is MODS, which may be initiated by different conditions associated with ARDS, such as VILI, refractory hypoxemia, RV dysfunction, sepsis. Understanding the risk factors for death in these patients is mandatory and could allow us to identify subsets of patients that should be assigned earlier to specific treatments (e. g., ECMO).

Patients who survive ARDS experience a lower QOL than the healthy population, with limited chances of improvement over time. Survivors with extrapulmonary ARDS, with a slower recovery of lung function and with periods of severe hypoxemia, are at greater risk for impaired QOL. An early observation of QOL reduction is likely to persist over time. Future research in ARDS should include routine evaluations of long-term outcome markers to identify specific interventions able to ameliorate quality of life.

References

1. Ashbaugh DG, Bigelow DB, Petty TL, Levine BE (1967) Acute respiratory distress in adults. Lancet 2:319–323
2. Cooke CR, Kahn JM, Caldwell E et al (2008) Predictors of hospital mortality in a population-based cohort of patients with acute lung injury. Crit Care Med 36:1412–1420
3. Vincent JL, Zambon M (2006) Why do patients who have acute lung injury/acute respiratory distress syndrome die from multiple organ dysfunction syndrome? Implications for management. Clin Chest Med 27:725–731
4. ARDS Definition Task Force (2012) Acute respiratory distress syndrome: the Berlin Definition. JAMA 307:2526–2533
5. Montgomery BA, Stager MA, Carrico J et al (1985) Causes of mortality in patients with the adult respiratory distress syndrome. Am Rev Respir Dis 132:485–491
6. Bersten AD, Edibam C, Hunt T, Moran J, Australian and New Zealand Intensive Care Society Clinical Trials Group (2002) Incidence and mortality of acute lung injury and the acute respiratory distress syndrome in three Australian States. Am J Respir Crit Care Med 165:443–448
7. Ferring M, Vincent JL (1997) Is outcome from ARDS related to the severity of respiratory failure? Eur Respir J 10:1297–1300

8. Estenssoro E, Dubin A, Laffaire E et al (2002) Incidence, clinical course, and outcome in 217 patients with acute respiratory distress syndrome. Crit Care Med 30:2450–2456
9. Stapleton RD, Wang BM, Hudson LD, Rubenfeld GD, Caldwell ES, Steinberg KP (2005) Causes and timing of death in patients with ARDS. Chest 128:525–532
10. Boussarsar M, Thierry G, Jaber S, Roudot-Thoraval F, Lemaire F, Brochard L (2002) Relationship between ventilatory settings and barotrauma in the acute respiratory distress syndrome. Intensive Care Med 28:406–413
11. Anzueto A, Frutos-Vivar F, Esteban A et al (2004) Incidence, risk factors and outcome of barotrauma in mechanically ventilated patients. Intensive Care Med 30:612–619
12. Ranieri VM, Suter PM, Tortorella C et al (1999) Effect of mechanical ventilation on inflammatory mediators in patients with acute respiratory distress syndrome: a randomized controlled trial. JAMA 282:54–61
13. Imai Y, Parodo J, Kajikawa O et al (2003) Injurious mechanical ventilation and end-organ epithelial cell apoptosis and organ dysfunction in an experimental model of acute respiratory distress syndrome. JAMA 289:2104–2112
14. Zhang H, Downey GP, Suter PM et al (2002) Conventional mechanical ventilation is associated with bronchoalveolar lavage-induced activation of polymorphonuclear leukocytes: a possible mechanism to explain the systemic consequences of ventilator-induced lung injury in patients with ARDS. Anesthesiology 97:1426–1433
15. Guérin C, Reignier J, Richard JC et al (2013) Prone positioning in severe acute respiratory distress syndrome. N Engl J Med 368:2159–2168
16. Forel JM, Voillet F, Pulina D et al (2012) Ventilator-associated pneumonia and ICU mortality in severe ARDS patients ventilated according to a lung-protective strategy. Crit Care 16:R65
17. Chastre J, Trouillet JL, Vuagnat A et al (1998) Nosocomialpneumonia in patients with acute respiratory distress syndrome. Am J Respir Crit Care Med 157:1165–1172
18. Bauer TT, Valencia M, Badia JR et al (2005) Respiratory microbiology patterns within the first 24 h of ARDS diagnosis: influence on outcome. Chest 128:273–279
19. Zapol WM, Snider MT (1977) Pulmonary hypertension in severe acute respiratory failure. N Engl J Med 296:476–480
20. Villar J, Blazquez MA, Lubillo S, Quintana J, Manzano JL (1989) Pulmonary hypertension in acute respiratory failure. Crit Care Med 17:523–526
21. Jardin F, Gueret P, Dubourg O, Farcot JC, Margairaz A, Bourdarias JP (1985) Two-dimensional echocardiographic evaluation of right ventricular size and contractility in acute respiratory failure. Crit Care Med 13:952–956
22. Vieillard-Baron A, Schmitt JM, Augarde R et al (2001) Acute cor pulmonale in acute respiratory distress syndrome submitted to protective ventilation: incidence, clinical implications, and prognosis. Crit Care Med 29:1551–1555
23. Monchi M, Bellenfant F, Cariou A et al (1998) Early predictive factors of survival in the acute respiratory distress syndrome. Am J Respir Crit Care Med 158:1076–1081
24. Rubenfeld GD, Caldwell E, Peabody E et al (2005) Incidence and outcomes of acute lung injury. N Engl J Med 353:1685–1693
25. Krafft P, Fridrich P, Pernerstorfer T et al (1996) The acute respiratory distress syndrome: definitions, severity and clinical outcome: an analysis of 101 clinical investigations. Intensive Care Med 22:519–529
26. Bernard GR, Artigas A, Brigham KL et al (1994) The American-European Consensus Conference on ARDS: definitions, mechanisms, relevant outcomes, and clinical trial coordination. Am J Respir Crit Care Med 149:818–824
27. Jardin F, Fellahi JL, Beauchet A et al (1999) Improved prognosis of acute respiratory distress syndrome 15 years on. Intensive Care Med 25:936–941
28. Kallet RH, Jasmer RM, Pittet JF et al (2005) Clinical implementation of the ARDS network protocol is associated with reduced hospital mortality compared with historical controls. Crit Care Med 33:925–929

29. Papazian L, Forel JM, Gacouin A et al (2010) Neuromuscular blockers in early acute respiratory distress syndrome. N Engl J Med 363:1107–1116

30. Zambon M, Vincent JL (2008) Mortality rates for patients with acute lung injury/ARDS have decreased over time. Chest 133:1120–1127

31. Phua J, Badia JR, Adhikari NK et al (2009) Has mortality from acute respiratory distress syndrome decreased over time? A systematic review. Am J Respir Crit Care Med 179:220–227

32. Zambon M, Vincent JL (2009) Are outcomes improving in patients with ARDS? Am J Respir Crit Care Med 180:1158–1159

33. Li G, Malinchoc M, Cartin-Ceba R et al (2011) Eight-year trend of acute respiratory distress syndrome: a population-based study in Olmsted County, Minnesota. Am J Respir Crit Care Med 183:59–66

34. Pierrakos C, Vincent JL (2012) The changing pattern of acute respiratory distress syndrome over time: a comparison of two periods. Eur Respir J 40:589–595

35. The ARDS Network (2000) Ventilation with lower tidal volumes as compared with traditional tidal volumes for acute lung injury and the acute respiratory distress syndrome. N Engl J Med 342:1301–1308

36. Kalhan R, Mikkelsen M, Dedhiya P et al (2006) Underuse of lung protective ventilation: analysis of potential factors to explain physician behavior. Crit Care Med 34:300–306

37. Erickson SE, Martin GS, Davis JL, Matthay MA, Eisner MD (2009) Recent trends in acute lung injury mortality: 1996–2005. Crit Care Med 37:1574–1579

38. Dowdy DW, Eid MP, Dennison CR et al (2006) Quality of life after acute respiratory distress syndrome: a meta-analysis. Intensive Care Med 32:1115–1124

39. Wilcox ME, Margaret SH (2011) Lung function and quality of life in survivors of the acute respiratory distress syndrome (ARDS). Presse Med 40(e595):e603

40. Cheung AM, Tansey CM, Tomlinson G et al (2006) Two-year outcomes, health care use, and costs of survivors of acute respiratory distress syndrome. Am J Respir Crit Care Med 174:538–544

41. Heyland DK, Groll D, Caeser M (2005) Survivors of acute respiratory distress syndrome: Relationship between pulmonary dysfunction and long-term health-related quality of life. Crit Care Med 33:1549–1556

42. Herridge MS, Tansey CM, Matté A et al (2011) Functional disability 5 years after acute respiratory distress syndrome. N Engl J Med 364:1293–1304

43. Hodgson CL, Hayes K, Everard T et al (2012) Long-term quality of life in patients with acute respiratory distress syndrome requiring extracorporeal membrane oxygenation for refractory hypoxaemia. Crit Care 16:R202

44. Kapfhammer HP, Rothenhäusler HB, Krauseneck T, Stoll C, Schelling G (2004) Posttraumatic stress disorder and health-related quality of life in long-term survivors of acute respiratory distress syndrome. Am J Psychiatry 161:45–52

45. Mikkelsen ME, Christie JD, Lanken PN et al (2012) The adult respiratory distress syndrome cognitive outcomes study: long-term neuropsychological function in survivors of acute lung injury. Am J Respir Crit Care Med 185:1307–1315

46. Tansey CM, Louie M, Loeb M et al (2007) One-year outcomes and health care utilization in survivors of severe acute respiratory syndrome. Arch Intern Med 167:1312–1320

47. Kim SJ, Oh BJ, Lee JS et al (2004) Recovery from lung injury in survivors of acute respiratory distress syndrome: difference between pulmonary and extrapulmonary subtypes. Intensive Care Med 30:1960–1963

48. Parker CM, Heyland DK, Groll D, Caeser M (2006) Mechanism of injury influences quality of life in survivors of acute respiratory distress syndrome. Intensive Care Med 32:1895–1900

49. Masclans JR, Roca O, Muñoz X et al (2011) Quality of life, pulmonary function, and tomographic scan abnormalities after ARDS. Chest 139:1340–1346

Part VI
Pulmonary Edema

Quantitative Evaluation of Pulmonary Edema

T. Tagami, S. Kushimoto, and H. Yokota

Introduction

Pulmonary edema is one of the most common problems in critically ill patients and has a profound effect on patient outcome [1]. Pulmonary edema is characterized by excess accumulation of fluid in the extravascular space of the lungs, namely extravascular lung water (EVLW). Because it is difficult to evaluate EVLW at the bedside in routine clinical practice, its existence and the severity of pulmonary edema are generally evaluated on the basis of patient history, physical examination (e. g., the presence of rales), laboratory examination, and chest radiographic findings [1]. However, the interpretation of these parameters (e. g., chest radiography) is often limited to a certain degree by subjectivity that may cause interobserver error, even among experts [2]. In addition, a recent study suggests that there is only a moderate positive correlation between chest radiographic findings and EVLW measurements [3].

The pathological condition of pulmonary edema develops by two mechanisms: An increase in the pulmonary capillary hydrostatic pressure (hydrostatic or cardiogenic pulmonary edema) and an increase in pulmonary capillary permeability (acute respiratory distress syndrome [ARDS]) [1]. However, it is often difficult to discriminate between edema caused by increased hydrostatic pressure in the course of cardiac disease, or by increased permeability associated with ARDS [1].

It is, therefore, difficult to evaluate pulmonary edema quantitatively in terms of its existence, its severity (the degree of pulmonary edema), and the nature of the disease (cardiogenic versus ARDS). However, recent studies suggest that

T. Tagami ✉ · H. Yokota
Departments of Emergency and Critical Care Medicine, Nippon Medical School, Tokyo, Japan
e-mail: t-tagami@nms.ac.jp

S. Kushimoto
Division of Emergency Medicine, Tohoku University Graduate School of Medicine, Miyagi, Japan

J.-L. Vincent (Ed.), *Annual Update in Intensive Care and Emergency Medicine 2014*, 257
DOI 10.1007/978-3-319-03746-2_20, © Springer International Publishing Switzerland 2014

transpulmonary thermodilution-derived variables, the extravascular lung water index (EVLWI) and the pulmonary vascular permeability index (PVPI), may be promising variables to overcome this clinical dilemma. In this review, we describe the value of EVLWI and PVPI in the quantitative evaluation of pulmonary edema in terms of the existence, severity, and type of the disease.

Difficulties in the Evaluation of Pulmonary Edema: Focusing on the ARDS Definition

Since the first description of ARDS by Ashbaugh et al. in 1967 [4], the definition was continuously reworked until the publication of the American-European Consensus Conference (AECC) definition in 1994 [5]. The AECC definition is based on: (a) acute onset; (b) the presence of bilateral pulmonary infiltrates on chest radiography; (c) a PaO_2/FiO_2 ratio < 300 mmHg (for acute lung injury [ALI]) or < 200 mmHg (for ARDS); and (d) a lack of evidence of left atrial hypertension [5]. Although the AECC criteria are simple and widely used, significant criticisms of these criteria have been reported [6–12]. First, the interpretation of chest radiography is often limited to a certain degree by subjectivity [2]. Second, the PaO_2/FiO_2 ratio depends on FiO_2, and the relationship between the numerator and denominator is non-linear [10]. In addition, the effect of positive end-expiratory pressure (PEEP) significantly impacts the PaO_2/FiO_2 ratio [11]. Third, the evidence for cardiac dysfunction does not imply causality: Patients with chronic cardiac disease also have abnormal cardiac function on echocardiography when they develop a lung injury [12]. Finally, and most importantly, studies of pathological-clinical correlations have shown only modest agreement between the pathologic findings of ARDS, diffuse alveolar damage (DAD), and the AECC diagnostic criteria [6–9].

Although the Berlin definition for ARDS was published in 2012 [13], it is still mainly based on bilateral pulmonary infiltrates on chest radiography and on PaO_2/FiO_2. It has been shown to have only slightly better predictive validity for mortality than the AECC definition; with an area under the receiver operating curve of 0.577 (95 % CI, 0.561–0.593) versus 0.536 (95 % CI, 0.520–0.553, p < 0.001). Although this result is 'statistically' significant, as stated in a recent editorial, this finding from the Berlin definition is "abysmal", and should not be considered to be progress [14]. Moreover, a recent autopsy study showed that histopathological findings of DAD were observed in only 45 % of patients identified as having ARDS according to the Berlin definition, suggesting very limited pathological-clinical validation [15, 16].

The panel that developed the Berlin definition [13] agreed in their conceptual model that ARDS has been described as a type of acute, diffuse, inflammatory lung injury leading to increased pulmonary vascular permeability, increased lung weight, and loss of aerated lung tissue. However, none of the suggested criteria evaluates the increase in pulmonary vascular permeability and increased EVLW, despite the fact that both are hallmarks of ARDS. Not only the AECC definition, but also the Berlin definition, may include an extensive range of respiratory insufficiencies without an increase in pulmonary microvascular permeability or pulmonary edema [17, 18].

Potential Variables for Evaluating Pulmonary Edema: EVLW and PVPI

The transpulmonary thermodilution-derived variables EVLW and PVPI are sensitive, specific, and conceptual markers for evaluating pulmonary edema [12, 14, 17–27] and can be easily, quickly, and repeatedly measured at the bedside. Previous studies in animal models suggest that in both increased permeability and hydrostatic pulmonary edema, measurement of EVLW using transpulmonary thermodilution with a single indicator is very closely correlated with gravimetric measurement of lung water [25], over a wide range of changes [28]. In humans, we observed a definite correlation between EVLW measured by the single-indicator transpulmonary thermodilution technique and post-mortem lung weight with a wide range of illnesses and injured lungs [29]. More recently, Venkateswaran et al. [30] reported a close correlation of the EVLW with gravimetric measurements of lung water in human brain-dead donors. The most reliable pathophysiological feature of ARDS is the development of DAD with increased permeability [31], which results in the accumulation of water in the lungs. We recently validated the pathologic-clinical relationship between EVLW and DAD using a pathological study and a nationwide autopsy database study [32].

In the Berlin definition, the measurement of EVLW was considered but not included in the current criteria [13, 33]. The authors stated that "EVLW does not distinguish between hydrostatic and inflammatory pulmonary edema", and for this reason it was not included [13, 33]. However, this statement is not rationally correct. The amount of EVLW represents the degree of the pulmonary edema, but it does not distinguish between hydrostatic or permeability pulmonary edema. It is PVPI that allows the distinction between these two types of pulmonary edema [25, 28]. Recent clinical studies have indicated that PVPI can be used to differentiate cardiogenic and non-cardiogenic (ARDS) pulmonary edema [20, 34].

Several clinical studies performed in patients with ARDS have suggested that EVLW and PVPI correlate with disease severity [17] and are independent risk factors for 28-day mortality [24]. Thus, these variables have significant clinical implications and may be the key 'bridge' for a pathological-clinical correlation [27, 32].

The Transpulmonary Thermodilution Technique

The introduction of the double-indicator thermodilution technique made it possible to measure EVLW, and demonstrated an excellent correlation between *in vivo* and postmortem gravimetric EVLW measurements [35]. However, this method was cumbersome and too technically challenging for application in routine clinical practice. For EVLW evaluation in a clinical setting, the double-indicator technique has been replaced by the single-indicator technique, which is implemented in the PiCCO™ monitoring system (Pulsion Medical Systems, Munich, Germany) [36]. The system uses a single thermal indicator technique to calculate cardiac output, global end-diastolic volume (GEDV), EVLW, PVPI, and other volumetric parameters [37]. After the insertion of a central venous catheter, the tip is placed near the right atrium, and a thermistor-tipped arterial catheter, the PiCCO™ catheter, is inserted into the femoral or brachial artery and connected to the monitoring system. A 15–20 ml bolus of cold ($<8\,^\circ$C), normal saline is injected through the central venous catheter. The mean value of at least three cold bolus injections reaches acceptable precision in clinical practice [38, 39]. The thermodilution curves are then recorded by the thermistor at the tip of the arterial catheter to allow for an estimation of cardiac output using the Stewart–Hamilton method [37]. Concurrently, the mean transit time and the exponential downslope time of the transpulmonary thermodilution curve are calculated. The product of the cardiac output and the mean transit time represents the intrathoracic thermal volume (ITTV) [36]. The product of the cardiac output and the exponential downslope time represents the pulmonary thermal volume (PTV). GEDV is calculated as the difference between the ITTV and PTV, and represents the combined end-diastolic volumes of the four cardiac chambers. This allows for the calculation of the intrathoracic blood volume (ITBV) from its linear relationship with GEDV: ITBV $= [1.25 \times$ GEDV$] - 28.4$ [36]. EVLW is the difference between the ITTV and the ITBV. The pulmonary blood volume is deduced from the difference between the PTV and the EVLW. The PVPI is calculated as the ratio between the EVLW and the pulmonary blood volume. A recent study by Belda et al. [40] suggested that use of the PiCCO™ catheter did not increase the risk of complications when compared to the commonly used short peripheral arterial or pulmonary artery catheters.

Several studies have suggested that indexing EVLW to the predicted body weight (PBW) instead of the actual body weight (ABW) could improve the predictive value of EVLW for survival and the correlation with markers of disease severity [22, 23, 41]. Indexing EVLW to the PBW instead of the ABW has been shown to improve the correlation between EVLW and lung injury score and the PaO_2/FiO_2 ratio [22]. The PBW is calculated as follows: men, PBW (kg) $= 50 + 0.91 \times$ (height in centimeters $- 152.4$); women, PBW (kg) $= 45.5 + 0.91 \times$ (height in centimeters $- 152.4$]. One must interpret the EVLWI value with caution, especially in studies reported earlier than the year 2008 [22, 41], because previously the EVLW was indexed only by ABW, not by PBW. The EVLW indexed by ABW may result in an underestimation, especially in obese patients [22, 41].

The accuracy of transpulmonary thermodilution EVLW has been validated against quantitative computed tomography (CT) scans [42] and gravimetry, which is considered to be the gold standard [25, 28–30, 35, 43]. EVLW and PVPI correlate with the level of a biological mediator that is thought to be related to increased pulmonary vascular permeability and the accumulation of lung water [44, 45]. Previous studies have also shown that the precision of these variables is clinically acceptable [38, 39].

EVLW: Existence and Degree of Pulmonary Edema

In 1983, Sibbald et al. [46] defined the normal mean EVLW value as 5.6 ml/kg (3.0 to 8.8 ml/kg) using the double-indicator technique. However, this study included only 16 patients, and all of the 'normal' patients were critically ill and mechanically ventilated without a pulmonary edema diagnosis on the basis of portable chest radiography findings. Similar observations were reported in 1986 by Baudendistel et al. [47]; a mean EVLW of 5.1 ml/kg (2.4 to 10.1 ml/kg) was obtained from 6 'normal' critically ill patients. These values have thus been considered as 'normal' for a long period; normal values of 3 to 7 ml/kg (indexed by ABW) have been reported, but without a robust, validated study.

Recently, our clinical-autopsy studies showed mean EVLW values of approximately 7.3 ± 2.8 ml/kg (indexed by PBW) to be the normal reference range for humans ($n = 534$) [29, 32]. This value was supported by Eichhorn et al. [48], who published a meta-analysis of clinical studies in which they found a mean EVLW of 7.3 ml/kg (95 % CI 6.8–7.6) in patients undergoing elective surgery ($n = 687$), who were believed not to have pulmonary edema. More recently, Wolf et al. [49] showed a similar result (8 ml/kg, interquartile range [IQR] 7–9) in 101 elective brain tumor surgery patients. In addition, an EVLWI > 10 ml/kg has been regarded as an increased EVLW in several clinical studies [12, 17, 20–22, 26, 43, 50]. Japanese nation-wide autopsy data ($n = 1688$) indicated that an EVLWI > 9.8 ml/kg represents the quantitative discriminating threshold for a diagnosis of pulmonary edema from normal lungs [32]. Several studies have suggested that an EVLWI > 10 ml/kg is an ideal value to include in a future definition of ARDS [12, 17, 18, 26]. Therefore, a normal EVLW value should be approximately 7 ml/kg and should not exceed 10 ml/kg.

Figure 1 clearly shows that EVLWI correlates with the severity of the lung injury [3, 19, 20, 23, 24, 29, 32, 34, 48, 49, 51, 52]. In addition, a recent multicenter prospective study suggested that EVLWI (and PVPI) was associated with the ARDS severity categories as described by the Berlin definition [17]. Therefore, quantitatively evaluating lung status may help physicians in making an accurate diagnosis. Moreover, evidence suggests that EVLWI relates to patient prognosis [24, 41, 53, 54]. A landmark study by Eisenberg et al. [55] suggested that EVLW-guided treatment reduced mortality rates in patients with permeability pulmonary edema. This study also indicated that patients with an initial EVLW of more than 14 ml/kg had a significantly greater mortality rate than those with a lower EVLW [55]. Sakka et al. [54] found that the mortality rate was approximately 65 % in patients with an EVLW level of 15 ml/kg, whereas the mortality rate was approximately 33 % in patients with an EVLW level of 10 ml/kg. Furthermore, two similar studies by Phillips et al. [41] and Craig et al. [23] demonstrated that an EVLW value > 16 ml/kg predicted intensive care unit (ICU) mortality in patients with ARDS. Recently, Jozwiak et al. [24] reported similar results with more severe and larger numbers of ARDS cases, and confirmed the results with multiple regression models.

The EVLWI value may also allow timely evaluation of pulmonary edema. This is in contrast to chest radiographic findings, which are not time effective and re-

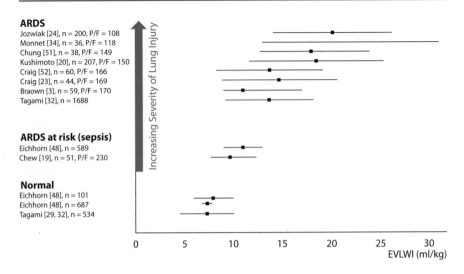

Fig. 1 The extravascular lung water index (EVLWI) and the degree of lung injury in individual studies. Individual studies with more than 30 patients were included. Data are presented as mean (SD) or median (interquartile range). P/F = PaO$_2$/FiO$_2$ ratio

sult in delays of several hours for detecting EVLW [56]. LeTourneau et al. [26] reported that EVLW could predict progression to ARDS in patients at risk for its development 2.6 days before the patients met the AECC criteria for ARDS. These 2.6 days may, therefore, represent a missed opportunity for therapeutic intervention and improved outcome [26]. Zeravik et al. [57] studied 20 patients with lung injury and suggested that EVLW may be useful in deciding when to switch from controlled mechanical ventilation to assisted spontaneous breathing mode (EVLWI < 11 ml/kg). Thus, EVLW may be helpful in guiding fluid management and could facilitate timely respiratory treatment.

PVPI: Differentiating the Types of Pulmonary Edema

It is a daily dilemma for the physician to determine which mechanism is responsible for an increase in EVLW: Extravasation of fluid toward the interstitium resulting from increased hydrostatic pressure in the pulmonary capillary bed, or increased permeability of the lung capillary membrane resulting from damage, as in ARDS. The concept that PVPI may reflect the permeability of the alveolocapillary barrier was first validated by Katzenelson et al. [25] in an animal model. Groeneveld and Verheij [58] demonstrated that lung vascular injury was associated with a rise in PVPI in mechanically ventilated patients with pneumonia or extrapulmonary sepsis-induced ARDS. Monnet et al. [34] reported in their retrospective single-center study that PVPI was a useful index for differentiating the two mechanisms of increased EVLW. Monnet et al. [34] reported that a PVPI ≥ 3 diagnosed ARDS

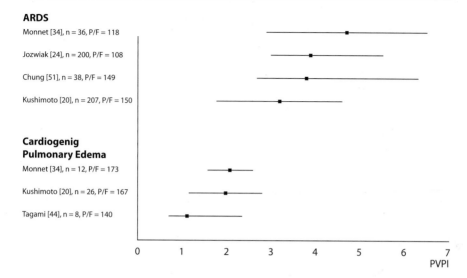

ARDS

Monnet [34], n = 36, P/F = 118

Jozwiak [24], n = 200, P/F = 108

Chung [51], n = 38, P/F = 149

Kushimoto [20], n = 207, P/F = 150

Cardiogenig Pulmonary Edema

Monnet [34], n = 12, P/F = 173

Kushimoto [20], n = 26, P/F = 167

Tagami [44], n = 8, P/F = 140

0 1 2 3 4 5 6 7

PVPI

Fig. 2 Comparisons of the pulmonary vascular permeability index (PVPI) in acute respiratory distress syndrome (ARDS) and cardiogenic pulmonary edema. Data are presented as mean (SD) or median (interquartile range). $P/F = PaO_2/FiO_2$ ratio

with a sensitivity of 85 % and a specificity of 100 %. We recently confirmed this finding in a large prospective, multicenter study [20], demonstrating that a PVPI value of 2.6 to 2.85 provided a definitive diagnosis of ARDS (specificity 0.90 to 0.95), and a value < 1.7 ruled out an ARDS diagnosis (specificity 0.95) [20]. Although this discrepancy may result from the difference in the studied patients' characteristics, further studies are needed to confirm the results because there were fewer cardiogenic pulmonary edema patients than ARDS patients in both studies (Fig. 2) [20, 34].

PVPI seems to be a better marker of disease severity in patients with a lung injury score > 2.5, implying that patients with severe ARDS have greater lung edema because of greater pulmonary permeability [19]. In addition, van der Heijden and Groeneveld [59] demonstrated that PVPI relates to pulmonary capillary permeability in non-septic patients on mechanical ventilation with or at risk for ARDS, and is largely unaffected by fluid loading and pressure forces. Normal ratios may help to exclude high permeability, independent of the clinical manifestations of permeability edema [59].

Examples: Interpretation of EVLW and PVPI Values

A patient admitted 2 days earlier with bacterial pneumonia and bilateral consolidations on a CT scan was ventilated with an FiO_2 of 60 %, a PEEP of 10 cm H_2O, and had an EVLW of 17 ml/kg, and a PVPI of 4.0. This patient must have moderate to severe ARDS with a high possibility of mortality. Early and aggressive intervention, in addition to lung-protective ventilation, may be required. On the other hand, despite a 2-day history of sepsis with fluid overload, 'white lungs' on portable radiograph, and ventilation with an FiO$_2$ of 60 % and a PEEP level of 10 cm H$_2$O, an EVLW of 8 ml/kg and a PVPI of 1.0 could indicate clinical conditions other than pulmonary edema, such as pleural effusion, atelectasis, or lobar/lung collapse. Appropriate therapies such as paracentesis, bronchoscopy, or addition of a higher PEEP may be required.

Limitations of Transpulmonary Thermodilution

Transpulmonary thermodilution has several limitations, mainly large vascular obstruction and focal lung injury, which clinicians must bear in mind when interpreting EVLW numbers. The amount of EVLW, the PaO$_2$/FiO$_2$ ratio, the tidal volume, and the PEEP level may slightly but significantly affect the estimation of EVLW by transpulmonary thermodilution [58]. Other limitations are discussed elsewhere in detail [60].

Conclusions

The transpulmonary thermodilution-derived variables, EVLW and PVPI, can quantitatively express the existence, severity, and nature of pulmonary edema at the bedside. The accuracy of this measurement has been validated against the gold standard method, and the precision is clinically acceptable. These values have significant clinical implications, predict the progression of disease, correlate with prognosis, and may be the key 'bridge' for a pathological-clinical correlation. EVLW and PVPI may open the door for future work to better define management algorithms for patients with pulmonary edema.

References

1. Ware LB, Matthay MA (2005) Clinical practice. Acute pulmonary edema. N Engl J Med 353:2788–2796
2. Meade MO, Cook RJ, Guyatt GH et al (2000) Interobserver variation in interpreting chest radiographs for the diagnosis of acute respiratory distress syndrome. Am J Respir Crit Care Med 161:85–90
3. Brown LM, Calfee CS, Howard JP, Craig TR, Matthay MA, McAuley DF (2013) Comparison of thermodilution measured extravascular lung water with chest radiographic assessment of pulmonary oedema in patients with acute lung injury. Ann Intensive Care 3:25
4. Ashbaugh DG, Bigelow DB, Petty TL, Levine BE (1967) Acute respiratory distress in adults. Lancet 2:319–323
5. Bernard GR, Artigas A, Brigham KL et al (1994) The American-European Consensus Conference on ARDS. Definitions, mechanisms, relevant outcomes, and clinical trial coordination. Am J Respir Crit Care Med 149:818–824

6. Esteban A, Fernandez-Segoviano P, Frutos-Vivar F et al (2004) Comparison of clinical criteria for the acute respiratory distress syndrome with autopsy findings. Ann Intern Med 141:440–445

7. de Hemptinne Q, Remmelink M, Brimioulle S, Salmon I, Vincent JL (2009) ARDS: a clinico-pathological confrontation. Chest 135:944–949

8. Ferguson ND, Frutos-Vivar F, Esteban A et al (2005) Acute respiratory distress syndrome: Underrecognition by clinicians and diagnostic accuracy of three clinical definitions. Crit Care Med 33:2228–2234

9. Sarmiento X, Guardiola JJ, Almirall J et al (2011) Discrepancy between clinical criteria for diagnosing acute respiratory distress syndrome secondary to community acquired pneumonia with autopsy findings of diffuse alveolar damage. Respir Med 105:1170–1175

10. Allardet-Servent J, Forel JM, Roch A et al (2009) FIO2 and acute respiratory distress syndrome definition during lung protective ventilation. Crit Care Med 37:202–207

11. Estenssoro E, Dubin A, Laffaire E et al (2003) Impact of positive end-expiratory pressure on the definition of acute respiratory distress syndrome. Intensive Care Med 29:1936–1942

12. Michard F, Fernandez-Mondejar E, Kirov MY, Malbrain M, Tagami T (2012) A new and simple definition for acute lung injury. Crit Care Med 40:1004–1006

13. Ranieri VM, Rubenfeld GD, Thompson BT et al (2012) Acute respiratory distress syndrome: the Berlin Definition. JAMA 307:2526–2533

14. Phillips CR (2013) The Berlin definition: real change or the emperor's new clothes? Crit Care 17:174

15. Thille AW, Esteban A, Fernandez-Segoviano P et al (2013) Comparison of the Berlin definition for acute respiratory distress syndrome with autopsy. Am J Respir Crit Care Med 187:761–767

16. Thompson BT, Matthay MA (2013) The Berlin definition of ARDS versus pathological evidence of diffuse alveolar damage. Am J Respir Crit Care Med 187:675–677

17. Kushimoto S, Endo T, Yamanouchi S et al (2013) Relationship between extravascular lung water and severity categories of acute respiratory distress syndrome by the Berlin definition. Crit Care 17:R132

18. Perel A (2013) Extravascular lung water and the pulmonary vascular permeability index may improve the definition of ARDS. Crit Care 17:108

19. Chew MS, Ihrman L, During J et al (2012) Extravascular lung water index improves the diagnostic accuracy of lung injury in patients with shock. Crit Care 16:R1

20. Kushimoto S, Taira Y, Kitazawa Y et al (2012) The clinical usefulness of extravascular lung water and pulmonary vascular permeability index to diagnose and characterize pulmonary edema: a prospective multicenter study on the quantitative differential diagnostic definition for acute lung injury/acute respiratory distress syndrome. Crit Care 16:R232

21. Martin GS, Eaton S, Mealer M, Moss M (2005) Extravascular lung water in patients with severe sepsis: a prospective cohort study. Crit Care 9:R74–82

22. Berkowitz DM, Danai PA, Eaton S, Moss M, Martin GS (2008) Accurate characterization of extravascular lung water in acute respiratory distress syndrome. Crit Care Med 36:1803–1809

23. Craig TR, Duffy MJ, Shyamsundar M et al (2010) Extravascular lung water indexed to predicted body weight is a novel predictor of intensive care unit mortality in patients with acute lung injury. Crit Care Med 38:114–120

24. Jozwiak M, Silva S, Persichini R et al (2013) Extravascular lung water is an independent prognostic factor in patients with acute respiratory distress syndrome. Crit Care Med 41:472–480

25. Katzenelson R, Perel A, Berkenstadt H et al (2004) Accuracy of transpulmonary thermodilution versus gravimetric measurement of extravascular lung water. Crit Care Med 32:1550–1554

26. LeTourneau JL, Pinney J, Phillips CR (2012) Extravascular lung water predicts progression to acute lung injury in patients with increased risk. Crit Care Med 40:847–854

27. Michard F (2013) The (pulmonary) watergate revisited. Crit Care Med 41:2234–2235

28. Kirov MY, Kuzkov VV, Kuklin VN, Waerhaug K, Bjertnaes LJ (2004) Extravascular lung water assessed by transpulmonary single thermodilution and postmortem gravimetry in sheep. Crit Care 8:R451–458

29. Tagami T, Kushimoto S, Yamamoto Y et al (2010) Validation of extravascular lung water measurement by single transpulmonary thermodilution: human autopsy study. Crit Care 14:R162

30. Venkateswaran RV, Dronavalli V, Patchell V et al (2013) Measurement of extravascular lung water following human brain death: implications for lung donor assessment and transplantation. Eur J Cardiothorac Surg 43:1227–1232

31. Corrin B, Nicholoson A (2011) Pathology of the Lungs. Churchill Livingstone, Edinburgh

32. Tagami T, Sawabe M, Kushimoto S et al (2013) Quantitative diagnosis of diffuse alveolar damage using extravascular lung water. Crit Care Med 41:2144–2150

33. Ferguson ND, Fan E, Camporota L et al (2012) The Berlin definition of ARDS: an expanded rationale, justification, and supplementary material. Intensive Care Med 38:1573–1582

34. Monnet X, Anguel N, Osman D, Hamzaoui O, Richard C, Teboul JL (2007) Assessing pulmonary permeability by transpulmonary thermodilution allows differentiation of hydrostatic pulmonary edema from ALI/ARDS. Intensive Care Med 33:448–453

35. Mihm FG, Feeley TW, Jamieson SW (1987) Thermal dye double indicator dilution measurement of lung water in man: comparison with gravimetric measurements. Thorax 42:72–76

36. Sakka SG, Ruhl CC, Pfeiffer UJ et al (2000) Assessment of cardiac preload and extravascular lung water by single transpulmonary thermodilution. Intensive care medicine 26:180–187

37. Sakka SG, Reuter DA, Perel A (2012) The transpulmonary thermodilution technique. J Clin Monit Comput 26:347–353

38. Monnet X, Persichini R, Ktari M, Jozwiak M, Richard C, Teboul JL (2011) Precision of the transpulmonary thermodilution measurements. Crit Care 15:R204

39. Tagami T, Kushimoto S, Tosa R et al (2012) The precision of PiCCO measurements in hypothermic post-cardiac arrest patients. Anaesthesia 67:236–243

40. Belda FJ, Aguilar G, Teboul JL et al (2011) Complications related to less-invasive haemodynamic monitoring. Br J Anaesth 106:482–486

41. Phillips CR, Chesnutt MS, Smith SM (2008) Extravascular lung water in sepsis-associated acute respiratory distress syndrome: indexing with predicted body weight improves correlation with severity of illness and survival. Crit Care Med 36:69–73

42. Patroniti N, Bellani G, Maggioni E, Manfio A, Marcora B, Pesenti A (2005) Measurement of pulmonary edema in patients with acute respiratory distress syndrome. Crit Care Med 33:2547–2554

43. Venkateswaran RV, Dronavalli V, Patchell V et al (2012) Measurement of extravascular lung water following human brain death; implications for lung donor assessment and transplantation. Eur J Cardiothorac Surg 43:1227–1232

44. Tagami T, Kushimoto S, Tosa R et al (2011) Plasma neutrophil elastase correlates with pulmonary vascular permeability: a prospective observational study in patients with pneumonia. Respirology 16:953–958

45. O'Kane CM, McKeown SW, Perkins GD et al (2009) Salbutamol up-regulates matrix metalloproteinase-9 in the alveolar space in the acute respiratory distress syndrome. Crit Care Med 37:2242–2249

46. Sibbald WJ, Warshawski FJ, Short AK, Harris J, Lefcoe MS, Holliday RL (1983) Clinical studies of measuring extravascular lung water by the thermal dye technique in critically ill patients. Chest 83:725–731

47. Baudendistel LJ, Kaminski DL, Dahms TE (1986) Evaluation of extravascular lung water by single thermal indicator. Crit Care Med 14:52–56

48. Eichhorn V, Goepfert MS, Eulenburg C, Malbrain ML, Reuter DA (2012) Comparison of values in critically ill patients for global end-diastolic volume and extravascular lung water measured by transcardiopulmonary thermodilution: a meta-analysis of the literature. Med Intensiva 36:467–474

49. Wolf S, Riess A, Landscheidt JF, Lumenta CB, Schurer L, Friederich P (2013) How to perform indexing of extravascular lung water: a validation study. Crit Care Med 41:990–998

50. Watanabe A, Tagami T, Yokobori S et al (2012) Global end-diastolic volume is associated with the occurrence of delayed cerebral ischemia and pulmonary edema after subarachnoid hemorrhage. Shock 38:480–485

51. Chung FT, Lin HC, Kuo CH et al (2010) Extravascular lung water correlates multiorgan dysfunction syndrome and mortality in sepsis. PLoS One 5:e15265

52. Craig TR, Duffy MJ, Shyamsundar M et al (2011) A randomized clinical trial of hydroxymethylglutaryl-coenzyme a reductase inhibition for acute lung injury (The HARP Study). Am J Respir Crit Care Med 183:620–626

53. Zhang Z, Lu B, Ni H (2012) Prognostic value of extravascular lung water index in critically ill patients: a systematic review of the literature. J Crit Care 27:420

54. Sakka SG, Klein M, Reinhart K, Meier-Hellmann A (2002) Prognostic value of extravascular lung water in critically ill patients. Chest 122:2080–2086

55. Eisenberg PR, Hansbrough JR, Anderson D, Schuster DP (1987) A prospective study of lung water measurements during patient management in an intensive care unit. Am Rev Respir Dis 136:662–668

56. Baudendistel L, Shields JB, Kaminski DL (1982) Comparison of double indicator thermodilution measurements of extravascular lung water (EVLW) with radiographic estimation of lung water in trauma patients. J Trauma 22:983–988

57. Zeravik J, Eckart J, Zimmermann G, Blumel G, Pfeiffer UJ, Wellhofer H (1989) Indications for combined high frequency ventilation in clinical use. Acta Anaesthesiol Scand Suppl 90:149–152

58. Groeneveld AB, Verheij J (2006) Extravascular lung water to blood volume ratios as measures of permeability in sepsis-induced ALI/ARDS. Intensive Care Med 32:1315–1321

59. van der Heijden M, Groeneveld AB (2010) Extravascular lung water to blood volume ratios as measures of pulmonary capillary permeability in nonseptic critically ill patients. J Crit Care 25:16–22

60. Michard F, Schachtrupp A, Toens C (2005) Factors influencing the estimation of extravascular lung water by transpulmonary thermodilution in critically ill patients. Crit Care Med 33:1243–1247

Distinguishing Between Cardiogenic and Increased Permeability Pulmonary Edema

O. Hamzaoui, X. Monnet, and J.-L. Teboul

Introduction

The differential diagnosis between cardiogenic pulmonary edema and increased permeability pulmonary edema or acute respiratory distress syndrome (ARDS) is a daily challenge for the intensive care unit (ICU) physician. Left atrial hypertension as the principal cause of cardiogenic pulmonary edema must be excluded in order to establish a diagnosis of ARDS [1]. Indeed, a pulmonary artery occlusion pressure (PAOP) greater than 18 mmHg is classically used as a marker of left atrial hypertension. PAOP measurement requires the insertion of a pulmonary artery catheter (PAC), an invasive and costly procedure, which has been associated with neutral [2] or potentially adverse clinical outcomes [3]. Nonetheless, distinction between cardiogenic pulmonary edema and ARDS is important, because the management and prognosis of these two pathological conditions are quite different [4]. In this review, we will go through the recent literature on various tools that enable differentiation of cardiogenic pulmonary edema and ARDS in critically ill patients.

Pathophysiology

ARDS has been described as passing through three pathological phases. An initial exudative phase begins with neutrophil-mediated damage to the alveolus, causing epithelial and endothelial damage. This leads to proteinaceous and markedly hem-

O. Hamzaoui
Hôpital Antoine Béclère, Service de Réanimation Médicale, Hôpitaux Universitaires Paris-Sud, 92141 Clamart, France

X. Monnet · J.-L. Teboul ✉
Hôpital de Bicêtre, Service de Réanimation Médicale, Hôpitaux Universitaires Paris-Sud, 94270 Le Kremlin-Bicêtre, France
Faculté de Médecine Paris-Sud, Université Paris-Sud, 94270 Le Kremlin-Bicêtre, France
e-mail: jean-louis.teboul@bct.aphp.fr

J.-L. Vincent (Ed.), *Annual Update in Intensive Care and Emergency Medicine 2014*,
DOI 10.1007/978-3-319-03746-2_21, © Springer International Publishing Switzerland
2014

orrhagic interstitial and alveolar edema [5]. A proliferative phase begins three to five days later and is characterized by organization of the exudate and by fibrosis. The capillary network is also damaged with development of intimal proliferation in many small vessels leading to a reduced luminal area. Alveolar type II cells proliferate in an attempt to cover the denuded epithelial surfaces and differentiate into type I cells. Fibroblasts become apparent in the interstitial space and later in the alveolar lumen. These processes result in narrowing or even obliteration of the airspaces. Fibrin and cell debris are progressively replaced by collagen fibrils [5]. A third fibrotic phase may develop later. The vasculature is markedly altered with vessels narrowed by myointimal thickening and mural fibrosis. There is a marked decline in neutrophils and a relative accumulation of lymphocytes and macrophages. Total lung collagen content may double within the first two weeks, however these alterations can be transient [5].

In contrast to ARDS, cardiogenic pulmonary edema is characterized by no substantial damage to the structure of the alveolus but rather by an increased pulmonary capillary hydrostatic pressure (i. e., lung filtration pressure). This latter phenomenon leads to an imbalance in transcapillary fluid movement, as predicted by the Starling equation [6]. At equilibrium, the transcapillary flow (from the capillaries to the interstitium) is continuously drained by the lymphatic system. However, when an acute increase in pulmonary hydrostatic pressure occurs via a generalized increase in blood volume or an acute redistribution of fluid (in case of acute heart failure), drainage systems are exceeded leading to airspace flooding [7]. Moreover the weak permeability of the alveolar epithelium and the interstitial distension due to fluids causing destruction of alveolar septa, results in alveolar edema.

Diagnostic Tools

Clinical Judgment

Some clinical elements may help in the differentiation between cardiogenic pulmonary edema and ARDS. History of cardiovascular disease or a recent cardiovascular event is in favor of cardiogenic pulmonary edema, whereas fever and cough may suggest ARDS. Nevertheless, the clinical examination is rarely discriminative and physicians are frequently unable to distinguish between cardiogenic and non-cardiogenic origins of pulmonary edema [6, 8]. Wheeze and widespread crepitations may occur in any form of pulmonary edema [6]. Important prognostic clinical signs of cardiogenic pulmonary edema, such as raised jugular venous pressure (JVP) or a third heart sound, may be difficult to assess with certainty in ICU patients [6, 9].

Pulmonary Artery Catheter

The PAC provides measurement of the PAOP, which reflects the pressure in a large pulmonary vein and thus the left atrial pressure. Although a PAOP value of 18 mmHg is classically considered as the cut-off value for distinguishing between cardiogenic pulmonary edema and increased permeability pulmonary edema, PAOP can be higher in 25–30 % cases of established acute lung injury (ALI) or ARDS [10]. Importantly, there are some sources of errors in measurement or interpretation of PAOP that deserve to be briefly reviewed.

The PAOP is obtained after inflation of the balloon at the tip of the PAC. Inflation of the distal balloon creates a continuous column of stagnant blood from the occluded branch of the pulmonary artery and the pulmonary vein where the blood flow resumes. However, if the PAC tip is in West zone 1 or 2, alveolar pressure interrupts the static blood column. In this case, which may occur with high positive end-expiratory pressure (PEEP) ventilation and/or hypovolemia, PAOP reflects alveolar pressure and not pulmonary venous pressure and left atrial pressure. Comparison of respiratory changes in pulmonary artery pressure with respiratory changes in PAOP allows identification of West zone 1 or 2 conditions [11].

In clinical practice, PAOP is assumed to estimate the pulmonary capillary pressure, which is an important determinant of lung filtration according to Starling's equation. However, the difference between pulmonary capillary pressure and PAOP is not constant because it depends on cardiac output and pulmonary venous resistance. This latter parameter can be abnormally elevated in patients with ARDS or congestive heart failure so that the PAOP cannot be a strong surrogate of pulmonary capillary pressure in pulmonary edema situations [12].

In the presence of PEEP or intrinsic PEEP, the value of end-expiratory PAOP overestimates the true left ventricular (LV) filling pressure. The difference between the two pressures is the end-expiratory intrathoracic pressure, which depends on PEEP and on the percentage of airway pressure transmission. Airway transmission can be estimated by dividing the respiratory changes in PAOP by the changes in alveolar pressure occurring at the same time [13].

All these potential errors in measurement and interpretation of PAOP, as well as the invasiveness of the PAC, the absence of proved benefit in clinical trials [2] and the development of less invasive technologies, are probably responsible for the current decline in PAC use in ICU patients.

Doppler-echocardiography

The LV filling pressure can be estimated non-invasively using Doppler-echocardiography. Although different methods have been proposed, all have limitations in terms of measurements as well as interpretation, so that Doppler-echocardiography provides a semi-quantitative estimation of LV filling pressure rather than an exact measure.

To assess LV filling pressure, pulsed-wave Doppler is performed in the apical 4-chamber view to obtain mitral inflow velocities [14], which consist of E (early diastolic) and A (late diastolic) velocities. A 1-mm to 3-mm sample volume is then placed in the mitral outflow 1 cm beyond the mitral leaflets to record a crisp velocity profile during diastole. Optimizing spectral gain and wall filter settings is important to clearly display the onset and cessation of LV inflow [14]. The E wave corresponds to the early LV filling phase and begins after the opening of the mitral valve, and the A wave corresponds to the left atrial contraction (Fig. 1). It is well established that the mitral E-wave velocity primarily reflects the left atrial-LV pressure gradient during early diastole and is thus influenced by preload and alterations in LV relaxation [15]. The mitral A-wave velocity reflects the left atrial-LV pressure gradient during late diastole, which is affected by LV compliance and left atrial contractility [15]. The E/A ratio was shown to be significantly correlated to PAOP [16]. Nevertheless, in cases of non-depressed LV ejection fraction (LVEF), the correlation is very weak [16]. It is thus recommended to pay attention to E/A as an estimate of left atrial pressure only in patients with a depressed LVEF [14]. In such cases, E/A < 1 suggests a non-elevated left atrial pressure, whereas E/A > 2 suggests a high left atrial pressure [14]. If the value of E/A is between 1 and 2, it is not sufficiently informative and measurement of other Doppler-echocardiographic indices is mandatory (see below) [14]. In addition, there are many limitations to use of E/A, such as atrial fibrillation, where no A-wave occurs, and sinus tachycardia with merging of the E and A waves.

The apical four-chamber view also allows tissue Doppler imaging of the mitral annulus to be obtained, which enables measurement of the early diastolic mitral annular velocity (E' or Ea). The E'-wave has been shown to be a load-independent measure of myocardial relaxation [17]. Combination of tissue Doppler imaging and pulsed Doppler transmitral flow, allows the E/E' ratio to be calculated, which is considered to be one of the best echocardiographic estimates of LV filling pressure irrespective of the LVEF [16].

An E/E' ratio < 8 is usually associated with normal LV filling pressure, whereas an E/E' ratio > 15 is associated with increased LV filling pressure [18]. When the E/E' ratio is between 8 and 15 (gray zone), it is not sufficiently informative to estimate LV filling pressure, so that measurements of other Doppler-echocardiographic indices are mandatory [14]. It should be stressed that, in the majority of ICU patients, the E/E' value is within this large gray zone and thus is inconclusive [19–23]. In this context, analysis of the pulmonary venous flow using pulsed wave Doppler can be performed in the apical 4-chamber view, although its feasibility is not optimal in the ICU patient. Measurements of pulmonary venous waveforms include the peak systolic velocity (S), the peak anterograde diastolic velocity (D), the S/D ratio and the peak Ar velocity in late diastole. Other useful measurements are the duration of the Ar wave and the time difference between Ar and mitral A-wave duration (Ar-A) [14]. Increased LV filling pressure is frequently associated with an increased Ar-A duration (> 30 ms) and an S/D ratio < 1 [24].

Another method to estimate LV filling pressure is to measure the color M-mode flow propagation velocity (Vp) in the apical 4-chamber view using color flow imag-

4-chamber apical view

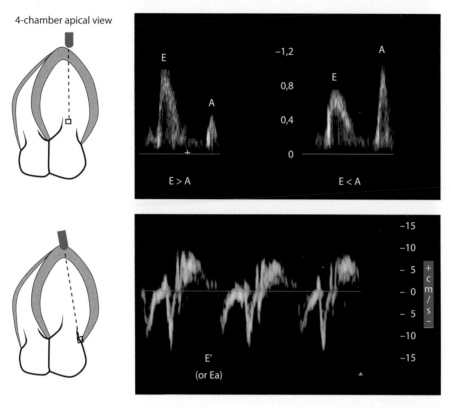

Fig. 1 Transmitral flow and tissue Doppler imaging of the mitral annulus. *Top*: With pulsed-wave Doppler, the sampling window is placed in the transmitral flow, beyond the mitral leaflets; this enables recording of the E and A waves. *Bottom*: With tissue Doppler imaging of the mitral annulus, the E′ (or Ea) and the A′ waves can be recorded

ing with a narrow color sector. The Vp is measured as the slope of the first aliasing velocity during early filling, measured from the mitral valve plane to 4 cm distally into the LV cavity [25]. The ratio of peak E velocity to Vp is directly proportional to left atrial pressure so that E/Vp has been proposed to estimate the LV filling pressure [25]. In patients with depressed LVEF, an E/Vp ≥ 2.5 was shown to predict a PAOP > 15 mmHg with reasonably good accuracy [26]. However, reproducibility of E/Vp in ICU patients is highly questionable [19]. Moreover, this method requires good echogenicity, which is often not present in critically ill patients.

In summary, a non-invasive semi-quantitative estimation of LV filling pressure is feasible at the bedside using Doppler-echocardiography. However, Doppler-echocardiography is an operator-dependent technique and measurement of these indices requires a high degree of knowledge of the operator [27]. This may explain the large variability in the cut-off echocardiographic estimates of LV filling pressure reported in studies conducted in ICU patients [19–23].

B-type Natriuretic Peptide and Amino-Terminal pro-BNP

B-type natriuretic peptide (BNP) is one of the members of the natriuretic peptide superfamily, synthesized and secreted by the ventricular cardiomyocytes in response to ventricular stretching [28, 29]. BNP secretion is markedly increased beyond the physiologic range by pathologic ventricular volume and/or pressure overload [30, 31]. Plasma BNP concentration is thus significantly elevated in patients with heart failure [32, 33] and is useful for the diagnostic approach to acute dyspnea [34, 35]. It has been suggested that BNP measurements could add to the clinical history, physical examination, and routine diagnostic data in order to exclude cardiogenic pulmonary edema in ICU patients with respiratory failure [8]. A low plasma concentration of BNP (< 200 pg/ml) was found to have a high specificity for the diagnosis of non-cardiogenic pulmonary edema and could reliably exclude the presence of cardiogenic pulmonary edema in a large number of patients [8]. However, a high BNP level cannot exclude a diagnosis of ARDS because factors other than myocardial stretch can elevate plasma BNP concentration. Septic shock is a condition in which release of BNP can be increased through enhancement of BNP gene transcription by pro-inflammatory cytokines [36]. Additionally, high plasma BNP levels could be also partially related to altered plasma BNP clearance pathway in septic shock patients [37]. Accordingly, elevated plasma BNP levels have been repeatedly reported in septic shock patients even in those without cardiac dysfunction [38–41]. In patients with renal failure, decreased BNP clearance can be responsible for an increased plasma BNP concentration independent of cardiac dysfunction [30, 42, 43]. Right ventricular dysfunction can also result in increased plasma BNP concentration [44].

The prohormone, NT-proBNP, which is the amino-terminal fragment of BNP, is also secreted by ventricular cardiomyocytes in response to ventricular stretching. However, it differs from BNP with regard to its biological half-life, *in vitro* stability, and mechanisms involved in its clearance [42]. NT-proBNP has been suggested to be a stronger discriminator of cardiac dysfunction in patients with significant comorbidities, preexisting cardiac dysfunction, and impaired renal function compared to BNP [45]. The proposed explanation for this difference is that NT-proBNP has much higher molar concentrations and steeper increases for any given degree of cardiac dysfunction. As such, NT-proBNP would be a more sensitive measure of cardiac dysfunction, particularly for milder degrees [45]. However, as with BNP, NT-proBNP does not correlate with PAOP [45]. Additionally, because NT-proBNP can also be increased in renal failure and in sepsis regardless of cardiac function, its utility to reliably discriminate cardiogenic pulmonary edema from ARDS remains debatable. As for BNP, a low value of NT-proBNP is suggestive of the absence of cardiogenic pulmonary edema, whereas a high value has a far less informative value. Finally, the longer biological half-life of NT-proBNP compared with BNP (70 min vs. 20 min) makes it less sensitive to short-term fluctuations in cardio-pulmonary status and less useful for short-term tests and/or evaluation of some therapies.

Lung Ultrasonography

Ultrasonography, traditionally used to explore plain organs, has recently been extended to the lungs in critically ill patients. Chest ultrasonography is becoming a bedside tool for the detection of thoracic disorders, in particular to diagnose the origin of acute respiratory failure [46–48]. Chest ultrasound is performed in the semi-recumbent position, or in the supine position in intubated patients. In a longitudinal scan, pleural lines, sought between two rib shadows, indicate the pleural layers. The horizontal lines arising from the pleural line and separated by regular intervals that are equal to the distance between the skin and the pleural line are called A-lines. The bilateral B profile including comet-tail artifacts (vertical B-lines) that arise strictly from the pleural line, characterizes pulmonary edema with high accuracy [47]. Whereas the A-line is a horizontal artifact indicating a normal lung surface, the B-line is a kind of comet-tail artifact indicating subpleural interstitial edema. In this regard, lung ultrasound was shown to be helpful in differentiating pulmonary edema from other types of respiratory failure, such as pneumonia, acute exacerbation of chronic obstructive pulmonary disease (COPD), pulmonary embolism, or asthma [47]. In a recent study [48], which included 75 patients admitted to the ICU for acute respiratory failure, the ultrasound approach was more accurate than a standard approach based on clinical, radiological, and biological data and associated with a significant improvement in the initial diagnostic accuracy [48].

In addition, some clinical studies have found that ultrasound evidence of elevated extravascular lung water (EVLW) (ultrasound comets or B-lines) correlated positively with radiographic and invasive methods of EVLW estimation [49–51]. In an experimental study, a significant increase in B-lines with time was observed after oleic acid infusion and a significant correlation was shown between the number of B-lines at the time of animal sacrifice and the wet/dry ratio using a gravimetric method [52]. This observation confirms that the presence of B-lines or ultrasound comets can be seen in the two types of pulmonary edema and thus cannot *per se* reliably differentiate cardiogenic pulmonary edema from increased permeability pulmonary edema. In this context, a comparison between lung ultrasound findings and PAOP (measured using a PAC) was performed in 102 mechanically ventilated patients [53]. The authors defined A-predominance as a majority of anterior A-lines and B-predominance as a majority of anterior B-lines. A PAOP > 18 mmHg was associated with B-predominance in 14/15 cases. However, a PAOP ≤ 18 mmHg was associated with A-predominance in 44 cases and with B-predominance in 43 cases [53] confirming that this technique cannot reliably differentiate between cardiogenic pulmonary edema and ARDS.

In summary, lung ultrasonography appears to be a good technique for diagnosing pulmonary edema but not for differentiating between the two main mechanisms of lung edema formation. In addition, this technique has some limitations: in particular, it is a user-dependent technique, which requires an advanced level of training. It is also important to note that B-lines can be detected in other diseases, such as pulmonary fibrosis, and may also be affected by other dynamic changes, such as the application of PEEP and the respiratory cycle [54].

Transpulmonary Thermodilution

The transpulmonary thermodilution method applies indicator dilution principles, using cold as the indicator. A known amount of cold solution with a known temperature is injected rapidly into the circulation through a central venous catheter (superior vena cava territory). This cold solution mixes with the surrounding blood, and the temperature is measured downstream at the level of the femoral artery through a thermistor-tipped arterial catheter. The mathematical analysis of the thermodilution curve (blood temperature vs. time) recorded by the device not only allows calculation of cardiac output but also of other relevant hemodynamic variables such as EVLW and the pulmonary vascular permeability index (PVPI).

The EVLW measured by transpulmonary thermodilution was found to be correlate well with the EVLW measured by gravimetry, the method of reference in animals [55], and with the post-mortem lung weight in humans [56]. The EVLW values measured by the PiCCO™ and the VolumeView™ monitors agree in animals [57] and in humans [58]. The normal range of indexed EVLW (EVLWI) values is between 3 and 7 mL/kg. Because of the potential errors in measurements, it is generally assumed that EVLWI is abnormally high (pulmonary edema) when it is above 10 ml/kg. A recent study suggests however, that EVLW can be between 10 and 14 ml/kg in dying patients with no evidence of lung edema at autopsy [59]. In cases of cardiogenic pulmonary edema or ARDS, values greater than 35 ml/kg can be measured [60]. The EVLW is thus considered a marker of pulmonary edema but cannot diagnose its origin. In contrast, the PVPI is highly valuable for differentiating between cardiogenic pulmonary edema and ARDS. This parameter is calculated automatically by transpulmonary thermodilution as the ratio of EVLW/pulmonary blood volume and as such is assumed to reflect the permeability of the lung capillary membrane. This was confirmed in an animal study in which PVPI increased when pulmonary edema was created by lung instillation of oleic acid but did not change when it was created by balloon inflation in the left atrium [55]. The discriminative value of PVPI was demonstrated in two clinical studies showing that a PVPI greater than 2.85 [61] or than 3 [62] could diagnose increased permeability edema with excellent accuracy. In these two studies, the diagnosis of reference was made *a posteriori* by experts, who considered the patient history, clinical presentation, chest computed tomography (CT) and X-ray, echocardiography, BNP level, and the time course of all preceding findings under hemodynamic and respiratory therapies [61, 62]. In a study including 200 patients with ARDS, the PVPI was shown to be an independent predictor of mortality, confirming its excellent clinical relevance [60]. However, using PVPI to differentiate between cardiogenic pulmonary edema and ARDS is limited to ICU patients and cannot be used practically in the emergency department since transpulmonary thermodilution measurements need insertion of both a central venous line and a femoral artery catheter.

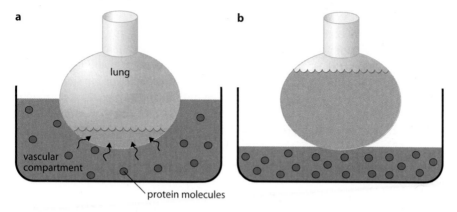

Fig. 2 Hemoconcentration during hydrostatic pulmonary edema. **a** In hydrostatic pulmonary edema, the increased pressure gradient between the pulmonary vascular compartment and the interstitial tissue leads to filtration of a significant volume of hypo-oncotic fluid, **b** which induces intravascular volume contraction and thus elevation of biochemical markers of hemoconcentration, such as plasma protein concentration

Biochemical Markers of Hemoconcentration

Hydrostatic pulmonary edema is accompanied by transfer of a hypo-oncotic fluid from the pulmonary capillary lumen toward the interstitium [63–65] (Fig. 2). When the amount of transferred fluid is large enough, hydrostatic pulmonary edema may result in hemoconcentration that can be detected on the basis of changes in plasma protein or hemoglobin concentrations or hematocrit [63–65]. Thus, measuring the changes in biochemical markers of hemoconcentration can help to differentiate between cardiogenic pulmonary edema and increased permeability pulmonary edema in patients who develop a sudden episode of pulmonary edema during their hospital stay. In this context, it has been demonstrated in critically ill patients who failed to be weaned from mechanical ventilation that an increase in plasma protein concentration and/or hemoglobin concentration $> 6\,\%$ during a weaning trial allowed a diagnosis of weaning-induced pulmonary edema with good sensitivity and specificity [66]. Detection of acute onset of hemoconcentration is more difficult in patients presenting to the hospital with pulmonary edema, because their normal plasma protein concentration and/or hemoglobin concentration are generally unknown. However, observation of abnormally high plasma protein and/or hemoglobin concentrations in patients with respiratory failure, suggests that acute cardiogenic pulmonary edema is developing and should encourage the physician to confirm this diagnosis.

Conclusions

Despite the availability of many tools to differentiate between cardiogenic pulmonary edema and ARDS, such as the PAC, Doppler-echocardiography, BNP, and others, this differentiation remains a difficult daily challenge for physicians. This difficulty is mainly related to the imperfection of these tools when used separately. Therefore, combining and multiplying the diagnostic methods may help to refine the correct diagnosis and improve patient management.

References

1. Ferguson ND, Fan E, Camporota L et al (2012) The Berlin definition of ARDS: an expanded rationale, justification, and supplementary material. Intensive Care Med 38:1573–1582
2. Shah MR, Hasselblad V, Stevenson LW et al (2005) Impact of the pulmonary artery catheter in critically ill patients: meta-analysis of randomized clinical trials. JAMA 294:1664–1670
3. Connors AF Jr, Speroff T, Dawson NV et al (1996) The effectiveness of right heart catheterization in the initial care of critically ill patients. SUPPORT Investigators. JAMA 276:889–897
4. Brower RG, Ware LB, Berthiaume Y, Matthay MA (2001) Treatment of ARDS. Chest 120:1347–1367
5. Bellingan GJ (2002) The pulmonary physician in critical care: the pathogenesis of ALI/ARDS. Thorax 57:540–546
6. Ware LB, Matthay MA (2005) Clinical practice. Acute pulmonary edema. N Engl J Med 353:2788–2796
7. Cleland JG, Yassin AS, Khadjooi K (2010) Acute heart failure: focusing on acute cardiogenic pulmonary oedema. Clin Med 10:1059–1064
8. Karmpaliotis D, Kirtane AJ, Ruisi CP et al (2007) Diagnostic and prognostic utility of brain natriuretic Peptide in subjects admitted to the ICU with hypoxic respiratory failure due to non cardiogenic and cardiogenic pulmonary edema. Chest 131:964–971
9. Drazner MH, Rame JE, Stevenson LW et al (2001) Prognostic importance of elevated jugular venous pressure and a third heart sound in patients with heart failure. N Engl J Med 345:574–581
10. Ferguson ND, Meade MO, Hallett DC, Stewart TE (2002) High values of the pulmonary artery wedge pressure in patients with acute lung injury and acute respiratory distress syndrome. Intensive Care Med 28:1073–1077
11. Teboul JL, Besbes M, Andrivet P et al (1992) A bedside index assessing the reliability of pulmonary occlusion pressure during mechanical ventilation with positive end-expiratory pressure. J Crit Care 7:22–29
12. Teboul JL, Andrivet P, Ansquer M et al (1992) Bedside evaluation of the resistance in large and medium pulmonary veins in various lung diseases. J Appl Physiol 72:998–1003
13. Teboul JL, Pinsky MR, Mercat A et al (2000) Estimating cardiac filling pressure in mechanically ventilated patients with hyperinflation. Crit Care Med 28:3631–3636
14. Nagueh SF, Appleton CP, Gillebert TC et al (2009) Recommendations for the evaluation of left ventricular diastolic function by echocardiography. Eur J Echocardiogr 10:165–193
15. Appleton CP, Hatle LK, Popp RL (1998) Relation of transmitral flow velocity patterns to left ventricular diastolic function: new insights from a combined hemodynamic and Doppler echocardiographic study. J Am Coll Cardiol 12:426–440
16. Nagueh SF, Mikati I, Kopelen HA, Middleton KJ, Quiñones MA, Zoghbi WA (1998) Doppler estimation of left ventricular filling pressure in sinus tachycardia. A new application of tissue Doppler imaging. Circulation 98:1644–1650

17. Nagueh SF, Middleton KJ, Kopelen HA, Zoghbi WA, Quiñones MA (1997) Doppler tissue imaging: a non invasive technique for evaluation of left ventricular relaxation and estimation of filling pressures. J Am Coll Cardiol 30:1527–1533
18. Ommen SR, Nishimura RA, Appleton CP et al (2000) Clinical utility of Doppler echocardiography and tissue Doppler imaging in the estimation of left ventricular filling pressures: a comparative simultaneous Doppler-catheterization study. Circulation 102:1788–1794
19. Bouhemad B, Nicolas-Robin A, Benois A, Lemaire S, Goarin JP, Rouby JJ (2003) Echocardiographic Doppler assessment of pulmonary capillary wedge pressure in surgical patients with postoperative circulatory shock and acute lung injury. Anesthesiology 98:1091–1100
20. Dokainish H, Zoghbi WA, Lakkis NM et al (2004) Optimal noninvasive assessment of left ventricular filling pressures: a comparison of tissue Doppler echocardiography and B-type natriuretic peptide in patients with pulmonary artery catheters. Circulation 109:2432–2439
21. Combes A, Arnoult F, Trouillet JL (2004) Tissue Doppler imaging estimation of pulmonary artery occlusion pressure in ICU patients. Intensive Care Med 30:75–81
22. Vignon P, AitHssain A, François B et al (2008) Echocardiographic assessment of pulmonary artery occlusion pressure in ventilated patients: a transoesophageal study. Crit Care 12:R18
23. Lamia B, Maizel J, Ochagavia A et al (2009) Echocardiographic diagnosis of pulmonary artery occlusion pressure elevation during weaning from mechanical ventilation. Crit Care Med 37:1696–1701
24. Kuecherer HF, Muhiudeen IA, Kusumoto FM et al (1990) Estimation of mean left atrial pressure from transesophageal pulsed Doppler echocardiography of pulmonary venous flow. Circulation 82:1127–1139
25. Kim YJ, Sohn DW (2000) Mitral annulus velocity in the estimation of left ventricular filling pressure: prospective study in 200 patients. J Am Soc Echocardiogr 13:980–985
26. Garcia MJ, Ares MA, Asher C et al (1997) An index of early left ventricular filling that combined with pulsed Doppler peak E velocity may estimate capillary wedge pressure. J Am Coll Cardiol 29:448–454
27. Vieillard-Baron A, Slama M, Cholley B, Janvier G, Vignon P (2008) Echocardiography in the intensive care unit: from evolution to revolution? Intensive Care Med 34:243–249
28. Mukoyama M, Nakao K, Hosoda K et al (1991) Brain natriuretic peptide as a novel cardiac hormone in humans. Evidence for an exquisite dual natriuretic peptide system, atrial natriuretic peptide and brain natriuretic peptide. J Clin Invest 87:1402–1412
29. Levin ER, Gardner DG, Samson WK (1998) Natriuretic peptides. N Engl J Med 339:321–328
30. De Lemos JA, McGuire DK, Drazner MH (2003) B-type natriuretic peptide in cardiovascular disease. Lancet 362:316–322
31. Sudoh T, Kangawa K, Minamino N, Matsuo H (1998) A new natriuretic peptide in porcine brain. Nature 332:78–81
32. Kazanegra R, Cheng V, Garcia A et al (2001) A rapid test for B-type natriuretic peptide correlates with falling wedge pressures in patients treated for decompensated heart failure: a pilot study. J Card Fail 7:21–29
33. Maeda K, Tsutamoto T, Wada A, Hisanaga T, Kinoshita M (1998) Plasma brain natriuretic peptide as a biochemical marker of high left ventricular end-diastolic pressure in patients with symptomatic left ventricular dysfunction. Am Heart J 135:825–832
34. Davis M, Espiner E, Richards G (1994) Plasma brain natriuretic peptide in assessment of acute dyspnoea. Lancet 343:440–444
35. Maisel AS, Krishnaswamy P, Nowak RM et al (2002) Rapid measurement of B-type natriuretic peptide in the emergency diagnosis of heart failure. N Engl J Med 347:161–167
36. Tanaka T, Kanda T, Takahashi T, Saegusa S, Moriya J, Kurabayashi M (2004) Interleukin-6-induced reciprocal expression of SERCA and natriuretic peptides mRNA in cultured rat ventricular myocytes. J Int Med Res 32:57–61
37. Pirracchio R, Deye N, Lukaszewicz AC et al (2008) Impaired plasma B-type natriuretic peptide clearance in human septic shock. Crit Care Med 36:2542–2546

38. Charpentier J, Luyt CE, Fulla Y (2004) Brain natriuretic peptide: A marker of myocardial dysfunction and prognosis during severe sepsis. Crit Care Med 32:660–665
39. Roch A, Allardet-Servent J, Michelet P et al (2005) NH2 terminal pro-brain natriuretic peptide plasma level as an early marker of prognosis and cardiac dysfunction in septic shock patients. Crit Care Med 33:1001–1007
40. Rudiger A, Gasser S, Fischler M, Hornemann T, von Eckardstein A, Maggiorini M (2006) Comparable increase of B-type natriuretic peptide and amino-terminal pro-B-type natriuretic peptide levels in patients with severe sepsis, septic shock, and acute heart failure. Crit Care Med 34:2140–2144
41. Maeder M, Fehr T, Rickli H, Ammann P (2006) Sepsis-associated myocardial dysfunction: diagnostic and prognostic impact of cardiac troponins and natriuretic peptides. Chest 129:1349–1366
42. Hall C (2004) Essential biochemistry and physiology of (NT-pro) BNP. Eur J Heart Fail 6:257–260
43. Potter LR, Abbey-Hosch S, Dickey DM (2006) Natriuretic peptides, their receptors, and cyclic guanosine monophosphate-dependent signaling functions. Endocr Rev 27:47–72
44. Yap LB, Mukerjee D, Timms PM, Ashrafian H, Coghlan JG (2004) Natriuretic peptides, respiratory disease, and the right heart. Chest 126:1330–1336
45. Jefic D, Lee JW, Jefic D, Savoy-Moore RT, Rosman HS (2005) Utility of B-type natriuretic peptide and N-terminal pro B-type natriuretic peptide in evaluation of respiratory failure in critically ill patients. Chest 128:288–295
46. Lichtenstein D, Mezière G, Biderman P, Gepner A, Barré O (1997) The comet-tail artifact, an ultrasound sign of alveolar-interstitial syndrome. Am J Respir Crit Care Med 156:1640–1646
47. Lichtenstein DA, Mezière GA (2008) Relevance of lung ultrasound in the diagnosis of acute respiratory failure: the BLUE protocol. Chest 134:1117–1125
48. Silva S, Biendel C, Ruiz J et al (2013) Usefulness of cardiothoracic chest ultrasound in the management of acute respiratory failure in critical care practice. Chest 144:859–865
49. Picano E, Frassi F, Agricola E, Gligorova S, Gargani L, Mottola G (2006) Ultrasound lung comets: a clinically useful sign of extravascular lung water. J Am Soc Echocardiogr 19:356–363
50. Jambrik Z, Monti S, Coppola V et al (2004) Usefulness of ultrasound lung comets as a nonradiologic sign of extravascular lung water. Am J Cardiol 93:1265–1270
51. Jambrik Z, Gargani L, Adamicza A et al (2010) B-lines quantify the lung water content: a lung ultrasound versus lung gravimetry study in acute lung injury. Ultrasound Med Biol 36:2004–2010
52. Agricola E, Bove T, Oppizzi M et al (2005) "Ultrasound comet-tail images": a marker of pulmonary edema: a comparative study with wedge pressure and extravascular lung water. Chest 127:1690–1695
53. Lichtenstein DA, Meziere GA, Lagoueyte JF, Biderman P, Goldstein I, Gepner A (2009) A-lines and B-lines: lung ultrasound as a bedside tool for predicting pulmonary artery occlusion pressure in the critically ill. Chest 136:1014–1020
54. Shyamsundar M, Attwood B, Keating L, Walden AP (2013) Clinical review: The role of ultrasound in estimating extra-vascular lung water. Crit Care 17:237
55. Katzenelson R, Perel A, Berkenstadt H et al (2004) Accuracy of transpulmonary thermodilution versus gravimetric measurement of extravascular lung water. Crit Care Med 32:1550–1554
56. Tagami T, Kushimoto S, Yamamoto Y et al (2010) Validation of extravascular lung water measurement by single transpulmonary thermodilution: human autopsy study. Crit Care 14:R162
57. Bendjelid K, Giraud R, Siegenthaler N, Michard F (2010) Validation of a new transpulmonary thermodilution system to assess global end-diastolic volume and extravascular lung water. Crit Care 14:R209
58. Kiefer N, Hofer CK, Marx G et al (2012) Clinical validation of a new thermodilution system for the assessment of cardiac output and volumetric parameters. Crit Care 16:R98

59. Tagami T, Sawabe M, Kushimoto S et al (2013) Quantitative diagnosis of diffuse alveolar damage using extravascular lung water. Crit Care Med 41:2144–2150

60. Jozwiak M, Silva S, Persichini R et al (2013) Extravascular lung water is an independent prognostic factor in patients with acute respiratory distress syndrome. Crit Care Med 41:472–480

61. Kushimoto S, Taira Y, Kitazawa Y et al (2012) The clinical usefulness of extravascular lung water and pulmonary vascular permeability index to diagnose and characterize pulmonary edema: a prospective multicenter study on the quantitative differential diagnostic definition for acute lung injury/acute respiratory distress syndrome. Crit Care 16:R232

62. Monnet X, Anguel N, Osman D et al (2007) Assessing pulmonary permeability by transpulmonary thermodilution allows differentiation of hydrostatic pulmonary edema from ALI/ARDS. Intensive Care Med 33:448–453

63. Sedziwy L, Thomas M, Shillingford J (1968) Some observations on haematocrit changes in patients with acute myocardial infarction. Br Heart J 30:344–349

64. Figueras J, Weil MH (1978) Increases in plasma oncotic pressure during acute cardiogenic pulmonary edema. Circulation 55:195–199

65. Henning RJ, Weil MH (1978) Effect of afterload reduction on plasma volume during acute heart failure. Am J Cardiol 42:823–827

66. Anguel N, Monnet X, Osman D et al (2008) Increase in plasma protein concentration for diagnosing weaning-induced pulmonary oedema. Intensive Care Med 34:1231–1238

Part VII
Early Goal-directed Therapy and Hemodynamic Optimization

Extravascular Lung Water as a Target for Goal-directed Therapy

M. Y. Kirov, V. V. Kuzkov, and L. J. Bjertnaes

Introduction

Accumulation of extravascular lung water (EVLW) is a hallmark of pulmonary edema and acute respiratory distress syndrome (ARDS) of various etiologies [1]. Increased EVLW is associated with a high mortality rate [1–3]. Thus, in critically ill patients, the balance and maintenance of cardiac preload and vital organ perfusion should be thoroughly weighed against the deleterious effects of worsening pulmonary edema, and quantification of EVLW may offer a valuable therapeutic guide to providers of intensive care.

The amount of edema fluid accumulated in the pulmonary tissue is, however, difficult to estimate at the bedside. Several techniques have been developed to assess EVLW. Clinical examination, including chest auscultation, blood gases, radiography, computed tomography (CT), positron emission tomography (PET), magnetic resonance imaging (MRI), bioimpedance, lung ultrasound, postmortem gravimetry and several other techniques have been introduced into clinical practice for quantification of pulmonary edema but with conflicting results [1, 4–7]. To date, among the various methods, thermal-dye dilution and single transpulmonary thermodilution have been used most frequently both in experimental and clinical studies [1, 2, 4, 6, 8]. In addition to EVLW, these techniques simultaneously display a number of hemodynamic variables that can give valuable guidance to the management of fluid balance and cardiopulmonary dysfunction. However, a debate is still going on regarding the value of EVLW for hemodynamic optimization during the peri-

M. Y. Kirov ✉ · V. V. Kuzkov
Department of Clinical Medicine (Anesthesiology), Faculty of Health Sciences, Northern State Medical University, 163000 Arkhangelsk, Russian Federation
e-mail: mikhail_kirov@hotmail.com

L. J. Bjertnaes
Department of Clinical Medicine (Anesthesiology), Faculty of Health Sciences, University of Tromsø, 9038 MH-Breivika, Tromsø, Norway

J.-L. Vincent (Ed.), *Annual Update in Intensive Care and Emergency Medicine 2014*,   285
DOI 10.1007/978-3-319-03746-2_22, © Springer International Publishing Switzerland 2014

Table 1 Potential indications for monitoring of extravascular lung water

Conditions	Indications [references]
Severe sepsis	Prevention or treatment of ARDS [1–4, 12–16, 18] Septic shock [6, 12, 22]
Respiratory failure	ARDS of any etiology [1–4, 12–14, 24–25] Pneumonia [12, 22]
Perioperative period	High-risk cardiac and non-cardiac surgery: coronary artery bypass grafting [31, 32], valve surgery [32, 33], pneumonectomy [35–37], esophagectomy [38, 39], major abdominal surgery [34], transplantation [48], other interventions accompanied by massive fluid shifts [6]
Trauma	Refractory shock [40] Blood loss > 50 % of circulating blood volume Chest trauma with pulmonary contusion Burns > 25–30 % of body surface area [41–43]
Cardiac failure	Cardiogenic shock [44] Pulmonary edema [26, 29, 44] Patients after cardiac arrest [44]
Neurological intensive care	Subarachnoid hemorrhage [45, 46] Neurogenic pulmonary edema [6]
Other critically ill patients	Necrotizing pancreatitis [47] Abdominal compartment syndrome [20] Multiple organ dysfunction syndrome [6, 9, 20] ICU patients receiving renal replacement therapy [49]

operative period and in intensive care. Thus, the aim of this chapter is to discuss the application of EVLW as a target for goal-directed therapy (GDT) in different categories of patients (Table 1).

Thermodilution Methods for the Determination of Extravascular Lung Water

Thermal-dye dilution and single thermodilution calculate cardiac output based on transpulmonary thermodilution curves according to the Stewart–Hamilton principle (Fig. 1).

Thermal-dye dilution determines the distribution volumes of the thermal and the dye indicators between the point of injection in the right atrium and the point of detection in the aorta by using a combination of thermal (ice-cold 5 % dextrose solution) and dye indicators (ice-cold indocyanine green [ICG] solution). This technique works by exchanging cold (temperature) extravascularly, whereas ICG binds to intravascular albumin. Therefore, the intrathoracic thermal volume (ITTV) and intrathoracic blood volume (ITBV) are calculated as cardiac output × mean transit time (MTt) of the thermal indicator and cardiac output × MTt of the dye indicator, respectively. The difference between ITTV and ITBV gives the EVLW value [4]. The thermal-dye dilution method has been validated versus postmortem gravime-

Thermal-dye dilution (TDD)

$ITTV = CO \cdot MTt_{TI}$

Single thermodilution (STD)

$ITTV = CO \cdot MTt_{TI}$

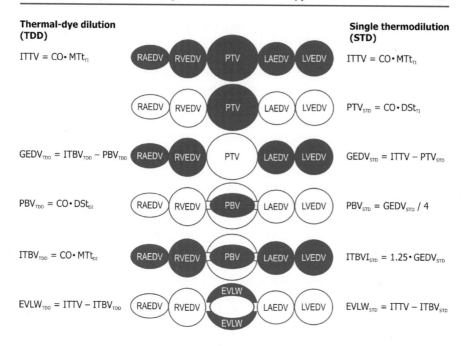

$PTV_{STD} = CO \cdot DSt_{TI}$

$GEDV_{TDD} = ITBV_{TDD} - PBV_{TDD}$

$GEDV_{STD} = ITTV - PTV_{STD}$

$PBV_{TDD} = CO \cdot DSt_{DI}$

$PBV_{STD} = GEDV_{STD} / 4$

$ITBV_{TDD} = CO \cdot MTt_{DI}$

$ITBVI_{STD} = 1.25 \cdot GEDV_{STD}$

$EVLW_{TDD} = ITTV - ITBV_{TDD}$

$EVLW_{STD} = ITTV - ITBV_{STD}$

Fig. 1 Methodology of transpulmonary thermodilution. TDD: thermal-dye dilution; STD: single thermodilution; MTt: indicator mean transit time; DSt: indicator downslope (exponential decay) time; TI: thermal indicator; DI: dye indicator. Calculated volumetric parameters: ITTV: intrathoracic thermal volume; ITBV: intrathoracic blood volume; GEDV: global end-diastolic volume; PTV: pulmonary thermal volume; PBV: pulmonary blood volume; EVLW: extravascular lung water. Heart volumes: RAEDV: right atrial end-diastolic volume; RVEDV: right ventricular end-diastolic volume; LAEDV: left atrial end-diastolic volume; LVEDV: left ventricular end-diastolic volume

try, which is supposed to be the 'gold standard' of EVLW measurements in animal models of lung edema [1, 6]. In critically ill patients, fluid management guided by measurements of EVLW with thermal-dye dilution has been associated with improved clinical outcome [9]. However, the thermal-dye dilution technique is relatively cumbersome and expensive. For these reasons, the method has not gained general clinical acceptance, triggering more widespread use of single thermodilution. Consequently, manufacturers have stopped producing thermal-dye dilution monitors and disposables.

Single transpulmonary thermodilution uses a temperature indicator only (usually ice-cold 5 % dextrose solution) that hampers direct assessment of ITBV, but calculates pulmonary thermal volume (PTV) by multiplying cardiac output and the down-slope time (duration of exponential thermodilution curve decay) assuming that PTV is the largest mixing volume for the thermal indicator made up of the pulmonary blood volume (PBV) and EVLW. The difference between ITTV and PTV gives the maximum end-diastolic volume of the four heart chambers, i.e., global end-diastolic volume (GEDV). Since single thermodilution assumes a constant relationship between PBV and GEDV = 1 : 4, ITBV is estimated as GEDV + PBV = 1.25 × GEDV (Fig. 1). The difference between ITTV and estimated ITBV gives EVLW [5, 8]. Multiple experimental and clinical studies have shown that EVLW assessed by single thermodilution demonstrates good reproducibility and close agreement with the double indicator technique and postmortem gravimetry [1, 6, 7, 10–12]. Moreover, single thermodilution provides the pulmonary vascular permeability index (PVPI) calculated as EVLW/PBV that may be useful to distinguish between cardiogenic and non-cardiogenic types of pulmonary edema and has a prognostic role [1, 3, 6, 12]. Compared with both thermal-dye dilution and right heart catheterization, single thermodilution has the advantage that it can be coupled with pulse contour analysis for continuous cardiac output monitoring. Moreover, it is simpler to apply, less invasive and more cost-effective, all factors making it more suitable for application at the bedside.

However, determination of EVLW using thermodilution methods can be influenced by changes in the pulmonary blood volume and perfusion distribution and by heat exchange between the thermal indicator and the myocardium and the vessels. Furthermore, inhomogeneous pulmonary edema, recirculation of the indicator, anatomical abnormalities (large aortic aneurysms, intracardiac shunts) and several other factors might disturb the readings [1, 6, 11]. The prognostic value of EVLW, particularly in obese patients, can be improved by indexing to predicted body weight (PBW) [13, 14]. Although most investigations use the normal limit of EVLW within 3–7 ml/kg [1, 6], Tagami et al., validating single thermodilution with postmortem gravimetry in a clinical study, recently noticed that the normal EVLW values indexed to PBW were 7.4 ± 3.3 ml/kg (7.5 ± 3.3 ml/kg for males and 7.3 ± 3.3 ml/kg for females) [7]. In another study, Tagami and colleagues demonstrated that the best EVLW cut-off value to discriminate between normal lungs and lungs with diffuse alveolar damage was around 10 ml/kg [15].

Summarizing this information, thermodilution methods for determination of EVLW are potentially promising in terms of their clinical application. Several categories of pediatric and adult ICU patients can benefit from monitoring EVLW. The main pathophysiological changes prompting a need to control EVLW include the risk of pulmonary edema, massive fluid shifts and severe changes in microvascular permeability [4]. The latter changes are among the hallmarks of critical conditions, including severe sepsis, ARDS, cardiogenic lung edema, multiple trauma with severe blood loss, burns, ischemia-reperfusion injury, etc. [1, 4, 6]. Thus, we can consider any critical illness resulting in shock and tissue hypoperfusion that is refractory to fluid resuscitation, as a valid subject for monitoring of EVLW together with other hemodynamic parameters, including cardiac output, preload, afterload, and oxygen transport. Importantly, the lungs are probably the only organ system in which edema can be relatively easily and accurately estimated at the bedside and might be assumed to be the 'mirror' of systemic capillary leakage in cases of non-cardiogenic edema. In addition, the method may be of value in patients undergoing major surgical procedures for perioperative hemodynamic optimization. In these settings, determination of EVLW in parallel with other volumetric variables can support the diagnosis with a potential to improve clinical outcomes when integrated into treatment protocols that are known to hasten the resolution of pulmonary edema [9].

Extravascular Lung Water in Sepsis

A number of studies have focused on the potential role of controlling hemodynamics and EVLW as a guide to the recognition and management in sepsis. Accumulation of EVLW triggered by systemic inflammation and increased vascular permeability occurs before any changes in blood gases, chest radiogram and, eventually, also in central venous pressure (CVP) and pulmonary artery occlusion pressure (PAOP) [4, 8, 12, 16]. Although still included in the international guidelines for sepsis treatment [17], CVP represents a non-specific diagnostic tool, influenced by a variety of factors and is indeed a poor indicator of pulmonary edema [4, 8, 12]. In sepsis, EVLW provides a valid estimate of the interstitial water content in the lungs and might become an alternative to filling pressures during fluid resuscitation. Since EVLW, but not CVP, correlates with lung injury score and its components, we suppose that assessment of this variable is valuable for the management of patients with severe sepsis complicated by ARDS [4, 12]. In addition, monitoring of EVLW can be useful in patients with severe sepsis at risk of developing ARDS, in whom EVLW predicts progression to ARDS 2.6 ± 0.3 days before they meet American European Consensus Committee criteria for this condition [18]. Notably, Martin and colleagues showed that more than 50 % of patients with severe sepsis but without ARDS have increased EVLW, possibly representing sub-clinical lung injury [16].

In septic shock, invasive cardiovascular monitoring facilitates the titration of fluids, vasopressor/inotrope agents, and adjustment of the ventilatory settings, and has been recommended by the Surviving Sepsis Campaign for the management of patients requiring vasopressor support [17]. The targets for therapy of sepsis include invasive arterial pressure and other indirect and direct hemodynamic determinants of cardiac output and fluid status. Fluid management during septic shock and ARDS requires a goal-oriented approach. On the one hand, restriction of fluids with the aim of counteracting organ edema positively influences the course of illness and improves cardiopulmonary function. On the other hand, these patients require volume resuscitation to achieve adequate oxygen transport and counteract systemic inflammation. Thus, a combination of adequate fluid load during the first 6 hours of severe sepsis, followed by a conservative fluid strategy (fluid restriction during 2 days minimally) decreases mortality compared with other therapeutic strategies [19]. In this context, inclusion of EVLW as a part of the hemodynamic management of septic shock can limit fluid resuscitation if EVLW increases by more than 10 % from baseline or exceeds 10 ml/kg [4, 20, 21]. In these patients, a resuscitation protocol aimed at decreasing EVLW serves as a useful addition to goal-directed therapy of severe sepsis and shortens the duration of mechanical ventilation and ICU stay and improves clinical outcomes [9, 21]. These findings were confirmed by our recent study, demonstrating that patients with a decrease in EVLW during the first 12 hours

Fig. 2 Effect of therapeutic interventions aimed at decreasing extravascular lung water (EVLW) on clinical outcome of septic shock and ARDS. * p < 0.01

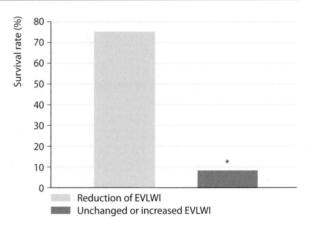

after the onset of septic shock and ARDS had a higher survival rate compared to those with unchanged or increased EVLW (Fig. 2) [22].

Extravascular Lung Water in ARDS

Monitoring of EVLW can be used in septic and in non-septic ARDS to evaluate the severity and prognosis of pulmonary edema and to optimize fluid balance during the course of ARDS. It has been shown that both EVLW and PVPI are increased in non-survivors of ARDS, peaking at days 3 and 4 from the onset of lung injury [1, 2, 12, 16]. Recently, Jozwiak and colleagues demonstrated that the mortality rate in ARDS patients with a maximum value of EVLW > 21 ml/kg and PVPI > 3.8 was as high as 70% [3]. In our study, EVLW exceeded 7 ml/kg in 74% of the patients with sepsis-induced ALI (in 95% of patients with a pulmonary source of ARDS, predominantly pneumonia, and in 50% of patients with non-pulmonary ARDS) [12]. Indexing EVLW to PBW can improve the diagnostic value of lung water, with EVLW > 10 ml/kg in 97% of ARDS patients [13, 14]. Thus, we suggest that, being a key marker of pulmonary edema as one of the main pathophysiological features of ARDS, EVLW > 10 ml/kg PBW could be an important addition to the current definition of ARDS [23]. This suggestion was also confirmed in a recent study by Kushimoto and colleagues [24], which demonstrated that increasing ARDS severity, according to the latest Berlin definition, was associated with an increase in EVLW to 14.7 ml/kg, 16.2 ml/kg, and 20.0 ml/kg in mild, moderate and severe ARDS, respectively, and the PVPI values followed the same pattern (2.6, 2.7, 3.5, respectively) [24].

In ARDS patients with cardiac comorbidities, EVLW and PVPI can distinguish between non-cardiogenic and cardiogenic pulmonary edema [3, 25]. In addition, EVLW is helpful in the differential diagnosis of the mechanisms of respiratory failure. Thus, recently it was shown that EVLW was greater in ARDS than in patients

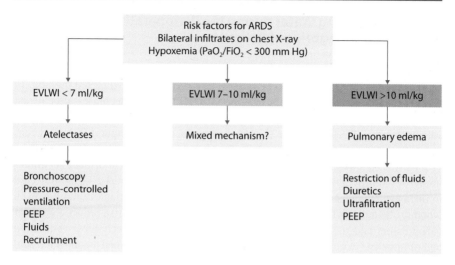

Fig. 3 Decision tree: Extravascular lung water in ARDS

with atelectasis or pleural effusion [25]. Therefore, depending on the EVLW value, we can provide different therapeutic interventions (Fig. 3).

When assessed in combination with other cardiopulmonary parameters, EVLW might provide useful guidance for the fluid management and the pharmacotherapy of ARDS including administration of albumin or furosemide. As far as mechanical ventilation is concerned, information about EVLW and other volumetric variables might support decisions associated with weaning the patient from the respirator, thereby decreasing the duration of respiratory support, and shortening ICU and hospital lengths of stay [6, 9, 20, 26–28]. Moreover, goal-directed therapy based on monitoring of EVLW can reduce mortality in critically ill patients with initially increased EVLW as compared to treatment guided by pulmonary artery catheter (PAC) [26]. In addition, EVLW can serve as a therapeutic target during mechanical ventilation in ARDS, helping to choose appropriate parameters of respiratory support including administration of positive end-expiratory pressure (PEEP) > 10 cmH$_2$O in case of increased EVLW [29]. The severity of pulmonary edema determines the response to recruitment maneuvers in ARDS: In patients with EVLW > 10 ml/kg, recruitment is less effective [28]. Evaluation of lung water is also useful before taking the decision to switch from mechanical ventilation to spontaneous breathing with EVLW > 11 ml/kg a predictor of unsuccessful weaning [27].

Extravascular Lung Water during the Perioperative Period and in Other Categories of Patients

During the perioperative period of cardiovascular interventions and major non-cardiac surgery, EVLW can also be one of the targets for goal-directed therapy. In off-pump coronary artery bypass grafting (CABG), EVLW decreases after revascularization in parallel with goal-directed therapy aimed at maintaining normal values of mean arterial pressure (MAP), heart rate, cardiac output, ITBV, and central venous saturation [30]. In a study by Goepfert and colleagues, maintenance of EVLW < 10 ml/kg was included in the algorithm for treatment of patients undergoing on-pump CABG. Patients with EVLW exceeding 12 ml/kg were subjected to intensive management of pulmonary edema and administration of diuretics [31]. Notably, the authors found that such goal-directed therapy led to a reduced need for vasopressors and inotropes, and shortened the duration of mechanical ventilation and of intensive care [31]. The same group recently also published a controlled trial of patients who underwent CABG and aortic valve surgery who were randomized either to a goal-directed therapy group with the aim to optimize GEDV or to a conventional therapy group guided by MAP and CVP [32]. The goal-directed therapy group received fluid load in response to stroke volume variations (SVV) > 10 % in parallel with observation of cardiac output and EVLW. Fluid resuscitation was stopped if cardiac output started to decrease or EVLW exceeded 12 ml/kg. Postoperative complications, time to fulfill all ICU discharge criteria and length of ICU stay were all reduced in the goal-directed therapy group [32]. Our randomized study demonstrated that goal-directed therapy based on transpulmonary thermodilution and oxygen transport parameters is also beneficial in high-risk cardiac patients with complex valve surgery. As compared to the PAC-guided algorithm, hemodynamic optimization using GEDV, EVLW and oxygen delivery increased the volume of fluid therapy, improved hemodynamics and oxygen transport, and reduced the duration of postoperative respiratory support [33]. The volumetric algorithm of goal-directed therapy modified from this study is shown in Fig. 4.

Lung water can increase perioperatively in major non-cardiac surgery. A study by Groeneveld and colleagues shows that subclinical pulmonary edema with EVLW > 7 ml/kg is relatively common after major vascular surgery and mainly caused by increased pulmonary capillary permeability in the absence of overt heart failure [34]. Thus, monitoring EVLW in patients requiring mechanical ventilation after aortic aneurysm repair or vascular reconstruction can help distinguish between ischemia-reperfusion lung injury, atelectasis or cardiogenic pulmonary edema, and support the choice of appropriate therapy [1, 34].

Assessment of EVLW could also be useful in major thoracic surgery for early diagnosis and management of postpneumonectomy pulmonary edema with ventilator-associated lung injury as one of its possible mechanisms [35, 36]. Both in experimental and clinical settings, EVLW decreased by 30 % immediately after pneumonectomy, a finding validated by thermal-dye dilution and single thermodilution techniques [35–37]. However, after lung removal, in contrast to lobe resection, EVLW increased significantly by 27 % in the postoperative period, peaking

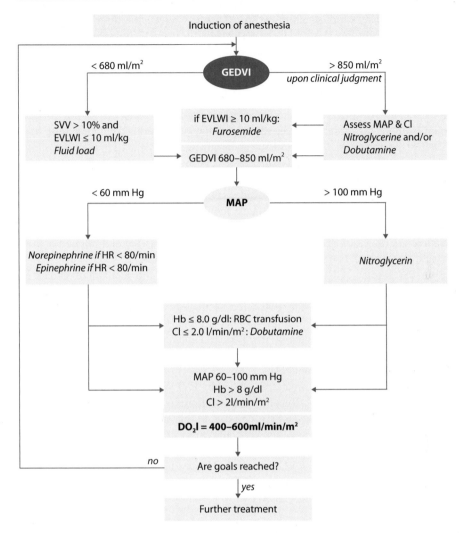

Fig. 4 Algorithm of goal-directed hemodynamic optimization using parameters of transpulmonary thermodilution. HR: heart rate; MAP: mean arterial pressure; SVV: stroke volume variations; CI: cardiac index; GEDVI: global end-diastolic volume index; EVLWI: extravascular lung water index; ScvO₂: central venous oxygen saturation; DO₂I: oxygen delivery index; Hb: hemoglobin concentration; RBC: red blood cell

36 hours after transfer of the patient to the ICU [37]. The increase in EVLW may be explained by redistribution and accumulation of pulmonary interstitial fluid due to augmented perfusion of the residual lung, which necessitates a conservative fluid strategy postoperatively [36, 37].

In addition to the condition after lung surgery, the level of EVLW may reflect the severity of postoperative pulmonary edema and predict pulmonary complications induced by esophagectomy with extended lymph node dissection [38, 39]. After esophagectomy, EVLW increased gradually from 12 hours postoperatively, and the changes correlated with oxygenation, respiratory compliance and lung injury score [38, 39]. Thus, the authors conclude that EVLW might become a useful additional parameter for evaluation of respiratory status in this type of surgery.

In trauma patients with arterial hypotension and hypoxemia, quantification of EVLW may also give rise to modifications of fluid and vasoactive therapy. These modifications may result in lower volume loading and improved outcome [40]. Volumetric parameters including EVLW can be advantageously used in burns involving more than 25–30 % of the body surface area both in adults and children [41, 42]. Pediatric patients from this study who underwent fluid resuscitation guided by cardiac output, ITBV, and EVLW received significantly smaller volumes of fluid and had significantly decreased fluid balance, better hemodynamic stability and a significantly lower incidence of cardiac and renal failure [42]. However, in burns, the traditional values of ITBV, EVLW, and cardiac output as the end-points for fluid resuscitation should be adjusted to avoid tissue edema [43].

In the cardiac ICU, monitoring EVLW should be the method of choice in patients with cardiogenic pulmonary edema and shock. Recently, Adler and colleagues demonstrated that goal-directed therapy guided by maintenance of $EVLWI \leq 10$ ml/kg, GEDV within 700–800 mL/m^2, and SVV and pulse pressure variations (PPV) < 10 % increased the fluid load and reduced the incidence of acute kidney injury in patients with circulatory shock after cardiac arrest treated with mild therapeutic hypothermia [44].

In the neurological ICU, treatment guided by EVLW can be used to avoid neurogenic pulmonary edema [6]. Recently, the monitoring of EVLW has been validated in subarachnoid hemorrhage (SAH) [45, 46]. In this situation, it is critical to minimize lung water, because patients with pulmonary complications are more likely to experience vasospasm, which can further increase their morbidity and mortality [45]. The increase in EVLW after SAH may have a biphasic course, with cardiogenic edema caused by low cardiac contractility immediately after SAH, and hydrostatic pulmonary edema caused by low cardiac contractility and hypervolemia from day 7 of SAH [46].

As a component of hemodynamic monitoring, assessment of EVLW can also be a guide for goal-directed therapy in acute necrotizing pancreatitis [47], organ transplantation [48], and multiple organ dysfunction syndrome including titration of fluid removal in patients receiving renal replacement therapy (RRT) [49]. It is important to note that the results of the goal-directed therapy studies, including those focusing on EVLW, are dependent on their protocols. Thus, in a study by Trof and colleagues, hemodynamic management in non-septic shock patients guided by the PiCCO system led to increased length of mechanical ventilation and ICU stay compared with a PAC-driven algorithm [50]. This difference may be attributed to a larger positive fluid balance with the use of single thermodilution; however, it could also be explained by the relatively 'liberal' end-points chosen for this particular protocol, because some patients received fluids even when EVLW exceeded 10 ml/kg.

Bedside monitoring of EVLW therefore appears to be an appropriate method for early diagnosis and management of pulmonary edema in many clinical situations. However, further clinical trials are warranted for in-depth evaluation of EVLW as a target for therapy in other categories of patients.

Conclusions

In many ICU patients, critical illness triggers inflammation in the lungs and increases microvascular pressure and permeability, thereby causing accumulation of EVLW and evolution of pulmonary edema. Thermodilution methods for the measurement of EVLW and PVPI can be successfully used at the bedside, taking into account their potential limitations. Lung water has a clear prognostic value for clinical outcome, especially in sepsis and ARDS, thus fluid resuscitation should be limited when EVLW exceeds 10 ml/kg. Being part of general patient monitoring, assessment of EVLW should be a target for goal-directed therapy aimed at improving clinical outcomes in conditions presenting an increased risk of pulmonary edema, e. g., severe sepsis, ARDS, high-risk cardiac and non-cardiac surgery, refractory shock, severe trauma and burns, cardiac arrest, SAH, and multiple organ dysfunction syndrome. Further randomized large-scale clinical trials are warranted to evaluate the potential of EVLW-based protocols for reduction of morbidity and mortality in different subgroups of critically ill patients.

References

1. Sakka SG (2013) Extravascular lung water in ARDS patients. Minerva Anestesiol 79:274–284
2. Sakka SG, Klein M, Reinhart K, Meier-Hellmann A (2002) Prognostic value of extravascular lung water in critically ill patients. Chest 122:2080–2086
3. Jozwiak M, Silva S, Persichini R et al (2013) Extravascular lung water is an independent prognostic factor in patients with acute respiratory distress syndrome. Crit Care Med 41:472–480
4. Kirov MY, Kuzkov VV, Bjertnaes LJ (2005) Extravascular lung water in sepsis. In: Vincent JL (ed) Yearbook of Intensive Care and Emergency Medicine. Springer-Verlag, Berlin, Heidelberg, New York, pp 449–461
5. Kuzkov VV, Suborov EV, Kirov MY et al (2010) Radiographic lung density assessed by computed tomography is associated with extravascular lung water content. Acta Anaesthesiol Scand 54:1018–1026
6. Brown LM, Liu KD, Matthay MA (2009) Measurement of extravascular lung water using the single indicator method in patients: research and potential clinical value. Am J Physiol Lung Cell Mol Physiol 297:L547–L558
7. Tagami T, Kushimoto S, Yamamoto Y et al (2010) Validation of extravascular lung water measurement by single transpulmonary thermodilution: human autopsy study. Crit Care 14:R162
8. Boussat S, Jacques T, Levy B et al (2002) Intravascular volume monitoring and extravascular lung water in septic patients with pulmonary edema. Intensive Care Med 28:712–718
9. Mitchell JP, Schuller D, Calandrino FS, Schuster DP (1992) Improved outcome based on fluid management in critically ill patients requiring pulmonary artery catheterization. Am Rev Respir Dis 145:990–998

10. Sakka SG, Ruhl CC, Pfeiffer UJ et al (2000) Assessment of cardiac preload and extravascular lung water by single transpulmonary thermodilution. Intensive Care Med 26:180–187
11. Kirov MY, Kuzkov VV, Kuklin VN, Waerhaug K, Bjertnaes LJ (2004) Extravascular lung water assessed by transpulmonary single thermodilution and postmortem gravimetry in sheep. Crit Care 8:R451–R458
12. Kuzkov VV, Kirov MY, Sovershaev MA et al (2006) Extravascular lung water determined with single transpulmonary thermodilution correlates with the severity of sepsis-induced acute lung injury. Crit Care Med 34:1647–1653
13. Berkowitz DM, Danai PA, Eaton S, Moss M, Martin GS (2008) Accurate characterization of extravascular lung water in acute respiratory distress syndrome. Crit Care Med 36:1803–1809
14. Phillips CR, Chesnutt MS, Smith SM (2008) Extravascular lung water in sepsis-associated acute respiratory distress syndrome: indexing with predicted body weight improves correlation with severity of illness and survival. Crit Care Med 36:69–73
15. Tagami T, Sawabe M, Kushimoto S, et al (2013) Quantitative diagnosis of diffuse alveolar damage using extravascular lung water. Crit Care Med 41:2144–2150
16. Martin GS, Eaton S, Mealer M, Moss M (2005) Extravascular lung water in patients with severe sepsis: a prospective cohort study. Crit Care 9:R74–R82
17. Dellinger RP, Levy MM, Rhodes A et al (2013) Surviving Sepsis Campaign: international guidelines for management of severe sepsis and septic shock: 2012. Crit Care Med 41:580–637
18. Le Tourneau JL, Pinney J, Phillips CR (2012) Extravascular lung water predicts progression to acute lung injury in patients with increased risk. Crit Care Med 40:847–854
19. Murphy CV, Schramm GE, Doherty JA et al (2009) The importance of fluid management in acute lung injury secondary to septic shock. Chest 136:102–109
20. Cordemans C, De Iaet I, Van Regenmortel N et al (2012) Fluid management in critically ill patients: the role of extravascular lung water, abdominal hypertension, capillary leak, and fluid balance. Ann Intensive Care 2(1):S1
21. Aman J, Groeneveld AB, van Nieuw Amerongen GP (2012) Predictors of pulmonary edema formation during fluid loading in the critically ill with presumed hypovolemia. Crit Care Med 40:793–799
22. Smetkin AA, Kuzkov VV, Suborov EV, Kulina IS, Kirov MY, Bjertnaes LJ (2009) The assessment of severity of pulmonary edema in patients with septic shock combined with direct and indirect acute lung injury. Intensive Care Med 35:246 (abst)
23. Michard F, Fernandez Mondejar E, Kirov M, Malbrain ML, Tagami T (2012) A new and simple definition for acute lung injury. Crit Care Med 40:1004–1007
24. Kushimoto S, Endo T, Yamanouchi S et al (2013) Relationship between extravascular lung water and severity categories of acute respiratory distress syndrome by the Berlin definition. Crit Care 17:R132
25. Kushimoto S, Tairo Y, Kitazawa Y et al (2012) The clinical usefulness of extravascular lung water and pulmonary vascular permeability index to diagnose and characterize pulmonary edema: a prospective multicenter study on the quantitative differential diagnostic definition for acute lung injury/acute respiratory distress syndrome. Crit Care 16:R232
26. Eisenberg PR, Hansbrough JR, Anderson D, Schuster DP (1987) A prospective study of lung water measurements during patient management in an intensive care unit. Am Rev Respir Dis 136:662–668
27. Zeravik J, Borg U, Pfeiffer UJ (1990) Efficacy of pressure support ventilation dependent on extravascular lung water. Chest 97:1412–1419
28. Smetkin AA., Kuzkov VV, Suborov EV, Bjertnaes LB, Kirov MY (2012) Increased extravascular lung water reduces the efficacy of alveolar recruitment maneuver in acute respiratory distress syndrome. Crit Care Res Pract: Article ID 606528
29. Fernández Mondéjar E, Vazquez Mata G, Cárdenas A, Mansilla A, Cantalejo F, Rivera R (1996) Ventilation with positive end-expiratory pressure reduces extravascular lung water and increases lymphatic flow in hydrostatic pulmonary edema. Crit Care Med 24:1562–1567

30. Smetkin AA, Kirov MY, Kuzkov VV et al (2009) Single transpulmonary thermodilution and continuous monitoring of central venous oxygen saturation during off-pump coronary surgery. Acta Anaesth Scand 53:505–514
31. Goepfert MS, Reuter DA, Akyol D, Lamm P, Kilger E, Goetz AE (2007) Goal-directed fluid management reduces vasopressor and catecholamine use in cardiac surgery patients. Intensive Care Med 33:96–103
32. Goepfert MS, Richter HP, Eulenburg CZ, et al (2013) Individually optimized hemodynamic therapy reduces complications and length of stay in the intensive care unit. Anesthesiology 119:824–836
33. Lenkin AI, Kirov MY, Kuzkov VV, et al (2012) Comparison of goal-directed hemodynamic optimization using pulmonary artery catheter and transpulmonary thermodilution in combined valve repair: a randomized clinical trial. Crit Care Res Pract 2012: article ID 821218
34. Groeneveld AB, Verheij J, van den Berg FG, Wisselink W, Rauwerda JA (2006) Increased pulmonary capillary permeability and extravascular lung water after major vascular surgery: effect on radiography and ventilatory variables. Eur J Anaesthesiol 23:36–41
35. Kuzkov VV, Suborov EV, Kirov MY et al (2007) Extravascular lung water after pneumonectomy and one-lung ventilation in sheep. Crit Care Med 35:1550–1559
36. Naidu BV, Dronavalli VB, Rajesh PB (2009) Measuring lung water following major lung resection. Interact Cardiovasc Thorac Surg 8:503–506
37. Kuzkov V, Uvarov D, Kruchkov D, Kirov M, Nedashkovsky E, Bjertnaes L (2007) Determination of extravascular lung water after pneumonectomy and lung resection. Acta Anaesth Scand 51:10 (abst)
38. Sato Y, Motoyama S, Maruyama K et al (2007) Extravascular lung water measured using single transpulmonary thermodilution reflects perioperative pulmonary edema induced by esophagectomy. Eur Surg Res 39:7–13
39. Oshima K, Kunimoto F, Hinohara H et al (2008) Evaluation of respiratory status in patients after thoracic esophagectomy using PiCCO system. Ann Thorac Cardiovasc Surg 14:283–288
40. Pino-Sanchez F, Lara-Rosales R, Guerrero-Lopez F et al (2009) Influence of extravascular lung water determination in fluid and vasoactive therapy. Trauma 67:1220–1224
41. Holm C, Mayr M, Hörbrand F et al (2005) Reproducibility of transpulmonary thermodilution measurements in patients with burn shock and hypothermia. J Burn Care Rehabil 26:260–265
42. Kraft R, Herndon DN, Branski LK, Finnerty CC, Leonard KR, Jeschke MG (2013) Optimized fluid management improves outcomes of pediatric burn patients. J Surg Res 181:121–128
43. Aboelatta Y, Abdelsalam A (2013) Volume overload of fluid resuscitation in acutely burned patients using transpulmonary thermodilution technique. J Burn Care Res 34:349–354
44. Adler C, Reuter H, Seck C, Hellmich M, Zobel C (2013) Fluid therapy and acute kidney injury in cardiogenic shock after cardiac arrest. Resuscitation 84:194–199
45. Mutoh T, Kazumata K, Ajiki M, Ushikoshi S, Terasaka S (2007) Goal-directed fluid management by bedside transpulmonary hemodynamic monitoring after subarachnoid hemorrhage. Stroke 38:3218–3224
46. Sato Y, Isotani E, Kubota Y, Otomo Y, Ohno K (2012) Circulatory characteristics of normovolemia and normotension therapy after subarachnoid hemorrhage, focusing on pulmonary edema. Acta Neurochir (Wien) 154:2195–2202
47. Huber W, Umgelter A, Reindl W et al (2008) Volume assessment in patients with necrotizing pancreatitis: a comparison of intrathoracic blood volume index, central venous pressure, and hematocrit, and their correlation to cardiac index and extravascular lung water index. Crit Care Med 36:2348–2354
48. Venkateswaran RV, Dronavalli V, Patchell V et al (2013) Measurement of extravascular lung water following human brain death: implications for lung donor assessment and transplantation. Eur J Cardiothorac Surg 43:1227–1232

49. Compton F, Hoffmann C, Zidek W, Schmidt S, Schaefer JH (2007) Volumetric hemodynamic parameters to guide fluid removal on hemodialysis in the intensive care unit. Hemodialysis Int 11:231–237
50. Trof RJ, Beishuizen A, Cornet AD et al (2012) Volume-limited versus pressure-limited hemodynamic management in septic and nonseptic shock. Crit Care Med 40:1177–1185

Real-life Implementation of Perioperative Hemodynamic Optimization

M. Biais, A. Senagore, and F. Michard

Introduction

Patients undergoing surgery may develop postoperative complications. The morbidity rate, defined as the proportion of patients developing at least 1 post-surgical complication, increases in the presence of co-morbidities (patient risk) and with the complexity and duration of the surgical procedure (procedure risk). Morbidity rates are often underestimated by clinicians when not measured from objective data. The principle post-surgical complications are listed in Table 1. A study by Ghaferi et al. [1] published in 2009 showed an average morbidity rate of 25 % in over 80,000 patients undergoing general and vascular surgery. Post-surgical complications are not exceptions.

Example 1: Calculation of the morbidity rate for a specific surgical population
If 200 patients had a colorectal resection last year in your institution and 60 developed at least 1 complication (e. g., 12 patients developed a urinary tract infection, 11 a prolonged paralytic ileus, 10 a wound infection, 9 hypotension, 7 nosocomial pneumonia, 6 acute renal insufficiency, 3 myocardial infarction, 1 an anastomotic leak, and 1 a pulmonary embolism), your morbidity rate was 60 / 200 = 30 %.

M. Biais ✉
Emergency and Critical Care Department, Pellegrin Hospital, CHU de Bordeaux and University Bordeaux Segalen, Bordeaux, France
e-mail: matthieu.biais@chu-bordeaux.fr

A. Senagore
Surgical Disciplines, Central Michigan University, Saginaw, MI USA

F. Michard
Critical Care, Edwards Lifesciences, Irvine, CA USA

J.-L. Vincent (Ed.), *Annual Update in Intensive Care and Emergency Medicine 2014*,
DOI 10.1007/978-3-319-03746-2_23, © Springer International Publishing Switzerland
2014

Table 1 List of most common post-surgical complications. Complications underlined were those used by Ghaferi et al. [1] to calculate the above mentioned morbidity rate

Infection	**Cardiovascular**
– Pneumonia	– Deep venous thrombosis
– Urinary tract infection	– Pulmonary embolism
– Superficial wound infection	– Myocardial infarction
– Deep wound infection	– Hypotension
– Organ-space wound infection	– Arrhythmia
– Systemic sepsis or septic shock	– Cardiogenic pulmonary edema
Gastrointestinal	– Cardiogenic shock
– Nausea and vomiting	– Infarction of GI tract
– Ileus (paralytic or functional)	– Distal ischemia
– Acute bowel obstruction	– Cardiac arrest (exclusive of death)
– Anastomotic leak	**Neuro**
– Gastro-intestinal bleeding	– Stroke or cerebrovascular accident
– Intraabdominal hypertension	– Coma
– Hepatic dysfunction	– Altered mental status or Cognitive
– Pancreatitis	dysfunction or Delirium
Respiratory	**Hemato**
– Prolonged mechanical ventilation (> 48 h)	– Bleeding requiring transfusion
– Unplanned intubation or reintubation	– Anemia
– Respiratory failure or ARDS	– Coagulopathy
– Pleural effusion	**Other**
Renal	– Vascular graft or flap failure
– Renal insufficiency (increase in creatinine	– Wound dehiscence
levels or decrease in urine output)	– Peripheral nerve injury
– Renal failure (requiring dialysis)	– Pneumothorax

The Clinical and Economic Burden of Post-Surgical Complications

On a short-term basis, complications increase hospital length of stay and hospital readmission rates [2, 3]. On a long-term basis, complications affect patient survival. An 8-year follow up study [4] in more than 100,000 surgical patients showed that the most important determinant of post-surgical survival was the occurrence, within 30 days post-surgery, of any complication. Independent of preoperative patient risk, the occurrence of a complication reduced median patient long-term survival by 69 % [4].

What is the Cost of Post-surgical Complications?

Treating post-surgical complications has a cost, which is related to the specific therapies needed to treat the complication (e. g., antibiotics, re-intervention, antico-agulation) and to the additional lab tests and investigations that are often necessary, as well as prolonged hospital length of stay. In the US, the average extra cost for treating a patient developing at least one complication is around $ 18,000 [2]. Any complication-related increase in length of stay or re-admission will also decrease

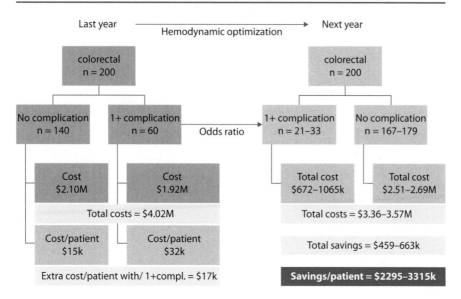

Fig. 1 Predicting the clinical and economic benefits of hemodynamic optimization. Example with a colorectal population of 200 patients and a current morbidity rate of 30 %

efficiency (i.e., the number of patients that can be treated and the related revenues every year).

Example 2: Calculation of the average extra cost per patient with at least one complication

Among 200 colorectal patients, 60 developed at least one complication (morbidity rate 30 %). If the total cost for the 60 patients with at least one complication was $ 1.92 M (i.e., $ 32 k per patient) and the total cost for the 140 remaining patients without any complication was $ 2.10 M (i.e., $ 15 k per patient), then the average extra cost per patient with at least one complication was $ 17 k (Fig. 1).

Example 3: Calculation of the economic burden of complications

The average extra cost per patient with at least one complication was $ 17 k. If 60 patients developed at least one complication, last year $ 1.02 M (60 × $ 17 k) was spent treating postoperative complications in this specific surgical population. If your budget is $ 4.02 M, this sum represents 25 % of that budget (Fig. 1).

Can You Prevent Post-surgical Complications?

Many post-surgical complications are related, at least in part, to insufficient or excessive fluid administration during the perioperative period [5]. A U shape relationship is classically described between the amount of fluid administered and

Table 2 Clinical benefits of hemodynamic optimization over standard fluid management

Reduction in	Average odds or risk ratio (confidence interval)	Author [ref]
Acute kidney injury	0.64 (0.50–0.83)	Brienza [9]
	0.71 (0.57–0.90)	Grocott [13]
	0.67 (0.46–0.98)	Corcoran [14]
Minor GI complications	0.29 (0.17–0.50)	Giglio [10]
Major GI complications	0.42 (0.27–0.65)	Giglio [10]
Surgical site infection	0.58 (0.46–0.74)	Dalfino [11]
	0.65 (0.50–0.84)	Grocott [13]
Urinary tract infection	0.44 (0.22–0.88)	Dalfino [11]
Pneumonia	0.71 (0.55–0.92)	Dalfino [11]
	0.74 (0.57–0.96)	Corcoran [14]
Respiratory failure	0.51 (0.28–0.93)	Grocott [13]
Total morbidity rate	0.44 (0.35–0.55)	Hamilton [12]
	0.68 (0.58–0.80)	Grocott [13]

GI: gastrointestinal

the morbidity rate [5]. Standard fluid management is usually based on clinical assessment, vital signs and/or central venous pressure (CVP) monitoring. However, clinical studies have shown that CVP is not able to predict fluid responsiveness [6] and that changes in blood pressure cannot be used to track changes in stroke volume (SV) or in cardiac output induced by volume expansion [7]. In patients at risk of developing complications, hemodynamic optimization with treatment protocols based on flow parameters (e. g., SV) and/or dynamic predictors of fluid responsiveness (e. g., SV variation [SVV]) is useful to decrease post-surgical morbidity [8]. Over 30 randomized controlled trials and several meta-analyses have demonstrated the superiority of hemodynamic optimization over standard fluid management to decrease renal, gastrointestinal, respiratory and infectious complications, as well as the overall morbidity rate [9–14]. Average reductions in post-surgical complications (odds or risk ratios) reported in meta-analyses [9–14] are summarized in Table 2. The decrease in post-surgical morbidity obtained with hemodynamic optimization was shown to be associated with a decrease in hospital length of stay ranging between 1 and 2 days [13, 14].

Example 4: Predicting the clinical benefits of hemodynamic optimization

Multiplying your current morbidity rate by the odds or risk ratio gives you an estimation of what your morbidity rate should be after the implementation of hemodynamic optimization. If your morbidity rate is currently 30 % for your 200 colorectal procedures, according to the odds ratio (0.35 to 0.55) reported in the meta-analysis of Hamilton et al. [11], it should range between 10.5 % (0.35 × 30 %) and 16.5 % (0.55 × 30 %) after the implementation of hemodynamic optimization (Fig. 1). If the average length of hospital stay for your 200 colorectal patients was 9 days, then you can expect it to range between 7 and 8 days after implementation of hemodynamic optimization.

Example 5: Predicting the economic benefits of hemodynamic optimization

If next year your morbidity rate drops from 30 % to somewhere between 10.5 % and 16.5 %, only 21 to 33 out of your next 200 colorectal patients should develop one or more complications. Last year, 60 patients developed at least one complication. With the implementation of hemodynamic optimization, you will then protect between 27 (60 – 33) and 39 (60 – 21) patients from complications (Fig. 1). We have previously estimated the extra cost related to the treatment of one or more complications to be $ 17 k. With the implementation of hemodynamic optimization, you should then save a total of $ 459–663 k next year for this surgical population, i. e., $ 2,295–3,315 per patient (Fig. 1).

Are there Official Recommendations and Guidelines?

Fuelled by the growing number of clinical studies and meta-analyses demonstrating the value of perioperative hemodynamic optimization, official recommendations have been published in the UK by the Enhanced Recovery Partnership (ERP) [15] and the Association of Surgeons of Great Britain & Ireland [16], in France by the French Society of Anesthesiology (SFAR) [17], and in Europe by the Enhanced Recovery After Surgery (ERAS) society [18]. In the UK, financial incentives have even been created by the National Health Service (NHS) to ensure that hospitals are going to implement hemodynamic optimization as standard of care for at least 80 % of eligible patients [19]. The Patient Safety Foundation of the European Society of Anesthesiology (ESA) recently released a Safety Kit which contains a booklet summarizing hemodynamic optimization treatment protocols [20].

Given the now well-established clinical and economic benefits of hemodynamic optimization and the above recommendations, more and more hospitals are interested in implementing hemodynamic optimization both to improve quality of care and to decrease costs.

The purpose of what follows is to provide a step-by-step guide for simple and successful implementation of hemodynamic optimization.

How to Implement Hemodynamic Optimization? A Phased Approach

Any classical implementation process comprises 4 phases: Assess, align, apply, and measure (Fig. 2). The 1st (assess) and the 4th (measure) phases are optional. The implementation itself is summarized in the 2nd (align) and the 3rd (apply) phases.

Phase 1: Assess

The objective of the 1st phase is to assess the current situation and to predict what should be the clinical and economic benefits of implementation.

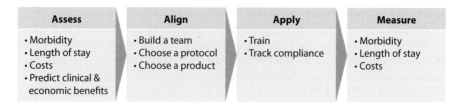

Fig. 2 How to implement perioperative hemodynamic optimization: A phased approach

Table 3 Non-cardiac surgical procedures, with corresponding International Classification of Diseases (ICD)-9 codes, part of positive randomized controlled trials demonstrating the value of perioperative hemodynamic optimization

Surgical procedure	ICD9 codes
Esophagectomy	42.40, 42.41, 42.42, 43.99
Gastrectomy	43.5, 43.6, 43.7, 43.81, 43.89, 43.91, 43.99
Partial hepatectomy	50.22, 50.3
Pancreatectomy and pancreaticoduodenectomy	52.51–52.53, 52.59, 52.6, 52.7
Colectomy	45.71–45.76, 45.79, 45.81–45.83, 48.41, 48.69
Resection of rectum	48.50–48.52, 48.59, 48.61–48.65, 48.69
Total cystectomy	57.71, 57.79
Femur & hip fracture repair	79.15, 79.25, 79.35, 79.85
Hip replacement	81.51–81.53
Abdominal aortic aneurysm	38.44
Aorto-iliac and peripheral bypass	39.25, 39.29

- Select one or several surgical procedures for which a benefit has been established (Table 3) and hence would also be expected in your institution. You can (but do not have to) restrict the implementation to a subgroup of patients who have a higher risk of developing complications (e. g., patients with specific co-morbidities, patients with American Society of Anesthesiologists [ASA] score > 1, or patients older than 65 yrs)
- Assess the current morbidity rate using the list of complications provided in Table 1 and following example 1 and/or assess the current hospital length of stay
- Predict the clinical benefits of your hemodynamic optimization program following example 4
- Predict the economic benefits of your hemodynamic optimization program following examples 2 and 5

Phase 2: Align

- Build a team. Changing standard of care is not a single person initiative. You need to work with a team, to understand and communicate the clinical and economic value of hemodynamic optimization, and be able to solve any technical, medical and human challenge you may encounter during the implementation phase. Your core team should be lead by a champion and include at least one representative of the surgical team, of the anesthesia team, of the anesthesia assistant and/or certified registered nurse anesthetist (CRNA) team, as well as your quality officer.

- Choose a treatment protocol. One of your first tasks will be to select the most appropriate hemodynamic optimization protocol for your surgical population. Several protocols have been shown to be effective and have been recently summarized by the European Society of Anesthesiology [20].
- Choose a product. Most hemodynamic optimization protocols are based on the monitoring of flow parameters and/or dynamic predictors of fluid responsiveness. Many techniques allowing the continuous (and sometimes non-invasive) monitoring of these parameters are now available on the market.

Phase 3: Apply

To ensure successful implementation of hemodynamic optimization, you need to provide appropriate training and track compliance.

- Training. All anesthesiologists and AA/CRNA who will perform hemodynamic optimization must be trained
- Ensure optimal compliance. Compliance to guidelines and recommendations is often suboptimal. To ensure hemodynamic optimization protocols are followed properly, several actions and tools are useful:
  - Standard operating procedure. Define hemodynamic optimization as an official and new standard operating procedure for hemodynamic management in your department
  - Surgical safety checklist. Adding a single item to the current "Sign In" section of the surgical safety checklist, such as "the patient's eligibility for hemodynamic optimization has been considered"
  - Compliance tools. Use tools specifically designed to quantify and track compliance to hemodynamic optimization protocols
  - Electronic data recording. Physiologic data can be downloaded from hemodynamic monitors in order to double-check that the optimization protocol has been followed and to quantify the time spent in target (e. g., $SVV < 12\%$)

Phase 4: Measure

Using the methods described in Phase 1 (assess), you can calculate the morbidity rate, hospital length of stay and real costs after implementation of your hemodynamic optimization program in order to confirm the clinical (reduction in morbidity and length of stay) and economic benefits (net savings).

Conclusions

To quote Dr. Pronovost, "the fundamental problem with the quality of medicine is that we have failed to view delivery of health care as a science. The tasks of medical science fall into three buckets. One is understanding disease biology. One is finding effective therapies. And one is ensuring those therapies are delivered effectively. That third bucket has been almost totally ignored by research funders, governments and academia. It is viewed as the art of medicine. That is a mistake, a huge mistake. And from a taxpayer perspective, this is outrageous" [21]. Perioperative hemodynamic optimization is an example of a clinical strategy that has been shown to be effective by many randomized controlled trials and several meta-analyses (evidence level 1A). Despite this level of evidence and official recommendations and guidelines, adoption of perioperative hemodynamic optimization is still poor [22]. The on-coming shift from a 'pay for service' to a 'pay for performance or P4P' health care system [23] is going to incite more and more clinicians and hospitals to improve quality of care. To do so, they should not forget that, according to Urbach and Baxter [24], "the immediate challenge to improving the quality of surgical care is not discovering new knowledge, but rather how to integrate what we already know into practice". Therefore, with simple and actionable implementation programs, like the one we describe in the present manuscript, clinicians and hospitals should be able to optimize care delivery, improve patient satisfaction and outcome, and decrease costs at the same time [25].

References

1. Ghaferi AA, Birkmeyer JD, Dimick JB (2009) Variation in hospital mortality associated with inpatient surgery. N Engl J Med 361:1368–1375
2. Boltz MM, Hollenbeak CS, Ortenzi G, Dillon PW (2012) Synergistic implications of multiple postoperative outcomes. Am J Med Qual 27:383–390
3. Lawson EH, Hall BL, Louie R et al (2013) Association between occurrence of a postoperative complication and readmission. Ann Surg 258:10–18
4. Khuri SF, Henderson WG, DePalma RG et al (2005) Determinants of long-term survival after major surgery and the adverse effect of post-operative complications. Ann Surg 242:326–343
5. Bellamy MC (2006) Wet, dry or something else? Br J Anaesth 97:755–757
6. Marik PE, Cavallazzi R (2013) Does the central venous pressure predict fluid responsiveness? An updated meta-analysis and a plea for some common sense. Crit Care Med 41:1774–1781
7. Le Manach Y, Hofer CK, Lehot JJ et al (2013) Can changes in arterial pressure be used to detect changes in cardiac output during volume expansion in the perioperative period? Anesthesiology 117:1165–1174
8. Michard F, Biais M (2012) Rational fluid management: dissecting facts from fiction. Br J Anaesth 108:369–371
9. Brienza N, Giglio MT, Marucci M, Fiore T (2009) Does perioperative hemodynamic optimization protect renal function in surgical patients? A meta-analytic study. Crit Care Med 37:2079–2090
10. Giglio MT, Marucci M, Testini M, Brienza N (2009) Goal-directed haemodynamic therapy and gastrointestinal complications in major surgery: a meta-analysis of randomized controlled trials. Br J Anesth 103:637–646

11. Dalfino L, Giglio MT, Puntillo F, Marucci M, Brienza N (2011) Haemodynamic goal-directed therapy and postoperative infections: earlier is better. A systematic review and meta-analysis. Crit Care 15:R154
12. Hamilton M, Cecconi M, Rhodes A (2011) A systematic review and meta-analysis on the use of preemptive hemodynamic intervention to improve outcomes in moderate and high-risk surgery. Anesth Analg 112:1392–1402
13. Grocott MPW, Dushiantan A, Hamilton MA et al (2013) Perioperative increase in global blood flow to explicit defined goals and outcomes after surgery: a Cochrane systematic review. Br J Anaesth 111:535–548
14. Corcoran T, Rhodes JEJ, Clarke S, Myles P, Ho KM (2012) Perioperative fluid management strategies in major surgery: a stratified meta-analysis. Anesth Analg 114:640–651
15. Mythen MG, Swart M, Acheson N et al (2012) Perioperative fluid management: Consensus statement from the enhanced recovery partnership. Perioperative Medicine 1:2
16. Powell-Tuck J, Gosling P, Lobo DN, et al (2011) British Consensus Guidelines On Intravenous Fluid Therapy For Adult Surgical Patients. Available at: . Accessed Nov 2013
17. Vallet B, Blanloeil Y, Cholley B, Orliaguet G, Pierre S, Tavernier B (2013) Guidelines for perioperative haemodynamic optimization. Ann Fr Anesth Reanim 32:454–62
18. Gustafsson UO, Scott MJ, Schwenk W et al (2013) Guidelines for perioperative care in elective colonic surgery: enhanced recovery after surgery (ERAS) society. World J Surg 37:259–284
19. Commissioning for quality and innovation (CQUIN): 2013/14 guidance. Available at: http://www.england.nhs.uk/wp-content/uploads/2013/02/cquin-guidance.pdf. Accessed Nov 2013
20. The Patient Safety Foundation of the European Society of Anesthesiology (ESA); Available at: http://html.esahq.org/patientsafetykit/resources/index.html. Accessed Nov 2013
21. Gawande A (2010) The Checklist Manifesto. How to Get Things Right? Metropolitan Books, New York
22. Miller TE, Roche AM, Gan TJ (2011) Poor adoption of hemodynamic optimization during major surgery: are we practicing substandard care? Anesth Analg 112:1274–1276
23. Eappen S, Lane BH, Rosenberg B et al (2013) Relationship between occurrence of surgical complications and hospital finances. JAMA 309:1599–1606
24. Urbach DR, Baxter NN (2005) Reducing variation in surgical care. BMJ 330:1401–1402
25. Pronovost P, Angus D (2000) Cost reduction and quality improvement: It takes two to tango. Crit Care Med 28:581–583

Update on Perioperative Hemodynamic Monitoring and Goal-directed Optimization Concepts

V. Mezger, M. Habicher, and M. Sander

Introduction

The prescription of perioperative fluids has been a persistent controversy among anesthesiologists, surgeons and intensivists. Interestingly, disagreements within each specialty as to the appropriative types and amounts of fluids required are just as intense as those seen among specialties. The challenge of navigating these waters is demanding because the safe harbor of optimal fluid administration is bounded by hypovolemia and end-organ hypoperfusion, resulting from inadequate fluid resuscitation, and the negative effects of edema formation on respiration and wound healing, resulting from excessive fluid administration.

Different strategies of fluid management have been implemented in the perioperative setting. The terms of 'liberal' or 'restrictive' fluid administration were used to define algorithms that used greater or lesser amounts of fluid for maintenance and substitution for losses caused by bleeding, preoperative fasting, and perspiration. With technological progress and the possibility of measuring hemodynamic variables, even with non-invasive technologies, a third fluid administration concept has become established in the perioperative setting – goal-directed fluid management. This therapy concept has been repeatedly shown to significantly improve both short-term and long-term outcomes. Goal-directed therapy is centered on the optimization of individually needed cardiac output and, thus, oxygen delivery (DO_2) by incremental fluid administration. The disadvantages of this concept are, in addition to the further invasiveness, the additional costs of these monitoring devices.

In clinical routine, intravascular measured pressures, e. g., central venous pressure (CVP) or mean arterial pressure (MAP), are often used to quantify the patient's volume status. Although these parameters are all important components of hemo-

V. Mezger · M. Habicher · M. Sander ✉
Department of Anesthesiology and Intensive Care Medicine, Campus Charité Mitte and Campus Virchow-Klinikum, Charité - University Medicine Berlin, 10117 Berlin, Germany
e-mail: michael.sander@charite.de

J.-L. Vincent (Ed.), *Annual Update in Intensive Care and Emergency Medicine 2014*, DOI 10.1007/978-3-319-03746-2_24, © Springer International Publishing Switzerland 2014

dynamic assessment, none has been shown to be a good predictor of the response of cardiac output to fluid administration [1]. The same applies to the more reliable preload parameters, such as left ventricular end-diastolic area (LVEDA) and global end-diastolic volume (GEDV). However, these static parameters are limited to predicting an increase (responders) or lack of increase (non-responders) in stroke volume (SV) and, thus, cardiac output in response to fluid loading. The inadequacy of commonly used hemodynamic parameters as predictors of the response to fluid stems from the fact that this response depends not only on the preload status, but also on the contractile state of the heart. In this context, dynamic variables like SV variation (SVV) and pulse pressure variation (PPV) are able to measure the change in cardiac output in response to a change in preload due to fluid administration [2].

However, in addition to the physiological variables mentioned above, this chapter aims to provide an update on perioperative hemodynamic monitoring and a brief overview of the different fluid administration concepts in the perioperative setting.

Monitoring Technology

Cardiac Output

Pulmonary artery catheter

The pulmonary artery catheter (PAC) is the classical invasive method for hemodynamic monitoring. It was the gold standard for goal-directed fluid management for many years. None of the other devices used for hemodynamic measurement has raised more controversy than the PAC.

The measurement of cardiac output follows the indicator transpulmonary thermodilution principle. After injection of a defined volume of a cold solution into the PAC's proximal lumen, the cooling of blood in the pulmonary artery is quantified via the PAC's distal catheter containing a thermistor. The variation in temperature over time is illustrated in an indicator dilution curve. The area under the curve (AUC) is inversely proportional to the cardiac output that can be calculated with the Stewart-Hamilton equation. The measured time/temperature curve is displayed on the cardiac output monitor. The smaller the decrease in temperature (the greater the cardiac output) the smaller is the AUC that is displayed. Modern catheters are fitted with a heating filament which intermittently heats and measures the thermodilution curve providing serial cardiac output measurement and making assessment of continuous cardiac output available. In this context the term 'continuous' should be considered carefully, because although there is a continuous serial heart rate (HR) triggered discharge of heat boluses, changes in cardiac output are detected with a clinically relevant mean delay of 8–10 minutes. Because of this interval, goal-directed volume therapy can be delayed and this technique may not be as useful and accurate as online measurements of stroke volume by other technology.

A further development of the volumetric thermodilution PAC is electrocardiogram (EKG)-triggered computation of the right ventricular end-diastolic volume

Table 1 Clinical advantages and disadvantages of the pulmonary artery catheter

Advantages	Disadvantages
Well-validated parameters	Interference by intrathoracic pressure
Measurement of pulmonary arterial pressures	Interference with valve disorders
Measurement of mixed venous oxygen saturation	Catheter-associated infections and thrombosis
Measurement of pulmonary artery occlusion pressure (PAOP)	Cardiac arrhythmias
Comprehensive computation of hemodynamic parameters	Valvular injury, rupture of the pulmonary artery, pulmonary infarction
Computation of oxygen supply and demand	

(RVEDV) and from this, the right ventricular ejection fraction (RVEF, %), using modern specialized monitors (e. g., Vigilance CEDV, Edwards Lifescience, Irvine, CA) and the following formula:

$$RVEDV \ (ml) = cardiac \ output \ (ml/min)/HR \ (b/min) \times RVEF(\%)$$

$$RVEF(\%) = RVEDV - RVESV/RVEDV \times 100$$

The RVEDV index (RVEDVI) connects the RVEDV with the body surface area and serves as an estimation of the RV, but limited LV, preload and enables conclusions to be drawn about a patient's circulatory status.

Measurement of the pulmonary artery occlusion pressure (POAP) enables estimation of the LV end-diastolic pressure (LVEP) and, thus, the LV preload. Limiting factors for interpretation of LV preload using the POAP are: Incorrect positioning of the PAC tip, mitral valve defects and reduced LV compliance, e. g., due to LV insufficiency. Therefore, when using POAP for hemodynamic therapy, several measurements should be compared over time. Furthermore, the POAP should not be used to determine SV responsiveness to fluid loading, because there is no evidence that this parameter enables any conclusions to be drawn regarding the increases in SV from fluid loading. For estimation of the above mentioned variables, further parameters like MAP, CVP and mixed venous oxygen saturation (SvO$_2$) are required. The advantages and disadvantages of the PAC are shown in Table 1.

Concerning the international literature, there is still controversy regarding the PAC. Because of higher costs and the availability of less invasive technology for determination of stroke volume, PAC use for hemodynamic monitoring has decreased in the USA. Furthermore, a recently published survey of leading physicians from 80 intensive care units (ICUs) in Germany treating patients after cardiothoracic surgery, showed that although availability of the PAC is 100 %, usage of PACs in patients had decreased to 48 % compared to data from 2005 in which 58 % of these patients were managed using a PAC [3]. Although a study by Tuman et al. [4] showed no benefit in terms of duration of ICU stay, mortality and incidence of postoperative myocardial ischemia using a PAC after coronary bypass surgery compared to clinical management using CVP, another study by Pölönen et al. showed a significantly shorter "median hospital stay" if hemodynamic therapy was targeted to reach $SvO_2 > 70\%$ and serum lactate levels ≤ 2.0 mmol/l [5]. Only a few studies have investigated perioperative PAC usage in patients not undergoing cardiac surgery. One of the most comprehensive analyses done in this patient cohort was a study by Sandham et al. using PAC for patients classified 3 and 4 by the American Society of Anesthesiologists (ASA). This study showed no benefit on duration of hospital stay or mortality rate after six months [6]. Jules-Elysee et al., who investigated the use of a PAC-compared to a CVP-based protocol for patients undergoing bilateral knee replacement, reported similar results [7].

It is presumed that the benefit of a PAC depends on its use for applying goal-directed hemodynamic therapy, implementing supranormal oxygen supply and stroke volume optimization, and not just as an instrument of observation. This hypothesis is reflected by the fact that all major retrospective or observational studies that have been performed showed no benefit of PAC use. In contrast, in a meta-analysis by Hamilton et al. [8], the PAC was the only technology that showed a benefit on morbidity and mortality if used in a goal-directed treatment algorithm.

In conclusion, there is need for further investigation to identify patient groups who can gain from using a PAC during the perioperative period.

Transpulmonal thermodilution technology

Transpulmonary thermodilution is a method to estimate intrathoracic and global end-diastolic volumes and is commercially available as a bedside monitoring device (PiCCO, Pulsion Medical Systems, Munich, Germany; EV1000, Volume View, Edwards Life Sciences). Placement of a central venous catheter and a modified arterial catheter equipped with both temperature and pressure sensors are required. The tip of the arterial catheter is positioned in a central artery through access from the femoral, brachial, axillary and radial arteries. The monitor offers recording of SV, cardiac index (CI), static volume parameters such as GEDV index (GEDVI) and extravascular lung water index (EVLWI), and dynamic volume parameters, such as SVV and PVV.

For cardiac output measurement, *in vivo* calibration has to be performed. A defined volume of a cold solution is injected into the central venous catheter. The blood temperature modulation is recorded via the thermistor placed at the tip of the arterial catheter. The recorded thermodilution curve is used to compute the cardiac output using the Stewart-Hamilton equation. Formerly, the volumetric parameter, the intrathoracic blood volume (ITBV), was calculated as the product of cardiac output and the mean transit time of a dye indicator. For clinical use, the previous, cumbersome method of transpulmonary double-indicator (cold and dye) dilution has been replaced by single-indicator thermodilution. The literature shows that the volumetric parameters, GEDV and ITBV, are superior to the CVP and POAP for assessing cardiac preload [9, 10].

The ability to estimate preload and volume reliably from these parameters has been studied by several authors. Transpulmonary thermodilution cardiac output shows good correlation with pulmonary arterial thermodilution cardiac output. In contrast to the many studies that have shown high validity and reliability of the transpulmonary thermodilution system during the perioperative period, especially following cardiac surgery [11, 12], only a few studies have investigated the use of transpulmonary thermodilution systems for intraoperative goal-directed volume management. Hence, transpulmonary thermodilution has been established in the intensive care setting, but not in the perioperative setting. This observation can be explained by the relative invasiveness of the transpulmonary thermodilution system, leading to less use of this method for intraoperative goal-directed volume management. Additionally, as mentioned above, the lack of clinical trials demonstrating an advantage of intraoperative volume therapy could explain these findings.

Uncalibrated and auto-calibrated pulse contour/ pulse wave technology

Because of the invasiveness of cardiac output measurements via the PAC or transpulmonary thermodilution technology, non-invasive systems have been developed to make intraoperative goal-directed fluid management more available and less invasive. One of these non-invasive systems is uncalibrated pulse-contour analysis. This technique is a further development of the original algorithm of pulse contour analysis described by Wesseling in which the relationship between arterial blood pressure and arterial blood flow that is determined by the vascular resistance is characterized. The cardiac output is calculated from the AUC of the arterial waveform. For uncalibrated pulse contour analysis, there are several devices available (e. g., Vigileo, Edwards Lifesciences LLC, Irvine, CA, USA; Pulsioflex, Pulsion Medical Germany). In some monitors, the cardiac output is calibrated using internal databases and adjusting for vascular resistance and compliance by demographic data; other devices use auto-calibration. In these latter devices, the calibration coefficient that adjusts for individual characteristics of vascular resistance and arterial compliance is auto-re-calculated every 10 minutes on the basis of demographic data and the arterial waveform analysis.

Clinical trials concerning the reliability and validity of uncalibrated pulse contour technology compared to established system, such as PAC thermodilution and transpulmonary thermodilution technology, show contrasting results. In one trial, a high bias and wide range of limits of agreement were found in cardiac output measurement using arterial waveform analysis [13]. Other studies confirmed these findings [14]. However, other studies showed no significant differences when comparing calibrated and uncalibrated pulse contour measurements [15]. These findings lead to the conclusion that a final assessment of this technology cannot be performed at this point in time. Nevertheless, although the validity of cardiac output determination compared to calibrated methods seems to be inferior, goal-directed volume administration using this monitoring technology appears to result in clinical benefits with decreased morbidity.

Bioimpedance and reactance technology

Another non-invasive procedure for cardiac output measurement is impedance cardiography. This technique is performed by attaching four electrodes on each side of the patient's neck, and on the left and right sides of the chest. Microelectric currents that flow through the patient's chest cavity are registered through these electrodes, and changes in impedance caused by the changes in thoracic aortic volume and blood flow are measured. Volumetric and static variables, such as SV, cardiac output, systemic vascular resistance (SVR) and thoracic fluid content can be observed by this technique [16]. Owing to limitations associated with its use, such as the various surgical manipulations undertaken, acute changes in patient fluid status and frequent electrocautery, impedance cardiography is interference-prone and, therefore, not widely used in the perioperative setting at the present stage of technical development [17].

Non-invasive cardiac output measurement devices

In addition to the above mentioned tools for non-invasive cardiac output measurements, there are considerable efforts being taken for the development of other non-invasive devices to make cardiac output determination easier and more available without having the disadvantages of invasive technologies. One of these recent devices is the Nexfin technology (BMEye, Edwards Life Sciences, Amsterdam, The Netherlands). This instrument provides a non-invasive estimation of cardiac output in two steps. First, the device enables continuous estimation of the arterial pressure curve using the volume-clamp method. For this purpose, the device includes an inflatable cuff that is wrapped around a finger. Additionally, a second device is included to measure the diameter of the finger's arteries by photoplethysmography. During measurement, the photoplethysmographic device senses the increase in the diameter of the finger's arteries at each systole and the cuff inflates immediately to keep the diameter constant and, thus, the cuff pressure reflects the arterial pressure. The continuous measurement allows estimation of the arterial pressure curve. During the second step, the cardiac output is computed from the arterial pressure curve by pulse contour analysis, which is included in the Nexfin device [18].

Since its launch, the Nexfin system has been the subject of many investigations showing divergent results. A large perioperative validation study for measuring arterial pressure showed positive results [19, 20], but contrasting results were reported in critically ill patients. Broch et al. showed that Nexfin was a reliable system for measuring cardiac output during and after cardiac surgery compared to the PiCCO system [21]. Other studies revealed similar results [18]. In contrast to these findings, a study by Fischer et al. showed higher percentage errors when comparing Nexfin with transpulmonary thermodilution. Furthermore, rapid changes in CI following a fluid challenge were detected less well compared to with the PiCCO system so that prediction of fluid responsiveness was reduced [22]. Similar results were shown for cardiac output by Monnet et al. in critically ill patients treated on the ICU [23].

As the Nexfin is a relatively new advice, further investigation is needed to substantiate its reliability and variability in the perioperative setting, including for surgeries other than cardiac. The Nexfin device is prone to error in cases of diminished peripheral perfusion, which might occur in critically ill patients. However, goal-directed volume therapy in high and intermediate risk surgery may prove to be an interesting indication for non-invasive monitoring. Another encouraging approach is the notion of external calibration to improve accuracy [22].

Venous and Tissue Saturation

Mixed venous versus central venous saturation

Advanced hemodynamic monitoring with determination of cardiac output and venous saturation measurements is widely used in the perioperative setting especially in cardiac surgical patients. SvO_2 and central venous oxygen saturation ($ScvO_2$) are different physiological variables. Both are parameters used to indicate the global ratio of oxygen supply and demand as well as tissue oxygenation. Consequently, it is possible to gather information on the adequacy of actual cardiac output in relation to demand from these parameters. SvO_2 measures the venous saturation in the pulmonary artery and thus a PAC is needed. In contrast, $ScvO_2$ is measured mostly in the venous blood of the superior vena cava, which makes this parameter easily available. In healthy subjects, oxygen saturation in the inferior vena cava, which contains blood from the upper and lower body, is higher than in the superior vena cava, which contains blood from the upper body only. In contrast to the situation described above, in clinical practice there is almost no mean difference between SvO_2 and $ScvO_2$ in a given patient population. It has been suggested that the difference between SvO_2 and $ScvO_2$ is not constant, but may be affected by conditions such as anesthesia and redistribution of blood; for example, following systemic inflammatory response syndrome (SIRS) or shock. $ScvO_2$ can exceed SvO_2 in critically ill patients. This difference between SvO_2 and $ScvO_2$ may be caused by increased cerebral blood flow owing to the vasodilating effect of inhalational anesthetics and reduced cerebral oxygen demand in anesthetized patients, both reducing cerebral oxygen extraction, which would lead to higher $ScvO_2$ in the superior vena cava. Increased oxygen extraction in the splanchnic region can also reverse the physiological difference between SvO_2 and $ScvO_2$. After hemodynamic deterioration, mesenteric blood flow decreases, resulting in venous de-saturation in the lower body. It, therefore, has to be assumed that the oxygen extraction rate is the major factor in the difference between SvO_2 and $ScvO_2$. Considering the above mentioned conditions, $ScvO_2$ and SvO_2 can be useful parameters for estimating cardiac output during surgery. It is important to mention that both variables, but especially $ScvO_2$, are limited when trying to exclude general or local hypoperfusion and for a more precise prediction both variables are needed, which narrows their use in the intraoperative setting [24]. Another limitation of the use of these parameters is that with reduced oxygen uptake in the periphery, high values of venous saturation do not exclude microcirculatory hypoperfusion.

Cerebral and tissue saturation

As described above, it is possible to draw indirect conclusions from tissue saturation about cardiac output and implement goal-directed, perioperative volume therapy. For monitoring tissue saturation there are several devices available. Near-infrared spectroscopy should be mentioned in this context. Using this technology, reduced tissue saturation, which can be caused by a discrepancy in oxygen supply and demand, can be measured non-invasively. The benefit of this technology has been shown in several studies, notably in vascular and cardiac surgery, but further investigation has to be performed to prove its clinical utility and its impact on outcome [25, 26].

Dynamic Parameters

Intermittent positive airway pressure during controlled mechanical ventilation in patients with regular heart rhythm results in intermittent variation of biventricular preload. This effect results in intermittent variation of SV and arterial pressure. Pulse contour algorithm-based quantification of SV and arterial pressure parameters and the availability of modern devices (Flotrac, Volume view, Edwards Life Systems; LidCO rapid, LIDCO, London, UK; and $PiCCO_2$, Pulsioflex, Pulsion Medical Systems, Munich, Germany) have introduced these dynamic parameters into clinical practice. High variation values can be indicative of hypovolemia and are used to monitor volume therapy by their assessment of volume responsiveness.

Systolic pressure variation

Systolic pressure variation (SPV) represents the difference between the maximum and minimum value of systolic arterial pressure during one mechanical breath. The SPV is composed of an early inspiratory increase in the systolic blood pressure, which reflects the inspiratory augmentation of the LV SV, and a later decrease in systolic blood pressure, which reflects the decreased SV due to the decrease in venous return. It has been shown experimentally and clinically that SPV reflects fluid responsiveness very well in a variety of different surgeries. Moreover, SPV can be easily and accurately estimated from visual examination of the arterial waveform tracing.

Pulse pressure variation

PPV also mirrors changes in pulse pressure induced by ventilation. It is calculated as the difference between maximum and minimum pulse pressure values during mechanical ventilation divided by their mean. PPV is an indicator of the position on the Frank-Starling curve and can predict the deleterious hemodynamic effects of fluid depletion. In the perioperative setting, patients who have reached the plateau of the Frank-Starling curve can be identified as patients in whom PPV is low. The clinical and intraoperative goal of maximizing SV by volume loading can, therefore, be achieved easily by minimizing PPV. These findings have been confirmed in various studies in cardiac as well bowel or other general surgery [27–29].

Stroke volume variation

SVV is the difference between the maximum and minimum SV during one mechanical breath divided by mean SV. Due to pulse contour measuring technology for cardiac output it is possible to provide continuous metering of SVV. High SVV is indicative of hypovolemia and differentiates responders from non-responders. The use of SVV for goal-directed fluid management has been investigated in various studies in the perioperative setting including cardiac and abdominal surgery as well as liver transplantation [2].

Pleth variability index

Variations in pulse oximeter waveform amplitude caused by respiration have been shown to be related to PPV. This measure is sensitive to changes in ventricular preload and is a good predictor of fluid responsiveness. The pleth variability index (PVI) provides automatic and continuous monitoring of respiratory variations in the pulse oximeter waveform amplitude. PVI was shown to be able to predict fluid responsiveness during cardiac and colorectal surgery [30, 31]. The limitation of these findings is that the majority of these studies were conducted in patients with a stable hemodynamic condition. A study by Monnet et al. showed that PVI was less reliable than PPV and SVV for predicting fluid responsiveness in patients receiving norepinephrine [32]. This technology is prone to error in cases of diminished peripheral perfusion, which may occur in unstable and critically ill patients. Due to conflicting findings in recent studies the advantage of PVI is still unclear.

Echocardiography and Doppler Technology

Esophageal Doppler monitoring

Esophageal Doppler monitoring is an easy to use, accurate and minimally invasive method for SV optimization. The CardioQ-System (Deltex Medical, Chichester, West Sussex, UK) is a device that utilizes a normogram incorporating age, weight and height and calculates descending aortic blood flow velocity directly based on the Doppler equation. The monitor displays a waveform of the velocity plotted against time. Because flow time depends on the heart rate, it is usually corrected automatically. The resulting corrected flow time (FTc) represents the systolic ejection time adjusted to one cardiac cycle per second. Further correction allows estimation of the SVR. SVR is inversely proportional to FTc, i.e., the higher the SVR, the shorter the FTc, and increased SVR is often associated with hypovolemia. Since FTc is an indicator of cardiac afterload, in hypovolemia, volume administration will lead to an increase in SV and FTc, because of increased cardiac preload. This effect can be interpreted as volume responsiveness and facilitates goal-directed volume therapy. In addition to being able to measure FTc, it is possible to draw inferences about LV inotropy, because myocardial contractility correlates with measured peak velocity.

In addition to the validity and reliability of esophageal Doppler monitoring compared to PAC-derived variables, several studies have demonstrated the benefit of this technique regarding postoperative complication rates and lengths of hospital stay [33]. It should be noted that interobserver differences because of lack of experience in using esophageal Doppler monitoring are limiting factors in the use of these systems [34, 35].

Transesophageal echocardiography

In current clinical practice, the LVEDA estimated by transesophageal echocardiography (TEE) is the preferred echocardiographic parameter for the assessment of preload. The simplicity of measurement and its reliability in reflecting the ventricle's loading status have led LVEDA to become the most popular choice in the intraoperative setting, especially in cardiac surgery. LVEDA is commonly measured in the transgastric midpapillary short-axis view. It has been shown that the LVEDA measured by TEE correlates quite well with ventricular volumes measured by nuclear medicine methods. The volumes identified by echocardiography give more detailed information about the volume status than parameters measured by PAC. In clinical routine, this parameter is mostly 'eyeballed'. Several studies have compared the end-diastolic area as an indicator for cardiac preload with conventional monitoring procedures. LVEDA was shown to be a sensitive method for detecting changes in preload after volume administration [36]. Moreover, ITBV and LVEDA were shown to be equivalent indices of cardiac preload [37]. Additionally, LVEDA is superior to static hemodynamic parameters, such as CVP or PAOP, in assessment of cardiac surgery patients' fluid responsiveness after fluid administration [38]. Furthermore, it is possible to measure the superior vena cava collapse index by TEE in mechanically ventilated patients. This index can predict a patient's fluid responsiveness because of a volume and ventilation-dependent collapse of the superior vena cava. The reliability of this index was shown by Viellard-Baron et al. in septic patients [39].

The main limitation of echocardiography is its relatively limited availability, high cost of the devices and the challenges in insuring adequate staff training. Diagnosis and treatment of acute hemodynamic instability are the main domains of echocardiography and it should be performed by trained experts in these conditions. Furthermore, echocardiographic parameters can be used to assess volume status and for goal-directed hemodynamic optimization if adequately trained staff and technology are available.

Optimization Concepts

Patient Selection

The health system's resources are limited. Therefore, it is clear that expensive and invasive, less-invasive and even non-invasive additional monitoring devices cannot be used in every patient for perioperative goal-directed fluid therapy. For this reason, high-risk patients who could benefit from this specialized therapy need to be identified preoperatively. Using the ASA classification, it is possible to assess a patient's preoperative physical condition; perioperative cardiac risk and intervention-based risk are not included in this classification. Nevertheless, the patient's risk

Table 2 Criteria for high-risk surgical patient (modified from Shoemaker et al. [40]). Presence of ≥ 1 criterion indicates high risk

1.	Severe cardiac or respiratory illness resulting in severe functional limitation (acute myocardial infarction, coronaropathy, dilated cardiomyopathy, ejection fraction < 40 %)
2.	Extensive surgery planned for carcinoma involving bowel anastomosis
3.	Acute massive blood loss (> 2.5 l)
4.	Age > 70 years with moderate functional limitation of one or more organ systems
5.	Septicemia (positive blood cultures or septic focus)
6.	Respiratory failure
7.	Acute abdominal catastrophe (e. g., pancreatitis, perforated viscous, gastro-intestinal bleeding)
8.	Acute renal failure (urea > 45 mg/dl, creatinine > 2.9 mg/dl)
9.	Diabetes (preoperative glycemia > 150 mg/dl)
10.	Chronic hepatopathy (Child B or C)
11.	Surgery for abdominal aortic aneurysm

depends not only on his/her preoperative health condition but also on intraoperative- and surgery-related factors as proposed by Shoemaker et al. (Table 2) [40]. Therefore, for identification of high-risk patients, a combination of variables to assess the patients risk due to the actual health status (e. g., ASA score, cardiac risk score) and the surgical risk (e. g., Physiological and Operative Severity Score for the enUmeration of Mortality and Morbidity [POSSUM] Score) are therefore needed. Most classifications, such as the POSSUM score, are not currently used in clinical practice but only for research purposes. Nevertheless, meta-analyses have shown positive effects of goal-directed fluid therapy and hemodynamic management in high-risk patients (using different definitions of risk) in the perioperative setting [8, 41–43].

Intraoperative Versus Postoperative Optimization

The main objective of goal-directed fluid management is to maintain tissue perfusion and assure organ function. Optimization of cardiac output, resulting in the optimization of oxygen supply and demand as well as tissue oxygenation, should be performed at an early stage prior to appearance of organ dysfunction. It is ineffective or even harmful when performed later. The oxygen debt that can result during surgery leads to a higher incidence of complications, such as infections, organ failure and, as a final consequence, death. Various studies and meta-analyses showed the benefit of intraoperative goal-directed fluid management [44, 45]. A review by Dalfino et al. [46] showed that goal-directed fluid therapy is an effective tool for reducing the incidence of infectious complications, and, more specifically, that goal-directed therapy significantly decreases the rate of surgical site infections, pneumonia and urinary tract infections. During surgery, goal-directed fluid therapy, by preserving or increasing cardiac output, may protect patients against severe gut ischemia-reperfusion injury and thus decrease the incidence of postoperative infections [46]. These findings were reported in a meta-analysis, which showed that goal-directed fluid therapy decreased the incidence of postoperative gastrointestinal dysfunction by maintaining an adequate systemic oxygenation in patients undergoing major surgery [47]. In addition to the benefits of intraoperative goal-directed fluid therapy, the benefit of this strategy during the immediate postoperative period included reductions in complications and duration of hospital stay [48]. Nevertheless, from a physiological point of view, it appears obvious that the patient will benefit from goal-directed fluid therapy that starts earlier in order to prevent intraoperative hypoperfusion, so that it should start intraoperatively.

Fluid Optimization Concepts

Apart from the benefits of goal-directed fluid therapy during major surgery discussed earlier, there are divergent opinions concerning whether liberal or restrictive fluid management leads to better outcome. The disadvantages of goal-directed fluid therapy are seen in excessive volume administration and consequently interstitial space overload, which might influence patient outcome. In a randomized, observer-blinded, multicenter trial, Brandstrup et al. showed that a restricted perioperative intravenous fluid regimen aimed at unchanged body weight reduced complications after elective colorectal resection [49]. Other studies in patients undergoing different kinds of surgery confirmed these findings. Nevertheless, it is difficult to make an objective decision as to whether goal-directed fluid therapy or restrictive fluid therapy is superior, because there are no studies comparing goal-directed fluid therapy with a standardized restrictive fluid therapy. Furthermore, the object of 'restrictive' fluid therapy is not clearly defined and is associated with different amounts of fluid administration in the current literature.

In addition to the amount of volume administration, the type of fluid used should not be disregarded. Whereas use of large amounts of crystalloids can lead to interstitial overload, as described above, or to iatrogenic hyperchloremic acidosis when using normal saline, a balanced use of different kinds of solution may help to prevent the disadvantages of liberal fluid therapy. Furthermore, the role of transfusion should not be ignored; especially in bleeding surgical patients, early fluid resuscitation with blood products seems to be advantageous [50].

Conclusions

Because of the increased numbers of high-risk patients undergoing surgery, the perioperative challenge to the anesthesiologist concerning monitoring and fluid management has increased and the benefits of goal-directed fluid therapy have become more evident. Technological advances in hemodynamic monitoring encourage the anesthesiologist to use extensive monitoring for this group of patients. However, further development of non-invasive monitoring devices will help customize goal-directed fluid therapy for a greater group of patients, to provide standardized fluid therapies in the perioperative setting. Nevertheless, there is still a lack of randomized controlled studies comparing the different concepts of fluid-management. Further trials are needed to study the benefits in lower risk patients and the long-term effects of perioperative, standardized fluid-management. Interesting research questions for the future will deal with the 'right' fluid for goal-directed volume optimization – crystalloids or colloids – and its effects on transfusion rates and coagulopathy, as well as implementation of a universal scoring system for patient characterization.

References

1. Marik PE, Cavallazzi R (2013) Does the central venous pressure predict fluid responsiveness? An updated meta-analysis and a plea for some common sense. Crit Care Med 41:1774–1781
2. Perel A, Habicher M, Sander M (2013) Bench-to-bedside review: Functional hemodynamics during surgery – should it be used for all high-risk cases? Crit Care 17:203
3. Kastrup M, Carl M, Spies C et al (2013) Clinical impact of the publication of S3 guidelines for intensive care in cardiac surgery patients in Germany: results from a postal survey. Acta Anaesthesiol Scand 57:206–213
4. Tuman KJ, McCarthy RJ, Spiess BD et al (1989) Effect of pulmonary artery catheterization on outcome in patients undergoing coronary artery surgery. Anesthesiology 70:199–206
5. Pölönen P, Ruokonen E, Hippeläinen M et al (2000) A prospective, randomized study of goal-oriented hemodynamic therapy in cardiac surgical patients. Anesth Analg 90:1052–1059
6. Sandham JD, Hull RD, Brant RF et al (2003) A randomized, controlled trial of the use of pulmonary-artery catheters in high-risk surgical patients. N Engl J Med 348:5–14
7. Jules-Elysee KM, YaDeau JT, Urban MK (2009) Pulmonary artery versus central venous catheter monitoring in the outcome of patients undergoing bilateral total knee replacement. HSS J 5:27–30
8. Hamilton MA, Cecconi M, Rhodes A (2011) A systematic review and meta-analysis on the use of preemptive hemodynamic intervention to improve postoperative outcomes in moderate and high-risk surgical patients. Anesth Analg 112:1392–1402
9. Sakka SG, Bredle DL, Reinhart K, Meier-Hellmann A (1999) Comparison between intrathoracic blood volume and cardiac filling pressures in the early phase of hemodynamic instability of patients with sepsis or septic shock. J Crit Care 14:78–83
10. Goedje O, Seebauer T, Peyerl M et al (2000) Hemodynamic monitoring by double-indicator dilution technique in patients after orthotopic heart transplantation. Chest 118:775–781
11. Button D, Weibel L, Reuthebuch O et al (2007) Clinical evaluation of the FloTrac/Vigileo system and two established continuous cardiac output monitoring devices in patients undergoing cardiac surgery. Br J Anaesth 99:329–336
12. Sander M, von Heymann C, Foer A et al (2005) Pulse contour analysis after normothermic cardiopulmonary bypass in cardiac surgery patients. Crit Care 9:R729–R734
13. Sander M, Spies CD, Grubitzsch H et al (2006) Comparison of uncalibrated arterial waveform analysis in cardiac surgery patients with thermodilution cardiac output measurements. Crit Care 10:R164
14. Østergaard M, Nielsen J, Nygaard E (2009) Pulse contour cardiac output: an evaluation of the FloTrac method. Eur J Anaesthesiol 26:484–489
15. Hofer CK, Senn A, Weibel L, Zollinger A (2008) Assessment of stroke volume variation for prediction of fluid responsiveness using the modified FloTrac and PiCCOplus system. Crit Care 12:R82
16. Woltjer HH, Bogaard HJ, de Vries PM (1997) The technique of impedance cardiography. Eur Heart J 18:1396–1403

17. Perrino AC, Lippman A, Ariyan C et al (1994) Intraoperative cardiac output monitoring: comparison of impedance cardiography and thermodilution. J Cardiothorac Vasc Anesth 8:24–29
18. Bogert LWJ, Wesseling KH, Schraa O et al (2010) Pulse contour cardiac output derived from non-invasive arterial pressure in cardiovascular disease. Anaesthesia 65:1119–1125
19. Hofhuizen CM, Lemson J, Hemelaar AEA et al (2010) Continuous non-invasive finger arterial pressure monitoring reflects intra-arterial pressure changes in children undergoing cardiac surgery. Br J Anaesth 105:493–500
20. Maggi R, Viscardi V, Furukawa T, Brignole M (2010) Non-invasive continuous blood pressure monitoring of tachycardic episodes during interventional electrophysiology. Europace 12:1616–1622
21. Broch O, Renner J, Gruenewald M et al (2012) A comparison of the Nexfin® and transcardiopulmonary thermodilution to estimate cardiac output during coronary artery surgery. Anaesthesia 67:377–383
22. Fischer M-O, Coucoravas J, Truong J et al (2013) Assessment of changes in cardiac index and fluid responsiveness: a comparison of Nexfin and transpulmonary thermodilution. Acta Anaesthesiol Scand 57:704–712
23. Monnet X, Picard F, Lidzborski E et al (2012) The estimation of cardiac output by the Nexfin device is of poor reliability for tracking the effects of a fluid challenge. Crit Care 16:R212
24. Sander M, Spies CD, Foer A et al (2007) Agreement of central venous saturation and mixed venous saturation in cardiac surgery patients. Intensive Care Med 33:1719–1725
25. Pennekamp CWA, Bots ML, Kappelle LJ et al (2009) The value of near-infrared spectroscopy measured cerebral oximetry during carotid endarterectomy in perioperative stroke prevention. A review. Eur J Vasc Endovasc Surg 38:539–545
26. Taillefer M-C, Denault AY (2005) Cerebral near-infrared spectroscopy in adult heart surgery: systematic review of its clinical efficacy. Can J Anaesth 52:79–87
27. Auler JO, Galas F, Hajjar L et al (2008) Online monitoring of pulse pressure variation to guide fluid therapy after cardiac surgery. Anesth Analg 106:1201–1206
28. Gan TJ, Soppitt A, Maroof M et al (2002) Goal-directed intraoperative fluid administration reduces length of hospital stay after major surgery. Anesthesiology 97:820–826
29. Sander M, Spies CD, Berger K et al (2007) Prediction of volume response under open-chest conditions during coronary artery bypass surgery. Crit Care 11:R121
30. Hood JA, Wilson RJT (2011) Pleth variability index to predict fluid responsiveness in colorectal surgery. Anesth Analg 113:1058–1063
31. Wyffels PAH, Durnez P-J, Helderweirt J et al (2007) Ventilation-induced plethysmographic variations predict fluid responsiveness in ventilated postoperative cardiac surgery patients. Anesth Analg 105:448–452
32. Monnet X, Guérin L, Jozwiak M et al (2013) Pleth variability index is a weak predictor of fluid responsiveness in patients receiving norepinephrine. Br J Anaesth 110:207–213
33. Walsh SR, Tang T, Bass S, Gaunt ME (2008) Doppler-guided intra-operative fluid management during major abdominal surgery: systematic review and meta-analysis. Int J Clin Pract 62:466–470
34. Roeck M, Jakob SM, Boehlen T et al (2003) Change in stroke volume in response to fluid challenge: assessment using esophageal Doppler. Intensive Care Med 29:1729–1735
35. Lefrant JY, Bruelle P, Aya AG et al (1998) Training is required to improve the reliability of esophageal Doppler to measure cardiac output in critically ill patients. Intensive Care Med 24:347–352
36. Tousignant CP, Walsh F, Mazer CD (2000) The use of transesophageal echocardiography for preload assessment in critically ill patients. Anesth Analg 90:351–355
37. Buhre W, Buhre K, Kazmaier S et al (2001) Assessment of cardiac preload by indicator dilution and transoesophageal echocardiography. Eur J Anaesthesiol 18:662–667
38. Wiesenack C, Fiegl C, Keyser A et al (2005) Continuously assessed right ventricular end-diastolic volume as a marker of cardiac preload and fluid responsiveness in mechanically ventilated cardiac surgical patients. Crit Care 9:R226–R233

39. Vieillard-Baron A, Chergui K, Rabiller A et al (2004) Superior vena caval collapsibility as a gauge of volume status in ventilated septic patients. Intensive Care Med 30:1734–1739
40. Shoemaker WC, Appel PL, Kram HB et al (1988) Prospective trial of supranormal values of survivors as therapeutic goals in high-risk surgical patients. Chest 94:1176–1186
41. Gurgel ST, do Nascimento P (2011) Maintaining tissue perfusion in high-risk surgical patients: a systematic review of randomized clinical trials. Anesth Analg 112:1384–1391
42. Kern JW, Shoemaker WC (2002) Meta-analysis of hemodynamic optimization in high-risk patients. Crit Care Med 30:1686–1692
43. Rhodes A, Cecconi M, Hamilton M et al (2010) Goal-directed therapy in high-risk surgical patients: a 15-year follow-up study. Intensive Care Med 36:1327–1332
44. Grocott MPW, Dushianthan A, Hamilton MA et al (2013) Perioperative increase in global blood flow to explicit defined goals and outcomes after surgery: a Cochrane Systematic Review. Br J Anaesth 111:535–548
45. Aya HD, Cecconi M, Hamilton M, Rhodes A (2013) Goal-directed therapy in cardiac surgery: a systematic review and meta-analysis. Br J Anaesth 110:510–517
46. Dalfino L, Giglio MT, Puntillo F et al (2011) Haemodynamic goal-directed therapy and postoperative infections: earlier is better. A systematic review and meta-analysis. Crit Care 15:R154
47. Giglio MT, Marucci M, Testini M, Brienza N (2009) Goal-directed haemodynamic therapy and gastrointestinal complications in major surgery: a meta-analysis of randomized controlled trials. Br J Anaesth 103:637–646
48. Pearse R, Dawson D, Fawcett J et al (2005) Early goal-directed therapy after major surgery reduces complications and duration of hospital stay. A randomised, controlled trial [ISRCTN38797445]. Crit Care 9:R687–R693
49. Brandstrup B, Tønnesen H, Beier-Holgersen R et al (2003) Effects of intravenous fluid restriction on postoperative complications: comparison of two perioperative fluid regimens: a randomized assessor-blinded multicenter trial. Ann Surg 238:641–648
50. Fouche Y, Sikorski R, Dutton RP (2010) Changing paradigms in surgical resuscitation. Crit Care Med 38:S411–S420

Macro- and Microcirculation in Systemic Inflammation: An Approach to Close the Circle

B. Saugel, C. J. Trepte, and D. A. Reuter

Introduction

Systemic inflammatory response syndrome (SIRS), sepsis, severe sepsis, and septic shock are common reasons for admission to the intensive care unit (ICU) and are still associated with high morbidity and mortality, because they are frequently associated with multiple organ dysfunction syndrome. SIRS is defined as the presence of certain physiological alterations, such as fever/hypothermia, leukocytosis/leukopenia, tachycardia, and tachypnea, and can be induced by various infectious and non-infectious conditions [1]. For example, early acute pancreatitis or the consequences of perioperative extracorporeal circulation in cardiac surgery are paradigms for SIRS in the absence of infection [1, 2]. In contrast, the definition of sepsis requires the presence of SIRS and clinical evidence of infection [1]. Severe sepsis and septic shock are defined as sepsis-induced organ dysfunction and sepsis-induced hypotension persisting despite adequate fluid resuscitation, respectively [1]. Septic shock is associated with inadequate tissue oxygenation.

A cornerstone of restoration of impaired end-organ function and pre-emptive organ protection during SIRS is the re-establishment and preservation of end-organ tissue perfusion. This, in the first instance, requires an adequate macrocirculation, which can be affected by hypovolemia, loss of vascular resistance, or impaired myocardial contractile function. Furthermore, an increasing number of findings from experimental and clinical studies demonstrate that, additionally, alterations in microcirculatory perfusion play a pivotal role in the development of organ dysfunction and are, therefore, also related to worse outcome [3–5]. When treating critically ill patients with SIRS/sepsis, it is therefore of paramount importance to initiate specific macrohemodynamic resuscitation by giving fluids, vasoactive or inotropic agents

B. Saugel ✉ · C. J. Trepte · D. A. Reuter
Department of Anesthesiology, Center of Anesthesiology and Intensive Care Medicine,
University Medical Center Hamburg-Eppendorf, Hamburg, Germany
e-mail: bernd.saugel@gmx.de

J.-L. Vincent (Ed.), *Annual Update in Intensive Care and Emergency Medicine 2014*, 325
DOI 10.1007/978-3-319-03746-2_25, © Springer International Publishing Switzerland
2014

based on the proper differential diagnosis of macrocirculatory failure as early as possible. However, if clinical signs of end-organ damage persist, assessment of the microcirculation, and appropriate treatment of microcirculatory dysfunction is desirable; however, both diagnostic and therapeutic options remain limited.

In this chapter, we review SIRS/sepsis-induced alterations in the systemic macro- and micro-circulations. We carve out the rationale for a comprehensive differential diagnostic approach which should be followed by individualized goal-directed therapeutic strategies for resuscitation of both the macro- and microcirculation, adapted to the specific clinical situation and the individual needs of a patient.

Alterations in Systemic Hemodynamics (macrocirculation) in Systemic Inflammation

The global hemodynamic state in patients with SIRS is characterized by a marked mediator-induced decrease in systemic vascular resistance and – given the absence of severe hypovolemia – normal or even elevated cardiac output/cardiac index (CI) (hyperdynamic circulatory state) [6]. However, often left ventricular (LV) systolic and diastolic myocardial dysfunction and right ventricular (RV) dysfunction can be observed in patients with severe systemic inflammation [6]. This holds true for both SIRS induced by infection and SIRS caused by other medical conditions, such as non-infectious acute pancreatitis, or perioperative extracorporeal circulation in cardiac surgery [2, 7]. Key mediators inducing the decrease in SIRS-associated systemic vascular resistance (SVR) are interleukin (IL)-1, tumor necrosis factor (TNF), and nitric oxide (NO), which is released excessively in SIRS [6, 7]. In the early stages of SIRS, severe sepsis, or septic shock, a hypovolemic intravascular state is often seen, which contributes to hypotension in addition to a reduced SVR and myocardial dysfunction. Various factors contribute to this hypovolemia. In addition to factors, such as venous pooling and decreased fluid intake, its main pathophysiological mechanism is a marked loss of fluid from the intravascular compartment into the interstitial space and the pleural and abdominal cavity as a result of a mediator-induced capillary leakage, i. e., increased microvascular permeability [6, 7].

Alterations in the Microcirculation in Systemic Inflammation

The microcirculation is the network of blood vessels with a diameter of $\leq 100\,\mu m$. Microcirculatory perfusion plays a key role in the delivery of oxygen to organ tissues. In SIRS/sepsis, an impairment of the microcirculation has been repeatedly demonstrated in both experimental and clinical studies [5] and the manifestation of microcirculatory failure is regarded as a crucial step in the development of organ failure [3].

In addition to a decrease in capillary density, heterogeneous capillary perfusion with perfused and non-perfused capillaries in close proximity seems to be characteristic of SIRS/sepsis-induced microcirculatory failure [5, 6, 8]. These characteristic changes have been identified in various models of sepsis in different animals [5, 6], as well as in patients with severe sepsis [9].

Different pathophysiological mechanisms may contribute to this impairment of the microcirculation. Inflammatory mediators can cause capillary leakage and changes in vasomotor tone by inducing dysregulation of the endothelium with impaired communication between endothelial cells and an imbalance between vasoconstrictive and vasodilatory substances [5, 8]. In this context, endothelial surface-cell interaction can be disturbed due to a modified composition and thickness or rupture of the glycocalyx, a layer located on the surface of vascular endothelial cells consisting of a proteoglycan, hyaluronan, and glycosaminoglycan [5, 8, 10]. In addition, plugs of platelets, leukocytes, and erythrocytes can obstruct the capillaries [5, 8]. Changes in the shape of erythrocytes and adhesion of erythrocytes to the endovascular surface can further contribute to an impairment of microcirculatory blood flow [5]. In systemic inflammatory states, the microcirculation can be additionally altered by an induction of pro-coagulatory cascades leading to further impairment of capillary perfusion [5].

Diagnosis, Management, and Monitoring of Macrocirculatory Dysfunction in Systemic Inflammation

Rationale for Differential Diagnosis

Because of the different types of cardiocirculatory failure that may require completely different treatment regimes (e. g., cardiogenic vs. distributive shock; hyperdynamic septic shock vs. septic shock accompanied by myocardial dysfunction), it is of crucial importance to quickly diagnose the underlying condition during the initial assessment and stabilization of a patient with suspected SIRS or sepsis. To be able to provide specific and adequate therapy in these patients, a systematic differential diagnostic approach for the assessment of the underlying inflammatory condition and cardiopulmonary impairment must precede therapeutic interventions. For this initial differential diagnostic procedure, clinical, laboratory, and radiographic findings as well as data obtained using technical devices need to be taken into account. In this early diagnostic phase, echocardiography, in particular, can provide information of tremendous importance for the identification of the underlying condition leading to the SIRS-induced cardiocirculatory failure. Echocardiography can be performed easily in the ICU or the operating room. There are standardized protocols for echocardiographic examinations (e. g., the focus-assessed transthoracic echocardiography [FATE] protocol) and echocardiography is recommended by the American Heart Association in surgery patients with persisting hemodynamic instability as a class I recommendation. After this initial differential diagnosis and determination of the treatment strategy, continuous monitoring of macrohemodynamics is essential for guiding further therapy and reassessment of therapeutic success.

Parameters for Monitoring the Macrocirculation

Over the last few decades, various methods for the assessment of hemodynamic parameters have been introduced and evaluated that can be applied to monitor patients with SIRS, severe sepsis, or septic shock in order to guide therapy. In general, monitoring the macrocirculation should provide the physician with data allowing a differential diagnostic procedure regarding the underlying hemodynamic alterations as well as a differentiated therapeutic hemodynamic management of these alterations. In addition, changes in macrocirculatory function requiring changes in therapeutic resuscitation strategies should be rapidly identified by a monitoring system.

Based on physiologic considerations, blood flow, cardiac preload/fluid responsiveness, and cardiac afterload need to be assessed. Despite the variety of technologies that are now available for hemodynamic monitoring, a cornerstone in the evaluation of a patient's hemodynamic state is still physical examination. However, the accuracy and reliability of clinical signs used to assess a patient's cardiocirculatory function, fluid status, and fluid responsiveness have been shown to be limited [11].

Blood flow, as determined by cardiac output, can be determined using a variety of techniques. Regarding indicator dilution techniques for cardiac output determination, the intermittent pulmonary artery thermodilution technique using a pulmonary artery catheter (PAC) is still considered to be the gold standard method [12]. Transpulmonary dye dilution methods and transpulmonary thermodilution methods are less invasive alternatives for intermittent cardiac output measurement [12]. Continuous cardiac output monitoring based on thermodilution can be performed with a PAC equipped with a dedicated electric filament [12]. In addition, continuous analysis of the pulse wave (pulse contour analysis) allows the estimation of cardiac output [13]. Different technologies providing pulse contour analysis-derived cardiac output calibrated to thermodilution or dye dilution cardiac output are available [13]. Uncalibrated cardiac output estimation derived from pulse contour analysis is provided by several different technologies but has been demonstrated to be less reliable as compared to calibrated systems [13].

Cardiac preload can be estimated by using cardiac filling pressures, volumetric parameters of preload, or functional preload parameters, i.e., variability parameters. Central venous pressure (CVP) is recommended as a target hemodynamic parameter for the initial resuscitation phase in patients with sepsis [14]. However, there are data demonstrating that CVP is an unreliable marker of intravascular fluid status and fluid responsiveness [15] and that targeting a CVP of 8–12 mmHg as recommended in current guidelines may result in indiscriminate fluid loading associated with increased mortality rates in septic patients [16]. Considering that there are overwhelming data questioning the value of cardiac filling pressures in the prediction of fluid responsiveness [17], alternative parameters for the assessment of cardiac preload have been proposed. Global end-diastolic volume (GEDV) can be determined using transpulmonary thermodilution techniques and has been shown to be a valuable volumetric parameter of cardiac preload [18]. In addition to this static transpulmonary thermodilution parameter, continuous pulse contour analysis allows the determination of dynamic functional parameters of cardiac preload, arising from the interactions between the heart and the lungs under mechanical ventilation, i. e., pulse pressure variation (PPV) and stroke volume variation (SVV) [19]. In addition to the hemodynamic parameters described earlier, there are functional tests that may help the intensivist to assess a patient's fluid status, e. g., cardiac preload or fluid responsiveness: A passive leg-raising test can be performed by elevating the patient's legs in order to evaluate whether the shift of blood from the lower extremities to the central circulation is able to improve central hemodynamics, which then can be detected by various monitoring techniques, such as transpulmonary thermodilution, pulse contour analysis, echocardiography, or esophageal Doppler [20].

Furthermore, to test whether fluid administration is beneficial for a patient in terms of hemodynamic improvement, a fluid challenge test following a structured protocol can be performed [21]. Because the fluid challenge maneuver directly assesses the actual hemodynamic response to fluid loading, it can be considered the criterion standard method for evaluation of fluid responsiveness. Surrogate parameters of cardiac afterload, e. g., mean arterial pressure (MAP) and SVR, can be continuously derived by analysis of the pulse wave.

To evaluate global oxygen transport/consumption and tissue oxygenation, central venous oxygen saturation ($ScvO_2$), mixed venous oxygen saturation (SvO_2), and blood lactate can be used. $ScvO_2$ – which is also part of the early-goal directed therapy algorithm [22] and of the current sepsis guidelines [14] – can also be determined easily at the bedside in the ICU. $ScvO_2$ which is a surrogate for SvO_2 can globally indicate (in)adequate oxygen delivery and has proven to be a useful parameter when used in resuscitation protocols for patients with severe sepsis or septic shock [23]. By using a PAC, (continuous) measurement of SvO_2 is possible. However, abnormal $ScvO_2$ and SvO_2 values non-specifically indicate tissue hypoxia, which may be caused by various reasons and do not enable identification of the specific underlying pathophysiological mechanisms. Blood lactate levels can help to identify patients with inadequate tissue oxygenation due to tissue hypoperfusion. Current sepsis guidelines, therefore, recommend that normalizing lactate should be a target of early resuscitation therapy in patients with severe sepsis or septic shock presenting with elevated serum lactate. However, although elevated serum lactate levels reliably (but non-specifically) indicate tissue damage caused by hypoperfusion, this laboratory parameter is not able to guide preemptive treatment strategies for preservation of tissue perfusion and organ function.

Evolving Individualized Goal-directed Hemodynamic Strategies

In critically ill patients, the early optimization of systemic hemodynamic parameters reflecting cardiac preload and afterload as well as cardiac contractility is of paramount importance. In this context, optimization of cardiac preload needs to go in parallel with avoiding indiscriminate volume expansion or inadequate administration of vasoactive agents, which has detrimental effects on pulmonary and cardiocirculatory function.

To accomplish these targets, different goal-directed therapeutic strategies have been proposed. However, in some of the previous studies, parameters that did not adequately reflect the hemodynamic state were used. In addition, other studies used undifferentiated and un-individualized goals for hemodynamic resuscitation. Shoemaker, a pioneer in the field of goal-directed hemodynamic approaches in critically ill patients, first suggested the since repeatedly questioned concept of targeting supranormal values of cardiac output and oxygen delivery in high-risk surgical patients [24].

Rivers et al. demonstrated in 2001 that in patients with severe sepsis or septic shock admitted to the emergency department, patient outcome could be improved by applying 'early goal-directed therapy' based on a simple algorithm including basic hemodynamic variables such as CVP, MAP, and $ScvO_2$ [22]. However, the protocol proposed by Rivers lacks a differentiated view of the underlying hemodynamic alterations, e. g., whether septic shock was complicated by myocardial dysfunction or not. In addition, as mentioned above, CVP, used as a key parameter in the Rivers' protocol, does not reliably reflect cardiac preload and fluid responsiveness [15] Therefore, the important beneficial effects observed in the trial by Rivers and colleagues may be largely due to the fact that patients were treated early rather than being treated according to adequate hemodynamic goals. Despite this shortcoming of this basic resuscitation protocol, the concept of 'early goal-directed therapy' with the need to monitor a patient's hemodynamic state was adopted in clinical sepsis guidelines for the treatment of critically ill septic patients [14].

In 2003, Sandham and co-workers published the results of a prospective randomized controlled study evaluating a goal-directed approach in high-risk surgery patients ≥ 60 years needing ICU treatment using – among others – the following parameters as targets: Hematocrit, MAP, and PAC-derived cardiac index (CI), pulmonary capillary wedge pressure, and oxygen delivery [25]. In comparison to the control group treated with standard care (i. e., CVP) without placement of a PAC, the authors reported no benefit with respect to hospital mortality or 6-month mortality in patients monitored using a PAC [25]. However, these findings might be due to the fact that the same therapeutic hemodynamic goals were used for a very heterogeneous group of patients and that the parameters applied in the study are of questionable value in the prediction of intravascular fluid status and fluid responsiveness.

To overcome these shortcomings, alternative algorithms based on more sophisticated advanced hemodynamic parameters have been proposed. Pearse et al. were able to demonstrate in high-risk general surgery patients that a postoperatively applied algorithm using oxygen delivery index as a target resulted in a reduction of hospital length of stay and postoperative complications [26]. In cardiac surgery patients, Goepfert and colleagues were able to demonstrate that a goal-directed treatment algorithm including CI, extravascular lung water (EVLW), and volumetric parameters of cardiac preload had beneficial effects in terms of reduced need for vasoactive agents, mechanical ventilation, and reduced length of stay in the ICU [27].

Benes and coworkers were able to improve intraoperative hemodynamics in parallel to a decrease in serum lactate and to reduce postoperative complications by using a SVV-based strategy for hemodynamic optimization in major abdominal surgery patients [28]. Recently, Trepte et al. demonstrated, in an experimental study using an animal model of SIRS induced by severe acute pancreatitis, that a goal-directed algorithm for fluid management based on functional cardiac preload assessment (SVV) and cardiac output resulted in improved survival, tissue oxygenation, and microcirculatory perfusion compared to management solely based on CVP and MAP [29]. In a multicenter study, Salzwedel et al. observed a decrease in postoperative complications in major abdominal surgery patients when using a goal-directed therapy approach based on PPV, CI trending and MAP [30].

It is important to mention that applying the same treatment goals to all patients suffering from certain diseases is most certainly an overly simplistic approach. Because individual patients may have their own individual hemodynamic normal values, future studies should rather try evaluating individualized goal-directed therapy approaches. In this context, Goepfert and colleagues recently published a prospective randomized controlled study in cardiac surgery patients [31]. In this study, a sophisticated goal-directed treatment algorithm using the functional cardiac preload parameter, SVV, to optimize cardiac preload and to define a patient's individual optimal GEDV index (GEDVI) was compared with a goal-directed algorithm using MAP and CVP. The results showed a statistically significant reduction in the total number of postoperative complications and the ICU length of stay in the individualized algorithm group.

The intriguing concept of combining different functional and volumetric cardiac preload parameters to be able to provide individualized hemodynamic optimization instead of using the same hemodynamic treatment goals for all patients should be further investigated in patients with SIRS caused by infectious and non-infectious conditions.

Monitoring the Microcirculation in Systemic Inflammation

Rationale for Monitoring the Microcirculation in Systemic Inflammation

As described earlier, it has been clearly demonstrated that multiple pathophysiological mechanisms lead to an impairment of the microcirculation in severe systemic inflammation. The rationale for monitoring these changes is that tissue perfusion and adequate tissue oxygenation are probably decisively related to microvascular perfusion. There is convincing evidence that sepsis-induced microcirculatory impairment and tissue hypoxia can be present despite optimization of systemic hemodynamics, i. e., despite normal or even increased cardiac output, normal blood flow to the end-organs, and normal global oxygen delivery. Therefore, changes in microcirculatory perfusion seem to be at least in part independent of systemic microcirculatory parameters, such as arterial pressure or cardiac output, and there is a marked and unpredictable inter-individual variability in the microcirculatory response to macrocirculatory changes in different patients [5, 32–34].

In addition, there are data showing that impairment of the microcirculation is associated with mortality and development of organ failure in septic patients [4, 8, 9]. In patients dying from septic shock or sepsis-related organ failure, persisting and therapy-refractory alterations in the microcirculation have been described [4, 8]. In accordance with these data, Trzeciak and colleagues demonstrated in septic shock patients that an improvement in microcirculatory flow as a consequence of resuscitation based on the principles of early-goal directed therapy resulted in reduced organ failure [3].

Monitoring the microcirculation in addition to systemic hemodynamic parameters seems, therefore, to be an opportunity to have a more differentiated view of sepsis-induced tissue hypoxia and organ dysfunction. In addition, considering the available data providing evidence that there is an association of microcirculatory perfusion and organ dysfunction and even mortality, monitoring microcirculatory perfusion and targeting it in sepsis resuscitation seems to be an intriguing approach.

Available Technologies for Monitoring the Microcirculation

Considering the importance of monitoring microcirculatory changes, different technologies have been introduced to monitor microcirculatory perfusion at the bedside in the ICU. In general, one has to distinguish methods providing indirect measures of tissue oxygenation and methods that enable direct visualization of tissue perfusion [35].

It has to be stressed that measuring the microcirculation at a specific site, e. g., the skin or the epithelial layer under the tongue, solely allows evaluation of perfusion of microvessels in this local area, which may or may not be representative of microcirculatory alterations at other sites [35].

A method that indirectly reflects tissue oxygenation/tissue perfusion is tissue carbon dioxide measurement [35]. By using electrode sensors, the partial pressure of carbon dioxide in the tissue can be evaluated using sublingual or buccal capnometry or capnometry at the earlobe [35]. In septic patients, the sublingual partial pressure of carbon dioxide gap, i. e., the difference between sublingual and arterial partial pressures of carbon dioxide, has been demonstrated to significantly correlate with microcirculatory perfusion determined using orthogonal polarization spectral (OPS) imaging [36].

Regarding methods that allow direct evaluation of microcirculatory perfusion, the following technologies have been developed: Laser doppler, videomicroscopy (including OPS and side-stream dark field [SDF] imaging), and near-infrared spectroscopy (NIRS) [35]. Advantages and disadvantages of the different technologies have been reviewed in detail [35].

In systemic inflammation characterized by heterogeneous microcirculatory impairment, the videomicroscopic SDF imaging technique is applicable for bedside assessment of microcirculatory perfusion. SDF imaging is based on the principle that tissue layers can be made translucent by applying light on the layer that is reflected by layers located deeper in the tissue [35, 37]. In ICU patients, SDF can be applied to the thin epithelial layer in the sublingual region by using handheld devices [37]. When using SDF, a semi-quantitative analysis regarding capillary density and heterogeneity of microvascular perfusion is recommended [37, 38]. Limiting the broad use of this technique, SDF can only be performed in sedated or cooperative patients. Furthermore, the technique is examiner-dependent and experience is necessary for correct SDF measurements and analysis of the obtained images. In addition, when using the sublingual region for SDF imaging, movement and pressure artifacts or secretions may influence SDF images [37].

Are we Ready to Specifically Target the Microcirculation in SIRS?

In a clinical setting, resuscitation of patients with SIRS and sepsis (fluid therapy and administration of vasoactive agents) is predominantly geared to the stabilization of systemic hemodynamics. However, most interventions for targeting macrocirculatory goals have been shown to also impact the microcirculation.

Regarding fluid therapy, there are data from an observational trial in patients with severe sepsis that the administration of crystalloids or albumin is able to improve microcirculatory perfusion measured with SDF imaging in the early phase of sepsis independently of macrocirculatory parameters, such as cardiac output or MAP [39]. In accordance, it has been demonstrated that in patients with severe sepsis or septic shock, a passive leg-raising test or fluid challenge maneuver can improve microcirculatory perfusion in the sublingual region [40]. A potential association of different types of fluid and improvement of the microcirculation still needs to be elucidated.

Although there are data on the effect of transfusion of red blood cell (RBC) concentrates on systemic hemodynamic parameters, the impact of RBC transfusion on the microcirculation is difficult to estimate. In two relatively small studies, microcirculation was globally not altered by RBC transfusion in patients with severe sepsis [41, 42].

Administration of norepinephrine can improve microcirculatory perfusion (assessed in muscle tissue using NIRS) in patients with severe sepsis-induced hypotension, probably by increasing the organ perfusion pressure [43]. However, administering norepinephrine in order to further increase MAP (above 65 mmHg) was not demonstrated to improve the microcirculation [33]. Further, as emphasized by the authors of this study, there was a considerable inter-individual variation in the response to norepinephrine resulting in harmful effects of norepinephrine administration in some patients. In contrast, in some patients with severely impaired microcirculation at baseline, norepinephrine seemed to have the most beneficial effect.

De Backer and colleagues reported an improvement in the microcirculation in septic shock patients following the administration of dobutamine [32]. Interestingly, the effects of dobutamine in this study were independent of the effects of the drug on the macrocirculation in septic shock patients. In contrast, Hernandez et al. recently presented the results of a randomized controlled double-blind crossover study showing that dobutamine did not improve the sublingual microcirculation despite an improvement in macrocirculatory parameters, such as CI or LV ejection fraction [44].

In addition to these interventions mainly targeting macrocirculatory parameters, in an experimental setting, several strategies for targeted resuscitation of the microcirculation in septic patients have been proposed and investigated.

First, hydrocortisone, which is – according to current sepsis guidelines [14] – useful as an adjunctive agent in patients with septic shock, has been demonstrated to have beneficial effects on sepsis-induced microcirculatory disturbances [45]

Second, several agents with vasodilating effects have been investigated. De Backer et al. demonstrated in severe sepsis patients with marked microcirculatory impairment, that topical administration of acetylcholine in high doses was able to improve microcirculatory perfusion failure [9]. Contradicting results exist on the effects of nitroglycerin in patients with septic shock, however [46, 47]. Boerma and colleagues failed to demonstrate a beneficial effect of nitroglycerin on the microcirculation in a double-blind randomized placebo-controlled trial in 70 septic shock patients [46].

Third, agents with anticoagulatory properties have been suggested to improve microcirculation in sepsis. Activated protein C was shown to improve sublingual microperfusion in patients with severe sepsis in a controlled study including 40 patients (20 treated with activated protein C) [48]. Although there are experimental data demonstrating beneficial effects of other anticoagulants, e. g., antithrombin [49], the underlying mechanisms for these effects are still unclear and need to be further assessed [5].

Finally, there are other agents, such as tetrahydrobioterin, which may be promising for microcirculatory resuscitation when considering available data from animal studies [50].

In summary, various therapeutic interventions can influence microvessel circulation in clinical and experimental settings. However, in the clinical setting, diagnostic and therapeutic approaches for microcirculatory assessment and restoration are limited by the fact that only the local microcirculation, with questionable representativeness for microvascular perfusion in other organ systems, can be assessed and targeted. Therefore, specific therapeutic approaches to restore microcirculatory failure are not yet available in clinical practice.

Concept for Rational Therapy of Systemic Inflammation-induced Hemodynamic Alterations in the Macro- and Microcirculations

As described in detail earlier, we are now able to identify and quantify alterations in the macrocirculation at the bedside in the ICU and are beginning to be able to do this also for the microcirculation. A variety of systemic hemodynamic parameters obtained using different clinical and apparative methods can be useful in the differ-

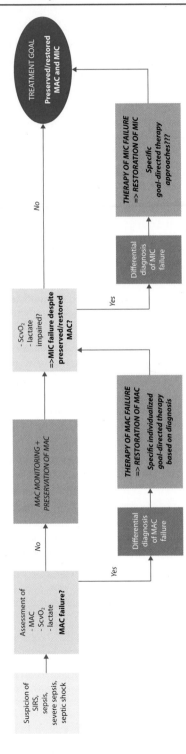

Fig. 1 Algorithm for the assessment and optimization of the macro- and microcirculation in sepsis/systemic inflammatory response syndrome (SIRS). MAC: macrocirculation; MIC: microcirculation; $ScvO_2$: central venous oxygen saturation

ential diagnosis procedure in patients with suspected SIRS/sepsis. Based on hemodynamic parameters reflecting the macrocirculation a rational management strategy
for optimization of intravascular fluid status can be established. The optimization of
macrocirculatory parameters is a prerequisite for the preservation or resuscitation of
microcirculatory perfusion. However, marked microcirculatory impairment can be
observed in patients with systemic inflammation despite normal or optimized systemic hemodynamics. Therefore, future concepts for hemodynamic optimization
in patients with severe inflammation should comprise individualized goal-directed
algorithms for resuscitation of the macrocirculation in parallel to strategies to optimize microcirculatory perfusion (Fig. 1).

Conclusions

A major goal in the treatment of patients with SIRS/sepsis is to preserve tissue
perfusion in order to avoid organ failure by providing early goal-directed therapy
for hemodynamic resuscitation. The differential diagnostic procedure based on assessment of macrocirculatory parameters followed by specific treatment strategies
and monitoring of systemic hemodynamics by measuring advanced hemodynamic
parameters has, therefore, become a cornerstone in the care of these patients. Various methods are available for determination of a patient's hemodynamic state.
There is evidence that macrocirculatory hemodynamic resuscitation should be performed following predefined individualized goal-directed treatment algorithms. As
well as alterations in systemic hemodynamics, i. e., macrocirculation, microcirculatory perfusion is also impaired in SIRS/sepsis. Recently developed handheld
devices now allow visualization of the microcirculation at the bedside. In sepsis, a decrease in capillary density and heterogeneous microvessel perfusion are
characteristic findings. These microcirculatory alterations are associated with mortality and development of organ failure in septic patients. However, impairment of
the microcirculation resulting in tissue hypoxia can be present despite normal systemic hemodynamics. Because of the importance of microcirculatory failure in the
development of organ dysfunction, monitoring of microcirculatory perfusion and
developing goal-directed strategies for the treatment of microcirculatory failure are
intriguing approaches. However, the link between microcirculatory impairment and
macrocirculatory failure needs to be further elucidated.

References

1. Levy MM, Fink MP, Marshall JC et al (2003) 2001 SCCM/ESICM/ACCP/ATS/SIS International Sepsis Definitions Conference. Intensive Care Med 29:530–538
2. Litmathe J, Boeken U, Bohlen G, Gursoy D, Sucker C, Feindt P (2011) Systemic inflammatory
response syndrome after extracorporeal circulation: a predictive algorithm for the patient at
risk. Hellenic J Cardiol 52:493–500

3. Trzeciak S, McCoy JV, Phillip Dellinger R et al (2008) Early increases in microcirculatory per-fusion during protocol-directed resuscitation are associated with reduced multi-organ failure at 24 h in patients with sepsis. Intensive Care Med 34:2210–2217
4. Sakr Y, Dubois MJ, De Backer D, Creteur J, Vincent JL (2004) Persistent microcirculatory alterations are associated with organ failure and death in patients with septic shock. Crit Care Med 32:1825–1831
5. De Backer D, Donadello K, Taccone FS, Ospina-Tascon G, Salgado D, Vincent JL (2011) Mi-crocirculatory alterations: potential mechanisms and implications for therapy. Ann Intensive Care 1:27
6. Vincent JL (1998) Cardiovascular alterations in septic shock. J Antimicrob Chemother 41(A):9–15
7. Yegneswaran B, Kostis JB, Pitchumoni CS (2011) Cardiovascular manifestations of acute pan-creatitis. J Crit Care 26:225 e211–225 e228
8. De Backer D, Ortiz JA, Salgado D (2010) Coupling microcirculation to systemic hemodynam-ics. Curr Opin Crit Care 16:250–254
9. De Backer D, Creteur J, Preiser JC, Dubois MJ, Vincent JL (2002) Microvascular blood flow is altered in patients with sepsis. Am J Respir Crit Care Med 166:98–104
10. Marechal X, Favory R, Joulin O et al (2008) Endothelial glycocalyx damage during endo-toxemia coincides with microcirculatory dysfunction and vascular oxidative stress. Shock 29:572–576
11. Saugel B, Kirsche SV, Hapfelmeier A et al (2013) Prediction of fluid responsiveness in patients admitted to the medical intensive care unit. J Crit Care 28:537 (e531–539)
12. Reuter DA, Huang C, Edrich T, Shernan SK, Eltzschig HK (2010) Cardiac output monitoring using indicator-dilution techniques: basics, limits, and perspectives. Anesth Analg 110:799–811
13. Alhashemi JA, Cecconi M, Hofer CK (2011) Cardiac output monitoring: an integrative per-spective. Crit Care 15:214
14. Dellinger RP, Levy MM, Rhodes A et al (2013) Surviving Sepsis Campaign: international guidelines for management of severe sepsis and septic shock: 2012. Crit Care Med 41:580–637
15. Marik PE, Baram M, Vahid B (2008) Does central venous pressure predict fluid responsive-ness? A systematic review of the literature and the tale of seven mares. Chest 134:172–178
16. Boyd JH, Forbes J, Nakada TA, Walley KR, Russell JA (2011) Fluid resuscitation in sep-tic shock: a positive fluid balance and elevated central venous pressure are associated with increased mortality. Crit Care Med 39:259–265
17. Osman D, Ridel C, Ray P et al (2007) Cardiac filling pressures are not appropriate to predict hemodynamic response to volume challenge. Crit Care Med 35:64–68
18. Michard F, Alaya S, Zarka V, Bahloul M, Richard C, Teboul JL (2003) Global end-diastolic volume as an indicator of cardiac preload in patients with septic shock. Chest 124:1900–1908
19. Reuter DA, Felbinger TW, Schmidt C et al (2002) Stroke volume variations for assessment of cardiac responsiveness to volume loading in mechanically ventilated patients after cardiac surgery. Intensive Care Med 28:392–398
20. Cavallaro F, Sandroni C, Marano C et al (2010) Diagnostic accuracy of passive leg raising for prediction of fluid responsiveness in adults: systematic review and meta-analysis of clinical studies. Intensive Care Med 36:1475–1483
21. Cecconi M, Parsons AK, Rhodes A (2011) What is a fluid challenge? Curr Opin Crit Care 17:290–295
22. Rivers E, Nguyen B, Havstad S et al (2001) Early goal-directed therapy in the treatment of severe sepsis and septic shock. N Engl J Med 345:1368–1377
23. Walley KR (2011) Use of central venous oxygen saturation to guide therapy. Am J Respir Crit Care Med 184:514–520

24. Shoemaker WC, Appel PL, Kram HB, Waxman K, Lee TS (1988) Prospective trial of supra-normal values of survivors as therapeutic goals in high-risk surgical patients. Chest 94:1176–1186
25. Sandham JD, Hull RD, Brant RF et al (2003) A randomized, controlled trial of the use of pulmonary-artery catheters in high-risk surgical patients. N Engl J Med 348:5–14
26. Pearse R, Dawson D, Fawcett J, Rhodes A, Grounds RM, Bennett ED (2005) Early goal-directed therapy after major surgery reduces complications and duration of hospital stay. A randomised, controlled trial [ISRCTN38797445]. Crit Care 9:R687–R693
27. Goepfert MS, Reuter DA, Akyol D, Lamm P, Kilger E, Goetz AE (2007) Goal-directed fluid management reduces vasopressor and catecholamine use in cardiac surgery patients. Intensive Care Med 33:96–103
28. Benes J, Chytra I, Altmann P et al (2010) Intraoperative fluid optimization using stroke volume variation in high risk surgical patients: results of prospective randomized study. Crit Care 14:R118
29. Trepte CJ, Bachmann KA, Stork JH et al (2013) The impact of early goal-directed fluid management on survival in an experimental model of severe acute pancreatitis. Intensive Care Med 39:717–726
30. Salzwedel C, Puig J, Carstens A et al (2013) Perioperative goal-directed hemodynamic therapy based on radial arterial pulse pressure variation and continuous cardiac index trending reduces postoperative complications after major abdominal surgery: a multi-center, prospective, randomized study. Crit Care 17:R191
31. Goepfert MS, Richter HP, Eulenburg CZ et al (2013) Individually optimized hemodynamic therapy reduces complications and length of stay in the intensive care unit: a prospective, randomized controlled trial. Anesthesiology 119:824–836
32. De Backer D, Creteur J, Dubois MJ et al (2006) The effects of dobutamine on microcirculatory alterations in patients with septic shock are independent of its systemic effects. Crit Care Med 34:403–408
33. Dubin A, Pozo MO, Casabella CA et al (2009) Increasing arterial blood pressure with nore-pinephrine does not improve microcirculatory blood flow: a prospective study. Crit Care 13:R92
34. Jhanji S, Stirling S, Patel N, Hinds CJ, Pearse RM (2009) The effect of increasing doses of norepinephrine on tissue oxygenation and microvascular flow in patients with septic shock. Crit Care Med 37:1961–1966
35. De Backer D, Donadello K, Cortes DO (2012) Monitoring the microcirculation. J Clin Monit Comput 26:361–366
36. Creteur J, De Backer D, Sakr Y, Koch M, Vincent JL (2006) Sublingual capnometry tracks microcirculatory changes in septic patients. Intensive Care Med 32:516–523
37. De Backer D, Ospina-Tascon G, Salgado D, Favory R, Creteur J, Vincent JL (2010) Monitoring the microcirculation in the critically ill patient: current methods and future approaches. Intensive Care Med 36:1813–1825
38. De Backer D, Hollenberg S, Boerma C et al (2007) How to evaluate the microcirculation: report of a round table conference. Crit Care 11:R101
39. Ospina-Tascon G, Neves AP, Occhipinti G et al (2010) Effects of fluids on microvascular perfusion in patients with severe sepsis. Intensive Care Med 36:949–955
40. Pottecher J, Deruddre S, Teboul JL et al (2010) Both passive leg raising and intravascular volume expansion improve sublingual microcirculatory perfusion in severe sepsis and septic shock patients. Intensive Care Med 36:1867–1874
41. Sakr Y, Chierego M, Piagnerelli M et al (2007) Microvascular response to red blood cell transfusion in patients with severe sepsis. Crit Care Med 35:1639–1644
42. Sadaka F, Aggu-Sher R, Krause K, O'Brien J, Armbrecht ES, Taylor RW (2011) The effect of red blood cell transfusion on tissue oxygenation and microcirculation in severe septic patients. Ann Intensive Care 1:46

43. Georger JF, Hamzaoui O, Chaari A, Maizel J, Richard C, Teboul JL (2010) Restoring arterial pressure with norepinephrine improves muscle tissue oxygenation assessed by near-infrared spectroscopy in severely hypotensive septic patients. Intensive Care Med 36:1882–1889
44. Hernandez G, Bruhn A, Luengo C et al (2013) Effects of dobutamine on systemic, regional and microcirculatory perfusion parameters in septic shock: a randomized, placebo-controlled, double-blind, crossover study. Intensive Care Med 39:1435–1443
45. Buchele GL, Silva E, Ospina-Tascon GA, Vincent JL, De Backer D (2009) Effects of hydrocortisone on microcirculatory alterations in patients with septic shock. Crit Care Med 37:1341–1347
46. Boerma EC, Koopmans M, Konijn A et al (2010) Effects of nitroglycerin on sublingual microcirculatory blood flow in patients with severe sepsis/septic shock after a strict resuscitation protocol: a double-blind randomized placebo controlled trial. Crit Care Med 38:93–100
47. Spronk PE, Ince C, Gardien MJ, Mathura KR, Oudemans-van Straaten HM, Zandstra DF (2002) Nitroglycerin in septic shock after intravascular volume resuscitation. Lancet 360:1395–1396
48. De Backer D, Verdant C, Chierego M, Koch M, Gullo A, Vincent JL (2006) Effects of drotrecogin alfa activated on microcirculatory alterations in patients with severe sepsis. Crit Care Med 34:1918–1924
49. Hoffmann JN, Vollmar B, Romisch J, Inthorn D, Schildberg FW, Menger MD (2002) Antithrombin effects on endotoxin-induced microcirculatory disorders are mediated mainly by its interaction with microvascular endothelium. Crit Care Med 30:218–225
50. He X, Su F, Velissaris D et al (2012) Administration of tetrahydrobiopterin improves the microcirculation and outcome in an ovine model of septic shock. Crit Care Med 40:2833–2840

Part VIII
Monitoring

Cardiac Ultrasound and Doppler in Critically Ill Patients: Does it Improve Outcome?

J. Poelaert and P. Flamée

Introduction

Contemporary hemodynamic bedside assessment and management necessitates a versatile tool, which offers instantaneous yet extensive information. Cardiac ultrasound with Doppler is generally considered to be an invaluable tool for assessing hemodynamically compromised patients. The morphology and function of cardiac chambers, including valves and the respective connective tissue, and major vessels can be evaluated and put into a pathophysiological perspective. Furthermore, hemodynamic monitoring, revealing ventricular function, insufficient preload or excessive afterload conditions, can often be fine-tuned using cardiac ultrasound and Doppler [1]. In postoperative mechanically ventilated as well as in non-ventilated critically ill patients, the non-invasive transthoracic mode is often the preferred technique of choice. Transesophageal Doppler echocardiography (TEE) is used in specific indications [2]. Although the transesophageal approach is more invasive, it remains a safe technique both in sick adults and children [3–5]. Less than 0.1 % of TEE interventions are associated with problems induced by the TEE probe, such as bleeding, hoarseness or sore throat. Recent guidelines from the European Society of Intensive Care Medicine (ESICM) strongly suggest this technique should form part of advanced echocardiography training [6].

Modern medicine is driven by endpoints and goals, such as outcome, morbidity and length of stay in the ICU and hospital. In the present chapter, we summarize how cardiac ultrasound and Doppler can improve outcomes of critically ill patients, in particular by the instantaneous and global information provided.

J. Poelaert ✉ · P. Flamée
Department of Anesthesiology and Perioperative Medicine, UZ Brussel, VUB,
1090 Brussels, Belgium
e-mail: jan.poelaert@uzbrussel.be

J.-L. Vincent (Ed.), *Annual Update in Intensive Care and Emergency Medicine 2014*,
DOI 10.1007/978-3-319-03746-2_26, © Springer International Publishing Switzerland
2014

Left Ventricular Function

Knowledge of left ventricular function is primordial in decision making in critically ill patients. An important difference between invasive hemodynamic monitoring and ingenious flow charts on goal-directed protocolized fluid management is knowledge of ventricular function. Cardiac index (CI) is often integrated in these flow charts, but this variable does not inform about ventricular function *per se*. A patient with extensive co-morbidities may have well-preserved left and right ventricular function, permitting easier hemodynamic management. In contrast, management of a patient with pronounced regional wall motion abnormalities, as a sign of myocardial infarction, will be hampered by more rapid limitation of filling capacity (reduced compliance of ventricles) and earlier need for inotropic or vasopressor support. Immediate information on both ventricular function and fluid status can be achieved with cardiac ultrasound and Doppler. One view at the level of the short axis permits evaluation of the global function of both the left and right ventricles [7]. Other views should be added to develop a comprehensive picture of ventricular function, segmental wall motion and morphology and valve function. This latter is important with respect to the evaluation of segmental wall motion analysis, because regurgitation at one level could be a warning sign of decreased or absent regional wall motion at the mitral valve level [8, 9]. The different tools of cardiac ultrasound and Doppler provide insight into functional hemodynamics in a few minutes; these data can be complemented with invasive data, to be incorporated into a physiological integration of all data.

Tissue Doppler imaging allows closer assessment of regional or global evaluation of the chamber function both during systole and diastole [10, 11]. A useful variable in daily clinical practice is the systolic velocity of the mitral annulus (Sm), assessed with tissue Doppler imaging. Velocities < 8 cm/s suggest decreased systolic function, whereas velocities > 12 cm/s imply normal left ventricular (LV) systolic function. Both preload [11] and afterload [12] appear to have an impact on the amplitude. In addition, diastolic function can be easily and rapidly assessed, as described in a recent overview [13]. Diastolic dysfunction is an early indicator that warns the clinician before systolic dysfunction appears. Some examples clarify the importance of determination of diastolic function variables. Acute ligation of a circumflex coronary artery in a rabbit model induced a decrease in early filling and atrial contraction waves after 1 h [14]. Three weeks later, this altered LV filling pattern was still present. In sepsis and septic shock, the role of diastolic dysfunction has been questioned for many years. Myocardial Doppler imaging provides insight into both systolic and diastolic function [15, 16]. An example is shown in Fig. 1, demonstrating a shift in transmitral early filling wave velocity as well as in the early annular velocity after administration of colloids in a septic rat model.

Various patterns can be recognized from normal through pseudonormalization to severe systolic-diastolic dysfunction [17]. Diastolic properties are an independent predictor of outcome in severe sepsis [18]. More recently, with the implementation of tissue Doppler, Sturgess et al. confirmed that the E/Em (early transmitral Doppler

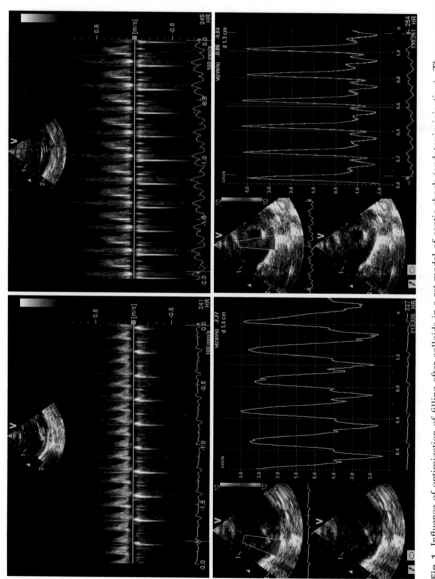

Fig. 1 Influence of optimization of filling after colloids in a rat model of septic shock (endotoxin injection). The *upper panels* show transmitral Doppler pattern before (*left*) and after (*right*) filling. The *lower panels* depict the tissue Doppler images with a clear shift from E′/A′ < 1 towards E′/A′ > 1

filling velocity/early mitral annular velocity during early diastole) ratio was an independent predictor of hospital survival in septic shock patients [19]

Right Ventricle

A similar differentiation can be made with respect to the right ventricle. A normal right ventricle at the level of the short axis is depicted as a crescent shaped structure. A dilated right ventricle (i. e., right ventricular [RV] diameter > 0.6 diameter of the left ventricle and stiffening of the interventricular septum, so called D shape of the right ventricle) most often suggests pressure overload (see below). Knowledge of the presence of a dilated right ventricle in conjunction with increased RV systolic pressure (RVSP), may be important in the direct management of ventilator settings [20], optimization of preload [21] and reduction in RV afterload conditions [22–24], with a direct impact on outcome.

Assessment of regurgitant flows across cardiac valves reveals transvalvular pressure gradients. Typically, from a tricuspid regurgitant flow, a pressure gradient can be determined to estimate RVSP if the right atrial pressure can be estimated [25, 26]. RVSP estimation is one of the most important direct measurements with echo-Doppler and readily assessed.

Before cardiac transplantation, the reversibility of pulmonary hypertension after acute nitroglycerin administration, with a significantly smaller right ventricle was related to a low mortality rate early after cardiac transplantation [27]. Similarly, in septic patients, cardiac ultrasound and Doppler provided significant advantages over right heart catheterization [28, 29]. Using tissue Doppler imaging, Sm, as a sign of RV dysfunction, was related to the severity of sepsis and mortality [30].

Intermittent dilation of the right ventricle during mechanical ventilation should alert the echocardiographer. Presence of intermittent tricuspid regurgitation should urge the attending physician to check the ventilator settings to abolish high positive end-expiratory pressure (PEEP) or inadvertent large tidal volumes to avoid development of acute cor pulmonale [20].

Fluid Responsiveness

Preload optimization is a daily problem perioperatively and in the ICU [31], and can improve outcomes when implemented early [32]. Fluid management protocols must be supplemented with the knowledge of ventricular function. In this context, fluid management has been related to improved outcomes [33, 34]. Clinically, the legs-up test or Trendelenburg positioning is preferable for evaluating optimal preloading conditions: it does no harm, is immediately reversible and provides instantaneous information about the filling status [35]. The only condition *sine qua non* is the knowledge of ventricular dimensions and function. In this respect, transthoracic echocardiography is an essential adjunct. From a short axis parasternal view, assessment of LV end-diastolic area (LVEDA) gives a direct indication of filling, only

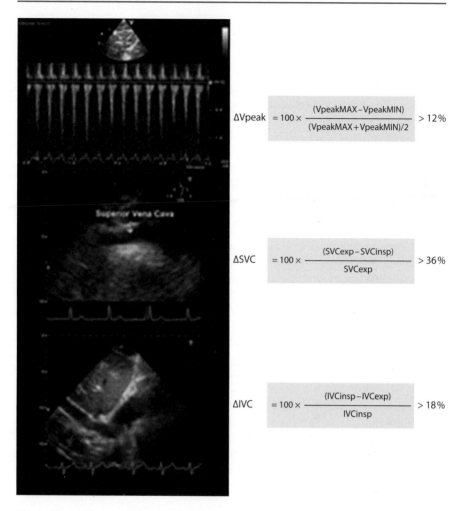

$$\Delta \text{Vpeak} = 100 \times \frac{(\text{VpeakMAX} - \text{VpeakMIN})}{(\text{VpeakMAX} + \text{VpeakMIN})/2} \; > 12\%$$

$$\Delta \text{SVC} = 100 \times \frac{(\text{SVCexp} - \text{SVCinsp})}{\text{SVCexp}} \; > 36\%$$

$$\Delta \text{IVC} = 100 \times \frac{(\text{IVCinsp} - \text{IVCexp})}{\text{IVCinsp}} \; > 18\%$$

Fig. 2 Three different methods to discriminate fluid responsiveness by means of cardiac ultrasound. *Upper panel*: peak velocity variation (*Vpeak*); *middle panel*: ventilation-induced variation of the diameter of the superior vena cava (*SVC*) during inspiration (*insp*) and expiration (*exp*); *lower panel*: variation of diameter of the inferior vena cava (*IVC*) during inspiration and expiration

when combined with a dynamic test, such as a legs-up test. LVEDAI $< 5.5 \, \text{cm}^2/\text{m}^2$ body surface area (BSA) is a sign of low preload conditions [36]. Nevertheless, static variables to describe filling state are not the first choice mainly because intrathoracic pressure may interfere with interpretation of these static variables in the critically ill.

Dynamic variables are, therefore, used in mechanically ventilated patients in the ICU or intraoperatively and rely on the ventilation-induced variation in intrathoracic pressures. Variation of stroke volume can be assessed through the variation of the time-velocity-integral [37]. On the right heart side, variations in inferior [38] and superior caval vein [39] diameters during changing intrathoracic pressures can be used (Fig. 2) by means of transthoracic and transesophageal approaches, respectively. Of note, these variables only provide insight into RV preload. Situations such as acute RV failure, intra-abdominal hypertension [40], open chest [41], arrhythmia [35], children, tidal volume < 8 ml/kg [42, 43], respiratory rate > 30 bpm, heart rate versus respiratory rate < 3.6 [44] and respiratory effort [35] hamper correct interpretation of fluid responsiveness assessed by means of alteration of the diameter of the caval veins.

Unexplained Hypotension

From a morphological point of view, cardiac ultrasound with Doppler in the perioperative care unit or ICU is particularly useful in patients with unresolved or unexplained hemodynamic instability and/or hypovolemia, unexpected or abrupt need for high doses of inotropic or vasopressor drugs or any situation where inadequate perfusion is present and not explainable [29, 45–47]. Echocardiography and Doppler often provide immediate insight into the physiological mechanism of the particular disease. Again, cardiac ultrasound is only performed after a full clinical assessment, which will often already reveal dyspnea, pulmonary crackles, murmurs, arrhythmias, etc. It should not be denied that additional tools, such as electrocardiogram (EKG), biomarkers (troponin, N-terminal pro-B-type natriuretic peptide [NT-BNP]) and the hemodynamic picture, may help fine-tune and confirm diagnosis to differentiate the various syndromes after a tentative diagnosis with echo-Doppler.

Acute LV dysfunction should be evaluated in terms of hyperkinesia or hypokinesia/dyskinesia (Box 1). The latter could be related to global or regional wall motion abnormalities. Often valvular involvement is present, either inducing acute LV dysfunction (aortic or mitral valve), or as a consequence of this acute ventricular failure (functional mitral regurgitation) [48].

Box 1:
Causes of acute left ventricular dysfunction: An echo-Doppler approach
1. hyperkinesia
   a. hypovolemia
   b. hyperdynamic left ventricular outflow obstruction
   c. diastolic dysfunction (often with normal fractional area contraction)
   d. stress cardiomyopathy
2. hypokinesia/dyskinesia
   a. global
      i. sepsis, septic shock
      ii. after cardiac arrest, resuscitation

iii. stress cardiomyopathy with high afterload (vasopressor overdose, acute hypertensive crisis, thyroid storm, cocaine, catecholamine burst during initial phase of brain death)
iv. tachyarrhythmias
b. regional
i. ischemic heart disease, acute coronary syndrome
ii. stress cardiomyopathy, in particular Taku Tsubo cardiomyopathy

A pathophysiologic approach to acute RV dysfunction refers to ischemic heart disease, volume or pressure overload (Box 2). Echocardiography allows immediate diagnosis of the etiology of RV dilation in conjunction with assessment of LV involvement. A dilated right ventricle in conjunction with a small left ventricle suggests acute pressure overload of the RV whereas a dilated LV rather suggests global RV/LV failure in terms of ischemic heart disease or septic cardiomyopathy.

Box 2:
Etiology of acute right ventricular dysfunction from an echo-Doppler perspective in acute illness
1. ischemic heart disease, acute coronary syndrome
2. volume overload
   a. atrial septum defect and altered pressure equilibrium;
   b. massive tricuspid regurgitation (pressure overload, endocarditis, deficient tricuspid repair/valve function)
   c. congenital
3. pressure overload
   a. acute pulmonary hypertension (pulmonary emboli, acute respiratory distress syndrome [ARDS], pulmonary edema with acute heart failure)
   b. inappropriate settings of mechanical ventilator (tidal volume, positive end-expiratory pressure [PEEP]-level, inspiratory-expiratory ratio)

Pericardial tamponade is the consequence of accumulation of effusion or blood. This prevents the ventricles from expanding fully and exerts a decrease in RV preload. Global tamponade (Box 3) refers to bleeding into the pericardial space, pericarditis or cancer. The degree of compression can be readily estimated by cardiac ultrasound and is life-saving [49, 50].

> **Box 3:**
> **Etiology of pericardial effusion in a critically ill patient**
> 1. bleeding into pericardium: typical fibrin strands, spontaneous contrast
>   a. myocardial injury
>   b. cardiac surgery
>   c. aortic dissection
>   d. ruptured cardiac muscle
> 2. pericarditis: sepsis
> 3. cancer

Immediate Bedside Hemodynamic Information

The difficulty with Doppler-echocardiography concerns both correct image capture and accurate interpretation: Knowledge and skills are both unequivocally important [51]. All data must be integrated into results obtained from routine hemodynamic monitoring. In a hypotensive patient, a quick investigation of cardiac function at the level of the short axis view permits differentiation between a cardiac and a non-cardiac cause of hypotension [2]. Additional optimization of preload conditions can be achieved by assessing the different variables of fluid responsiveness.

When a dilated right ventricle is found on a short axis level, other views will again confirm or deny the initial finding, complemented with tissue Doppler data, suggesting decreased systolic function. In view of the hemodynamic picture, a rapid decision for further evaluation or investigation could be taken, such as ultra-fast computed tomography (CT) scan, to exclude pulmonary emboli.

Conclusions

Doppler echocardiography provides immediate insight into the morphological and hemodynamic functioning of the heart and circulation. Performing a complete echocardiogram offers a full picture of the heart as cardiac muscle and pump of the circulation. As with every other (invasive) hemodynamic monitoring tool, all tricks and flaws must be recognized to permit a comprehensive integrative evaluation of a hemodynamically unstable patient. Further decision making can then be related to the findings of this ultrasound assessment. Clinicians involved in the daily management of hemodynamic instability should be aware of the value of cardiac ultrasound and Doppler and apply this powerful tool, ensuring it is used in the correct physiological context.

References

1. Vignon P (2005) Hemodynamic assessment of critically ill patients using echocardiography Doppler. Curr Opin Crit Care 11:227–234
2. Poelaert JI, Schupfer G (2005) Hemodynamic monitoring utilizing transesophageal echocardiography: the relationships among pressure, flow, and function. Chest 127:379–390
3. Colreavy FB, Donovan K, Lee KY et al (2002) Transesophageal echocardiography in critically ill patients. Crit Care Med 30:989–996
4. Daniel WG, Erbel R, Kasper W et al (1991) Safety of transesophageal echocardiography. A multicenter survey of 10,419 examinations. Circulation 83:817–821
5. Stevenson J (1999) Incidence of complications in pediatric transesophageal echocardiography: experience in 1650 cases. J Am Soc Echocardiogr 12:527–532
6. Expert Round Table on Ultrasound in ICU participants (2011) International expert statement on training standards for critical care ultrasonography. Intensive Care Med 37:1077–1083
7. Leung JM, Levine EH (1994) Left ventricular end-systolic cavity obliteration as an estimate of intraoperative hypovolemia. Anesthesiology 81:1102–1109
8. Flynn M, Curtin R, Nowicki ER et al (2009) Regional wall motion abnormalities and scarring in severe functional ischemic mitral regurgitation: A pilot cardiovascular magnetic resonance imaging study. J Thorac Cardiovasc Surg 137:1063–1070 e2
9. Kamp O, de Cock CC, van Eenige MJ et al (1994) Influence of pacing-induced myocardial ischemia on left atrial regurgitant jet: a transesophageal echocardiographic study. J Am Coll Cardiol 23:1584–1591
10. Edvardsen T, Urheim S, Skulstad H et al (2002) Quantification of left ventricular systolic function by tissue doppler echocardiography: Added value of measuring pre- and postejection velocities in ischemic myocardium. Circulation 105:2071–2077
11. Amà R, Segers P, Roosens C et al (2004) Effects of load on systolic mitral annular velocity by tissue Doppler imaging. Anesth Analg 99:332–338
12. Borlaug BA, Melenovsky V, Redfield MM et al (2007) Impact of arterial load and loading sequence on left ventricular tissue velocities in humans. J Am Coll Cardiol 50:1570–1577
13. Poelaert J, Osipowska E, Verborgh C (2008) Diastolic dysfunction and cardiac failure in the ICU. In: Vincent J-L (ed) Update in Emergency and Intensive Care Medicine. Springer, Heidelberg, pp 76–87
14. Pennock GD, Yun DD, Agarwal PG et al (1997) Echocardiographic changes after myocardial infarction in a model of left ventricular diastolic dysfunction. Am J Physiol 273:H2018–H2029
15. Oki T, Tabata T, Mishiro Y et al (1999) Pulsed tissue Doppler imaging of left ventricular systolic and diastolic wall motion velocities to evaluate differences between long and short axes in healthy subjects. J Am Soc Echocardiogr 12:308–313
16. Yu CM, Chan JY, Zhang Q et al (2009) Impact of cardiac contractility modulation on left ventricular global and regional function and remodeling. JACC Cardiovasc Imaging 2:1341–1349
17. Poelaert J, Declerck C, Vogelaers D et al (1997) Left ventricular systolic and diastolic function in septic shock. Intensive Care Med 23:553–560
18. Munt B, Jue J, Gin K et al (1998) Diastolic filling in human severe sepsis: an echocardiographic study. Crit Care Med 26:1829–1833
19. Sturgess DJ, Marwick TH, Joyce C et al (2010) Prediction of hospital outcome in septic shock: a prospective comparison of tissue Doppler and cardiac biomarkers. Crit Care 14:R44
20. Vieillard-Baron A, Prin S, Chergui K et al (2002) Echo-Doppler demonstration of acute cor pulmonale at the bedside in the medical intensive care unit. Am J Respir Crit Care Med 166:1310–1319
21. Vieillard-Baron A, Chergui K, Augarde R et al (2003) Cyclic changes in arterial pulse during respiratory support revisited by Doppler echocardiography. Am J Respir Crit Care Med 168:671–676

22. Jardin F, Vieillard-Baron A (2003) Right ventricular function and positive pressure ventilation in clinical practice: from haemodynamic subsets to respirator settings. Intensive Care Med 29:1426–1434
23. Schmitt J, Vieillard-Baron A, Augarde R et al (2001) Positive end-expiratory pressure titration in acute respiratory distress syndrome: impact on right ventricular outflow impedance evaluated by pulmonary artery Doppler flow velocity measurements. Crit Care Med 29:1154–1158
24. Poelaert J, Visser C, Everaert J et al (1993) Acute hemodynamic changes of inverse ratio ventilation in adult respiratory distress syndrome. A transesopahgeal echo Doppler study. Chest 104:214–249
25. Sagie A, Schwammenthal E, Padial LR et al (1994) Determinants of functional tricuspid regurgitation in incomplete tricuspid valve closure: Doppler color flow study of 109 patients. J Am Coll Cardiol 24:446–453
26. Yock P, Popp R (1984) Noninvasive estimation of right ventricular systolic pressure by Doppler ultrasound in patients with tricuspid regurgitation. Circulation 70:657–662
27. Gavazzi A, Ghio S, Scelsi L et al (2003) Response of the right ventricle to acute pulmonary vasodilation predicts the outcome in patients with advanced heart failure and pulmonary hypertension. Am Heart J 145:310–316
28. Jardin F, Bourdarias JP (1995) Right heart catheterization at bedside: a critical view. Intensive Care Med 21:291–295
29. Poelaert JI, Trouerbach J, De Buyzere M et al (1995) Evaluation of transesophageal echocardiography as a diagnostic and therapeutic aid in a critical care setting. Chest 107:774–779
30. Harmankaya A, Akilli H, Gul M, et al (2013) Assessment of right ventricular functions in patients with sepsis, severe sepsis and septic shock and its prognostic importance: A tissue Doppler study. J Crit Care 1111.e7-1111.e11
31. Benes J, Chytra I, Altmann P et al (2010) Intraoperative fluid optimization using stroke volume variation in high risk surgical patients: results of prospective randomized study. Crit Care 14:R118
32. Rivers E, Nguyen B, Havstad S et al (2001) Early goal-directed therapy in the treatment of severe sepsis and septic shock. N Engl J Med 345:1368–1377
33. Feissel M, Michard F, Faller JP et al (2004) The respiratory variation in inferior vena cava diameter as a guide to fluid therapy. Intensive Care Med 30:1834–1837
34. Michard F, Teboul JL (2000) Using heart-lung interactions to assess fluid responsiveness during mechanical ventilation. Crit Care 4:282–289
35. Monnet X, Rienzo M, Osman D et al (2006) Passive leg raising predicts fluid responsiveness in the critically ill. Crit Care Med 34:1402–1407
36. Skarvan K, Lambert A, Filipovic M et al (2001) Reference values for left ventricular function in subjects under general anaesthesia and controlled ventilation assessed by two-dimensional transoesophageal echocardiography. Eur J Anaesthesiol 18:713–722
37. Slama M, Masson H, Teboul JL et al (2002) Respiratory variations of aortic VTI: a new index of hypovolemia and fluid responsiveness. Am J Physiol Heart Circ Physiol 283:H1729–H1733
38. Barbier C, Loubieres Y, Schmit C et al (2004) Respiratory changes in inferior vena cava diameter are helpful in predicting fluid responsiveness in ventilated septic patients. Intensive Care Med 30:1740–1746
39. Vieillard-Baron A, Augarde R, Prin S et al (2001) Influence of superior vena caval zone condition on cyclic changes in right ventricular outflow during respiratory support. Anesthesiology 95:1083–1088
40. Mahjoub Y, Touzeau J, Airapetian N et al (2010) The passive leg-raising maneuver cannot accurately predict fluid responsiveness in patients with intra-abdominal hypertension. Crit Care Med 38:1824–1829
41. Wyffels PA, Sergeant P, Wouters PF (2010) The value of pulse pressure and stroke volume variation as predictors of fluid responsiveness during open chest surgery. Anaesthesia 65:704–709

42. De Backer D, Heenen S, Piagnerelli M et al (2005) Pulse pressure variations to predict fluid responsiveness: influence of tidal volume. Intensive Care Med 31:517–523
43. Suehiro K, Okutani R (2011) Influence of tidal volume for stroke volume variation to predict fluid responsiveness in patients undergoing one-lung ventilation. J Anesth 25:777–780
44. De Backer D, Taccone FS, Holsten R et al (2009) Influence of respiratory rate on stroke volume variation in mechanically ventilated patients. Anesthesiology 110:1092–1097
45. Heidenreich PA, Stainback RF, Redberg RF et al (1995) Transesophageal echocardiography predicts mortality in critically ill patients with unexplained hypotension. J Am Coll Cardiol 26:152–158
46. Reichert CL, Visser CA, Koolen JJ et al (1992) Transesophageal echocardiography in hypotensive patients after cardiac operations. Comparison with hemodynamic parameters. J Thorac Cardiovasc Surg 104:321–326
47. Vignon P, Mentec H, Terre S et al (1994) Diagnostic accuracy and therapeutic impact of transthoracic and transesophageal echocardiography in mechanically ventilated patients in the ICU. Chest 106:1829–1834
48. Poelaert J (2009) Functional mitral regurgitation in the critically ill. In: Vincent JL (ed) Yearbook Update in Emergency and Intensive Care Medicine. Springer, Heidelberg, pp 543–551
49. Schmidlin D, Schuepbach R, Bernard E et al (2001) Indications and impact of postoperative transesophageal echocardiography in cardiac surgical patients. Crit Care Med 29:2143–2148
50. Subramaniam B, Talmor D (2007) Echocardiography for management of hypotension in the intensive care unit. Crit Care Med 35:S401–S407
51. Poelaert J, Mayo P (2007) Education and evaluation of knowledge and skills in echocardiography: how should we organize? Intensive Care Med 33:1684–1686

The Hemodynamic Puzzle: Solving the Impossible?

K. Tánczos, M. Németh, and Z. Molnár

Introduction

Development of multiorgan dysfunction is often the result of hypoperfusion, which severely affects outcomes of medical and surgical patients and substantially increases the utilization of resources and costs [1]. Therefore, the use of early and efficient strategies to detect tissue hypoperfusion and to treat the imbalance between oxygen consumption and delivery is of particular importance [2]. Traditional endpoints, such as heart rate, blood pressure, mental status and urine output, can be useful in the initial identification of inadequate perfusion, but are limited in their ability to identify ongoing, compensated shock [3]. Therefore, more detailed assessment of global macrohemodynamic indices, such as cardiac output and derived variables and measures of oxygen delivery and uptake, may be necessary to guide treatment [4–5]. Furthermore, after optimization of these parameters, indicators of tissue perfusion should also be assessed to verify the effectiveness of therapy [6]. This multimodal approach can be translated into the individualized use of target endpoints for hemodynamic stabilization instead of treating 'normal' values, and can help to achieve adequate oxygen supply and tissue oxygenation in order to avoid under- or over-resuscitation, which are equally harmful.

Physiological Issues

The primary goal of the cardiorespiratory system is to deliver adequate oxygen to the tissues to meet their metabolic requirements. The adequacy of tissue oxygenation is determined by the balance between the rate of oxygen transport to the tissues (oxygen delivery, DO_2) and the rate at which the oxygen is used by the tissues (oxy-

K. Tánczos · M. Németh · Z. Molnár ✉
Department of Anesthesiology and Intensive Care, University of Szeged, 6725 Szeged, Hungary
e-mail: zsoltmolna@gmail.com

J.-L. Vincent (Ed.), *Annual Update in Intensive Care and Emergency Medicine 2014*, 355
DOI 10.1007/978-3-319-03746-2_27, © Springer International Publishing Switzerland 2014

gen consumption, VO_2) [7]. Standard formulae to determine DO_2 and VO_2 are:

$$DO_2 = SV \times HR \times [Hb \times 1.34 \times SaO_2 + 0.003 \times PaO_2] = CO \times [CaO_2]$$

$$VO_2 = CO \times [CaO_2 - (Hb \times 1.34 \times SvO_2 + 0.003 \times PvO_2)]$$
$$= CO \times [CaO_2 - CvO_2]$$

where, SV = stroke volume, HR = heart rate, Hb = hemoglobin, SaO_2 = hemoglobin arterial oxygen saturation, PaO_2 = arterial oxygen partial pressure, CO = cardiac output, CaO_2 = arterial oxygen content, SvO_2 = hemoglobin mixed venous oxygen saturation, PvO_2 = venous oxygen partial pressure, CvO_2 = venous oxygen content

$$Oxygen\ extraction\ (O_2ER) = VO_2/DO_2 \times 100$$
$$\approx 250\,ml/min/1{,}000\,ml/min \times 100 = 25\,\%$$

In the critically ill and in the perioperative period there is often an imbalance between DO_2 and VO_2. DO_2 may be inadequate considering that CaO_2 content and/or cardiac output may be reduced [8, 9]. The circulation can compensate to some extent, and VO_2 is usually independent over a wide range of DO_2. If CaO_2 decreases, cardiac output increases to maintain the same DO_2 levels, but, after a critical threshold or in low cardiac output states, the O_2ER increases to maintain adequate VO_2/DO_2. After exhausting compensatory resources, VO_2 becomes dependent on DO_2 and anaerobic metabolism begins, leading to metabolic acidosis and oxygen debt [10].

The principle task of acute care is to avoid or correct oxygen debt by optimizing DO_2 and VO_2. Furthermore, it is just as important to recognize that DO_2 and tissue perfusion have normalized, because any further measures to increase DO_2 may do harm by unnecessary over-resuscitation.

Pieces of the 'Hemodynamic Puzzle'

There is mounting evidence that conventional parameters, such as blood pressure, central venous pressure (CVP), heart rate are poor indicators of cardiac index (CI) or DO_2 [11, 12], and there is also increasing evidence that, for example in high risk surgery, perioperative care algorithms based on advanced hemodynamic monitoring are beneficial [13, 14]. There are several hemodynamic endpoints without a universally accepted gold standard for this 'hemodynamic puzzle' (Fig. 1). Fundamentally they can be grouped into flow-based and oxygen extraction based indices.

Flow-based Resuscitation

There are various commercially available devices for blood flow measurement. Cardiac output and the driven variables can be determined by several methods:

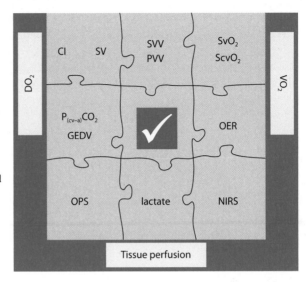

Fig. 1 The hemodynamic puzzle. $ScvO_2$: central venous oxygen saturation; SvO_2: mixed venous oxygen saturation; DO_2: oxygen delivery; VO_2: oxygen consumption; SVV: stroke volume variation; PPV: pulse pressure variation; GEDV: global-end-diastolic volume; CI: cardiac index; P(cv-a)CO_2: venous-to-arterial CO_2 gap; NIRS: near infrared spectroscopy; OPS: orthogonal polarization spectral

Thermodilution with a pulmonary artery catheter (PAC), transpulmonary indicator dilution (PiCCO®, LiDCO®, VolumeView®); less invasive, non-calibrated devices utilizing pulse contour analysis of the arterial pressure signal (Vigileo®, ProAQT®); and esophageal Doppler [5, 15, 16]. Each monitor has advantages and disadvantages and can be used in most clinical scenarios if the underlying principles and the inherent limitations are well understood, but the discussion of that goes well beyond the scope of this article.

Cardiac output/stroke volume as a resuscitation endpoint

Several clinical investigations have reported that optimization of cardiac output calculated from thermodilution or pulse contour analysis and used as a therapeutic goal seems appropriate to monitor goal-directed hemodynamic strategies and has been shown to have positive effects on overall outcome after surgery [17, 18]. However, there is no consensus on a universally accepted parameter as resuscitation target.

In two recent animal experiments, we tested the effects of cardiac output- and stroke volume (SV)-guided hemorrhage and fluid resuscitation [19, unpublished data]. After baseline measurements (t_{bsl}), animals were bled until CI (n = 9) or SV index (SVI-group, n = 12) decreased by 50 %; measurements were then repeated (t_0), after which animals were resuscitated during 60 minutes with lactated Ringer's solution until baseline CI and SVI values were reached, then final measurements were recorded (t_{end}).

In both experiments, CI and SVI targets were reached at t_0 and t_{end} alike (Table 1). In the CI-group all parameters changed significantly during the bleeding phase, as expected (Table 1). However, SV, global end-diastolic volume (GEDV), and central venous oxygen saturation ($ScvO_2$) remained significantly lower, whereas SV variation (SVV) and central venous-to-arterial carbon dioxide

Table 1 Hemodynamic changes during cardiac index or stroke volume based algorithms

	CI-group			SVI-group		
	t_{bsl}	t_0	t_{end}	t_{bsl}	t_0	t_{end}
SVI (ml/m^2)	33.6 ± 6.2	$14.6 \pm 10.1^*$	$23.4 \pm 7.9^{*\#}$	26.8 ± 4.7	$13.4 \pm 2.3^*$	$26.6 \pm 4.1^\#$
CI (l/min/m^2)	2.88 ± 0.42	$1.79 \pm 0.53^*$	2.73 ± 0.35	2.6 ± 0.4	$1.8 \pm 0.3^*$	$2.9 \pm 0.5^{*\#}$
Mean arterial pressure (mmHg)	127 ± 13.07	$75 \pm 25^*$	$85 \pm 22^{*\#}$	112 ± 23	$74 \pm 18^*$	$91 \pm 19^{*\#}$
Heart rate (beats/min)	87 ± 16	$140 \pm 40^*$	$124 \pm 37^*$	95 ± 12	$131 \pm 27^*$	$107 \pm 16^{*\#}$
Global end-diastolic volume (ml/m^2)	317 ± 36	$198 \pm 57^*$	$249 \pm 46^{*\#}$	309 ± 57	$231 \pm 61^*$	$287 \pm 49^{*\#}$
Stroke volume variation (%)	10.8 ± 5.5	$17.3 \pm 5.1^*$	$16.4 \pm 8.2^*$	13.6 ± 4.3	$22.6 \pm 5.6^*$	$12.2 \pm 4.3^\#$

CI: cardiac index; SVI: stroke volume index; bsl: baseline; * significantly different from t_{bsl}; # significantly different from t_0

difference ($P(cv\text{-}a)CO_2$) were significantly higher by the end of resuscitation compared to baseline, indicating that fluid resuscitation may have been inadequate and the normalization of CI was mainly due to the persistently elevated heart rate, rather than to restoration of the circulating blood volume (Tables 1, 2).

In contrast, in the SVI-group, although there were similar changes during bleeding as in the CI-group, SV, SVV, $ScvO_2$, and $P(cv\text{-}a)CO_2$ had all improved significantly or returned to their baseline values by the end of the experiment (Tables 1, 2). Although $ScvO_2$ returned to the normal range at the end of the experiment, it remained significantly lower than at baseline with an average difference of 5 %, possibly due to a hemodilution-related decrease in DO_2. It is, therefore, important to bear in mind that using baseline $ScvO_2$ values as a resuscitation target, for example, in the intraoperative period, may result in fluid overload by the end of surgery.

In conclusion, in these experiments the SVI-based algorithm resulted in better hemodynamic and oxygenation indices as compared to the CI-based approach. The latter was mainly affected by the elevated heart rate, possibly due to the sympathetic response to bleeding. Therefore, normalization of CI may mask hypovolemia in conditions when strong sympathetic activation is present, such as acute bleeding. It is also important to note that conventional parameters, such as heart rate and mean arterial pressure (MAP), did not follow the changes in SVI; therefore, our results do not support the routine use of these measures as resuscitation endpoints. These observations are in agreement with several recent clinical studies [12].

Table 2 Oxygenation changes during cardiac index or stroke volume based algorithms

	CI-group			SVI-group		
	t_{bsl}	t_0	t_{end}	t_{bsl}	t_0	t_{end}
Oxygen delivery (DO$_2$) index (ml/min/m^2)	335 ± 63	158 ± 62*	238 ± 52*#	419 ± 62	272 ± 56*	341 ± 62*#
Oxygen consumption (VO$_2$) index (ml/min/m^2)	44 ± 25	62 ± 38	76 ± 34	77 ± 26	96 ± 19*	82 ± 27
Oxygen extraction (VO$_2$/DO$_2$)	0.13 ± 0.08	0.38 ± 0.19*	0.32 ± 0.14*	0.20 ± 0.07	0.36 ± 0.05*	0.24 ± 0.09*
pH	7.43 ± 0.05	7.41 ± 0.07	7.43 ± 0.05	7.50 ± 0.63	7.45 ± 0.7	7.45 ± 0.43
Central venous oxygen saturation (%)	81 ± 8	58 ± 18*	64 ± 15*	78 ± 7	61 ± 5*	73 ± 9*#
Venous to arterial carbon dioxide gap (mm Hg)	3.3 ± 3.1	8.9 ± 3.3*	7.8 ± 4.8*	5.3 ± 2	9.6 ± 2.3*	5.1 ± 2.6#
Lactate (mmol/L)	3.6 ± 1.1	5.0 ± 1.6	4.6 ± 2.0	1.62 ± 0.43	3.86 ± 1.49*	3.54 ± 1.9*
Hemoglobin (g/L)	9.0 ± 0.7	8.0 ± 2.7	6.9 ± 1.3*	12.05 ± 1.37	11.22 ± 1.39*	8.45 ± 1.1*#

CI: cardiac index; SVI: stroke volume index; bsl: baseline; *significantly different from t_{bsl}; # significantly different from t_0

Stroke volume variation and pulse pressure variation as resuscitation endpoints

Recently, less invasive devices assessing cardiac output by pulse contour analysis based on the radial artery pressure signal have been introduced. Although these devices show lower precision compared to the gold standard of thermodilution, there is some evidence that these methods can adequately show changes in the trend of cardiac output [20]. As PPV and SVV are well established indicators of fluid responsiveness [21], these devices seem to be simple and useful alternatives to invasive hemodynamic monitoring. Furthermore, in various studies, fluid therapy guided by SVV and PPV proved to be more accurate than static preload indicator-based approaches and was also shown to improve patient outcome [22]. However, use of PPV and SVV is limited to patients who are fully ventilated and have no arrhythmias [23, 24].

Venous-to-arterial CO_2 gap as a therapeutic endpoint

Another easily obtainable blood flow related blood gas parameter is the $P(cv-a)$ CO_2. Several authors have reported increased $P(cv-a)CO_2$ in different low flow states [25–27]. In oxygen debt causing anaerobic metabolism, hydrogen ions are generated in two ways: 1) Hydrolysis of adenosine triphosphate to adenosine diphosphate and 2) increased production of lactic acid [28]. These hydrogen ions are buffered by bicarbonate presented in the cells, a process that will generate CO_2 production [29]. Although arterial $PaCO_2$ is variable and dependent on pulmonary gas exchange, central venous $PvCO_2$ is dependent on the ability of the flow (i. e., cardiac output) to wash out CO_2 from the tissues. The Fick principle adapted to carbon dioxide, demonstrates the inverse relationship between the cardiac output and $P(cv-a)$ CO_2 [30]. Thus, it has been postulated that increased $P(cv-a)CO_2$ reflects decreased flow. It has been shown that in sepsis, heart failure, and severe hypovolemia, $P(cv-a)$ CO_2 can be increased [31, 32]. In the results of our experimental animal study, $P(cv-a)CO_2$ returned to its initial baseline value in the SVI-group, and there was also a strong, significant correlation between $P(cv-a)CO_2$ and SVI ($r^2 = -0.591$, $p < 0.001$), which lends further support to this theory [19]. Furthermore, adding the $P(cv-a)CO_2$ to the $ScvO_2$ to identify $VO_2/DO_2 > 30\%$ improved specificity, positive predictive and negative predictive values [33].

In situations (e. g., severe sepsis) in which oxygen uptake is insufficient due to microcirculatory and/or mitochondrial defects, $ScvO_2$ may be elevated (i. e., false negative). Previous studies have suggested that under such circumstances, the increased value of $P(cv-a)CO_2$ (> 5 mmHg), may help the clinician in detecting inadequate DO_2 to the tissues, hence the complementary use of $ScvO_2$ and $P(cv-a)$ CO_2 is recommended [34–36].

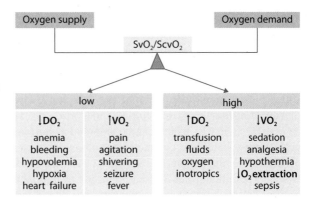

Fig. 2 Mixed venous saturation in the critically ill patient. ScvO$_2$: central venous oxygen saturation; SvO$_2$: mixed venous oxygen saturation; DO$_2$: oxygen delivery; VO$_2$: oxygen consumption

Oxygen Extraction-based Resuscitation

Perhaps the most commonly used methods to assess global VO$_2$/DO$_2$ are SvO$_2$ and its surrogate, ScvO$_2$. ScvO$_2$ is easily obtained via the central venous catheter already *in situ* in most critically ill patients and is often used as a marker of the balance between oxygen delivery and consumption. Because of the different level of measurement (entire body in the case of SvO$_2$ versus brain and the upper part of the body with ScvO$_2$) there has been considerable debate about the interpretation of ScvO$_2$ values compared to SvO$_2$. Most of the studies that have analyzed the relationship between ScvO$_2$ and SvO$_2$ have shown that ScvO$_2$ is an average of 5 % higher than SvO$_2$ and is considered a reasonable surrogate marker in the clinical setting [37–39]. However, recent clinical trials, mainly in septic patients, did not show satisfactory agreement between ScvO$_2$ and SvO$_2$. This observation may in part be explained by modifications of blood flow distribution and oxygen extraction by brain and splanchnic tissues [40]. It seems that ScvO$_2$ and SvO$_2$ are not numerically equivalent but the variations in these two parameters usually occur in a parallel manner [41].

The main factors that influence ScvO$_2$, are hemoglobin, SaO$_2$, cardiac output and VO$_2$. Theoretically, if three of these factors are kept constant, the value of ScvO$_2$ reflects changes in VO$_2$. The multiple physiologic, pathologic and therapeutic factors that influence venous oxygen saturation are summarized in Fig. 2 [42].

One of the important features of venous saturation is that it can be pathologic both if it is high and when it is low. In a recent large cohort of septic patients in the emergency department it was found that mortality was 40 % in patients admitted with an ScvO$_2$ < 70 % but it was almost as high, 34 %, in patients with high initial ScvO$_2$ of > 90 %, probably due to impaired oxygen utilization [43]. High ScvO$_2$ values may thus represent an inability of the cells to extract oxygen or microcirculatory shunting in sepsis [44]. Therefore, additional measures are necessary to help evaluate high ScvO$_2$ values, such as for example P(cv-a)CO$_2$, or use of advanced, invasive hemodynamic monitoring.

Targets of Tissue Oxygenation at the Microcirculatory Level

Lactate, the end product of anaerobic metabolism, has been thoroughly investigated in critical illness over the last few decades. It has good prognostic value in several clinical scenarios, including trauma, sepsis, and high-risk surgical patients [45]. Changes over time (determined by production and clearance) seem an even better marker of adequate resuscitation and outcome [46]. However, lactate kinetics are assessed 2–6 hourly, which can be regarded as far too long considering that acute resuscitation should be conducted as soon as possible. Indeed, in our animal experiments, lactate remained significantly elevated by the end of resuscitation while $ScvO_2$, $P(cv-a)CO_2$ and SVI had returned to normal (Tables 1, 2). These results suggest that these latter parameters are more rapid markers of adequate resuscitation than absolute values of lactate. Furthermore, in our experiments high lactate levels at t_{end} may have indicated inadequate resuscitation, but had it been treated, it would inevitably have led to fluid overload. However, there was an almost 10 % decrease in lactate levels in both experiments within 60 minutes, which should be regarded as a reasonable value over such a short period of time. Hence our results provide further support for the concept that lactate kinetics rather than absolute values should be followed as resuscitation endpoints.

In addition to biochemical monitoring, there are also several devices that measure changes in tissue oxygenation percutaneously or can detect changes in microcirculatory flow. Changes in tissue O_2 saturation (StO_2) and total hemoglobin (HbT) during vascular occlusion tests assessed by near infrared spectroscopy (NIRS) proved to be good markers of VO_2 and cardiovascular reserve [47].

Orthogonal polarization spectral (OPS) and sidestream dark field (SDF) imaging are currently the devices most often used for *in vivo* evaluation of the microcirculation. They have the advantage of permitting direct, dynamic and real time *in vivo* illustration of red blood cell (RBC) velocity or capillary perfusion rate in the microcirculation. The technique is non-invasive, and no fluorescent material is required for imaging [48]. These techniques are, therefore, well accepted for evaluation of the microcirculation in different scenarios where altered microcirculation is present. The major limitations of these devices are the off-line evaluation, the limited availability and operator-dependent evaluation of the results.

Conclusion

Solving the hemodynamic puzzle in our patients is an everyday challenge and there are several hemodynamic indices in use. Discussing all the elements of this puzzle and their advantages and limitations is an impossible task within the frame of an article. Our aim was to provide a deeper insight into the controversies, particularly regarding stroke volume and cardiac output as resuscitation endpoints, and to highlight some practical issues about indices of oxygen delivery and consumption at global and tissue levels. However, regardless of which device is used, one must remember that there is not, and will never be, one single parameter with a set value, that one should treat or follow as a target. Multimodal, individualized care is required and nothing can ever replace the thoughtful physician who draws together all the pieces of the puzzle and uses his/her knowledge and experience to make a treatment decision.

References

1. Shoemaker WC, Appel PL, Kram HB (1992) Role of oxygen debt in the development of organ failure sepsis, and death in high-risk surgical patients. Chest 102:208–215
2. Shoemaker WC, Appel PL, Kram HB (1988) Tissue oxygen debt as determinant of lethal and nonlethal postoperative organ failure. Crit Care Med 16:1117–1120
3. (2006) Endpoints of resuscitation: what should we be monitoring? AACN Adv. Crit Care 17(3):306–316
4. Donati A, Pelaia P, Pietropaoli P et al (2011) Do use ScvO$_2$ and O$_2$ER as therapeutical goals. Minerva Anestesiol 77:483–484
5. Marik PE, Desai H (2012) Goal directed fluid therapy. Curr Pharm Des 18:6215–6224
6. Benes J, Pradl R, Chyrta I (2012) Perioperative hemodynamic optimization: A way to individual goals. In: Vincent JL (ed) Annual Update in Intensive Care and Emergency Medicine 2012. Springer, New York, pp 357–367
7. Vallet B, Tavernier B, Lund N (2000) Assessment of tissue oxygenation in the critically ill. Eur J Anaesthesiol 17:221–229
8. Perner A (2009) Diagnosing Hypovolemia in the critically ill. Crit Care Med 37:2674–2675
9. Sakr Y, Dubois MJ, De Backer D et al (2004) Persistent microcirculatory alterations are associated with organ failure and death in patients with septic shock. Crit Care Med 32:1825–1831
10. Vincent JL (1990) The relationship between oxygen demand, oxygen uptake, and oxygen supply. Intensive Care Med 16:145–148
11. Marik PE, Baram M, Vahid B (2008) Does central venous pressure predict fluid responsiveness? A systematic review of the literature and the tale of seven mares. Chest 134:172–178
12. Osman D, Ridel C, Ray P et al (2007) Cardiac filling pressures are not appropriate to predict hemodynamic response to volume challenge. Crit Care Med 35:64–68
13. Kern JW, Shoemaker WC (2002) Meta-analysis of hemodynamic optimization in high-risk patients. Crit Care Med 30:1686–1692
14. Gurgel ST, do Nascimento P Jr. (2011) Maintaining tissue perfusion in high-risk surgical patients: a systematic review of randomized clinical trials. Anesth Analg 112:1384–1391
15. Alhashemi JA, Cecconi M, Hofer CK (2011) Cardiac output monitoring: an integrative perspective. Crit Care 15:214
16. Donati A, Nardella R, Gabbanelli V et al (2008) The ability of PiCCO versus LiDCO variables to detect changes in cardiac index: a prospective clinical study. Minerva Anestesiol 74:367–374
17. Benes J, Chytra I, Altmann P et al (2010) Intraoperative fluid optimization using stroke volume variation in high risk surgical patients: results of prospective randomized study. Crit Care 14:R118
18. Cecconi M, Fasano N, Langiano N et al (2011) Goal-directed haemodynamic therapy during elective total hip arthroplasty under regional anaesthesia. Crit Care 15:R132
19. Nemeth M, Demeter G, Kaszaki J et al (2012) Venous-arterial CO$_2$ gap (DCO$_2$) can be complementary of central venous oxygen saturation (ScvO$_2$) as target end points during fluid resuscitation. Intensive Care Med 38:S0030
20. Michard F, Teboul JL (2000) Using heart-lung interactions to assess fluid responsiveness during mechanical ventilation. Crit Care 4:282–289

21. Marik PE, Cavallazzi R, Vasu T et al (2009) Dynamic changes in arterial waveform derived variables and fluid responsiveness in mechanically ventilated patients: a systematic review of the literature. Crit Care Med 37:2642–2647
22. Marik PE, Baram M, Vahid B (2008) Does central venous pressure predict fluid responsiveness? A systematic review of the literature and the tale of seven mares. Chest 134:172–178
23. Michard F, Teboul JL (2002) Predicting fluid responsiveness in ICU patients: A critical analysis of the evidence. Chest 121:2000–2008
24. Monnet X, Osman D, Ridel C et al (2009) Predicting volume responsiveness by using the end-expiratory occlusion in mechanically ventilated intensive care unit patients. Crit Care Med 37:951–956
25. Weil MH, Rackow EC, Trevino R et al (1986) Arterionvenous carbon dioxide and pH gradients during cardiac arrest. Circulation 74:1071–1074
26. Cuschieri J, Rivers EP, Donnino MW et al (2005) Central venous-arterial carbon dioxide difference as an indicator of cardiac index. Intensive Care Med 31:818–822
27. Benjamin E, Paluch TA, Berger SR et al (1987) Venous hypercarbia in canine hemorrhagic shock. Crit Care Med 15:516–518
28. Weil MH (1986) Difference in acid-base state between venous and arterial blood during cardiopulmonary resuscitation. N Engl J Med 315:1616–1618
29. Vallet B, Teboul JL, Cain S et al (2000) Venoarterial CO(2) difference during regional ischemic or hypoxic hypoxia. J Appl Physiol 89:1317–1321
30. Lamia B, Monnet X, Teboul JL (2006) Meaning of arterio-venous PCO_2 difference in circulatory shock. Minerva Anestesiol 72:597–604
31. Mecher CE, Rackow EC, Astiz ME et al (1990) Venous hypercarbia associated with severe sepsis and systemic hypoperfusion. Crit Care Med 18:585–589
32. Adrogué HJ, Rashad MN, Gorin AB et al (1989) Assessing acid-base status in circulatory failure. Differences between arterial and central venous blood. N Engl J Med 320:1312–1316
33. Kocsi Sz, Demeter G, Erces D, et al (2013) Central venous-to-arterial CO_2 gap is a useful parameter in monitoring hypovolemia-caused altered oxygen balance: animal study. Crit Care Res Pract Article ID 583598
34. Vallée F, Vallet B, Mathe O et al (2006) Central Venous-to-arterial Carbon Dioxide Difference: an Additional Target for Goal-directed Therapy in Septic Shock? Intensive Care Med 34:2218–2225
35. Futier E, Robin E, Jabaudon M et al (2010) Central venous O_2 saturation and Venous-to-arterial CO_2 difference as complementary tools for goal-directed therapy during high-risk surgery. Crit Care 14:R193
36. Vallet B, Lebuffe G (2007) How to titrate vasopressors against fluid loading in septic shock. Adv Sepsis 6:34–40
37. Chawla LS, Zia H, Gutierrez G et al (2004) Lack of equivalence between central and mixed venous oxygen saturation. Chest 126:1891–1896
38. Reinhart K, Kuhn HJ, Hartog C et al (2004) Continuous central venous and pulmonary artery oxygen saturation monitoring in the critically ill. Intensive Care Med 30:1572–1578
39. Varpula M, Karlsson S, Ruokonen E et al (2006) Mixed venous oxygen saturation cannot be estimated by central venous oxygen saturation in septic shock. Intensive Care Med 32:1336–1343
40. van Beest PA, van Ingen J, Boerma EC et al (2010) No agreement of mixed venous and central venous saturation in sepsis, independent of sepsis origin. Crit Care 14:R219
41. Rivers E (2006) Mixed versus central venous oxygen saturation may be not numerically equal, but both are still clinically useful. Chest 129:507–508
42. van Beest PA, Wietasch G, Scheeren T (2011) Clinical review: use of venous oxygen saturations as a goal– a yet unfinished puzzle. Crit Care 15:232
43. Pope JV, Jones AE, Gaieski DF et al (2010) EMShockNet. Multicenter study of central venous oxygen saturation ($ScvO_2$) as a predictor of mortality in patients with sepsis. Ann Emerg Med 55:40–46

44. Ince C, Sinaasappel M (1999) Microcirculatory oxygenation and shunting in sepsis and shock. Crit Care Med 27:1369–1377
45. Meregalli A, Oliveira RP, Friedman G (2004) Occult hypoperfusion is associated with increased mortality in hemodynamically stable, high-risk, surgical patients. Crit Care 8:R60–R65
46. Nguyen HB, Rivers EP, Knoblich BP et al (2004) Early lactate clearance is associated with improved outcome in severe sepsis and septic shock. Crit Care Med 32:1637–1642
47. Gómez H, Torres A, Polanco P et al (2008) Use of non-invasive NIRS during a vascular occlusion test to assess dynamic tissue O(2) saturation response. Intensive Care Med 34:1600–1607
48. De Backer D, Ospina-Tascon G, Salgado D et al (2010) Monitoring the microcirculation in the critically ill patient: current methods and future approaches. Intensive Care Med 36:1813–1825

A New Generation Computer-controlled Imaging Sensor-based Hand-held Microscope for Quantifying Bedside Microcirculatory Alterations

G. Aykut, Y. Ince, and C. Ince

Introduction

The microcirculation is the final station for oxygen transport to the tissues and plays a key role in the cardiovascular system [1]. The microcirculation includes all the vessels that are smaller than 100 micrometer in diameter and has a crucial role in blood and tissue interactions in physiological and pathophysiological states. Many studies have demonstrated that persistent microcirculatory alterations that are unresponsive to therapy are independently associated with adverse outcome, especially in septic patients (e. g., [1–5]). Additionally, these microcirculatory alterations are independent of systemic hemodynamic variables; therefore, microcirculatory observations are a potentially important extension of conventional systemic hemodynamic monitoring of critically ill patients [3,4]. These findings have been made possible by introduction of hand-held microscopes to surgery and intensive care and in this chapter we present the latest generation of these hand-held devices.

The first generation of these devices was based on the implementation of orthogonal polarization spectral (OPS) imaging into a hand-held microscope, which enabled the first observations of human internal organ microcirculation during surgery [6, 7]. This technique was improved upon by our development of a second generation of hand-held microscopes based on sidestream dark field (SDF) imaging [8]. These devices, however, have remained research tools, mainly because of the technological limitations imposed by the analog video cameras used and the inability to achieve automatic analysis of the microcirculation needed for clinical evaluation. Additionally, analysis of the images to extract relevant functional microcirculatory parameters required time consuming off-line analyses limiting the use of these first and second generation devices to research [9]. In this chapter,

G. Aykut · Y. Ince · C. Ince ✉
Department of Intensive Care, Erasmus MC University Hospital Rotterdam,
3000 Rotterdam, Netherlands
e-mail: c.ince@erasmusmc.nl

J.-L. Vincent (Ed.), *Annual Update in Intensive Care and Emergency Medicine 2014*,   367
DOI 10.1007/978-3-319-03746-2_28, © Springer International Publishing Switzerland
2014

we present a third generation hand-held microscope based on incident dark field (IDF) imaging [10]. Incorporation of a computer-controlled image sensor and illumination in a hand-held microscope together with specialized software enables automatic and instant analysis of images. We anticipate that this technological advancement will move microcirculatory monitoring from the research environment to bedside applications, where it may be used as a clinical platform for microcirculatory diagnoses and to guide therapy.

The Microcirculation in Critically Ill Patients

The microcirculation is a physiological compartment in which blood components (e. g., circulating cells, plasma and coagulation factors), the vessels lined by the endothelium, the glycocalyx and the smooth muscle cells function together to transport the oxygen and nutrients needed for respiring parenchymal cells to perform their functional activities in support of organ function. The vessels of the microcirculation have diameters of less than 100 micrometers and include arterioles, metarterioles, capillaries and post-capillary venules [11]. In some tissue beds, especially in the skin where they are involved in thermoregulation, there are short low-resistance connections between the arterioles and the veins, called arteriovenous shunts. Microcirculatory structures are tailor-made to the oxygen and functional requirements of the different organs they exist in and exhibit considerable heterogeneity [12]. This is especially the case for endothelial cells and their gel-like lining, the glycocalyx. These structures play a key role in hemostasis, vascular regulation and in protecting tissues from edema [13]. A multiplicity of factors influence the blood flow in the (micro)vascular tree, including local and metabolic control mechanisms (autoregulation), endothelium-derived factors, the autonomic nervous system and circulating hormones. Equally important is smooth muscle tone regulation by mechanosensor stimulation, which occurs through the sheer stress of flowing blood via the glycocalyx. The microcirculation provides a total surface area of approximately $700 \, m^2$, which enables the exchange of oxygen, nutrients, hormones and waste products between the circulating blood and parenchymal cells. The exchange of these substances occurs primarily in the capillaries and postcapillary venules.

Diffusion is the principal mechanism of microvascular exchange. The diffusion rate is dependent on the solubility of the substance, the temperature and the available surface area and is inversely related to the molecular size and the distance it must diffuse across (e. g., [14]). The hydrostatic pressure difference across the endothelium leads to filtration. The presence of large molecules in the blood creates oncotic pressure which counteracts filtration. The Starling hypothesis holds that the balance between filtration and water reabsorption depends on the hydrostatic and oncotic pressure differences between the blood and tissues as well as on the vessel permeability. This concept, however, must be revised due to the recent identification and appreciation of the functional importance of the endothelial glycocalyx layer [15].

Microcirculatory Failure and its Importance in Critically Ill Patients

Shock is the failure of the microcirculation to deliver adequate oxygen to the tissue cells [16]. It may arise due to cardiogenic, hypovolemic, obstructive or distributive failure. In an intensive care setting, sepsis is the most studied condition in relation to microcirculatory alterations in critical illness [11]. Sepsis and septic shock are considered as systemic inflammatory responses to infection [17]. Severe sepsis exists where there is organ dysfunction or generalized hypoperfusion. Septic shock is defined as sepsis associated with hypotension and signs of hypoperfusion despite adequate fluid resuscitation. It is usually characterized by inadequate tissue perfusion and widespread cellular dysfunction. Moreover, it is generally recognized that microcirculatory alterations form a key hemodynamic characteristic of this condition, defining its pathophysiology and outcome [1, 2]. Sepsis treatments are based on infection control and eradication, hemodynamic resuscitation to allow adequate perfusion and oxygenation, maintenance and supportive treatment of complications. It is becoming increasingly clear, however, that the normalization of systemic hemodynamics is inadequate, if it is not matched by normalization of microcirculatory function.

The introduction of the pulmonary artery catheter (PAC) [18] enabled cardiac output measurements at the bedside using the thermodilution technique. Additionally, cardiac output normalization has been a prime target in critically ill patient management [19]. Shoemaker pioneered the use of therapeutic targets based on oxygen availability (DO_2) and consumption (VO_2) by the measurement of cardiac output [20, 21]. Following these studies, Hayes et al. observed increased mortality in patients treated with supranormal target values [22] and new targets like central venous oxygen saturation ($ScvO_2$) and oxygen extraction ratio (O_2ER) were introduced. Currently, new and less invasive monitoring tools for cardiac output measurements such as the PiCCO system, LiDCO system, EV 1,000/VolumeView system, the pressure analytical method (PRAM), and thoracic or esophageal Doppler devices are in use.

Even after evaluating immediate interventions with the optimized macro-hemodynamic device parameters, high organ failure and mortality rates have persisted [11]. It is thought that this condition only occurs when the oxygen supply cannot effectively meet the needs of the cells and when oxygen extraction deficits persist due to microcirculatory alterations and shunting [23]. Dr Weil played a key role in our understanding of shock by classifying it into four states: hypovolemic, obstructive, cardiogenic and distributive shock [16]. The first three forms of shock are associated with a reduction in cardiac output. In contrast, distributive shock can occur in the presence of normal or even elevated cardiac outputs. This defect occurs if the cardiac output distribution to and within organs results in an inability of the (micro)circulation to supply the necessary oxygen to the cells. This condition is characterized by persistent signs of regional dysoxia (as indicated by high lactate levels and disturbed acid-base balance) despite normalized systemic hemodyanamics. This condition is further characterized by functional shunting of the microcirculation, leaving weak microcirculatory units hypoxemic and prone to reperfusion injury [23]. This phenomenon explains the oxygen extraction defect that is the key circulatory defect associated with sepsis. Microcirculatory observations at the bedside of septic patients have enabled direct observations of this phenomenon. Additionally, heterogeneous microcirculatory perfusion is the most sensitive and specific circulatory defect associated with organ function and mortality in the critically ill patient [2–5].

In addition to the importance of evaluating microcirculatory defects during distributive shock (such as in sepsis), hand-held microscopes are also used to assess cardiogenic, hypovolemic and obstructive shock (e. g., [24–26]). The main difference between these types of shock and distributive shock is that the microcirculatory changes found in cardiogenic, hypovolemic and distributive shock are often associated with a reduction in cardiac output, whereas distributive shock can occur with normal or even elevated cardiac output levels. Following the realization that microcirculatory alterations were a significant risk parameter in critically ill patients, many studies were performed that investigated the effects of different therapeutic interventions on the microcirculation (for reviews see [11, 27]). Recently, Pranskanus et al. observed that lack of microcirculatory perfusion was a successful means of predicting which patients with clinical symptoms of hypovolemia would respond to fluid therapy [25]. This study indicated that reduced microcirculatory perfusion and its increased flow response to fluids might indeed be a fluid therapy target. In a second key study, Xu et al. showed that resuscitation of pigs with fluid and blood following hemorrhagic shock based on normalization of microcirculatory parameters required no blood and 170 ml of Ringer's lactate, whereas targeting blood pressure required 303 ml of blood and 834 ml of Ringer's lactate for normalization of blood pressure. Both groups had a 100 % survival rate and the same neurological awareness score, indicating that microcirculation targeting required less fluid volumes for identical outcomes. This study shows that targeting the microcirculation in resuscitation may avoid administering unnecessary volumes of fluid and blood [28]. Together these studies suggest that the microcirculation can be used to diagnose states of shock and guide therapy and that doing so may result in a more optimal resuscitation than targeting systemic hemodynamic or clinical variables in critically ill patients.

Previous Methods and Limitations of Direct Observation of the Microcirculation

Galen's classical theories of the circulation lasted for many centuries, until Ibn Al-Nafis, Michael Servetus and William Harvey adapted Galen's concepts [29]. In 1628, William Harvey first described the closed circuit circulation theory [30]. By the end of the 16th century, Jansen had invented the compound microscope which led to intravital microscopy. It was Malpighi, however, who first observed animal capillaries with the use of microscopy [31]. In 1688, Van Leeuwenhoek observed the microcirculation using *in vivo* studies [32]. After achromatic lenses were introduced in 1830, microscopy became a widely adopted research tool.

In the early 19th century, direct intravital observation of the human microcirculation was limited to the use of bulky capillary microscopes which were mainly applied to the nailfold capillary bed. In 1964, Krahl used incident light directed at an oblique angle to the study tissue surfaces [33]. In 1971, Sherman et al. introduced a new method for microcirculation observations, called IDF illumination microscopy. This method enabled observations of the organ surface microcirculation using epi-illumination, without the need for transilluminating the tissue from below [10]. An alternative method to observe the microcirculation using epi-illumination was introduced by Slaaf et al., which enabled the imaging of subsurfaces using cross polarized light microscopy [34]. In the late 1990s, Groner et al. used the Slaaf et al. method and adapted this technique to a hand-held microscope [6]. This method was called OPS imaging. We validated and introduced this technique and were able to produce for the first time organ surface microcirculation images in surgical patients [7, 35]. This technique opened the field for studying the human microcirculation in organ and tissue surfaces at the bedside. OPS imaging can be regarded as the first generation hand-held bedside imaging instruments to be applied to critically patients, and resulted in the recognition that the microcirculation is an important physiological compartment that is compromised during critical illness [36, 37].

OPS imaging is based on cross polarization of polarized green light (548 nm wavelength) illuminating the tissue embedding the microcirculation. Backscattered and depolarized light is projected onto an analog video camera after it passes through an analyzer. By only imaging the backscattered light, the microcirculation can be observed. The use of green light ensures optical absorption by the (de)oxyhemoglobin-containing red blood cells (RBCs) with respect to the lack of absorption by the tissue, therefore, creating contrast. The OPS imaging device was called the Cytoscan and was introduced by Cytometrics (Philadelphia, USA). A limitation of OPS imaging was that it required high powered illumination light sources; thus, there was a need to develop a low powered device that would allow battery operation. To this end, we developed a second-generation microcirculation device based on SDF imaging, which enabled battery operation of the devices [38]. In SDF imaging, the illumination is provided by surrounding a central light guide with concentrically placed light emitting diodes (LEDs), which thus provide SDF illumination. The lens system in the light guide core is optically isolated from the illuminating outer ring thus preventing tissue surface reflections to enter the center of the light guide. Both first generation OPS imaging and second generation SDF imaging make use of green light illumination absorption by the RBC hemoglobin. These techniques, therefore, only display RBC filled microvessels. Both device types are fitted with an analog video camera that needs to be digitalized by separate analog to digital convertor devices for off-line image analysis using specialized software [39]. Analog cameras have the disadvantage of alternatively scanning odd and even video lines, resulting in loss of resolution in the time domain. SDF imaging was commercially introduced by MicroVision Medical (Amsterdam, The Netherlands) and called MicroScan. Later a newer version of this device was introduced by KK Technology (Honiton, UK) called the Capiscope and was essentially a similar device to the Microscan; however, the video output provided a digital signal that could be connected to a laptop via a USB cable so there was no need for analog to digital conversion.

First and Second Generation Hand-held Bedside Imaging: OPS and SDF Imaging

OPS and SDF devices are fitted with a 5× objective lens system and the analog cameras can be directly connected to a television monitor. Illumination intensity and image focus are hand operated by dials on the devices and have to be manually adjusted to obtain focus and illumination. This process requires skill, causes movement artifacts, is operator dependent, can result in inter-operator differences in image quality, and does not allow automatic on-line image analysis (e. g., [9, 40]), as well as being time consuming to produce images of sufficient quality for off-line computer analysis. Covered by a sterile disposable cap, the probes can be placed on organ and tissue surfaces for microcirculatory observations. To obtain good image quality following focus and illumination optimization, the probe needs to be kept very still for 5 to 10 seconds to obtain stable images fit for analysis. It is essential to avoid artifacts induced by manual pressure or pressure exerted by the weight of the devices (first and second generation devices weigh ± 0.5 kg) and saliva bubbles that could interfere with the image quality. Recently a scoring system was introduced by Massey and co-workers to quantify the quality of these recordings. This system gives an objective measure of the image quality as an entry criterion for computer analysis and quantification [41].

Quantifying Microcirculatory Images

Tissue perfusion is dependent on capillary number and distribution of the capillaries and on the blood flow. There are two main mechanisms that govern oxygen transport to tissues. These mechanisms define the microcirculatory functional parameters. The first is convection, based on RBC flow and the second is diffusion, which is the distance oxygen must travel from the capillary RBCs to the respiring mitochondria in the parenchymal cells [14]. Convection is quantified by the flow measurements in the microvessels, and diffusion is quantified by the perfused microvessel density, also referred to as the functional capillary density (FCD). In 2005, a round-table conference was organized to prepare microcirculation scoring guidelines [42]. Microvascular density (total or perfused vessel density) and microvascular perfusion (the proportion of perfused vessels and the microcirculatory flow index [MFI]) parameters were identified. These parameters answered three questions:

1) how many vessels are perfused;
2) what is the quality of the flow; and
3) are there non-perfused areas next to well-perfused areas?

Following tissue imaging, the microcirculation parameters have to be determined for quantification to take place. These parameters can be analyzed off-line manually or aided by specialized computer software [39, 42]. Two parameters can determine microvascular density. These parameters include the total vessel density (TVD) and the perfused vessel density (PVD). PVD is defined as the total perfused capillary length divided by the total analyzed surface area. However, measuring the total vessel length in the area of interest is time consuming even with the aid of available software.

The microvascular perfusion parameters are quantified by the proportion of perfused vessels and the microcirculatory flow. The flow can be described by a semi-quantitative score referred to as the MFI [43] or by quantitative measurement of flow using space time diagrams (e. g., [4]). The MFI is based on the determination of the average or predominant flow type in the field of view. To determine the MFI, the image is divided into four quadrants in which blood flow assessments are categorized based on vessel diameter: Small (10–25 µm), medium (26–50 µm), large (51–100 µm). A number is then assigned for each quadrant according to the predominant flow type (0: no flow; 1: intermittent; 2: sluggish; 3: continuous flow). The proportion of perfused vessels is defined as the number of perfused vessels divided by the total vessel number. This method is performed by visual image inspection.

The tissue perfusion heterogeneity is another parameter for identifying the presence of microcirculatory distributive alterations and shunting related to the oxygen extraction deficit characteristic of septic shock [23, 44]. For that reason, a flow heterogeneity index was introduced and is defined as the difference between the highest MFI and the lowest MFI divided by the mean MFI [5, 43].

Technical Limitations of the First and Second Generation Devices

Three basic technical limitations of these devices were defined by Lindert et al. [45]. Lindert and colleagues criticized the fact that undesirable pressure of the probe affected blood flow, lateral movement of the device with respect to the tissue precluded continuous investigation of the selected microvascular region, and blood flow velocities > 1 mm/s were difficult to measure. In addition to the fact that relatively strong light sources are required for OPS imaging, these high-powered light sources limit the portability and clinical applicability of this method. An important limiting factor for SDF imaging is the pressure-induced microcirculatory alterations that are caused by probe application onto the tissue surfaces. This alteration is predominantly caused by the large weight of these first and second generation devices (± 0.5 kg). These effects may lead to false interpretation of the actual perfusion. A further limitation of these devices is that they require hand-operated focusing, which may result in lengthy procedures for obtaining images of sufficient quality and length. The major short-coming of OPS and SDF imaging devices imposed by their hardware, however, is their inability to implement automatic image analysis. These analyses are needed to identify the functional microcirculatory parameters needed to identify the microcirculatory alterations necessary for clinical decision making and to guide therapy [9]. Despite the fact that we developed software modalities that can automatically analyze the images, the hardware offered by these first and second generation devices did not allow for their use in on-line microcirculatory image quantification [46]. From this work, it was clear that if microcirculatory imaging was to proceed from a research tool into a clinical device, devices based on computer control of pixel-based digital imaging sensors, image acquisition and illumination together with high quality optics had to be developed.

Third Generation Hand-held Microscopes Using Computer-controlled Imaging Sensors and Illumination Based on IDF Imaging

OPS and SDF imaging devices can be regarded as first and second generation hand-held microscopes. Recently a third generation hand-held microscope has been clinically introduced that overcomes many of the limitations of the first and second generation analog devices [47]. Based on the IDF principle that was introduced by Sherman and Cook [10], this device is a novel lightweight computer-controlled imaging sensor-based hand-held microscope, called the Cytocam (Fig. 1).

The Cytocam (Braedius Medical, Huizen, The Netherlands) is a state of the art microscopy method, which incorporates a digital imaging sensor camera that can be used for bedside visualization of organ surface microcirculation. This device uses an IDF imaging illumination system with high brightness LEDs able to provide a very short pulse time of 2 ms. This combination results in a high penetration and sharp contours of fast moving RBCs. The Cytocam is constructed of aluminum and titanium and is light weight and easy to handle. The low weight of the device (120 gram) minimizes the pressure artifact problems that were present in the earlier heavy devices. The camera is fully digital and contains a high resolution sensor, which can be used in binning mode, resulting in a 3.5 megapixel frame size. The combination of a high quality custom designed lens of 4× optical magnification with the large sensor image area provides a 1.55×1.16 mm field of view, which is almost twice as large as the field of view of earlier devices. As seen in Fig. 1, this device is pen-like and is held as such. The optical system has been designed for the purpose of microcirculation imaging and provides an optical resolution of more than 300 lines/mm, which is a 50 % improvement over earlier devices and provides a significant improvement in image quality (e. g., Figs. 1b and 2)

A completely new feature of the Cytocam is the quantitative focusing mechanism. This feature uses a piezo linear motor with an integrated distance measuring system, which positions the sensor within 2 microns. Furthermore it significantly eases the focusing problem. Once the focus depth for a specific patient has been established, repeated measurements can be made without the need for subsequent

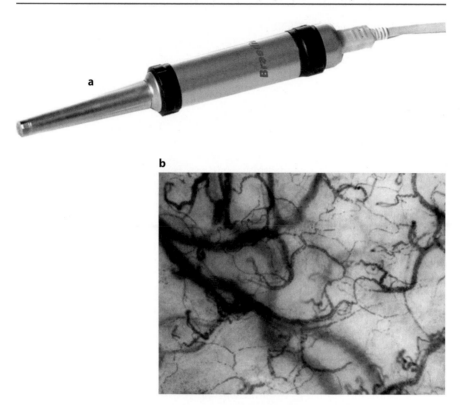

Fig. 1 The Cytocam is shown (**a**), with an example sublingual image (**b**)

measurement focus adjustments, which significantly reduces the measurement time allowing serial measurements to be easily made to determine response to therapy without the need to readjust the focus. Figure 3 shows an example of repeated measurements at time intervals without having to readjust the focus depth. Initial results identify the focus depth as being specific to each patient and as being constant in different sublingual areas [48]. The camera is connected to a device controller based on a powerful medical grade computer, which is used for image storage and analysis. The device controller includes a camera adapter with a dedicated microprocessor for controlling the camera. Additionally, the camera adapter enables high speed data transfer between the camera and controller. Importantly, the Cytocam is equipped with an application for direct microcirculation assessment with which the images are recorded digitally and analyzed automatically (Fig. 4). As demonstrated in the screen shots, the vessels are automatically detected and specialized software is able to quantitatively assess the vessel diameters and the flow velocity of RBCs in the different vessels. Current studies are under way to validate this automatic software system. Additionally, there is also the possibility of analyzing the recorded files using off-line software developed for the earlier generation devices (e. g., [39]).

Fig. 2 The improved optics of the Cytocam device gives good resolution images in other locations for measurement, including **a** buccal, **b** labial, and **c** skin microcirculation

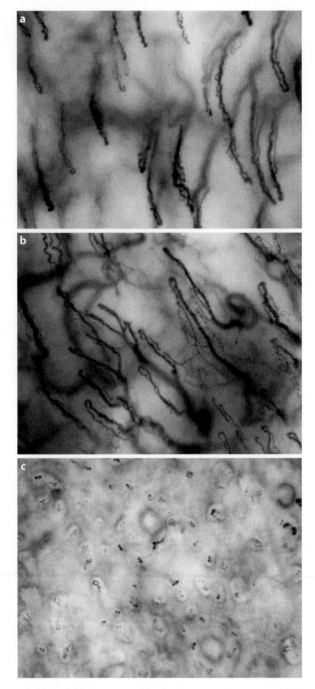

Fig. 3 The quantitative focus mechanism allows repeated measurement to be made without the need to re-adjust focus. In this example, focus depth was determine sublingually at t = 0 (**a**) and images were taken at 15 minute intervals: **b** (15 min), **c** (30 min), and **d** (45 min) without readjusting the focus

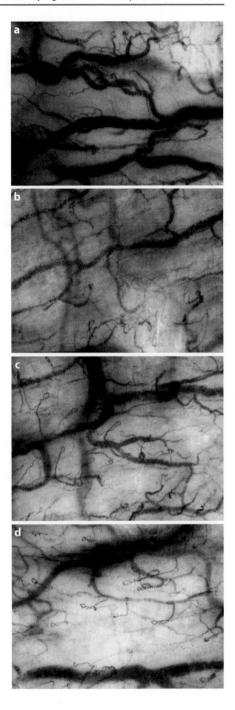

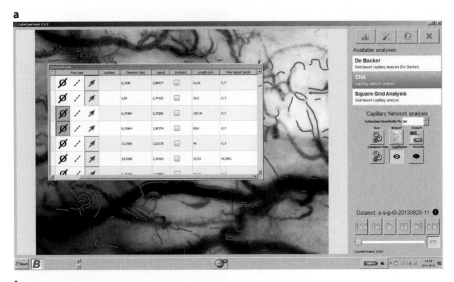

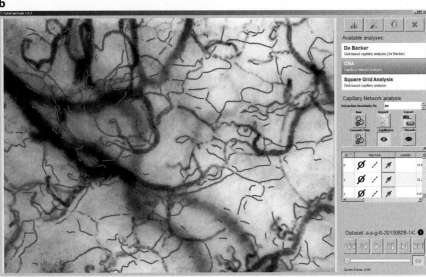

Fig. 4 This figure shows a screen shot of the automatic analysis module of the Cytocam. In **a**, the *blue lines* indicate the automatic recognition (segmentation) of the vessels of the sublingual microcirculatory image. In panel **b**, the flow velocity has been calculated in the different generation vessels and classified into flow, no flow, and intermittent flow

Conclusion

In conclusion, hand-held microscopy has extended the area of hemodynamic monitoring to the level of the microcirculation [49]. This technology has identified the microcirculation as an important clinical compartment, dysfunction of which is highly correlated to adverse outcomes in critically ill patients. These findings were made possible by first and second generation hand-held microscopes over the last decade. The technical limitations of these first and second generation devices have, however, limited the application of these devices to research tools only. The increasing realization that hand-held microscopy may become an important clinical diagnostic tool for circulatory dysfunction and to guide therapies, has led to improved technical developments and to the realization of automatic microcirculatory image analysis to calculate clinically relevant microcirculatory parameters at the bedside. Hence, the Cytocam computer-controlled image sensor and illumination platform based on IDF imaging was realized. We anticipate that this third generation device will open up a new era of clinical monitoring enabling patient-tailored diagnoses and therapies at the microcirculatory and cellular levels.

References

1. Ince C (2005) The microcirculation is the motor of sepsis. Crit Care 9:S13–S19
2. De Backer D, Donadello K, Sakr Y et al (2013) Microcirculatory alterations in patients with severe sepsis: impact of time of assessment and relationship with outcome. Crit Care Med 41:791–799
3. Top AP, Ince C, de Meij N, van Dijk M, Tibboel D (2011) Persistent low microcirculatory vessel density in nonsurvivors of sepsis in the pediatric intensive care. Crit Care Med 39:8–19
4. Edul VS, Enrico C, Laviolle B, Vazquez AR, Ince C, Dubin A (2012) Quantitative assessment of the microcirculation in healthy volunteers and in patients with septic shock. Crit Care Med 40:1443–1448
5. Trzeciak S, Dellinger RP, Parrillo JE et al (2007) Early microcirculatory perfusion derangements in patients with severe sepsis and septic shock: relationship to hemodynamics, oxygen transport, and survival. Ann Emerg Med 49:88–98
6. Groner W, Winkelman JW, Harris AG et al (1999) Orthogonal polarization spectral imaging: a new method for study of the microcirculation. Nat Med 5:1209–1212
7. Mathura KR, Bouma GJ, Ince C (2001) Abnormal microcirculation in brain tumours during surgery. Lancet 358:1698–1699
8. Goedhart PT, Khalilzada M, Bezemer R, Merza J, Ince C (2007) Sidestream dark field (SDF) imaging: a novel stroboscopic LED ring-based imaging modality for clinical assessment of the microcirculation. Opt Express 15:15101–15114
9. Mik EG, Johannes T, Fries M (2009) Clinical microvascular monitoring: a bright future without a future? Crit Care Med 37:2980–2981
10. Sherman H, Klausner S, Cook WA (1971) Incident dark-field illumination: a new method for microcirculatory study. Angiology 22:295–303
11. Donati A, Tibboel D, Ince C (2013) Towards integrative physiological monitoring of the critically ill: from cardiovascular to microcirculatory and cellular function monitoring at the bedside. Crit Care 17:5
12. Klijn E, Den Uil CA, Bakker J, Ince C (2009) The heterogeneity of the microcirculation in critical illness. Clin Chest Med 29:643–654
13. van Golen RF, van Gulik TM, Heger M (2012) Free Mechanistic overview of reactive species-induced degradation of the endothelial glycocalyx during hepatic ischemia/reperfusion injury. Free Rad Biol Med 52:1382–1402

14. Boerma EC, Ince (2010) The role of vasoactive agents in the resuscitation of microvascular perfusion and tissue oxygenation in critically ill patients. Intensive Care Med 36:2004–2018

15. Levick JR, Michel CC (2010) Microvascular fluid exchange and the revised Starling principle. Cardiovasc Res 87:198–210

16. Vincent JL, Ince C, Bakker J (2012) Clinical review: Circulatory shock – an update: a tribute to Professor Max Harry Weil. Crit Care 16:239–243

17. American College of Chest Physician, Society of Critical Care Medicine Consensus Conference (1992) Definitions for sepsis and organ failure and guidelines for the use of innovative therapies in sepsis. Crit Care Med 20:864–874

18. Swan HJ, Ganz W, Forrester J, Marcus H, Diamond G, Chonette D (1970) Catheterization of the heart in man with use of a flow-directed balloon-tipped catheter. N Engl J Med 283:445–447

19. Ganz W, Donoso R, Marcus HS, Forrester JS, Swan HJC (1971) A new technique for measurement of cardiac output by thermodilution in man. Am J Cardiol 27:392–396

20. Bland RD, Shoemaker WC, Abraham E, Cobo JC (1985) Hemodynamic and oxygen transport patterns in surviving and nonsurviving postoperative patients. Crit Care Med 13:85–90

21. Shoemaker WC, Appel PL, Kram HB, Waxman K, Lee TS (1988) Prospective trial of supranormal values of survivors as therapeutic goals in high-risk surgical patients. Chest 94:1176–1186

22. Hayes MA, Timmins AC, Yau EHS, Palazzo M, Hinds CJ, Watson D (1994) Elevtion of systemic oxygen delivery in the treatment of critically ill patients. N Engl J Med 330:1717–1722

23. Ince C, Sinaasappel M (1999) Microcirculatory oxygenation and shunting in sepsis and shock. Crit Care Med 277:H1532–H1539

24. De Backer D, Creteur J, Dubois MJ, Sakr Y, Vincent JL (2004) Microvascular alterations in patients with acute severe heart failure and cardiogenic shock. Am Heart J 147:91–99

25. Pranskunas A, Koopmans M, Koetsier PM, Pilvinis V, Boerma EC (2013) Microcirculatory blood flow as a tool to select ICU patients eligible for fluid therapy. Intensive Care Med 39:612–619

26. Atasever B, Boer C, Speekenbrink R et al (2011) Cardiac displacement during off-pump coronary artery bypass grafting surgery: effect on sublingual microcirculation and cerebral oxygenation. Interact Cardiovasc Thorac Surg 13:573–577

27. Hernandez G, Bruhn A, Ince C (2013) Microcirculation in sepsis: new perspectives. Curr Vasc Pharmacol 11:161–169

28. Xu J, Ma L, Sun S, Lu X, Wu X, Li Z, Tang W (2013) Fluid resuscitation guided by sublingual partial pressure of carbon dioxide during hemorrhagic shock in a porcine model. Shock 39:361–365

29. Schultz SG (2002) William Harvey and the circulation of the blood: the birth of a scientific revolution and modern physiology. News Physiol Sci 17:175–180

30. Harvey W (1628) Exercitato anatomica de motu cordis et sanguinis in animalibus. Sumptibus Gvilielmi Fitzeri, Frankfurt

31. Malpighi M (1661) De pulmonibus observationes anatomicae. Baptistae Ferronii, Bologna

32. Ford BJ (1995) First steps in experimental microscopy, Leeuwenhoek as practical scientist. The Microscope 43:47–57

33. Krahl VE (1962) Observations on the pulmonary alveolus and its capillary circulation in the living rabbit. Anat Rec 142:350

34. Slaaf DW, Tangelder GJ, Reneman RS, Jaeger K, Bollinger A (1987) A versatile incident illuminator for intravital microscopy. Int J Microcirc Clin Exp 6:391–397

35. Mathura KR, Vollebrecht KC, Boer K, de Graaf JC, Ubbink DT, Ince C (2001) Comparison of OPS imaging to intravital capillarosopy of nail fold microcirculation. J Appl Physiol 91:74–78

36. De Backer D, Creteur J, Preiser JC, Dubois MJ, Vincent JL (2002) Microvascular blood flow is altered in patients with sepsis. Am J Respir Crit Care Med 166:98–104

37. Spronk PE, Ince C, Gardien MJ, Mathura KR, Oudemans-van Straaten HM, Zandstra DF (2002) Nitroglycerin in septic shock after intravascular volume resuscitation. Lancet 360:1395–1396
38. Goedhart PT, Khalilzada M, Bezemer R, Merza J, Ince C (2007) Sidestream dark field (SDF) imaging: a novel stroboscopic LED ring-based imaging modality for clinical assessment of the microcirculation. Opt Express 15:15101–15114
39. Dobbe JGG, Streekstra GJ, Atasever B, van Zijderveld R, Ince C (2008) Measurement of functional microcirculatory geometry and velocity distributions using automated image analysis. Med Biol Eng Comput 46:659–670
40. Sallisalmi M, Oksala N, Pettilä V, Tenhunen J (2012) Evaluation of sublingual microcirculatory blood flow in the critically ill. Acta Anaesthesiol Scand 56:298–306
41. Massey M, LaRochelle E, Najarro G et al (2013) The microcirculation image quality score: development and preliminary evaluation of a proposed approach to grading quality of image acquisition for bedside videomicroscopy. J Crit Care 28:913–917
42. De Backer D, Hollenberg S, Boerma C et al (2007) How to evaluate the microcirculation: report of a round table conference. Crit Care 11:R101
43. Boerma EC, Mathura KR, van der Voort PHJ, Spronk PE, Ince C (2005) Quantifying bedside-derived imaging of microcirculatory abnormalities in septic patients: a prospective validation study. Critical Care 9:R601–R606
44. Elbers PE, Ince C (2006) Mechanisms of critical illness: Classifying microcirculatory flow abnormalities in distributive shock. Crit Care 10:221–299
45. Lindert J, Werner J, Redlin M, Kuppe H, Habazettl H, Pries AR (2002) OPS imaging of human circulation: a short technical report. J Vasc Res 39:368–372
46. Bezemer R, Dobbe JG, Bartels SA et al (2011) Rapid automatic assessment of microvascular density in sidestream dark field images. Med Biol Eng Comput 49:1269–1278
47. Bezemer R, Bartels SA, Bakker J, Ince C (2012) Clinical review: Clinical imaging of the sublingual microcirculation in the critically ill– where do we stand? Crit Care 16(3):224
48. Milstein DMJ, Romay E, Ince C (2012) A novel computer-controlled high resolution video microscopy imaging system enables measuring mucosal subsurface focal depth for rapid acquisition of oral microcirculation video images. Intensive Care Med 38:S271
49. Weil MH, Tang W (2007) Welcoming a new era of hemodynamic monitoring: expanding from the macro to the microcirculation. Crit Care Med 35:1204–1205

Part IX
Fluid Therapy

Pulse Pressure Variation in the Management of Fluids in Critically Ill Patients

A. Messina and P. Navalesi

Introduction

In healthy, spontaneously breathing subjects, arterial blood pressure decreases during inspiration. This reduction is commonly slight and unimportant, though it may become more relevant in certain conditions, such as volume depletion and large inspiratory intrathoracic pressure swings. Kussmaul first described the abnormal progression of this phenomenon in patients affected by constrictive pericarditis, observing "pulse disappearing during inspiration and returning during expiration", despite no modification in cardiac activity throughout inspiration and expiration, the so-called pulsus paradoxus [1]. Pulsus paradoxus is considered to occur when the systolic arterial blood pressure decreases by more than 10 mmHg during inspiration. In addition to pericardial tamponade of any etiology, pulsus paradoxus is also observed in situations in which intrathoracic (pleural) pressure swings are exaggerated or the right ventricle is distended, such as acute severe asthma, exacerbations of chronic obstructive pulmonary disease (COPD), and any clinical condition leading to acute pulmonary hypertension [1].

Decades later, a reverse phenomenon to that reported by Kussmaul was observed and described in patients receiving application of positive pressure to the airways through a mechanical ventilator: Arterial blood pressure was found to increase during ventilator insufflation and then decrease during the expiratory phase, initially referred to as reversed pulsus paradoxus [2], paradoxical pulsus paradoxus [3], respirator paradox [4] and, later on, pulse pressure variation (PPV) [5].

A. Messina
Anesthesia and Intensive Care Medicine, Maggiore della Carità University Hospital, Novara, Italy

P. Navalesi ✉
Department of Translational Medicine, Università del Piemonte Orientale "Amedeo Avogadro", Alessandria-Novara-Vercelli, Italy
Anesthesia and Intensive Care Medicine, Sant'Andrea Hospital (ASL VC), Vercelli, Italy
CRRF Mons. L. Novarese, Moncrivello (VC), Italy
e-mail: paolo.navalesi@med.unipmn.it

J.-L. Vincent (Ed.), *Annual Update in Intensive Care and Emergency Medicine 2014*, 385
DOI 10.1007/978-3-319-03746-2_29, © Springer International Publishing Switzerland 2014

From Physiology to Clinical Application

Many studies have investigated the physiological basis of this phenomenon. Following the intuition of Rick and Burke, who first suggested its relationship with a patient's volemic status [4], several animal studies clarified the physiologic determinants of PPV [6–8]. However, despite progress in the comprehension of the underlying physiological mechanisms, the clinical use of PPV remained marginal for many years. At the end of the 1990s, a survey reported that only 1 % of physicians in Germany considered the arterial blood pressure swings through the respiratory cycle in the decision-making process regarding volume expansion [9].

An accurate approach to fluid management is essential to avoid both depletion and overload of fluids. For this reason, the routine use of validated indicators of a patient's position on the Frank-Starling curve is crucial, especially in specific clinical conditions. Although aggressive fluid therapy is helpful in the early phase of septic shock [10], patients receiving large amounts of fluid in the emergency room without a specific hemodynamic target or limit are exposed to an increased risk of fluid overload once renal function gets worse. Therapeutic strategies founded on fluid restriction can improve the outcome of patients with acute respiratory failure associated with a shorter duration of mechanical ventilation and reduced intensive care unit (ICU) lengths of stay [11]. Nonetheless, volemic status is still often only approximately estimated. For example, in critically ill patients undergoing continuous hemofiltration, the balance between the ultrafiltrated plasma water and the infused replacement volume is often determined by measuring body weight and then adjusting when hypotension occurs.

Assessing Volemic Status

The possibility of defining *a priori* whether or not fluid therapy is indicated and to properly guide its titration is of paramount importance for the management of critically ill patients. For this reason, ICU physicians have been continuously seeking indicators able to predict a patient's response to fluids. Although decades ago physicians based their clinical judgment primarily on physical examination and urine output, subsequently they relied predominantly on static indexes requiring invasive procedures. These static indexes share a number of assumptions and their use is based on a simplified approach, i. e., the lower the value, the greater the need for fluid replacement. Because of the complex physiological interactions between cardiac preload and afterload, ventricular interdependence, and thoracic and pulmonary compliance, however, this approach may result in erroneous evaluations of volemic status and potentially lead to inappropriate fluid administration in several clinical conditions.

Central Venous Pressure

Interestingly, despite many published studies in various clinical conditions showing no relationship between fluid responsiveness and central venous pressure (CVP), either in absolute value or rate of variation [12], according to a recent European survey, most (up to 90 %) ICU physicians use CVP to guide fluid management. Concomitantly, a Canadian survey also reported that 90 % of intensivists utilize CVP to monitor fluid replacement in patients with septic shock [13].

CVP provides a good approximation of the right atrial (RA) pressure, which is a determinant of right ventricular (RV) preload and, consequently, of left ventricular (LV) filling. Consequent to these considerations, for decades CVP has been assumed to provide a reliable, though indirect, estimation of LV preload. According to this dogma, patients with a low CVP are volume depleted, whereas patients with high CVP are overloaded. Unfortunately, changes in venous tone, intrathoracic pressures, LV and RV compliance, and interventricular septum geometry make the relationship between the CVP and RV end-diastolic volume inconsistent. Poor sensitivity and specificity of CVP in predicting the improvement in cardiac output following rapid fluid infusion [12, 14] make CVP unhelpful for guiding fluid management in the ICU, operating room, or emergency room [14].

Pulmonary Artery Occlusion Pressure

Another static index that has received high consideration for guiding fluid management in critically ill patients is the pulmonary artery occlusion pressure (PAOP) or wedge pressure, which requires positioning of a pulmonary artery catheter (PAC). Although the PAC remains the 'gold standard' for determining cardiac output in critically ill patients, its use has markedly decreased [15, 16] because of the results of recent randomized trials and meta-analyses suggesting little or no clinical benefit [15, 17–19]. The elevated risk of inaccurate measurements and the need for highly trained specialists for correct interpretation of the numerous parameters obtained make the use of PACs problematic [15, 16]. Specific indications for PAC monitoring in the ICU remain diagnosis and treatment of acute RV failure and pulmonary hypertension [20], as occurs in significant proportions of patients with acute respiratory distress syndrome (ARDS), and weaning failure of cardiac origin [20]. The PAC also remains indicated in ICU patients with severe heart failure, with or without shock, necessitating inotropic, vasopressor, and/or vasodilator therapy [20].

The aforementioned German survey [9] also showed that in the late 1990s more than half the intensivists used PAOP to guide fluid therapy, considering as hypovolemic patients with low PAOP (< 10 mmHg) and hypervolemic those with high PAOP (> 18 mmHg). More recently, PAOP has also been regarded as a poor indicator of preload and its use to predict fluid responsiveness is limited to the extremes values only [21]. In fact, the relationship between PAOP and LV end-diastolic volume (LVEDV) is not linear and may be quite different among subjects.

Moreover, even assuming it approximates left atrial pressure, PAOP poorly reflects LV end-diastolic pressure (LVEDP) because it does not consider either the diastolic pressure rise induced by the atrial contraction or by the pericardial pressure surrounding the heart, which opposes LV distension. Cardiac tamponade, pulmonary hyperinflation, active inspiratory and expiratory muscle efforts, determining rapid and potentially remarkable changes in intrathoracic pressure, may all alter pericardial pressure, LV diastolic function, and then LVEDV, without necessarily affecting PAOP. Finally, even without considering these limitations, LV diastolic compliance may rapidly vary, consequent to several clinical events occurring over a few heart beats, such as myocardial ischemia, arrhythmias, and acute RV dilation, thereby changing the relationship between LV filling pressure and end-diastolic volume.

PAOP may also be affected by the position of the PAC tip within the pulmonary vessels. PAC tip balloon occlusion stops blood flow distally to the catheter. Considering a continuous column of blood from the catheter tip to the left atrium, PAOP then measures pulmonary venous pressure. When the pressure inside the alveoli exceeds that of the pulmonary vessels, however, the occlusion pressure may actually reflect the former rather than the latter. This condition occurs when the catheter tip ends in West zone 1 and, less frequently, in zone 2 [22]. The PAC tip, nonetheless, commonly ends in the vessels of the dependent lung regions (West zone 3), where the ventilation/perfusion ratio is lower [22].

Pulse Pressure Variation Estimation

PPV is calculated as follows:

$$\frac{PP_{max} - PP_{min}}{1/2(PP_{max} + PP_{min})} \times 100$$

Pulse pressure is the difference between systolic and diastolic arterial pressure. Maximal (PP_{max}) and minimal (PP_{min}) pulse pressures are calculated over a single respiratory cycle. Additionally, it has been observed that PP_{max} and PP_{min} occur during the inspiratory and expiratory phases, respectively. A cut-off PPV value of 12–13 % is considered to predict fluid responsiveness [14, 23].

Although the physiological determinants of PPV were clarified in the 1980s, its use was limited for decades by the lack of commercially available devices automatically detecting PPV for clinical applications [24]. The first available monitoring device providing PPV was the PiCCO system (Pulsion Medical Systems, Germany). Unfortunately, the first algorithm used by PiCCO had technical limitations, mostly related to the decline in PPV reliability consequent to sudden hemodynamic variations or artifacts. These limitations were largely overcome by the first non-proprietary algorithm for automatic PPV determination, available since 2004. This algorithm was proved to be as valid as the gold standard represented by manual PPV assessment [25, 26] and was then adopted by other monitoring

Table 1 Limitations of pulse pressure variation (PPV)

Variable	Implication
Ventilator mode	PPV accurately predicts fluid responsiveness in the ICU setting only during controlled mechanical ventilation
Breathing pattern	PPV sensitivity and specificity worsen when tidal volume is less than 8 ml/kg. High respiratory rates decrease the number of cardiac beats per respiratory cycle, reducing the ability of PPV to detect respiratory variations in stroke volume.
Cardiac function	Need for sinus rhythm. Arrhythmias cause beat-to-beat variations in stroke volume and blood pressure unrelated to mechanical ventilation. Heart failure may modify the response to the variations in cardiac preload and afterload consequent to mechanical ventilation.
Respiratory mechanics	PPV specificity is reduced when lung compliance is severely reduced, in particular when chest wall impedance is normal or near-normal.
Miscellaneous	Increased adrenergic tone in response to conditions such as pain, anxiety, noise, or dyspnea. Open chest. Air bubbles, kinks, clot formation, excessively long and/or compliant tubing of the arterial monitoring system.

ICU: intensive care unit

devices. Since 2009, two new algorithms have been proposed for PPV calculation that use either a state-space model or a nonlinear analysis technique, based on entropy [24].

The Achilles' heel of pulse pressure variation

PPV has limitations and drawbacks that must be considered. In mechanically ventilated ICU patients, PPV derives from the interaction between the positive pressure applied by the ventilator and cardiac function. This interaction is also responsible for most of PPV's limitations (Table 1).

During controlled mechanical ventilation, RV preload and afterload are both affected by the inspiratory increase in pleural pressure, which reduces venous return, and increases transpulmonary pressure [27]; as a consequence, ventilator insufflation determines a reduction in RV stroke volume. The subsequent reduction in LV filling (evident after a lag of two or three heart beats due to the blood pulmonary transit time) leads in turn to LV stroke volume reduction. Worth mentioning, these cyclic changes in RV and LV stroke volume are related to the operating portion of both ventricles on the Frank-Starling curve [14, 27, 28]. The magnitude of these reductions caused by mechanical ventilation is greater when the right and left ventricles operate on the steeper part of the curve, and is reduced when they operate on the flat part [27]. The variations in LV stroke volume are associated with pulse pressure (i. e., the difference between systolic and diastolic pressure), which is directly proportional to LV stroke volume and inversely related to arterial compliance. Because mechanical ventilation does not affect pulse pressure *per se,* because the rise in pleural pressure affects both diastolic and systolic pressures at the same time, the modifications in peripheral pulse pressure are determined by LV stroke volume variations consequent to peripheral pulse pressure changes throughout the respiratory cycle [27].

A review article recently compared the diagnostic accuracy of PPV obtained by different studies with the results of other static and dynamic indexes of fluid responsiveness [23]. The area under the curve (AUC) was 0.94 for PPV, which out-performed other dynamic indexes, such as systolic pressure variation (AUC 0.86) and stroke volume variation (SVV, AUC 0.84). This difference was even larger when comparing PPV with static indexes; in fact the AUCs of the LV end-diastolic area index (LVEDAI), as obtained by transesophageal echocardiography, the global end-diastolic volume index (GEDVI), as obtained by transpulmonary thermodilution, and the CVP were 0.64, 0.56 and 0.55, respectively [23].

Unfortunately, the excellent performance of PPV in predicting fluid responsiveness during mechanical ventilation is limited to the ventilatory modes of total support, so-called controlled modes, in which the respiratory muscles are passive and do not contribute at all to the generation of the ventilatory output. In fact, PPV accuracy decreases when applied in patients undergoing mechanical ventilation with modes of partial assistance in which the effort exerted by the inspiratory muscles interacts with the machine to generate ventilation [29]. While the forms of total support, associated or not with blocking agents, were widely used in the past, today the early use of partial ventilatory support, such as pressure support ventilation (PSV), has become a cornerstone in the management of mechanically ventilated ICU patients [30]. PSV is commonly used in the weaning process, which encompasses up to 40 % of the whole duration of mechanical ventilation [31]. The risk of inappropriate fluid therapy during partial ventilatory support is thus significantly higher, since the performance of the best available dynamic index is limited [23, 29]. Heenen et al. [32] found poor correlation between PPV and fluid responsiveness (AUC 0.64 ± 0.26) in nine patients ventilated with pressure support, and Monnet et al. [33] reported a sensitivity of 75 % and a specificity of 46 % for PPV $\geq 12\,\%$ in a heterogeneous group of 19 patients with spontaneous breathing activity (5 patients receiving PSV and 14 assist/control mode).

This finding may have different explanations. The physiological basis of the dynamic indices of preload relies on the changes in stroke volume induced by the variations in intrathoracic pressure. The ability of PPV to properly predict fluid responsiveness is influenced by both cardiovascular and respiratory mechanisms [34, 35]. PPV is reliable during controlled mechanical ventilation when the cyclic changes in both intrathoracic (pleural) and transpulmonary pressures are large enough to remarkably affect RV stroke volume and LV stroke volume [34, 35]. Patients receiving PSV may be characterized by reduced tidal volume (V_T) [29], because of a low inspiratory support level, and by a concomitant elevated respiratory rate (RR). A limited increase in lung volume may be insufficient to increase pleural pressure enough to decrease venous return and then RV preload [34]. In addition, the role of V_T with respect to PPV reliability has been recently confirmed by several clinical investigations in ARDS patients, mechanically ventilated according to the currently recommended lung protective strategy ($V_T \leq 6\,ml/kg$). In this setting, a PPV > 10–12 % maintains a good predictive value, whereas a PPV < 10 % is less specific of fluid unresponsiveness because of the increased rate of false-negative cases [36]. In this specific condition, protective ventilation of ARDS patients, a low PPV may be consequent to relatively small swings in pleural pressure during insufflation when lung compliance is very low with normal or near normal chest wall impedance, without truly reflecting the volemic status [36].

During partial ventilatory support, because of the active inspiration [29] sometimes associated with expiratory muscles recruitment [32], the cyclic changes in alveolar pressure may become irregular; moreover, because of abrupt changes in abdominal pressure, RV preload can be increased consequent to squeezing of blood from the abdomen to the thorax [37].

PPV is not helpful during spontaneous unassisted breathing. Increased adrenergic tone in response to conditions such as pain, anxiety, noise, or dyspnea, may play a role [32]. In a study including 32 hemodynamically unstable ICU patients breathing spontaneously with no ventilator assistance, sensitivity and specificity of PPV (> 12 %) were 63 % and 92 %, respectively [38]. In addition, when the patients were asked to perform a deep inspiration followed by a forced expiration, sensitivity actually further decreased down to 21 %, while specificity remained unchanged. This maneuver was performed with the purpose of enhancing PPV sensitivity by expanding the variation in intrathoracic pressure. Actually, the increased magnitude of V_T determined an artificial and transient variation in RV stroke volume, changing the operating portion of the RV Frank-Starling curve and leading the patient to a preload dependency unrelated to the true volemic status [38].

The effects of a deep inflation followed by forced expiration have been evaluated in spontaneously breathing patients with hemodynamic instability, but no published study has so far assessed the effects of an inspiratory maneuver against a quasi-closed airway, as occurs when the patient's inspiratory muscles exert an effort not followed by ventilator assistance, the so-called ineffective or wasted inspiratory effort. Ineffective or wasted efforts represent the most common form of patient ventilator dyssynchrony during PSV and have recently been shown to be more frequent than previously considered, reaching up to 25 % of the total number of breaths in patients mechanically ventilated for more than 24 hours [39, 40]. By determining a negative swing in intrathoracic pressure associated with little or no V_T, the ineffective or wasted effort might generate an irregular and variable increase in venous return and RV filling that, consequent to the ventricular diastolic interdependence, makes the LV stiffer, hampering its filling, reducing pulse pressure and, ultimately, increasing PPV [41].

RV and LV failure may also impair PPV effectiveness in predicting fluid responsiveness. When RV output is compromised, the inspiratory increase in transpulmonary pressure may accentuate the reduction in RV stroke volume due to the compromised systolic function. Moreover, because of LV failure, pulmonary venous pressure increases, which expands the size of the West zones III, where the pressure in the alveoli is less than in the pulmonary vessels. In this condition, ventilator insufflation increases pulmonary venous flow and LV preload. Also, the increased pleural pressure induced by the insufflation reduces LV transmural pressure and, consequently, LV afterload. Finally, a failing ventricle works on the flat portion of the Frank-Starling curve and is, therefore, less influenced by the changes in preload and afterload produced by mechanical ventilation [34–36, 42]. Of note, a small, though significant, increase in PPV (from 5.3 % to 6.9 %) was recently described by Keyl et al. during ventricular resynchronization, which improves LV contractility [43].

PPV is also affected by other conditions not related to heart-lung interaction. PPV is useless in the presence of cardiac arrhythmias [36]. Heart rate (HR) also plays a role. HR to RR ratio (HR/RR) has recently been identified as a determinant of PPV's success in detecting fluid responsiveness. With HR/RR values < 3.6, PPV does not reliably predict fluid responsiveness, likely because when HR is low the pulmonary transit time is too long relative to the respiratory cycle [44]. A high RR decreases the chance of detecting variations in stroke volume throughout the respiratory cycle because of the reduced number of heart beats occurring during each breath [32]. Differences between central (e. g., femoral) and peripheral (e. g., radial) systolic and pulse pressures have been reported in septic patients and after cardiopulmonary bypass, which may potentially affect PPV calculation [36]. The stiffness of the arterial tree, as occurs in elderly patients, alters systolic and pulse pressure and causes large variations in arterial pressure in spite of relatively small changes in LV stroke volume [36]. Finally, air bubbles, kinks, clot formation, excessively long and/or compliant tubing may all affect the dynamic response of the invasive arterial monitoring system and should be carefully excluded. The dynamic response of the monitoring system can be assessed by a fast-flush test [36].

Conclusions and Future Perspectives

PPV is currently an excellent means of predicting fluid responsiveness in ICU patients without major impairment in respiratory mechanics and heart function, and undergoing controlled mechanical ventilation with $V_T \geq 8$ ml/kg. PPV's effectiveness in ascertaining fluid responsiveness is reduced when the patient receives modes of partial support, such as PSV. Improved knowledge of the mechanisms underlying this limitation might lead to application of PPV in a large subgroup of patients receiving PSV and other forms of partial assistance, such as proportional assist ventilation (PAV), neutrally-adjusted ventilatory assist (NAVA), and noisy-PSV [45], designed to improve patient-ventilator interactions and synchrony.

References

1. Bilchick KC, Wise RA (2002) Paradoxical physical findings described by Kussmaul: pulsus paradoxus and Kussmaul's sign. Lancet 359:1940–1942
2. Massumi RA, Mason DT, Vera Z, Zelis R, Otero J, Amsterdam EA (1973) Reversed pulsus paradoxus. N Engl J Med 289:1272–1275
3. Vaisrub S (1974) Editorial: Paradoxical pulsus paradoxus. JAMA 229:74
4. Rick JJ, Burke SS (1978) Respirator paradox. South Med J 71:1376–1378

5. Michard F, Chemla D, Richard C et al (1999) Clinical use of respiratory changes in arterial pulse pressure to monitor the hemodynamic effects of PEEP. Am J Respir Crit Care Med 159:935–939
6. Perel A, Pizov R, Cotev S (1987) Systolic blood pressure variation is a sensitive indicator of hypovolemia in ventilated dogs subjected to graded hemorrhage. Anesthesiology 67:498–502
7. Preisman S, DiSegni E, Vered Z, Perel A (2002) Left ventricular preload and function during graded haemorrhage and retranfusion in pigs: analysis of arterial pressure waveform and correlation with echocardiography. Br J Anaesth 88:716–718
8. Preisman S, Pfeiffer U, Lieberman N, Perel A (1997) New monitors of intravascular volume: a comparison of arterial pressure waveform analysis and the intrathoracic blood volume. Intensive Care Med 23:651–657
9. Boldt J, Lenz M, Kumle B, Papsdorf M (1998) Volume replacement strategies on intensive care units: results from a postal survey. Intensive Care Med 24:147–151
10. Dellinger RP, Levy MM, Annane D, Rhodes A et al (2013) Surviving sepsis campaign: international guidelines for management of severe sepsis and septic shock: 2012. Crit Care Med 41:580–637
11. Wiedemann HP, Wheeler AP, Bernard GR et al (2006) Comparison of two fluid-management strategies in acute lung injury. N Engl J Med 354:2564–2575
12. Marik PE, Baram M, Vahid B (2008) Does central venous pressure predict fluid responsiveness? A systematic review of the literature and the tale of seven mares. Chest 134:172–178
13. McIntyre LA, Hebert PC, Fergusson D et al (2007) A survey of Canadian intensivists' resuscitation practices in early septic shock. Crit Care 11:R74
14. Marik PE, Monnet X, Teboul JL (2011) Hemodynamic parameters to guide fluid therapy. Ann Intensive Care 1:1
15. Rajaram SS, Desai NK, Kalra A, et al (2013) Pulmonary artery catheters for adult patients in intensive care. Cochrane Database Syst Rev 2:CD003408
16. Pinsky MR, Vincent JL (2005) Let us use the pulmonary artery catheter correctly and only when we need it. Crit Care Med 33:1119–1122
17. Sandham JD, Hull RD, Brant RF et al (2003) A randomized, controlled trial of the use of pulmonary-artery catheters in high-risk surgical patients. N Engl J Med 348:5–14
18. Richard C, Warszawski J, Anguel N et al (2003) Early use of the pulmonary artery catheter and outcomes in patients with shock and acute respiratory distress syndrome: a randomized controlled trial. JAMA 290:2713–2720
19. Harvey S, Harrison DA, Singer M et al (2005) Assessment of the clinical effectiveness of pulmonary artery catheters in management of patients in intensive care (PAC-Man): a randomised controlled trial. Lancet 366:472–477
20. Vincent JL, Pinsky MR, Sprung CL et al (2008) The pulmonary artery catheter: in medio virtus. Crit Care Med 36:3093–3096
21. Pinsky MR (2003) Clinical significance of pulmonary artery occlusion pressure. Intensive Care Med 29:175–178
22. Pinsky MR (2003) Pulmonary artery occlusion pressure. Intensive Care Med 29:19–22
23. Marik PE, Cavallazzi R, Vasu T, Hirani A (2009) Dynamic changes in arterial waveform derived variables and fluid responsiveness in mechanically ventilated patients: a systematic review of the literature. Crit Care Med 37:2642–2647
24. Cannesson M, Aboy M, Hofer CK, Rehman M (2011) Pulse pressure variation: where are we today? J Clin Monit Comput 25:45–56
25. Cannesson M, Slieker J, Desebbe O et al (2008) The ability of a novel algorithm for automatic estimation of the respiratory variations in arterial pulse pressure to monitor fluid responsiveness in the operating room. Anesth Analg 106:1195–1200
26. Aboy M, Crespo C, Austin D (2009) An enhanced automatic algorithm for estimation of respiratory variations in arterial pulse pressure during regions of abrupt hemodynamic changes. IEEE Trans Biomed Eng 56:2537–2545

27. Michard F, Teboul JL (2000) Using heart-lung interactions to assess fluid responsiveness during mechanical ventilation. Crit Care 4:282–289
28. Magder S (2011) Hemodynamic monitoring in the mechanically ventilated patient. Curr Opin Crit Care 17:36–42
29. De Backer D, Pinsky MR (2007) Can one predict fluid responsiveness in spontaneously breathing patients? Intensive Care Med 33:1111–1113
30. McConville JF, Kress JP (2012) Weaning patients from the ventilator. N Engl J Med 367:2233–2239
31. Branson RD (2012) Modes to facilitate ventilator weaning. Respir Care 57:1635–1648
32. Heenen S, De Backer D, Vincent JL (2006) How can the response to volume expansion in patients with spontaneous respiratory movements be predicted? Crit Care 10:R102
33. Monnet X, Rienzo M, Osman D et al (2006) Passive leg raising predicts fluid responsiveness in the critically ill. Crit Care Med 34:1402–1407
34. Feihl F, Broccard AF (2009) Interactions between respiration and systemic hemodynamics. Part I: basic concepts. Intensive Care Med 35:45–54
35. Feihl F, Broccard AF (2009) Interactions between respiration and systemic hemodynamics. Part II: practical implications in critical care. Intensive Care Med 35:198–205
36. Michard F (2005) Changes in arterial pressure during mechanical ventilation. Anesthesiology 103:419–428
37. Takata M, Beloucif S, Shimada M, Robotham JL (1992) Superior and inferior vena caval flows during respiration: pathogenesis of Kussmaul's sign. Am J Physiol 262:H763–H770
38. Soubrier S, Saulnier F, Hubert H et al (2007) Can dynamic indicators help the prediction of fluid responsiveness in spontaneously breathing critically ill patients? Intensive Care Med 33:1117–1124
39. Chao DC, Scheinhorn DJ, Stearn-Hassenpflug M (1997) Patient-ventilator trigger asynchrony in prolonged mechanical ventilation. Chest 112:1592–1599
40. Thille AW, Rodriguez P, Cabello B, Lellouche F, Brochard L (2006) Patient-ventilator asynchrony during assisted mechanical ventilation. Intensive Care Med 32:1515–1522
41. Messina A, Colombo D, Cammarota G, De Lucia M, Della Corte F, Navalesi P (2013) Fluid responsiveness in pressure support ventilation: role of asynchrony. Crit Care 17:P202 (abst)
42. Michard F, Lopes MR, Auler JO Jr (2007) Pulse pressure variation: beyond the fluid management of patients with shock. Crit Care 11:131
43. Keyl C, Stockinger J, Laule S, Staier K, Schiebeling-Romer J, Wiesenack C (2007) Changes in pulse pressure variability during cardiac resynchronization therapy in mechanically ventilated patients. Crit Care 11:R46
44. De Backer D, Taccone FS, Holsten R, Ibrahimi F, Vincent JL (2009) Influence of respiratory rate on stroke volume variation in mechanically ventilated patients. Anesthesiology 110:1092–1097
45. Navalesi P, Costa R (2003) New modes of mechanical ventilation: proportional assist ventilation, neurally adjusted ventilatory assist, and fractal ventilation. Curr Opin Crit Care 9:51–58

Albumin: Therapeutic Role in the Current Era

A. Farrugia and M. Bansal

Introduction: Albumin's Historical Position

The development of albumin as a blood substitute and plasma expanding agent has been reviewed [1]. This role appeared unquestioned over the first four decades of its use, although the tenets of current evidence-based assessment were lacking. The application of one of these tenets, through the generation of a Cochrane review in 1998 [2], threw doubts on the safety of albumin and had a drastic effect on usage [3]. It is probable that this contributed to the rapid ascendancy of hydroxyethyl starch solutions (HES) as the predominant colloid fluid therapy in the 2000s [4], despite the already established adverse events associated with these compounds. The obviation of much of the evidence base for HES through the Boldt scandal [5], coupled with the increasing body of evidence that all types of HES were associated with serious adverse effects [6], has led the regulatory agencies of the United States [7] and Europe [8] to severely restrict the use of these products in critical illness. It seems unlikely that HES will regain a significant position in fluid replacement therapy and the position of albumin as the colloid least associated with adverse events [9] has undergone a remarkable evolution since the questions raised by the Cochrane review. The usage of albumin has increased to levels exceeding those in the pre-Cochrane review period (Fig. 1) and a huge increase in usage has occurred in Asia, because of a heavy demand for albumin in China (Fig. 2).

Given that albumin continues to be an important product, the purpose of this chapter is to review its basic biological properties and assess their role in albumin's current and potential use in clinical therapeutics.

A. Farrugia ✉
School of Surgery, University of Western Australia, Crawley, Australia
e-mail: albert.farrugia@uwa.edu.au

M. Bansal
Plasma Protein Therapeutics Association, Annapolis, Maryland USA

J.-L. Vincent (Ed.), *Annual Update in Intensive Care and Emergency Medicine 2014*, 395
DOI 10.1007/978-3-319-03746-2_30, © Springer International Publishing Switzerland
2014

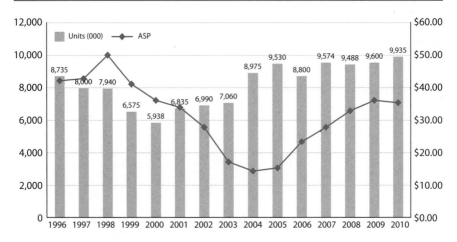

Fig. 1 The albumin market in the USA. Data from the Market Research Bureau. ASP: average sales price

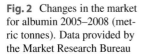

Fig. 2 Changes in the market for albumin 2005–2008 (metric tonnes). Data provided by the Market Research Bureau

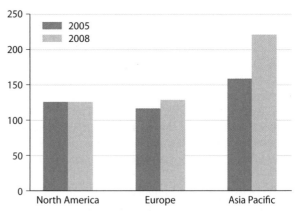

Basic Physiology

Structure/Function Relationships

Human albumin accounts for approximately 55 % of total serum protein content (40 g/l or 0.601 mmol/l) and 80 % of plasma oncotic pressure. Albumin is specifically synthesized by hepatocytes following transcription of the albumin gene on chromosome 4. Analbuminemia is a rare congenital defect in which lack of albumin synthesis is compensated by production of other proteins to maintain oncotic function, and is accompanied by severe morbidity, mortality and pre-term death [10]. Albumin is synthesized at a rate of 12–25 g/day, accounting for 50 % of the energy consumption of the hepatocytes [11]. The total body albumin pool measures about

Fig. 3 Structure of the albumin molecule

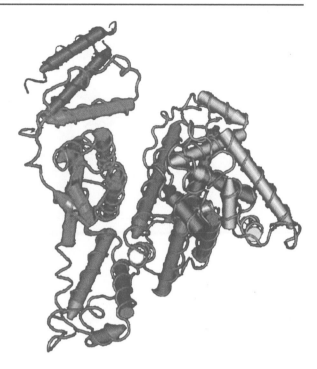

250–300 g for a healthy 70 kg adult. The distribution of albumin between plasma and extravascular compartments has been described previously [12].

Albumin consists of a single polypeptide chain of 585 amino acids with a molecular weight of 66,500 Da. Its three-dimensional structure is composed of three domains that are linked through 17 S-S bonds between 35 cysteine residues. The Cys-34 residue is the only free cysteine in the whole molecule. Albumin has a heart-shaped tertiary structure, but in solution is ellipsoid. Albumin is composed of 3 homologous domains (I–III), each containing two sub-domains (A and B) composed of 4 and 6 α-helices respectively. The sub-domains move relative to one another by means of flexible loops provided by proline residues. This, together with the flexibility provided by domain-linking disulfide bridges assists the binding of substances (below). The *in vivo* architecture [13] (Fig. 3) results in the formation of hydrophobic pockets with exposure of amino acid residues that affect the non-oncotic properties of albumin [14]. Three structural characteristics are of major importance in relation to albumin's possible role in pathophysiological processes:

- The presence of an exposed −SH (thiol) group over cysteine residue at position 34 (Fig. 4), which provides extracellular antioxidant activity [15], binds to nitric oxide (NO) and generates S-nitrosothiols [16];
- Albumin domains I and II enable the transport of various endogenous (fatty acids, toxins, metals) and exogenous (drugs) molecules (Fig. 5), some of which may show competition for binding sites.
- Albumin is relatively very soluble in water through its high content of ionizable amino acids. Ionizable groups may be present in the dissociated (ionized) or

Fig. 4 The exposed thiol residue in the albumin molecule

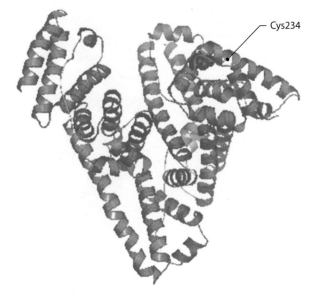

Fig. 5 Drug binding sites in the albumin molecule

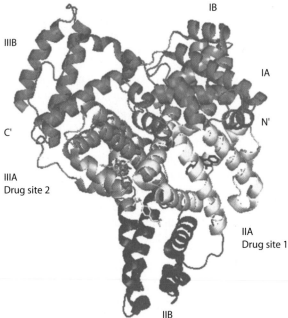

non-dissociated form (non-ionized) and constitute the amino-terminal residues. At physiological pH, the –NH$_2$ residues of lysine and arginine (pK $\approx$ 10–12) contribute positive charge whereas the –COOH carboxylic residues of aspartate and glutamate contribute negative charge. A net negative fixed charge equal to

–21 Eq/mol ensues, independent of pH values. In addition to the fixed charges, albumin contains 16 histidine residues, the imidazole groups of which may react with H^+ at a given pH [17]. This gives albumin buffering capacity which may play an important role in the extravascular space.

Therapeutic Application

Figure 6 depicts the breakdown of usage of albumin in the USA. The traditional approved indication for correcting hypovolemia when this is clinically indicated still constitutes the majority of usage. Other emerging areas of usage draw on the pharmacologic properties of albumin, reflecting the biochemical aspects reviewed above. We will assess some of these areas.

Volume Replacement/Substitution

The position of albumin as the major contributor of plasma oncotic pressure makes it the natural choice for volume replacement and represents its initial and historical use. This position is part of the constant debate on whether crystalloids or colloids should be used for fluid replacement; a debate which we feel is beyond our scope in this article. We note the constant iterations of the relevant Cochrane review [18], now moderated to reflect the latest findings on HES solutions, the use of which is now severely restricted in most areas of critical care as discussed earlier. Demonstrations of the superiority of colloids in maintaining hemodynamic parameters and clinical outcomes in volume replacement during cardiac [19] and

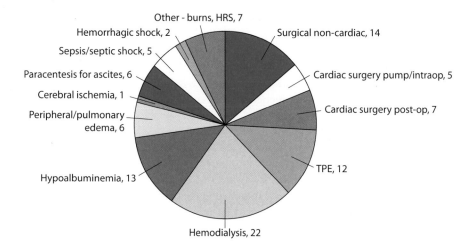

Fig. 6 Percentage share of indications in the US albumin market, 2011. Data from the Market Research Bureau. HRS: hepato-renal syndrome; TPE: therapeutic plasma exchange

general [20] surgery and in treating the progressive anemia of hemorrhage [21] must, therefore, be evaluated with this in mind, and albumin's role in these areas, previously diminished relative to HES because of cost issues, will likely be reinforced.

Hypoalbuminemia is well established as a prognostic indicator in many disease states and, despite a paucity of evidence that albumin administration improves survival, analysis of dose-dependency in controlled trials of albumin therapy suggested that complication rates may be reduced when the serum albumin level attained during albumin administration exceeds 30 g/l [22]. This observation may explain the continuing use of albumin in this condition, including a substantial usage in correcting hypoalbuminemia-related hypotension in hemodialysis patients [23], despite the Cochrane Review's conclusion [24]. Trials supporting the use of HES [25] are subject to the same qualification discussed above, particularly in view of the renal injury which may be more serious for these susceptible patients. Albumin is superior to artificial colloids in this setting [26], through mechanisms which, intriguingly, include a specific reduction in oxidative stress by albumin [27]. Despite conflicting clinical trial evidence [28, 29], the strong relationship between hypoalbuminemia and hypotension in this condition [30] argues for continuing investigation into the use of albumin.

The use of albumin for volume replacement/expansion in coronary artery bypass graft (CABG) surgery, both as a pump priming fluid and postoperatively, is well reflected in current usage (Fig. 6). Albumin maintains a less positive fluid balance then crystalloids when used as a priming agent [31]. Albumin levels are a strong predictor of morbidity and mortality [32, 33] and albumin administration maintains hemodynamic stability [34] and decreases mortality [35], through mechanisms which may include albumin's role in suppressing inflammation [36] and endothelial activation [37], which are both pathological outcomes in CABG [38, 39].

Pharmacological Effects

The concept of albumin as a drug has gained credence as the biochemical features outlined above have been recognized as having potential therapeutic effects independent of volume expansion [40]. In fact, as observed in the hemodialysis and cardiac environments, volume effects can also be mediated through pharmacological action, and it is likely that the two aspects work in tandem. Of primary importance is the well-characterized anti-oxidant capacity of albumin contributed by the single exposed thiol group at position 34 (Fig. 4), which is the principal extracellular antioxidant and chiefly responsible for maintaining the redox state of plasma. Free thiols have been shown to be important in potentially influencing processes that determine cellular fate or apoptosis (Fig. 7).

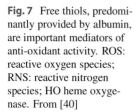

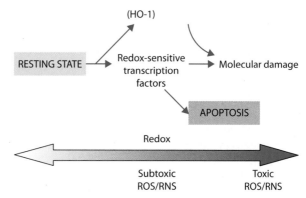

Fig. 7 Free thiols, predominantly provided by albumin, are important mediators of anti-oxidant activity. ROS: reactive oxygen species; RNS: reactive nitrogen species; HO heme oxygenase. From [40]

Sepsis

Sepsis has been proposed as a disease of the microcirculation [41] and several facets of this pathological concept may be modulated by albumin (Fig. 8). These include the inhibition of endothelial activation [37], decreased edema formation through inhibiting sepsis-induced capillary permeability [42] and preservation of normal blood rheology [43]. In a subgroup analysis of the SAFE study [44] and a subsequent meta-analysis [45] a survival benefit was apparent when treating septic patients with albumin. It is possible that the anti-oxidant process outlined earlier contributes to this effect. Albumin administered to patients with sepsis results in increased plasma thiol levels which are sustained after the albumin is cleared from the circulation [46]. This may initiate cascades of thiol oxidative-reductive reactions and influence cellular signaling processes. Despite the increased capillary

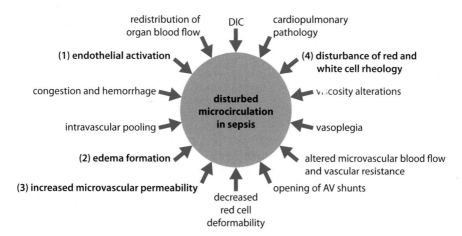

Fig. 8 Microcirculatory pathology in sepsis showing areas (1–4) of possible moderation by albumin. DIC: disseminated intravascular coagulation. From [41]

permeability seen in sepsis, albumin administered to septic patients expands the plasma volume [47] and exerts a hemodynamic effect [44]. Preliminary results from a major trial confirm the benefits of albumin in septic shock [48]. These findings suggest cumulatively that the Surviving Sepsis Campaign's recommendation of albumin as the fluid of choice when colloid resuscitation is needed is based on evidence [49].

Summary and Conclusions

Fluid replacement in critical care has undergone considerable turmoil over the past 20 years, as, in addition to the crystalloid versus colloid debate, issues about the safety of fluids have contributed to the questions, "Which crystalloid?" and "Which colloid?". The extraordinary claims of the Cochrane review were rapidly dismissed through evidence, but not before they contributed to the grip of HES on the fluid market. The pendulum has now swung to the virtual exclusion of these compounds because of their adverse effects, and a renewed interest in albumin. The clinical benefits described in this work are a reflection of unique biochemical features resulting from albumin's position as an essential human protein. Other clear benefits in areas such as hepatology are beyond our current scope but are also the result of these features combining volume and pharmacological effects. The considerable ongoing basic and clinical research into the therapeutic effects of albumin will continue to ensure this protein's role in the therapeutic armamentarium for intensive care physicians.

References

1. Farrugia A (2010) Albumin usage in clinical medicine: tradition or therapeutic? Transf Med Rev 24:53–63
2. Reviewers CIGA (1998) Human albumin administration in critically ill patients: systematic review of randomised controlled trials. BMJ 317:235–240
3. Roberts I, Edwards P, McLelland B (1999) More on albumin. BMJ 318:1214
4. Finfer S, Liu B, Taylor C et al (2010) Resuscitation fluid use in critically ill adults: an international cross-sectional study in 391 intensive care units. Crit Care 14:R185
5. Wise J (2013) Boldt: the great pretender. BMJ 346:f1738
6. Myburgh J, McIntyre L (2013) New insights into fluid resuscitation. Intensive Care Med 39:998–1001
7. Food and Drug Administration (2013) FDA Safety Communication: Boxed warning on increased mortality and severe renal injury, and additional warning on risk of bleeding, for use of hydroxyethyl starch solutions in some settings. Available at: http://www.fda.gov/BiologicsBloodVaccines/SafetyAvailability/ucm358271.htm. Accessed September 2013
8. European Medicines Agency (2013) PRAC confirms that hydroxyethyl-starch solutions (HES) should no longer be used in patients with sepsis or burn injuries or in critically ill patients. Available at: http://www.ema.europa.eu/ema/index.jsp?curl=pages/news_and_events/news/2013/10/news_detail_001917.jsp&mid=WC0b01ac058004d5c1 Accessed Nov 2013
9. Farrugia A (2011) Safety of plasma volume expanders. J Clin Pharmacol 51:292–300
10. Toye JM, Lemire EG, Baerg KL (2012) Perinatal and childhood morbidity and mortality in congenital analbuminemia. Paediatr Child Health 17:e20–e23

11. Schomerus H, Mayer G (1975) Synthesis rates of albumin and fibrinogen in patients with protein-losing enteropathy and in a patient recovering from protein malnutrition. Digestion 13(4):201–208
12. Weil MH, Henning RJ, Puri VK (1979) Colloid oncotic pressure: clinical significance. Crit Care Med 7:113–116
13. Carter DC, Ho JX (1994) Structure of serum albumin. Adv Protein Chem 45:153–203
14. Doweiko JP, Nompleggi DJ (1991) Role of albumin in human physiology and pathophysiology. JPEN J Parenter Enteral Nutr 15:207–211
15. King TP (1961) On the sulfhydryl group of human plasma albumin. J Biol Chem 236:PC5
16. Stamler JS, Jaraki O, Osborne J, Simon DI, Keaney J, Vita J (1992) Nitric oxide circulates in mammalian plasma primarily as an S-nitroso adduct of serum albumin. Proc Natl Acad Sci 89:7674–7677
17. Reeves RB (1976) Temperature-induced changes in blood acid-base status: Donnan rCl and red cell volume. J Appl Physiol 40:762–767
18. Perel P, Roberts I, Ker K (2013) Colloids versus crystalloids for fluid resuscitation in critically ill patients. Cochrane Database Syst Rev 2:CD000567
19. Magder S, Potter BJ, Varennes BD et al (2010) Fluids after cardiac surgery: a pilot study of the use of colloids versus crystalloids. Crit Care Med 38:2117–2124
20. Hiltebrand LB, Kimberger O, Arnberger M, Brandt S, Kurz A, Sigurdsson GH (2009) Crystalloids versus colloids for goal-directed fluid therapy in major surgery. Crit Care 13:R40
21. Schebesta K, Kimberger O (2012) Crystalloids versus colloids during acute normovolemic anemia: the quest continues. Crit Care 16:131
22. Vincent J-L, Dubois M-J, Navickis RJ, Wilkes MM (2003) Hypoalbuminemia in acute illness: is there a rationale for intervention? A meta-analysis of cohort studies and controlled trials. Ann Surg 237:319–334
23. Maher FT, Broadbent JC, Callahan JA, Daugherty GW (1958) Hypotension during hemodialysis: its prevention using human serum albumin. Proc Staff Meet Mayo Clin 33:641–646
24. Fortin PM, Bassett K, Musini VM (2010). Human albumin for intradialytic hypotension in haemodialysis patients. Cochrane Database Syst Rev CD006758
25. Van der Sande FM, Luik AJ, Kooman JP, Verstappen V, Leunissen KM (2000) Effect of intravenous fluids on blood pressure course during hemodialysis in hypotensive-prone patients. J Am Soc Nephrol 11:550–555
26. Rostoker G, Griuncelli M, Loridon C, Bourlet T, Illouz E, Benmaadi A (2011) A pilot study of routine colloid infusion in hypotension-prone dialysis patients unresponsive to preventive measures. J Nephrol 24:208–217
27. Rostoker G, Griuncelli M, Loridon C, Bourlet T, Illouz E, Benmaadi A (2011) Modulation of oxidative stress and microinflammatory status by colloids in refractory dialytic hypotension. BMC Nephrol 12:58
28. Jardin F, Prost JF, Ozier Y, Margairaz A (1982) Hemodialysis in septic patients: improvements in tolerance of fluid removal with concentrated albumin as the priming fluid. Crit Care Med 10:650–652
29. Knoll GA, Grabowski JA, Dervin GF, O'Rourke K (2004) A randomized, controlled trial of albumin versus saline for the treatment of intradialytic hypotension. J Am Soc Nephrol 15(2):487–492
30. Nakamoto H, Honda N, Mimura T, Suzuki H (2006) Hypoalbuminemia is an important risk factor of hypotension during hemodialysis. Hemodialysis Int 10:S10–S15
31. Himpe D (2003) Colloids versus crystalloids as priming solutions for cardiopulmonary bypass: a meta-analysis of prospective, randomised clinical trials. Acta Anaesthesiol Belg 54:207–215
32. Bhamidipati CM, LaPar DJ, Mehta GS, Kern JA, Upchurch GR Jr, Kron IL (2011) Albumin is a better predictor of outcomes than body mass index following coronary artery bypass grafting. Surgery 150:626–634
33. De la Cruz KI, Bakaeen FG, Wang XL et al (2011) Hypoalbuminemia and long-term survival after coronary artery bypass: a propensity score analysis. Ann Thorac Surg 91:671–675

34. Arya VK, Nagdeve NG, Kumar A, Thingnam SK, Dhaliwal RS (2006) Comparison of hemodynamic changes after acute normovolemic hemodilution using Ringer's lactate versus 5 % albumin in patients on beta-blockers undergoing coronary artery bypass surgery. J Cardiothorac Vasc Anesth 20:812–818
35. Sedrakyan A, Gondek K, Paltiel D, Elefteriades JA (2003) Volume expansion with albumin decreases mortality after coronary artery bypass graft surgery. Chest 123:1853–1857
36. Rhee P, Wang D, Ruff P et al (2000) Human neutrophil activation and increased adhesion by various resuscitation fluids. Crit Care Med 28:74–78
37. Nohé B, Dieterich HJ, Eichner M, Unertl K (1999) Certain batches of albumin solutions influence the expression of endothelial cell adhesion molecules. Intensive Care Med 25:1381–1385
38. Karu I, Taal G, Zilmer K, Pruunsild C, Starkopf J, Zilmer M (2010) Inflammatory/oxidative stress during the first week after different types of cardiac surgery. Scand Cardiovasc J 44:119–124
39. Vallely MP, Bannon PG, Bayfield MS, Hughes CF, Kritharides L (2010) Endothelial activation after coronary artery bypass surgery: comparison between on-pump and off-pump techniques. Heart Lung Circ 19:445–452
40. Evans TW (2002) Review article: albumin as a drug-biological effects of albumin unrelated to oncotic pressure. Aliment Pharmacol Ther 16(5):6–11
41. Spronk PE, Zandstra DF, Ince C (2004) Bench-to-bedside review: sepsis is a disease of the microcirculation. Crit Care 8:462–468
42. Jacob M, Bruegger D, Rehm M, Welsch U, Conzen P, Becker BF (2006) Contrasting effects of colloid and crystalloid resuscitation fluids on cardiac vascular permeability. Anesthesiology 104:1223–1231
43. Sakai H, Sato A, Okuda N, Takeoka S, Maeda N, Tsuchida E (2009) Peculiar flow patterns of RBCs suspended in viscous fluids and perfused through a narrow tube (25 microm). Am J Physiol Heart Circ Physiol 297:H583–H589
44. The SAFE Study Investigators (2010) Impact of albumin compared to saline on organ function and mortality of patients with severe sepsis. Intensive Care Medicine 37:86–96
45. Delaney AP, Dan A, McCaffrey J, Finfer S (2011) The role of albumin as a resuscitation fluid for patients with sepsis: A systematic review and meta-analysis. Crit Care Med 39:386–391
46. Quinlan GJ, Margarson MP, Mumby S et al (1998) Administration of albumin to patients with sepsis syndrome: A possible beneficial role in plasma thiol repletion. Clin Sci 95:459–465
47. Ernest D, Belzberg AS, Dodek PM (1999) Distribution of normal saline and 5 % albumin infusions in septic patients. Crit Care Med 27:46–50
48. Taverna M, Marie AL, Mira JP, Guidet B (2013) Specific antioxidant properties of human serum albumin. Ann Intensive Care 3:4
49. Dellinger RP, Levy M, Rhodes A, Annane D, Gerlach H, Opal S (2013) Surviving Sepsis Campaign: International guidelines for management of severe sepsis and septic shock: 2012. Crit Care Med 41:580–637

Part X
Cardiac Concerns

Inotropic Support in the Treatment of Septic Myocardial Dysfunction: Pathophysiological Implications Supporting the Use of Levosimendan

A. Morelli, M. Passariello, and M. Singer

Introduction

Myocardial dysfunction is a frequent organ manifestation during septic shock and the subsequent impairment in cardiac output may result in organ hypoperfusion, requiring prompt and adequate treatment to restore cardiovascular function and reverse shock [1]. Current sepsis guidelines recommend resuscitation with intravascular fluid administration in association with inotropes and vasopressors to maintain organ perfusion [2]. Dobutamine is recommended as first-line inotropic agent and should be administered when low cardiac output or signs of hypoperfusion persist after adequate fluid resuscitation and perfusion pressure have been achieved [2]. However, the efficacy of dobutamine in patients with heart failure has not been fully demonstrated and concerns on its use are still present [3]. Although dobutamine improves perfusion and increases oxygen delivery (DO_2), its impact on survival in septic shock patients is limited, with guideline recommendations based mainly on the landmark study by Rivers et al. [4]. Recently, Wilkman et al. [5] reported that the use of inotropes, particularly dobutamine, in septic shock was associated with increased 90-day mortality. In explaining the lack of outcome benefit [3, 5], several aspects need to be taken into account. First, the need of inotropic support may simply represent an expression of disease severity rather than the cause of a poor outcome. Second, whereas the treatment of impaired cardiac output should be tailored based on the etiological mechanism of the cardiovascular dysfunction, the current guidelines recommend the use of inotropes without differentiating the un-

A. Morelli ✉ · M. Passariello
Department of Cardiovascular, Respiratory, Nephrological, Anesthesiological and Geriatric
Sciences, University of Rome, La Sapienza, Italy
e-mail: andrea.morelli@uniroma1.it

M. Singer
Bloomsbury Institute of Intensive Care Medicine, University College London, London, UK

J.-L. Vincent (Ed.), *Annual Update in Intensive Care and Emergency Medicine 2014*, 407
DOI 10.1007/978-3-319-03746-2_31, © Springer International Publishing Switzerland
2014

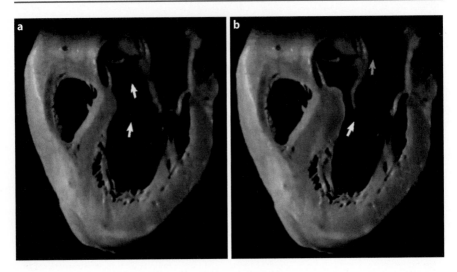

Fig. 1 Left ventricular outflow tract. **a** normal; **b** significant left ventricular outflow tract obstruction due to systolic anterior motion of the mitral apparatus. In presence of this alteration, the administration of inotropes may worsen systemic hemodynamics

derlying causes of impaired left ventricular (LV) stroke volume [2, 6]. In addition, the majority of cardiovascular monitoring instruments provide data almost exclusively on cardiac output and pressures. This approach may potentially increase the number of patients who may be harmed by inotrope administration (Fig. 1). Finally, the beneficial short-term effect of enhanced contractility by cAMP-increasing drugs (e. g., dobutamine, milrinone) is, at least partly, abolished by the increased energy consumption, the worsening of ventricular relaxation and the direct cardiomyocyte toxicity [1, 7–10].

On this basis, a wider use of echocardiography to better define septic myocardial dysfunction and an alternative to catecholaminergic inotropes with less harmful effects may contribute to improving septic myocardial dysfunction. Promising new inotropes that have been developed for patients with heart failure are of potential interest for patients with sepsis-related myocardial dysfunction, although future studies are needed before these drugs can be considered for clinical use (Table 1). In recent years, much attention has been paid to the use of the calcium sensitizer, levosimendan, in the treatment of septic myocardial dysfunction [11–16]. The aim of this chapter is, therefore, to provide an overview on the pathophysiology of sepsis-induced cardiac dysfunction and how it may support the use of levosimendan in the clinical management of affected patients.

Table 1 Inotropes currently used in clinical practice and new drugs under investigation

Inotropic mechanism	Drugs
Sodium-potassium-ATPase inhibition	Digoxin
β-adrenoceptor stimulation	Dobutamine, dopamine, epinephrine
Phosphodiesterase inhibition	Enoximone, milrinone
Calcium sensitization	Levosimendan
Sodium-potassium-ATPase inhibition plus SERCA activation	Istaroxime
Acto-myosin cross-bridge activation	Omecamtiv mecarbil
SERCA activation	Gene transfer
SERCA activation plus vasodilation	Nitroxyl donor; CXL-1020
Ryanodine receptor stabilization	Ryanodine receptor stabilizer; S44121
Energetic modulation	Etomoxir, pyruvate

SERCA: sarcoendoplasmic reticulum calcium ATPase

Mechanisms of Action and Clinical Implications

Inotropism

The underlying mechanisms of sepsis-induced cardiac dysfunction and the pharmacological features of levosimendan [1, 16] both suggest that this alternative inodilator might be a useful drug in the presence of depressed contractility, with potential advantages compared with conventional catecholamines. One of the key feature of the early phase of septic shock is massive sympathetic activation leading to tachycardia, vasoconstriction and increased inotropism, in a physiologic attempt to maintain vital organ perfusion [17, 18]. In this phase, high levels of circulating catecholamines are also produced at the level of gut, lymphocyte, macrophages and neutrophils [18]. Despite increased sympathetic outflow, the septic heart is characterized by depressed contractility due to the attenuation of the adrenergic response at the cardiomyocyte level. This impaired adrenergic response is mediated by cytokines and nitric oxide (NO), which cause downregulation of β-adrenergic receptors and depression of post-receptor signaling pathways [18]. Adrenergic response is further blunted by neuronal apoptosis in the cardiovascular autonomic centers and by catecholamine inactivation by reactive oxygen species (ROS) [18]. Because 75–80 % of myocardial adrenergic receptors are β_1, the attenuation of the adrenergic response represents a major mechanism of sepsis-induced cardiac dysfunction.

In addition to impaired adrenergic response, suppression of L-type calcium currents, decreases in ryanodine receptor density and activity, as well as changes in calcium re-uptake into the sarcoplasmic reticulum have all been demonstrated in experimental sepsis and constitute another cause of septic myocardial dysfunction [18]. Down-regulation of β-adrenergic receptors and altered intracellular calcium trafficking with decreased myofilament responsiveness to calcium are among the main underlying mechanisms of septic myocardial dysfunction but also account for the attenuated hemodynamic effects of dobutamine infusion in septic shock compared with less severe sepsis and non-septic heart failure [12, 18, 19]. Incremental doses of dobutamine may, therefore, be required to achieve therapeutic goals. Nevertheless, in the presence of elevated endogenous sympathetic outflow, such as in septic shock, incremental doses of dobutamine may dramatically increase the risk of adverse effects and lead to myocardial structural damage [1, 5, 7, 9]. In a state of oxygen delivery and consumption mismatching, such as septic shock, enhancing muscle contraction with dobutamine by increasing intracellular calcium concentration and subsequently myocardial oxygen consumption, may further deteriorate myocardial performance. Not surprisingly, Schmittinger et al. [9] observed histologic lesions indicative of stress-induced cardiotoxicity in most patients dying from septic shock. Furthermore, it has also been demonstrated that catecholaminergic inotropic support in sepsis is among the leading causes of LV apical ballooning in patients admitted to the intensive care unit (ICU) [10].

In the light of these pathological mechanisms, the strong rationale for administration of levosimendan to improve septic myocardial dysfunction is related to the ability of this compound to exert positive inotropic effects independent of interactions with β-adrenergic receptors and cAMP production, thereby leaving intracellular calcium concentrations unaffected [20, 21]. In the cardiac myocyte, levosimendan selectively binds to the N-domain of cardiac troponin C (cTnC), thereby stabilizing the calcium-dependent interaction between cTnC and cTnI. The conformational change in cTnC is an essential condition for the interaction between actin and myosin microfilaments necessary to generate contractile force [20, 21]. Because decreased myofilament responsiveness to calcium is a major determinant of septic myocardial depression, calcium sensitization may be more effective, compared to just increasing intracellular calcium concentrations (e. g., with dobutamine), in counteracting septic myocardial depression [12, 22]. An additional advantage of this mechanism is that in parallel to improving cardiac performance, levosimendan decreases sympathetic activity leading to a reduction in catecholamine concentrations [23]. In the presence of septic myocardial depression, levosimendan may, therefore, improve cardiac performance without promoting tachyarrhythmia or relevant increases in myocardial oxygen consumption [11–16, 18, 20, 21].

Effects on systolic function
Oldner et al. [24] demonstrated a marked improvement in cardiac index (CI) and systemic DO_2 following the administration of levosimendan in an experimental model of sepsis. Nevertheless, in parallel with the increase in CI, the authors observed a decrease in mean arterial pressure (MAP) and systemic vascular resistance index (SVRI). Other studies confirmed these preliminary findings. In isolated guinea pig hearts, incremental concentrations of levosimendan improved systolic function, with positive effects following concentrations > 0.03 μM [25]. An increase in LV contractility was observed in two rabbit endotoxic models with animals receiving levosimendan at doses of 3.0 or 3.3 μg/kg/min (with no loading dose) [26, 27]. In a study by Barraud et al. [27], changes were noticed in preload and load independent measurements, thus suggesting a direct increase in contractility inde-

pendent of volume status or changes in vascular properties [21, 27]. Improved cardiac efficiency was indirectly confirmed by the ability of levosimendan to increase systemic DO_2 as well as mixed venous oxygen saturation (SvO_2) [24, 26, 28]. In two recent studies, addition of levosimendan to arginine-vasopressin (AVP) improved global hemodynamics and resulted in a survival benefit compared to AVP infusion alone or placebo in animals with septic shock secondary to generalized peritonitis [29, 30].

In contrast to the experimental models, extensive clinical data on levosimendan to treat septic myocardial depression are still lacking and are mainly restricted to small single center trials with its use described for the first time in a case report in 2005 [11]. Our research group [12] performed the first clinical trial aimed at evaluating the effects of levosimendan in septic shock patients. Patients with septic shock with persistent LV ejection fraction (LVEF) < 45 % after 48 h of standard therapy

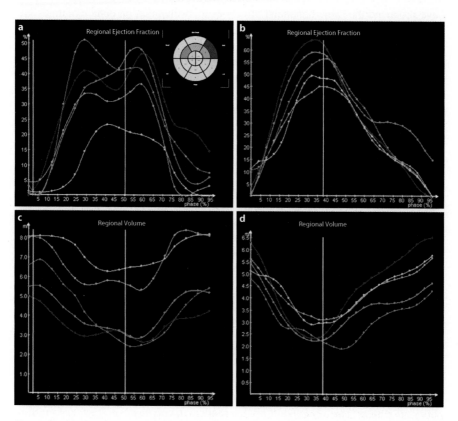

Fig. 2 Regional left ventricular ejection fraction and end diastolic volume. Regional ejection fraction and end-diastolic volume after switching dobutamine 5 µg/kg/min (**a, c**) to levosimendan 0.2 µg/kg/min (**b, d**). The different lines represent different regions of the left ventricle. The figure shows the improvements in regional myocardial kinetics leading to a better cardiac performance following levosimendan infusion

(volume substitution, norepinephrine and dobutamine) were randomized to receive levosimendan (0.2 μg/kg/min infusion without preceding bolus) or dobutamine infusion (5 μg/kg/min) for 24 h. Norepinephrine was titrated to maintain MAP at 70–80 mmHg. In this study, we observed an increase in CI and LVEF following levosimendan infusion. Levosimendan was also superior to dobutamine in improving end-diastolic and end-systolic volume index and LV stroke work index (LVSWI). Although we did not perform a direct evaluation of cardiac contractility, our findings suggest that overall myocardial function was improved (Fig. 2). This assumption is also supported by the observed increases in oxygen delivery and consumption (vs. baseline) and the decrease in arterial lactate (vs. baseline and dobutamine) observed 24 h after levosimendan infusion, indicating an improvement in global tissue oxygenation. Importantly, we did not find a decrease in MAP or an increase in norepinephrine requirements [12]. Although one could anticipate that a higher dose of dobutamine (10, 15, or 20 μg/kg/min as suggested by current guidelines) would have produced the same beneficial effects as levosimendan on hemodynamics, the increased risk of adverse effects also needs to be taken into account. An improvement in global hemodynamics following levosimendan infusion was observed by the same group in patients with acute respiratory distress syndrome (ARDS) and septic shock [13] and by Powell and De Keulenaer [14] in a case series of septic shock patients. More recently, Busani et al. [31] reported an increase in myocardial contractility after switching from dobutamine (up to 8 μg/kg/min) to levosimendan (0.1 μg/kg/min) in a case of fulminant peri-myocarditis associated with influenza A/H1N1 virus.

Effects on diastolic function

Diastolic dysfunction is strongly associated with age, hypertension, diabetes mellitus, and coronary artery disease. In view of the growing elderly and morbid patient population treated in modern ICUs, the number of septic patients who will suffer from diastolic dysfunction is likely to increase in the future [32]. Patients with septic shock frequently have both systolic and diastolic dysfunction. Whereas patients with systolic dysfunction have better survival and myocardial dysfunction recovers if patients survive the septic course [18], diastolic dysfunction does not improve and is associated with high mortality [33]. Although it is conceivable that diastolic dysfunction is a pre-existing condition in the majority of septic patients [33], one cannot exclude that in these patients diastolic dysfunction can be aggravated not only by the disease per se but also by the treatment, especially if echocardiography is not performed. Correct hemodynamic management is crucial to prevent worsening of diastolic dysfunction in septic shock. As a consequence of down-regulation of β-adrenergic receptors, dobutamine loses its lusitropic effect due to hyperphosphorylation of troponin I, a condition that renders the myocytes refractory to further phosphorylation in response to dobutamine [27]. More importantly, dobutamine, by increasing heart rate and inducing tachyarrhythmia, may dramatically worsen diastolic dysfunction. Conversely, levosimendan binds to cTnC in a calcium-dependent manner. It dissociates from cTnC when calcium concentration decreases during diastole, thereby acting only during systole and not impairing diastolic myocardial relaxation [20, 21]. In addition, since levosimendan causes a significant decrease in sympathetic nervous system activity, its administration is not associated with an increase in heart rate, allowing better ventricular filling during diastole. In this regard, Barraud et al. [27] demonstrated that in contrast to dobutamine, levosimendan produced a parallel enhancement of myocardial contractility and improvement in LV diastolic function in experimental septic shock.

Vasodilation

Levosimendan not only increases myocardial contractility, but also induces arterial and venous vasodilation [20, 21]. Vasodilation is the result of the opening of potassium channels, including K_{ATP} channels in small resistance vessels and Ca^{2+}-activated and voltage-gated K^+ channels in large conductance vessels. This action is linked to hyperpolarization of the membrane with subsequent inhibition of the inward Ca^{2+} current and activation of the Na^+-Ca^+ exchanger to extrude Ca^{2+}. The resultant decrease in intracellular Ca^{2+} ions then contributes to vasorelaxation [20, 21]. The vasodilatory effect of levosimendan has been demonstrated in several vasculatures including coronary and pulmonary arteries, systemic arteries, and veins [20].

Vasodilation and its effects on cardiac performance

The vasodilatory effects of levosimendan may play a pivotal role in improving cardiac performance in patients with septic myocardial dysfunction. The matching between the ventricle and arterial load is crucial to provide adequate blood flow to the peripheral tissues. A sufficient cardiac output is the net result of various combinations of myocardial contractility (stroke volume) and afterload (systemic vascular resistance) and the cardiovascular system chooses any combination of these to optimize coupling between the ventricle and the arterial system [6, 34]. The maximum efficiency of the cardiovascular system with the lowest energy costs is obtained when the whole pulsating energy produced by the left heart is transmitted downstream to the peripheral regions [6, 34]. Ventriculo-arterial coupling, the ratio between arterial elastance and ventricular elastance, has therefore been, recognized as an accurate index of cardiovascular performance. When this ratio is near unity, the efficiency of the system is optimal. In this case, the left ventricle provides an adequate stroke volume with the lowest possible energy consumption [6, 34]. Patients with septic myocardial dysfunction may present some degree of ventriculo-arterial uncoupling, because of an imbalance between increased arterial elastance induced by pharmacological vasoconstriction and decreased ventricular elastance depending on the reduction in myocardial contractility [6]. Ventriculo-arterial uncoupling may, therefore, worsen or contribute to septic myocardial dysfunction. This assumption is supported by an echocardiographic evaluation performed in a series of septic shock patients [35]. Among the 67 patients investigated, 14 patients without global LV hypokinesia at admission, developed the condition after 24 hrs or 48 hrs of continuous norepinephrine infusion. Although this change could have been related to the progression of the disease, one cannot exclude that increasing LV afterload with norepinephrine impaired ventriculo-arterial coupling, leading to myocardial failure. According to guidelines [2], the secondary LV hypokinesia observed in these patients was corrected by addition of dobutamine to the hemodynamic support [35]. Because dobutamine may restore the ratio between arterial elastance and ventricular elastance by increasing only the latter, the cardiac energetics of such a strategy may be unfavorable, especially if prolonged. Furthermore, frequency potentiation of contractile function is a major mechanism for the increase in myocardial performance thanks to an improvement in ventricular-arterial coupling. Conversely, in the failing heart, such as the septic heart, this positive force-frequency relation is impaired with ventricular-arterial coupling that becomes negatively affected by tachycardia [34]. Therefore, in septic myocardial dysfunction, dobutamine may further worsen ventricular-arterial coupling by inducing tachycardia [6, 34]. By contrast, levosimendan improves ventriculo-arterial coupling by acting on both myocardial and arterial elastance. Due to the enhancement of calcium sensitivity to contractile proteins, this drug also restores the positive force-frequency relation and prevents tachycardia-induced adverse effects on venticular-arterial coupling [34]. Thus, levosimendan repairs ventriculo-arterial uncoupling better than dobutamine because of greater inotropic effects with less energy expenditure and additional vasodilatory effects [6, 35]. With the same mechanisms, levosimendan, by positively affecting right ventriculo-arterial coupling, improves right ventricular (RV) performance and pulmonary hemodynamics. This effect may be of great importance because patients with septic shock may develop an increase in RV afterload leading to RV dysfunction. In the experimental setting, it has been reported that levosimendan decreased mean pulmonary artery pressure as well as pulmonary vascular resistance, without impairing arterial blood oxygenation [24, 28–30, 36]. In 35 patients with ARDS and septic shock, levosimendan infusion contributed to a decrease in pulmonary vascular resistance. The subsequent reduction in RV afterload was associated with a significant increase in RVEF compared to the control group, suggesting an improvement in RV systolic function also [13]. In harmony with our previous study [12], global hemodynamics were improved following levosimendan infusion [13]. A decrease in pulmonary vascular resistance was also noted in case series from Noto et al. [11] and Powell and De Keulenaer [14].

Vasodilation and its effects on regional hemodynamics

The vasodilatory effects of levosimendan may also be effective in improving regional blood flow. Maintaining adequate splanchnic perfusion, particularly of the gastrointestinal mucosa, is crucial because splanchnic hypoperfusion is implicated in the activation of the inflammatory response and subsequent multiple organ failure [17]. Several vasoactive drugs have been used in an attempt to prevent hepatosplanchnic ischemia and to improve intestinal perfusion. Nevertheless, the efficacy of vasoactive agents in preserving splanchnic blood flow or preventing gastrointestinal mucosal ischemia has not been demonstrated. Levosimendan, by increasing cardiac output and simultaneously redistributing perfusion toward splanchnic regions by its additional vasodilatory activity, might be a prophylactic or therapeutic option to support the integrity of the gastrointestinal mucosa and to preserve splanchnic perfusion during septic shock. In animal models of septic shock, levosimendan was associated with reduced gut vascular resistance, increased portal venous blood flow, increased splanchnic oxygen delivery and consumption, as well as increased mucosal O_2 saturation and reduced intramucosal partial pressure of carbon dioxide ($PiCO_2$) [24, 28, 36]. These effects were more pronounced following levosimendan administration when compared with dobutamine [28]. Our research group previously demonstrated that levosimendan compared to dobutamine (5 µg/kg/min) increased gastric mucosal perfusion, decreased the PCO_2 gradient and increased capillary blood flow in patients with septic myocardial depression [12]. In a study by Memiş et al. [37], levosimendan improved liver perfusion to a greater extent than dobutamine (10 µg/kg/min) in a series of septic shock patients. Of note, previous studies [12, 38] reported that levosimendan decreased serum lactate more than dobutamine did, although there was no difference between the two drugs with regard to their effects on central venous oxygen saturation ($ScvO_2$) [38]. These findings suggest an improvement in regional hemodynamics following levosimendan infusion. On the other hand, Hernandez et al. [39] very recently demonstrated that dobutamine (5 µg/kg/min) failed to improve metabolic, hepatosplanchnic or peripheral perfusion parameters despite inducing a significant increase in systemic hemodynamic variables in septic shock patients without low cardiac output but with persistent hypoperfusion. Kidney dysfunction is common among septic shock patients and may be associated with poor outcome. Levosimendan induces vasodilation, preferentially of the pre-glomerular resistance vessels, increasing both renal blood flow and glomerular filtration rate (GFR) without jeopardizing renal oxygenation [40]. We previously reported that in addition to the effects on gastric mucosal flow, levosimendan increased creatinine clearance and urinary output [12, 40].

Vasodilation and its effects on the microcirculation

Microvascular dysfunction plays a pivotal role in the pathophysiology of septic shock and may occur even in the presence of normal systemic oxygen supply and MAP [15, 17, 41]. In this regard, inotropes have been investigated to improve microcirculatory blood flow in patients with septic shock. De Backer et al. [41] reported that dobutamine improved the microcirculation in a series of septic shock patients. In contrast, in a very recent study, similar dobutamine doses (5 µg/kg/min) failed to improve microcirculatory blood flow [39]. Interestingly, in the study by De Backer et al. [41], the subsequent addition of a topical vasodilator, acetylcholine, completely restored sublingual capillary perfusion, supporting the hypothesis that stronger vasodilatory compounds, such as levosimendan, may be more effective than dobutamine in improving microcirculatory blood flow. The physiological implication is that because of their vasodilatory effects, such compounds may improve microcirculatory blood flow by increasing the driving pressure of blood flow at the entrance of the microcirculation [41]. In line with this assumption, we demonstrated that compared to a standard dose of 5 µg/kg/min of dobutamine, levosimendan at 0.2 µg/kg/min improved microcirculatory blood flow in patients with septic shock [15]. Interestingly, the improvement in microvascular perfusion was independent of changes in cardiac output. This finding suggests that effects of levosimendan at the level of the endothelium, such as the ability to decrease cytokine synthesis, plasma levels of endothelin-1, intercellular adhesion molecule (ICAM)-1 and vascular cell adhesion molecule (VCAM)-1 [20], may have contributed to the improvement in the microcirculation.

Mitochondria K_{ATP} Channel-opening and Organ Protection

Evidence supports the hypothesis that mitochondrial dysfunction and consequent cellular energetic failure may play a key role in the development of sepsis-related organs failure and thus myocardial dysfunction [17, 42]. The mechanisms of such mitochondrial dysfunction are extremely complex and involve an excessive production of ROS, such as superoxide, peroxynitrite and NO, directly inhibiting activities of the respiratory chain complexes [42]. Compounds that have the ability to open the K_{ATP} channels in the plasma membrane of smooth cells, such as levosimendan, may also act on the K_{ATP} channels located at the level of mitochondria. This latter activity may be particularly relevant, because the stimulation of K^+ flux through mitochondrial K_{ATP} has been demonstrated to maintain cellular energy homeostasis and to protect mitochondria from oxidative injury [20]. In this regard, all available clinical data show an increase in SvO_2 following levosimendan administration, which may be related not only to an improvement in systemic hemodynamics but also to a better energetic substrate utilization by mitochondria. Evidence also suggests that levosimendan exerts antioxidant activity and ischemic preconditioning [20, 43]. Whether levosimendan may protect mitochondria and improve energy failure in the presence of multifactorial damage, such as the septic insult, is still unclear. By performing muscle biopsies in a series of septic shock patients, we found that 24 h levosimendan administration at a dose of 0.2 µg/kg/min increased antioxidant defense and was able to enhance the protein level of two defective respiratory chain enzymes, complex I and III (unpublished data). These preliminary unpublished data suggest that levosimendan may protect mitochondria from oxidative stress during septic shock and, potentially, confront the bioenergetic defect through stimulation of mitochondrial biogenesis.

Clinically Relevant Adverse Effects

Opening of K_{ATP} channels in response to levosimendan administration typically is associated with significant vasodilation increasing the risk of hypotension. Nevertheless, in the presence of an adequate volume status, the decrease in blood pressure may be limited by a simultaneous increase in cardiac output [21]. In this context, it is especially important to underline that the vasodilatory effects of levosimendan are dose-dependent and most pronounced if a loading bolus is administered. In the presence of septic shock, levosimendan should, therefore, only be given when adequate fluid resuscitation can be assured. Since the majority of patients suffering from septic myocardial dysfunction do not require an immediate increase in myocardial contractility, it is reasonable to continuously infuse levosimendan without a preceding loading bolus dose [44]. Data from the available clinical studies suggest that in the presence of adequate volume status and maintained perfusion pressure with norepinephrine, use of levosimendan is a safe and effective alternative to increasing dobutamine doses in treating the failing heart of septic shock patients. Notably, levosimendan is the only inotrope that is not associated with increased mortality in patients with septic shock [5]. This finding assumes importance in light of the fact that levosimendan is used rather as a last resort treatment than as a first-line agent. In most cases, levosimendan is administered in shock states refractory to conventional inotropes, in a final attempt to save a patient's life. For many such patients, however, this may be too late to adequately reverse organ failure, as underlined by Bollen Pinto et al. [21].

Conclusion

As an inodilator, levosimendan (at low energy expenditure) may improve cardiac performance in the presence of septic myocardial dysfunction by optimizing the ratio between arterial and myocardial elastance, rather than by increasing myocardial contractility itself. Due to its mechanism of action, levosimendan lowers catecholamine concentrations and thus reduces cardiotoxicity. By its vasodilating properties, levosimendan may improve both cardiac performance and regional hemodynamics. In addition to these hemodynamic properties, non-hemodynamic effects of levosimendan may further contribute to improvements in microvascular blood flow and thus organ perfusion. Moreover, levosimendan has no significant effect on platelets and does not affect blood coagulation [45]. Finally, levosimendan may positively affect several other pathophysiological pathways, such as ischemia-reperfusion injuries, apoptosis, inflammation and oxidative stress, which all contribute to worsen septic myocardial dysfunction. Taking into account these effects, levosimendan seems to be the closest available drug to an ideal vasoactive agent for improving septic myocardial dysfunction. Although extensive clinical data are still lacking, the efficacy of levosimendan in treating septic myocardial dysfunction is strengthened by the evidence of increasing use of this drug by ICU physicians for the hemodynamic management of septic shock [46].

References

1. Rudiger A, Singer M (2007) Mechanisms of sepsis-induced cardiac dysfunction. Crit Care Med 35:1599–1608
2. Dellinger RP, Levy MM, Rhodes A et al (2013) Surviving sepsis campaign: international guidelines for management of severe sepsis and septic shock: 2012. Crit Care Med 41:580–637

3. Tacon CL, McCaffrey J, Delaney A (2012) Dobutamine for patients with severe heart failure: a systematic review and meta-analysis of randomised controlled trials. Intensive Care Med 38:359–367
4. Rivers E, Nguyen B, Havstad S et al (2001) Early goal-directed therapy in the treatment of severe sepsis and septic shock. N Engl J Med 345:1368–1377
5. Wilkman E, Kaukonen KM, Pettilä V, Kuitunen A, Varpula M (2013) Association between inotrope treatment and 90-day mortality in patients with septic shock. Acta Anaesthesiol Scand 57:431–442
6. Guarracino F, Baldassarri R, Pinsky MR (2013) Ventriculo-arterial decoupling in acutely altered hemodynamic states. Crit Care 17:213
7. Dünser MW, Hasibeder WR (2009) Sympathetic overstimulation during critical illness: adverse effects of adrenergic stress. J Intensive Care Med 24:293–316
8. Parissis JT, Rafouli-Stergiou P, Stasinos V, Psarogiannakopoulos P, Mebazaa A (2010) Inotropes in cardiac patients: update 2011. Curr Opin Crit Care 16:432–441
9. Schmittinger CA, Dünser MW, Torgersen C et al (2013) Histologic pathologies of the myocardium in septic shock: A prospective, observational study. Shock 39:329–335
10. Park JH, Kang SJ, Song JK et al (2005) Left ventricular apical ballooning due to severe physical stress in patients admitted to the medical ICU. Chest 128:296–302
11. Noto A, Giacomini M, Palandi A, Stabile L, Reali-Forster C, Iapichino G (2005) Levosimendan in septic cardiac failure. Intensive Care Med 31:164–165
12. Morelli A, De Castro S, Teboul JL et al (2005) Effects of levosimendan on systemic and regional hemodynamics in septic myocardial depression. Intensive Care Med 31:638–644
13. Morelli A, Teboul JL, Maggiore SM et al (2006) Effects of levosimendan on right ventricular afterload in patients with acute respiratory distress syndrome: A pilot study. Crit Care Med 34:2287–2293
14. Powell BP, De Keulenaer BL (2007) Levosimendan in septic shock: A case series. Br J Anaesth 99:447–448
15. Morelli A, Donati A, Ertmer C et al (2010) Levosimendan for resuscitating the microcirculation in patients with septic shock: a randomized controlled study. Crit Care 14:R232
16. Papp Z, Édes I, Fruhwald S et al (2012) Levosimendan: Molecular mechanisms and clinical implications: consensus of experts on the mechanisms of action of levosimendan. Int J Cardiol 159:82–87
17. Parillo JE (1993) Pathogenetic mechanisms of septic shock. N Engl J Med 328:1471–1477
18. Rudiger A, Singer M (2013) The heart in sepsis. Curr Vasc Pharmacol 11:187–195
19. Cariou A, Pinsky MR, Monchi M et al (2008) Is myocardial adrenergic responsiveness depressed in human septic shock? Intensive Care Med 34:917–922
20. Papp Z, Édes I, Fruhwald S et al (2012) Levosimendan: Molecular mechanisms and clinical implications: consensus of experts on the mechanisms of action of levosimendan. Int J Cardiol 159:82–87
21. Bollen Pinto B, Rehberg S, Ertmer C, Westphal M (2008) Role of levosimendan in septic shock. Curr Opin Anesthesiol 21:168–177
22. Bonnemeier H, Weidtmann B (2010) Mechanisms of myocardial depression in sepsis: association of L-type calcium current density and ventricular repolarization duration. Crit Care Med 38:724–725
23. Despas F, Trouillet C, Franchitto N et al (2010) Levosimedan improves hemodynamics functions without sympathetic activation in severe heart failure patients: direct evidence from sympathetic neural recording. Acute Card Care 12:25–30
24. Oldner A, Konrad D, Weitzberg E, Rudehill A, Rosse P, Wanecek M (2001) Effects of levosimendan, a novel inotropic calcium-sensitizing drug, in experimental septic shock. Crit Care Med 29:2185–2193
25. Behrends M, Peters J (2003) The calcium sensitizer levosimendan attenuates endotoxin-evoked myocardial dysfunction in isolated guinea pig hearts. Intensive Care Med 29:1802–1807

26. Faivre V, Kaskos H, Callebert J et al (2005) Cardiac and renal effects of levosimendan argi-nine vasopressin, and norepinephrine in lipopolysaccharide treated rabbits. Anesthesiology 103:514–521
27. Barraud D, Faivre V, Damy T et al (2007) Levosimendan restores both systolic and diastolic cardiac performance in lipopolysaccharide-treated rabbits: Comparison with dobutamine and milrinone. Crit Care Med 35:1376–1382
28. Dubin A, Murias G, Sottile JP et al (2007) Effects of levosimendan and dobutamine in ex-perimental acute endotoxemia: a preliminary controlled study. Intensive Care Med 33:485–494
29. Rehberg S, Ertmer C, Vincent JL et al (2010) Effects of combined arginine vasopressin and levosimendan on organ function in ovine septic shock. Crit Care Med 38:2016–2023
30. Ji M, Li R, Li GM et al (2012) Effects of combined levosimendan and vasopressin on pul-monary function in porcine septic shock. Inflammation 35:871–880
31. Busani S, Pasetto A, Ligabue G, Malavasi V, Lugli R, Girardis M (2012) Levosimendan in a case of severe peri-myocarditis associated with influenza A/H1N1 virus. Br J Anaesth 109:1011–1013
32. Marik PE (2006) Management of the critically ill geriatric patient. Crit Care Med 34:S176–S182
33. Landesberg G, Gilon D, Meroz Y et al (2012) Diastolic dysfunction and mortality in severe sepsis and septic shock. Eur Heart J 33:895–903
34. Masutani S, Cheng HJ, Tachibana H, Little WC, Cheng CP (2011) Levosimendan restores the positive force-frequency relation in heart failure. Am J Physiol Heart Circ Physiol 301:H488–H496
35. Vieillard-Baron A, Caille V, Charron C, Belliard G, Page B, Jardin F (2008) Actual incidence of global left ventricular hypokinesia in adult septic shock. Crit Care Med 36:1701–1706
36. García-Septien J, Lorente JA, Delgado MA et al (2010) Levosimendan increases portal blood flow and attenuates intestinal intramucosal acidosis in experimental septic shock. Shock 34:275–280
37. Memiş D, Inal MT, Sut N (2012) The effects of levosimendan vs dobutamine added to dopamine on liver functions assessed with noninvasive liver function monitoring in patients with septic shock. J Crit Care 27:318.e1–318.e6
38. Alhashemi JA, Alotaibi QA, Abdullah GM, Shalabi SA (2009) Levosimendan vs dobutamine in septic shock. J Crit Care 24:e14–e15
39. Hernandez G, Bruhn A, Luengo C et al (2013) Effects of dobutamine on systemic, regional and microcirculatory perfusion parameters in septic shock: a randomized, placebo-controlled, double-blind, crossover study. Intensive Care Med 39:1435–1443
40. Yilmaz MB, Grossini E, Silva Cardoso JC, et al (2013) Renal effects of levosimendan: A con-sensus report. Cardiovasc Drugs Ther 27:581–590
41. De Backer D, Creteur J, Dubois MJ et al (2006) The effects of dobutamine on microcirculatory alterations in patients with septic shock are independent of its systemic effects. Crit Care Med 34:403–408
42. Carré JE, Orban JC, Re L et al (2010) Survival in critical illness is associated with early activation of mitochondrial biogenesis. Am J Respir Crit Care Med 182:745–751
43. Hasslacher J, Bijuklic K, Bertocchi C et al (2011) Levosimendan inhibits release of reactive oxygen species in polymorphonuclear leukocytes in vitro and in patients with acute heart fail-ure and septic shock: a prospective observational study. Crit Care 15:R166
44. Morelli A, Ertmer C, Westphal M (2008) Calcium sensitizing in sepsis: is levosimendan on the right path? Crit Care Med 36:1981–1982
45. Bent F, Plaschke K (2013) Levosimendan's effect on platelet function in a rat sepsis model. Platelets 24:189–193
46. Torgersen C, Dünser MW, Schmittinger CA et al (2011) Current approach to the haemody-namic management of septic shock patients in European intensive care units: a cross-sectional, self-reported questionnaire-based survey. Eur J Anaesthesiol 28:284–290

Supraventricular Dysrhythmias in the Critically Ill: Diagnostic and Prognostic Implications

E. Brotfain, M. Klein, and J. C. Marshall

Introduction

The systemic inflammatory response to infection or tissue injury is the leading cause of morbidity and mortality for critically ill patients. Systemic inflammation has been associated with the development of refractory tissue hypoperfusion [1], and with the pathogenesis of the impaired vital organ function of the multiple organ dysfunction syndrome (MODS) [2]; progressive cardiovascular dysfunction plays a central role in the pathogenesis of MODS [3]. The cardiovascular dysfunction of sepsis is most commonly described as hypotension and the use of vasoactive therapy [4, 5]. However the spectrum of sepsis-related myocardial dysfunction is extensive (Fig. 1) and incompletely characterized.

The focus of this brief chapter is atrial arrhythmias; however it is instructive to first consider the spectrum of derangements in normal cardiac function that has been described in the critically ill patient.

Cardiac Dysfunction in the Critically Ill Patient

Deranged cardiovascular physiology has been recognized as contributing to the pathophysiology of sepsis for more than sixty years [6]. Early descriptions of cardiovascular dysfunction in sepsis and septic shock focused on the cardinal role of reduced peripheral vascular resistance, and the concomitant increase in car-

E. Brotfain · M. Klein
Department of Anesthesiology and Critical Care, Soroka Medical Center, Ben Gurion University of the Negev, Beer-Sheva, Israel

J. C. Marshall ✉
Departments of Surgery and Critical Care Medicine, and the Keenan Research Centre of the Li Ka Shing Knowledge Institute, St. Michael's Hospital, Toronto, Canada
Department of Critical Care Medicine, University of Toronto, Toronto, Canada
e-mail: marshallj@smh.ca

J.-L. Vincent (Ed.), *Annual Update in Intensive Care and Emergency Medicine 2014*,   421
DOI 10.1007/978-3-319-03746-2_32, © Springer International Publishing Switzerland 2014

Myocardial depression   *Autonomic dysregulation*

Cytokine-mediated biventricular   Sympathetic hyperactivity and loss of
dysfunction   heart rate variability

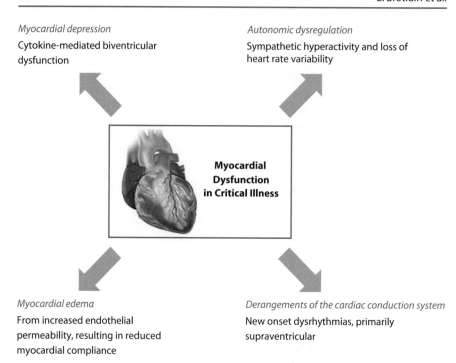

Myocardial edema   *Derangements of the cardiac conduction system*

From increased endothelial   New onset dysrhythmias, primarily
permeability, resulting in reduced   supraventricular
myocardial compliance

Fig. 1 The spectrum of cardiac dysfunction in critical illness. Cardiac dysfunction in the critically ill patient includes abnormalities of autonomic regulation and of the conduction system, as well as of myocardial function. Myocardial edema contributes to these derangements

diac output, producing the classic hyperdynamic profile of resuscitated sepsis [7]. However, it became apparent that despite the increased cardiac output, myocardial function is compromised [8, 9]. Myocardial dysfunction in sepsis is a biventricular phenomenon [8, 10, 11], involving both systolic [12] and diastolic [13] dysfunction. Its causes are multifactorial and include the direct effects of cytokines on the myocardium [5] and myocardial edema secondary to increased vascular permeability [14, 15].

Autonomic dysfunction is a prominent feature of cardiac dysfunction in sepsis [16, 17]. Normal heart rate variability is reduced [18, 19]. A reduction in heart rate variability frequently precedes other clinical manifestations of sepsis [20] and presages a worse clinical prognosis [17]. Reduced variability is associated with decreased responsiveness of pacemaker cells to cholinergic stimuli [21], and with enhanced sympathetic tone that overrides normal vagal activity [22]. Reduced neural regulation of cardiac function may also result from the nitric oxide (NO)-induced apoptotic death of neurons in cardiovascular autonomic centers [23].

Disorders of normal cardiac rhythm are common in septic patients [24]. These arrhythmias commonly arise *de novo*, in the absence of a prior history of arrhythmia [25, 26], and may contribute to significant cardiovascular morbidity [27]. They cannot be explained exclusively by autonomic dysfunction, but likely involve impairment of the cardiac conduction system [28, 29]. Whereas cardiac dysrhythmias are a well-recognized manifestation of sepsis, abnormalities of the cardiac conduction system in sepsis have not been well-described. We will review what is currently known about new heart rate disturbances related to acute severe illness, addressing both the mechanisms of cardiac conduction system dysfunction in sepsis, and the diagnostic and therapeutic implications of new onset dysrhythmias in this high-risk patient population.

Normal Physiology of the Cardiac Conduction System

The normal cardiac conduction system comprises five elements: The sinoatrial node, the atrioventricular node, the bundle of His, the left and right bundle branches and the Purkinje fibers (Fig. 2).

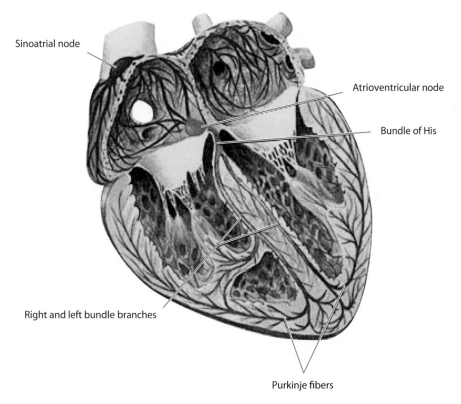

Sinoatrial node

Atrioventricular node

Bundle of His

Right and left bundle branches

Purkinje fibers

Fig. 2 The conduction system of the heart. The conduction system of the heart includes the sinoatrial and atrioventricular nodes, the Bundle of His that branches into right and left bundles, and the Purkinje fibers that deliver stimuli to the cardiomyocytes

The sinoatrial node serves as the pacemaker of the heart. It is located in a subepi-cardial position at the junction of the superior vena cava and right atrium, and consists histologically of a mass of specialized myocardial cells. The sinoatrial node in the adult is 3–5 mm thick and 10–15 mm long [30], and releases electrical stimuli at a rate of approximately 60–100 beats/minute. The electrical signal so generated passes through Bachmann's bundle to the left atrium, leading to the co-ordinated contraction of both atria. The electrical stimulus passes simultaneously along internodal pathways towards the atrioventricular node, then, after a brief de-lay of 60 to 70 msec that enables closure of the tricuspid and mitral valves, through the atrioventricular node to the right and left Bundles of His and into the Purk-inje fibers. The Purkinje fibers disseminate the electrical stimulus in a coordinated fashion throughout ventricular myocardium, causing the ventricles to contract. The tricuspid and mitral valves close at the end of atrial contraction, allowing the atria to refill, and the action potential of the sinoatrial node is restored, enabling the next cardiac contraction. The potential difference of the atrioventricular node is restored while the ventricles are refilling. The entire process takes less than one third of a second and consists of three different stages: Atrial depolarization, ventricular depolarization and atrial and ventricular repolarization. These processes create the characteristic elements of an electrocardiographic (EKG) tracing: the P wave re-flecting the passage of the electrical impulse through the atria, the QRS complex the depolarization of the ventricles, and the T wave the repolarization of the ventricles. The PR interval reflects the delay in passage of the signal through the atrioventric-ular node, while the QT interval reflects the duration of ventricular depolarization and repolarization.

This process is described physiologically by the progress of the action potential across the cellular membrane (Fig. 3); this too can be divided into 5 phases. During the first stage, Phase 4, the nodal cells are resting. With the onset of the second stage, Phase 0, the resting cell receives an electrical impulse triggering rapid de-polarization and the contraction of the myocardial cell. The third stage, Phase 1, involves a rapid, partial repolarization of the cell, and corresponds to progression of myocardial contraction. Phase 2, the fourth stage, is a plateau phase corresponding to the completion of myocardial contraction, and the beginning of slow repolariza-tion of the cell, and during the final stage or Phase 3, repolarization is complete.

The rapid depolarization during Phase 0 reflects the opening of the membrane voltage-gated sodium (Na^+) channels, resulting in Na^+ influx into the cell with dissipation of the transmembrane potential. The opening of the Na^+ channels in pacemaker cells in the sinoatrial node and atrioventricular node is significantly slower than in other cardiomyocytes, suggesting that these channels do not play an important role in the depolarization of pacemaker cells. Rather, slow-inward, L-type calcium channels appear to be responsible for the entry of calcium into the cell during phase 0 [31].The elevation of intracellular Ca^{2++} is sensitive to β adren-ergic catecholamine stimulation, and plays a mechanistic role in the latter third of diastolic depolarization (phase 0).

Closure and inactivation of the fast Na^+ channels occurs during phase 1. At the same time, the fast transient voltage gated outward K^+ currents are opened, initiat-

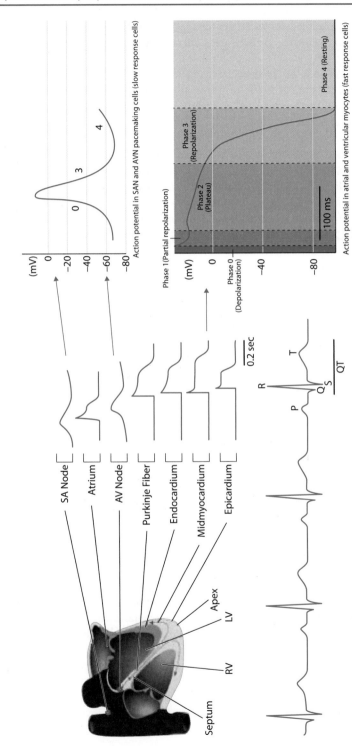

Fig. 3 Progress of the cardiac action potential. Cardiomyocytes comprise two distinct subtypes – the fast response cells of the atria, ventricles, and Purkinje fibers, and the slow response cells of the sinoatrial (SAN) and atrioventricular (AVN) nodes. From [30] with permission

ing repolarization of the cardiac cell membrane. During the plateau phase (phase 2), voltage-gated Ca^{2++} currents are activated, and result in a balance between the influx of Ca^{2++} through L-type Ca^{2++} channels and the efflux of potassium; this electrostatic neutrality creates the 'plateau' on the action potential graph (Fig. 3).

During the rapid repolarization of phase 3, ion channels are completely closed resulting in a loss of electrical balance between the influx of Ca^{2+} through L-type Ca^{2++}channels and the efflux of K^+. K^+ efflux is responsible for restoration of the membrane voltage potential back to its baseline resting state, characterized by a transmembrane potential of –80 to –94 mV and a delayed outward potassium current (Fig. 3) [30, 32].

Within the pacemaker cells of the sinoatrial and atrioventricular nodes, however, phase 4 is characterized by slow depolarization of the membrane until the threshold for firing of another action potential is reached. This slow depolarization is associated with activation during diastole of the hyperpolarization activated current (If), a key element in the generation of sinoatrial node pacemaker activity [33]. The pacemaker current, If, regulates the duration of diastolic depolarization of cells of the sinoatrial node and, as a consequence, directly regulates cardiac rate, and is effected through f-channels encoded by genes of the hyperpolarization-activated cyclic nucleotide-gated gene (HCN) family [34]. Importantly, If current is accelerated by increased sympathetic output and decreased by vagal activity [35].

The conduction of electrical impulses throughout the heart, and particularly in the specialized conduction system, is influenced by autonomic nerve activity. This autonomic control is most apparent at the atrioventricular node. Sympathetic activation increases conduction velocity in the atrioventricular node by increasing the rate of depolarization of the action potential, leading in turn to more rapid depolarization of adjacent cells, and to a more rapid conduction of action potentials (positive dromotropy). Sympathetic activation of the atrioventricular node reduces the normal delay of conduction through the atrioventricular node, thereby reducing the time between atrial and ventricular contraction. Sympathetic stimulation is mediated through the release of norepinephrine that binds to β receptors, resulting in an increase in intracellular cAMP. Parasympathetic (vagal) activation decreases conduction velocity (negative dromotropy) at the atrioventricular node, resulting in slower depolarization of adjacent cells, and reduced velocity of conduction. Increased vagal tone shifts pacemaker dominance to areas with low responsiveness to both transmitters, whereas a high sympathetic tone shifts pacemaker dominance to areas with high responsiveness to both transmitters [36].

Disorders of Cardiac Rhythm and Rate in Critically Ill Patients

Incidence and Risk Factors

Arrhythmias are common in a mixed medical surgical intensive care unit (ICU) population. Supraventricular arrhythmias, including sinus tachycardia, atrial fibrillation, atrial flutter, and atrioventricular-nodal reentrant tachycardia with rapid ventricular response, are the most common, however ventricular tachyarrhythmias are also encountered. Bradyarrhythmias, on the other hand, are rare. A multicenter European study found that sustained atrial dysrhythmias occurred in 8 % of patients, and were associated with a doubling of mortality risk [37]. Other authors have reported incidence rates ranging from 5 to 19 % depending in part on the numbers of patients admitted with a primary cardiac diagnosis.

Patients admitted to an ICU with a diagnosis of sepsis are at particular risk for the development of atrial dysrhythmias. Walkey and colleagues used administrative data and ICD-9-CM codes to assess rates of new-onset atrial fibrillation in a cohort of 3,144,787 hospitalized patients [27]. They reported that atrial fibrillation developed in 5.9 % of patients with severe sepsis, but only 0.65 % of patients without sepsis (OR 6.8, 95 % CI 6.5–7.1). In a separate study of more than 60,000 Medicare beneficiaries, these authors documented an incidence of atrial fibrillation of 25.5 %, the majority of cases occurring in patients with a prior history of atrial fibrillation; rates of new onset atrial fibrillation were 10.7 % in patients with sepsis who had been admitted to an ICU [38]. Meierhenrich et al. reported new onset atrial fibrillation in 23 of 50 patients (46 %) with septic shock, compared to 26 of 579 patients without septic shock (4.5 %) [26]. A retrospective study of Norwegian patients with *Escherichia coli* or *Streptococcus pneumoniae* bacteremia revealed that 15.4 % (104/672) had coincident new onset atrial fibrillation [39]. Similarly a case-control study of patients developing acute tachyarrhythmias (primarily atrial fibrillation) in the ICU showed the presence of sepsis or systemic inflammation to be the strongest predictor for the development of an arrhythmia (OR 36.5, 95 % CI 11.5–115.5).

Although sepsis is a risk factor for new onset atrial fibrillation in the critically ill patient, the relative roles of microbial products, the endogenous host inflammatory response, and iatrogenic factors in the development of arrhythmias is unclear. Moreover pre-existing cardiac disease and other co-morbid conditions may contribute to the risk, though this is controversial [38]. Arora and colleagues identified increased age, increased illness severity, and an admission diagnosis of sepsis as independent risk factors for new onset atrial fibrillation [40]. Seguin and colleagues in a study of new onset atrial fibrillation in 293 trauma patients identified catecholamine use, increased illness or trauma severity, age, and the presence of systemic inflammatory response syndrome (SIRS) as independent risk factors [41]. The same authors, in a study of 460 patients in a surgical ICU reported that age, pre-existing cardiovascular disease, and prior use of calcium channel blockers independently increased the risk of atrial fibrillation [42]. They commented that patients with atrial fibrillation received more fluids and more catecholamines; however it is unclear whether these were risk factors for the arrhythmias or a therapeutic response to the resulting cardiovascular instability. The largest study of new onset atrial fibrillation [27] identified a large number of factors associated with the development of dysrhythmias (Table 1).

Table 1 Risk factors for new onset atrial fibrillation

Variable	Odds ratio (95 % CI)
Age, per 10 years	1.52 (1.47–1.56)
Female sex	0.83 (0.76–0.90)
Race/Ethnicity	
White	1
Black	0.67 (0.58–78)
Hispanic	0.58 (0.50–0.63)
Other	0.78 (0.69–0.87)
Comorbidities	
Hypertension	0.88 (0.81–0.95)
Diabetes mellitus	0.82 (0.75–0.90)
Obesity	1.20 (1.03–1.40)
Congestive heart failure	1.61 (1.41–1.83)
Metastatic malignancy	1.23 (1.09–1.39)
Prior stroke	1.64 (1.35–2.01)
Acute organ dysfunction	
Respiratory failure	2.81 (2.43–3.19)
Renal failure	1.40 (1.26–1.56)
Hematologic failure	1.50 (1.34–1.68)
Acidosis	0.87 (0.77–0.97)
Right heart catheterization	2.25 (1.87–2.70)
Infection (Site)	
None	1.0
Respiratory tract	1.27 (1.14–1.40)
Urinary tract	0.89 (0.81–0.99)
Abdominal	1.77 (1.59–1.97)
Primary bacteremia	1.17 (1.02–1.36)
Infection (Microbiology)	
None	1.0
Gram positive	1.29 (1.18–1.55)
Fungi	1.59 (1.27–2.00)

Modified from [27]

Clinical Significance

Arrhythmias develop in patients with greater severity of illness, and so the attributable contribution of the acute arrhythmia to ultimate clinical outcome is difficult to evaluate. In the largest available study of new onset atrial fibrillation in hospitalized patients, 49,082 of whom had severe sepsis by ICD-9-CM codes, atrial fibrillation increased the risk of in-hospital death from 39 % to 56 % (RR 1.07, 95 % CI 1.04–1.11, $p < 0.001$) [27]. Strikingly, these same authors also reported that new onset dysrhythmias increased the risk of new stroke from 0.6 % to 2.6 % (OR 2.7, 95 % CI 2.1–3.6), a finding echoed by other reports [37]. Others have found increased mortality and prolonged duration of ICU stay in patients with supraventricular arrhythmias [25, 26, 43].

The prognostic impact of new onset arrhythmias is difficult to ascertain precisely, given the small number of published studies, and the small sample sizes reported within them. It is entirely possible that estimates of the burden of illness are exaggerated, confounded by unmeasured co-morbid processes that are driving the mortality risk. On the other hand, it is clear that new onset atrial fibrillation should prompt a search for a treatable cause. Occult infection is one of the more important of these, but the clinician should also consider the potential causative role of electrolyte disorders, volume overload, excessive catecholamine stimulation, atrial irritation by a central line, or medications such as propofol.

Pathogenesis

The mechanisms underlying new onset supraventricular dysrhythmias in the critically ill are incompletely understood, although multiple mechanisms are plausible. Sustained atrial tachycardia during sepsis further increases calcium influx through L-type Ca^{2+} channels; increased intracellular calcium load leads to marked shortening of the atrial refractory period and so may predispose to atrial fibrillation [44]. Clinical studies show that the onset of atrial fibrillation in critically ill patients is related to increased circulating levels of tumor necrosis factor (TNF), interleukin (IL)-6 and C-reactive protein (CRP) [45].

Studies in animal models show that inflammatory stimuli such as endotoxin (lipopolysaccharide [LPS]) can alter the expression or function of ion channels in atrial myocytes. For example, the administration of intraperitoneal endotoxin to a guinea pig results in a shortened duration of atrial action potential and reduced current through L-type calcium channels; these alterations are NO dependent, for they can be blocked by NO inhibition by L-NAME [46]. Although these authors found no change in channel expression, Okazaki and colleagues reported that endotoxin reduced transcription of the L-type calcium channel gene in rat myocytes [47]. Endotoxin also inhibits the pacemaker current, If, and slows down current activation in isolated human myocytes; in doing so, it may reduce responsiveness to sympathetic or vagal stimulation [28].

Insights from animal studies must be interpreted with caution, however; studies in human volunteers receiving a single bolus of endotoxin reveal that although endotoxin elicited a systemic cytokine response, there was no evidence of new onset atrial fibrillation in the volunteers [48], although endotoxin did reduce heart rate variability [49].

Management

The optimal management of new onset atrial dysrhythmias in the acutely ill patient is unclear. Emergent chemical or electrical cardioversion is indicated if there is associated hemodynamic instability. More commonly, however, hemodynamic stability is maintained; for these patients, it is not known whether control of cardiac rate, rhythm, both, or neither impacts outcome. Observational studies report that successful restoration of normal cardiac rhythm is associated with increased survival [26]; however a systematic review of four randomized trials was unable to document clear evidence of clinical benefit for any discrete strategies [50]. Given the frequency with which arrhythmias arise in critically ill patients, this is clearly a priority for future research.

Conclusions

Supraventricular arrhythmias are a common complication of critical illness. Their development is associated with an increased risk of complications, such as stroke, and with increased ICU mortality. However, it remains unclear whether they are the cause of this increased risk or a consequence of the state of being critically ill. Multiple factors – consequent to both systemic inflammation and clinical management strategies – contribute to this increased risk. Optimal management strategies are poorly characterized, but given the potential for increased morbidity in the form of stroke or increased mortality, further study is warranted.

References

1. Hotchkiss RS, Karl IE (2003) The pathophysiology and treatment of sepsis. N Engl J Med 348:238–250
2. Annane D, Bellissant E, Cavaillon JM (2005) Septic shock. Lancet 365:63–78
3. Muller-Werdan U, Buerke M, Ebelt H et al (2006) Septic cardiomyopathy – A not yet discovered cardiomyopathy? Exp Clin Cardiol 11:226–236
4. Vincent JL, Moreno R, Takala J et al (1996) The sepsis-related organ failure assessment (SOFA) score to describe organ dysfunction/failure. Intensive Care Med 22:707–710
5. Zanotti-Cavazzoni SL, Hollenberg SM (2009) Cardiac dysfunction in severe sepsis and septic shock. Curr Opin Crit Care 15:392–397
6. Waisbren BA (1951) Bacteremia due to gram-negative bacilli other than the Salmonella; a clinical and therapeutic study. Arch Intern Med 88:467–488
7. Maclean LD, Mulligan WG, Mclean APH, Duff JH (1967) Patterns of septic shock in man – a detailed study of 56 patients. Ann Surg 166:543–562
8. Parker MM, Shelhamer JH, Bacharach SL et al (1984) Profound but reversible myocardial depression in patients with septic shock. Ann Intern Med 100:483–490
9. Merx MW, Weber C (2007) Sepsis and the heart. Circulation 116:793–802
10. Ognibene FP, Cunnion RE (1992) Mechanisms of myocardial depression in sepsis. Crit Care Med 20:6–8
11. Ognibene FP, Parker MM, Natanson C, Shelhamer JH, Parrillo JE (1988) Depressed left ventricular performance. Response to volume infusion in patients with sepsis and septic shock. Chest 93:903–910
12. Natanson C, Fink MP, Ballantyne HK, Macvittie TJ, Conklin JJ, Parrillo JE (1986) Gram-negative bacteremia produces both severe systolic and diastolic cardiac dysfunction in a canine model that simulates human septic shock. J Clin Invest 78:259–270
13. Stahl TJ, Alden PB, Ring WS, Madoff RC, Cerra FB (1990) Sepsis-induced diastolic dysfunction in chronic canine peritonitis. Am J Physiol 258:H625–H633

14. Yu P, Boughner DR, Sibbald WJ, keys J, Dunmore J, Martin CM (1997) Myocardial collagen changes and edema in rats with hyperdynamic sepsis. Crit Care Med 25:657–662
15. Chagnon F, Bentourkia M, Lecomte R, Lessard M, Lesur O (2006) Endotoxin-induced heart dysfunction in rats: assessment of myocardial perfusion and permeability and the role of fluid resuscitation. Crit Care Med 34:127–133
16. Annane D, Trabold F, Sharshar T et al (1999) Inappropriate sympathetic activation at onset of septic shock: a spectral analysis approach. Am J Respir Crit Care Med 160:458–465
17. Schmidt H, Hoyer D, Hennen R et al (2008) Autonomic dysfunction predicts both 1 – and 2-month mortality in middle-aged patients with multiple organ dysfunction syndrome. Crit Care Med 36:967–970
18. Winchell RJ, Hoyt DB (1996) Spectral analysis of heart rate variability in the ICU: a measure of autonomic function. J Surg Res 63:11–16
19. Schmidt HB, Werdan K, Muller-Werdan U (2001) Autonomic dysfunction in the ICU patient. Curr Opin Crit Care 7:314–322
20. Ahmad S, Ramsay T, Huebsch L et al (2009) Continuous multi-parameter heart rate variability analysis heralds onset of sepsis in adults. PLoS ONE 4:e6642
21. Gholami M, Mazaheri P, Mohamadi A et al (2012) Endotoxemia is associated with partial uncoupling of cardiac pacemaker from cholinergic neural control in rats. Shock 37:219–227
22. Stein PK, Kleiger RE (1999) Insights from the study of heart rate variability. Annu Rev Med 50:249–261
23. Sharshar T, Gray F, de la Lorin Grandmaison G et al (2003) Apoptosis of neurons in cardiovascular autonomic centres triggered by inducible nitric oxide synthase after death from septic shock. Lancet 362:1799–1805
24. Goodman S, Weiss Y, Weissman C (2008) Update on cardiac arrhythmias in the ICU. Curr Opin Crit Care 14:549–554
25. Christian SA, Schorr C, Ferchau L, Jarbrink ME, Parrillo JE, Gerber DR (2008) Clinical characteristics and outcomes of septic patients with new-onset atrial fibrillation. J Crit Care 23:532–536
26. Meierhenrich R, Steinhilber E, Eggermann C et al (2010) Incidence and prognostic impact of new-onset atrial fibrillation in patients with septic shock: a prospective observational study. Crit Care 14:R108
27. Walkey AJ, Wiener RS, Ghobrial JM, Curtis LH, Benjamin EJ (2011) Incident stroke and mortality associated with new-onset atrial fibrillation in patients hospitalized with severe sepsis. JAMA 306:2248–2254
28. Zorn-Pauly K, Pelzmann B, Lang P et al (2007) Endotoxin impairs the human pacemaker current If. Shock 28:655–661
29. Zhong J, Hwang TC, Adams HR, Rubin LJ (1997) Reduced L-type calcium current in ventricular myocytes from endotoxemic guinea pigs. Am J Physiol 273:H2312–H2324
30. Park DS, Fishman GI (2011) The cardiac conduction system. Circulation 123:904–915
31. Mangoni ME, Nargeot J (2008) Genesis and regulation of the heart automaticity. Physiol Rev 88:919–982
32. Nerbonne JM, Kass RS (2005) Molecular physiology of cardiac repolarization. Physiol Rev 85:1205–1253
33. DiFrancesco D (2010) The role of the funny current in pacemaker activity. Circ Res 106:434–446
34. Baruscotti M, Barbuti A, Bucchi A (2010) The cardiac pacemaker current. J Mol Cell Cardiol 48:55–64
35. DiFrancesco D, Noble D (2012) The funny current has a major pacemaking role in the sinus node. Heart Rhythm 9:299–301
36. Opthof T (2000) The normal range and determinants of the intrinsic heart rate in man. Cardiovasc Res 45:177–184
37. Annane D, Sebille V, Duboc D et al (2008) Incidence and prognosis of sustained arrhythmias in critically ill patients. Am J Respir Crit Care Med 178:20–25

38. Walkey AJ, Greiner MA, Heckbert SR et al (2013) Atrial fibrillation among Medicare beneficiaries hospitalized with sepsis: incidence and risk factors. Am Heart J 165:949–955
39. Kindem IA, Reindal EK, Wester AL, Blaasaas KG, Atar D (2008) New-onset atrial fibrillation in bacteremia is not associated with C-reactive protein, but is an indicator of increased mortality during hospitalization. Cardiology 111:171–180
40. Arora S, Lang I, Nayyar V, Stachowski E, Ross DL (2007) Atrial fibrillation in a tertiary care multidisciplinary intensive care unit-incidence and risk factors. Anaesth Intensive Care 35:707–713
41. Seguin P, Laviolle B, Maurice A, Leclercq C, Malledant Y (2006) Atrial fibrillation in trauma patients requiring intensive care. Intensive Care Med 32:398–404
42. Seguin P, Signouret T, Laviolle B, Branger B, Malledant Y (2004) Incidence and risk factors of atrial fibrillation in a surgical intensive care unit. Crit Care Med 32:722–726
43. Salman S, Bajwa A, Gajic O, Afessa B (2008) Paroxysmal atrial fibrillation in critically ill patients with sepsis. J Intensive Care Med 23:178–183
44. Aldhoon B, Melenovsky V, Peichl P, Kautzner J (2010) New insights into mechanisms of atrial fibrillation. Physiol Res 59:1–12
45. Engelmann MD, Svendsen JH (2005) Inflammation in the genesis and perpetuation of atrial fibrillation. Eur Heart J 26:2083–2092
46. Aoki Y, Hatakeyama N, Yamamoto S et al (2012) Role of ion channels in sepsis-induced atrial tachyarrhythmias in guinea pigs. Br J Pharmacol 166:390–400
47. Okazaki R, Iwasaki YK, Miyauchi Y et al (2009) lipopolysaccharide induces atrial arrhythmogenesis via down-regulation of L-type Ca_2^+ channel genes in rats. Int Heart J 50:353–363
48. Boos CJ, Lip GY, Jilma B (2007) Endotoxemia, inflammation, and atrial fibrillation. Am J Cardiol 100:986–988
49. Godin PJ, Fleisher LA, Eidsath A et al (1996) Experimental human endotoxemia increases cardiac regularity: Results from a prospective, randomized, crossover trial. Crit Care Med 24:1117–1124
50. Kanji S, Stewart R, Fergusson DA, McIntyre L, Turgeon AF, Hebert PC (2008) Treatment of new-onset atrial fibrillation in noncardiac intensive care unit patients: a systematic review of randomized controlled trials. Crit Care Med 36:1620–1624

The Pros and Cons of Epinephrine in Cardiac Arrest

J. Rivers and J. P. Nolan

Introduction

Cardiac arrest is defined as the sudden cessation of the mechanical pumping activity of the heart, most often caused by arrhythmia or electromechanical dissociation and will, unless rapidly reversed, lead to end-organ damage and, ultimately, death. Cardiac massage, defibrillation, drug therapy and assisted ventilation may be successful in achieving return of spontaneous circulation (ROSC) and, subsequently, recovery. Cardiopulmonary resuscitation (CPR) is highly protocolized. Guidelines are provided and continually updated by national and international organizations based on the best available evidence. Epinephrine remains the primary drug recommended for administration during CPR and has been since the inception of modern advanced life support (ALS): It appeared in guidelines written in 1961, in which doses of 10 mg intravenously or 0.5 mg intracardiac were advised [1]. Despite being in almost universal usage, the risks and benefits of epinephrine injected during cardiac arrest remain controversial; even if the benefits outweigh the risks, the optimal dose and timing are unknown.

Historical Perspectives

In 1874, Pellicani showed that injecting animals with aqueous extract of the adrenal gland was generally fatal; in contrast, Oliver and Schäfer found that this extract produced marked cardiovascular effects including arteriolar contraction and an increase in blood pressure [2]. In 1906, Crile and Dolley documented a potential role for epinephrine in resuscitation by showing that in dogs and cats asphyxiated with chloroform or ether, its vasoactive properties increased aortic pressure sufficiently

J. Rivers · J. P. Nolan ✉
Dept of Anesthesia and Intensive Care Medicine, Royal United Hospital, Bath, UK
e-mail: jerry.nolan@nhs.net

J.-L. Vincent (Ed.), *Annual Update in Intensive Care and Emergency Medicine 2014*,
DOI 10.1007/978-3-319-03746-2_33, © Springer International Publishing Switzerland
2014

to enable ROSC to be achieved [3]. They suggested that a coronary perfusion pressure of at least 30 to 40 mm Hg was required.

Current Guidelines

The International Liaison Committee on Resuscitation (ILCOR) 2010 Consensus on CPR Science concluded that vasopressors (epinephrine or vasopressin) may improve ROSC and short-term survival, but there was insufficient evidence to indicate that vasopressors improve survival to discharge and neurological outcome [4]. There was also insufficient evidence to suggest the optimal dose of vasopressor for the treatment of cardiac arrest.

Despite the lack of evidence, epinephrine appears in resuscitation guidelines: The 2010 European Resuscitation Council (ERC) guidelines advise injecting 1 mg epinephrine after the third shock in cardiac arrest secondary to ventricular fibrillation/pulseless ventricular tachycardia (VF/VT) and as soon as intravenous access is obtained in pulseless electrical activity (PEA) [5].

Rationale for Using Epinephrine

The pharmacological effects of epinephrine are diverse and are mediated via its effects on alpha- and beta-adrenoceptors. The effect of stimulation of beta-adrenoceptors by epinephrine includes activation of Gs-proteins, which increases the activity of adenyl cyclase and increases production of cyclic adenosine monophosphate (cAMP). In cardiac myocytes, this increases intracellular calcium concentration and improves contractility (positive inotropic effect). An increase in heart rate (positive chronotropy) also occurs. Alpha-1 receptor stimulation, acting via Gq, phospholipase C, and an increase in intracellular inositol phosphates and diacyl glycerol, induces smooth muscle contraction and consequently peripheral arterial vasoconstriction. Coronary perfusion pressure, estimated by aortic diastolic minus right atrial diastolic pressure, and generated in cardiac arrest by external chest compressions, may be augmented by epinephrine. An adequate coronary circulation during CPR is dependent on achieving coronary perfusion pressures of greater than 15 mmHg, (somewhat less than estimated by Crile and Dolley) with pressures lower than this associated with reduced rates of ROSC [6]. In animal studies, epinephrine increases both cerebral and coronary blood flow during cardiac arrest [7]. However, there are both theoretical and experimentally demonstrable adverse effects of injecting epinephrine during CPR.

Potential Adverse Effects of Epinephrine

Combined Alpha and Beta Stimulation

The major benefit of exogenous epinephrine during CPR is mediated via its effects on alpha-adrenoceptors: By increasing aortic diastolic pressure, epinephrine increases coronary perfusion pressure and blood flow. The effects of beta-receptor stimulation are generally considered to be undesirable. Beta-receptor stimulation causes tachycardia, increased tendency to arrhythmia, and an increase in myocardial oxygen demand. The results of animal studies performed in the 1970s suggested that alpha-blockade was associated with failure of resuscitation from cardiac arrest whereas beta-blockade was not [8]. Three groups (alpha-blocked, beta-blocked, and unblocked) of dogs were studied. All dogs achieved ROSC after five minutes in the beta-blocked group resuscitated with phenylephrine and the unblocked group resuscitated with epinephrine, but only 27 % of alpha-blocked animals resuscitated with isoproterenol were successfully revived. The peripheral vasoconstriction produced by epinephrine appears to be beneficial during CPR; the cardiac stimulation is not.

Adverse Effects on Myocardial Oxygen Balance and Cerebral Microvascular Blood Flow

Despite the increase in coronary blood flow, an adverse effect on oxygen supply-demand has been demonstrated in a dog model of CPR: Epinephrine was associated with a reduction in myocardial adenosine triphosphate (ATP) and increased myocardial lactate values [9]. This might be caused by the positive inotropic effect of epinephrine, which increases oxygen demand more than oxygen delivery.

Undesirable effects of epinephrine on the microcirculation have been documented in a pig model of CPR [10]. Despite increased mean aortic pressure, flow through the cerebral microcirculation was decreased and cerebral ischemia increased (demonstrated by increased cerebral PCO_2 and decreased PO_2). The reduction in microvascular flow occurring during CPR persisted after ROSC. By this action, epinephrine might contribute to an increase in the duration and severity of cerebral ischemia following arrest. In a further pig model, carotid arterial flow was reduced (despite an increase in cerebral perfusion pressure) in the presence of epinephrine, although coronary blood flow was increased [11].

Epinephrine Increases Cardiovascular Instability

Epinephrine has been linked to increased cardiovascular instability once ROSC has been achieved. In a Norwegian CPR study, a higher rate of re-arrest following ROSC occurred in patients given epinephrine compared with those who were not [12]. Further evidence of instability and myocardial dysfunction secondary to epinephrine has been provided by animal studies, including a rat model in which temperature-dependent myocardial dysfunction was observed following epinephrine administration [13]. When epinephrine was injected during CPR at 34°C, the increase in severity of post-arrest myocardial ischemia that was seen following normothermic CPR with epinephrine was not observed; however, the vasopressor effects of epinephrine were maintained. The authors suggest that mild hypothermia may offset some of the increase in metabolic demand caused by epinephrine, and there was also thought to be some change in the sensitivity of beta-adrenoceptors at lower temperatures.

Immune and Inflammatory Effects and Infective Complications

Modulation of the immune system occurs via the sympathetic nervous system. Beta-adrenoceptors are expressed on many cells of the immune system including neutrophils, macrophages, and T-lymphocytes. Stimulation by beta-agonists may be harmful to these cells and may reduce neutrophil chemotaxis [14], degranulation and oxidative burst [15]. Beta-adrenergic stimulation also alters cytokine profile by increasing anti-inflammatory and decreasing pro-inflammatory cytokines [16].

The early period following out-of-hospital cardiac arrest (OHCA) is commonly complicated by infection, particularly pneumonia, which is associated with worse outcomes [17]. Therapeutic hypothermia, now commonly used after OHCA, increases the risk of infection. In one series, 97.8 % of patients admitted to the intensive care unit (ICU) following OHCA had evidence of infection, and the provision of early antibiotics was associated with improved outcome (mortality 30/53 [56.6 %] compared with 64/85 [75.3 %], p = 0.025) [18]. Given that infections are common and are a major source of morbidity following OHCA, any reduction in immune function caused by epinephrine may impact significantly on outcome.

Acute coronary syndromes are a common cause of OHCA [19]. Epinephrine activates platelets and promotes thrombogenesis [20], which might increase the risk of coronary occlusion and myocardial ischemia in cardiac arrest caused by an acute coronary syndrome.

Metabolic Effects

Epinephrine is associated with the development of both lactic acidosis and hyperglycemia. A high blood lactate concentration and low lactate clearance have been associated with poor outcome following arrest [21]. Stress hyperglycemia is also associated with poor outcome following arrest [22].

Improved Rate of ROSC Following Epinephrine during CPR

A randomized, double-blinded, placebo controlled trial of epinephrine in OHCA was undertaken in Western Australia [23]. The original intention of the investigators in this study was to recruit 5,000 patients to provide sufficient statistical power to study survival to hospital discharge as the primary endpoint. Unfortunately, only 601 out of 4,103 patients screened for inclusion were randomized, with 534 being included in the final analysis. ROSC was achieved in 64 of 272 (23.5 %) patients given epinephrine versus 22 of 262 (8.4 %) patients given placebo (odds ratio [OR] 3.4; 95 % confidence interval [CI] 2.0–5.6). This threefold increase in ROSC did not translate into an increased survival to hospital discharge: Epinephrine 11 (4.0 %) versus placebo 5 (1.9 %, OR 2.2, 95 % CI 0.7–6.3).

A Norwegian study randomized OHCA patients to intravenous cannulation and drug therapy before ROSC versus no cannula or drugs until after ROSC was achieved [24]. In this way, the impact of all drug therapy versus no drug therapy, and not epinephrine alone, was studied. ROSC was higher in the intravenous group (40 versus 25 %; OR 1.99, 95 % CI 1.48–2.67, p<0.001), although in this study the higher ROSC rate was seen only in patients whose initial rhythm was non-shockable (PEA or asystole) – a three-fold increase was seen in these patients (p<0.001). In patients with VF or VT as the presenting rhythm, the rate of ROSC was 75/142 versus 85/144 (59 versus 53 %, p=0.35).

The effect of epinephrine injected during resuscitation has been examined in several observational studies. Results from observational studies need to be interpreted with caution. Investigators may use statistical methods such as propensity matching and logistic regression in an attempt to reduce the effects of unmeasured confounders, but they are unlikely to be removed completely. For example, epinephrine is given relatively late during CPR; patients who achieve ROSC rapidly are unlikely to receive epinephrine and are likely to have a better outcome. Patients undergoing prolonged resuscitation are more likely to receive epinephrine and in repeated doses, thus selection bias is introduced.

The largest observational study to date was undertaken in Japan between 2005 and 2008 and involved 417,188 patients [25]. Following propensity matching to adjust for potential confounders, the use of epinephrine was associated with a ROSC rate of 2.5 times that when epinephrine had not been given (adjusted OR 2.51, 95 % CI 2.24–2.80; p=0.001).

Long-term Survival Following Epinephrine during CPR

The Western Australian randomized controlled trial (RCT) of epinephrine in cardiac arrest did not demonstrate improved survival to hospital discharge, despite the increase in ROSC [23]. The Norwegian RCT also found no significant difference in survival to hospital discharge (44/418 [10.5 %] versus 40/433 [19.2 %]; OR 1.16, 95 % CI 0.74–1.82, p=0.61), survival at one year (10 % versus 8 %, p=0.53) or survival with favorable neurological outcome (cerebral performance category [CPC] 1-2 = 9.8 versus 8.1 %; OR 1.24, 95 % CI 0.77–1.98, p = 0.45) between the group receiving intravenous therapy and the group that did not [24]. As the Norwegian study was a trial of intravenous access and drug therapy rather than just of epinephrine use, and the results were based on intention-to-treat analysis, many of the patients in the intravenous access and drugs group did not actually receive epinephrine. A *post hoc* analysis of this study was undertaken according to whether epinephrine had actually been given [26]. Patients who were given epinephrine (n = 367) were more likely to be admitted to hospital (OR 2.5, 95 % CI 1.9–3.4); however, the chance of survival to hospital discharge was reduced in the epinephrine group (24/367 [7 %] versus 60/481 [13 %]; OR 0.5, 95 % CI 0.3–0.8), as were the chances of surviving with CPC 1-2 (19/367 [5 %] versus 57/481 [11 %]; OR 0.4, 95 % CI 0.2–0.7).

In the Japanese observational study, the one-month survival rate of patients given epinephrine was roughly half that of patients not given epinephrine (adjusted OR 0.54; 95 % CI 0.43–0.68, p = 0.001) [25]. A multivariate analysis of a Swedish ambulance cardiac arrest registry (n = 10,966) revealed a lower one-month survival in patients who received epinephrine [27]. The Ontario Prehospital Advanced Life Support (OPALS) study used a before-and-after design to investigate the effect of adding tracheal intubation and drug therapy to an optimized basic life support (BLS) and defibrillation system [28]. There was no change in the rate of survival to hospital discharge (69 [5.0 %] versus 217 [5.1 %], p = 0.831), despite an increase in the rate of hospital admission; epinephrine was given to 95.8 % of the patients in the ALS group. A before-and-after design was also used in Singapore to investigate the impact of epinephrine on survival to hospital discharge after OHCA between 2002 and 2004 [29]. There was no significant difference in survival to discharge between the pre-epinephrine and epinephrine phases (1.0 % versus 1.6 %; OR 1.7, 95 % CI 0.6–4.5) but a major limitation was that less than half of the patients in the epinephrine phase actually received the drug.

The results of prospective controlled trials and observational studies of standard-dose epinephrine versus no epinephrine (control) are summarized in Table 1.

The combination of epinephrine and vasopressin during CPR and corticosteroid supplementation during and after CPR (study group) versus epinephrine alone (control), was studied in a pilot RCT (n = 100) [30]. The authors documented increased ROSC and survival to hospital discharge in the study group. A subsequent three-center RCT (of in-hospital cardiac arrest patients requiring vasopressors) compared epinephrine, vasopressin, and methylprednisolone (vasopressin-steroids-epinephrine [VSE]) during CPR and hydrocortisone during post-resuscitation shock with epinephrine and saline placebo (control) [31]. Two hundred and sixty-eighty patients were allocated randomly to receive vasopressin (20 IU/CPR cycle) plus epinephrine (1 mg/CPR cycle; cycle duration approximately 3 minutes; VSE group n = 130) or saline placebo plus epinephrine (1 mg/CPR cycle; cycle duration approximately 3 minutes; control group n = 138) for the first 5 CPR cycles after randomization, followed by additional epinephrine if required. Patients in the VSE group also received methylprednisolone (40 mg) and patients in the control group saline, during the first CPR cycle. Post-resuscitation shock was treated with hydro-

Table 1 Studies comparing standard-dose epinephrine (1 mg) given during cardiopulmonary resuscitation (CPR) compared with control group receiving no epinephrine

Author, year [ref]	Design	N	ROSC, %				Survival to discharge, %				Neurological outcome (CPC 1-2), %			
			Epine-phrine	Control	OR (95 % CI)	p	Epine-phrine	Control	OR (95 % CI)	p	Epine-phrine	Control	OR (95 % CI)	p
Ong, 2007 [29]	Before/after	1,296	15.7	17.9	0.9 (0.6–1.2)		1.6	1	1.7 (0.6–4.5)		1.3	0.7		
Hagihara, 2012 [25]	Before/after	417,188	18.5	5.7	3.75 (3.59–3.91)	<0.001					1.4	2.2	0.61 (0.53–0.70)	<0.001
Olasveengen, 2009 [24]	RCT*	851	40	25	1.99 (1.48–2.67)	<0.001	10.5	9.2	1.16 (0.74–1.82)	0.61	9.8	8.1	1.24 (0.77–1.98)	0.45
Jacobs, 2011 [23]	RCT	535	23.5	8.4	3.4 (2.0–5.6)	<0.001	4	1.9	2.2 (0.7–6.3)	0.15	3.3	1.9		0.31
Olasveengen, 2012 [26]	Post-hoc RCT	848	29	24	1.3 (0.9–1.8)	0.12	7	13	0.5 (0.3–0.8)		5	11	0.4 (0.2–0.7)	
Stiell, 2004 [28]	Before/after	5,638	18.0	12.9		<0.001	5.1	5.0		0.83				

ROSC: return of spontaneous circulation; RCT: randomized controlled trial; OR: odds ratio; CI: confidence interval; CPC: cerebral performance category.
* This study compared intravenous drugs (not just epinephrine) with no intravenous drugs

cortisone (300 mg daily for 7 days and gradual taper) in the VSE group (n = 76) or saline in the control group (n = 73). The rate of survival to hospital discharge with favorable neurological status (CPC 1-2) was significantly higher in the VSE group (18/130 [13.9 %] versus 7/138 [5.1 %]; OR 3.28, 95 % CI 1.17–9.20, p = 0.02). Assessment of outcomes at one year was not included in the study. Although this result appears promising, and is one of few prospective studies to show an increase in survival associated with drugs injected during cardiac arrest, the combination of drugs, and the use of epinephrine (rather than saline placebo) in the control group (when the benefits of epinephrine alone are in question) are limitations. Potentially, all three drugs may be of benefit, or one or two may simply be offsetting some of the harm of the other one or two.

Mode of Death Following ROSC from CPR

A retrospective observational study of patients admitted to the ICU following OHCA and surviving for more than one hour documented the mode of death among those failing to survive to hospital discharge [32]. Neurological injury was the commonest cause of death following cardiac arrest (accounting for approximately two thirds of deaths); thus any detrimental effect of epinephrine on cerebral perfusion, despite its beneficial effect on increasing ROSC, could be significant. Post-cardiac arrest shock was the second most common mode of death.

Timing of Epinephrine Administration

The unpredictable nature of cardiac arrest means that there is much variation in the time when patients first receive epinephrine – a fact that complicates many studies. The more controlled nature of animal studies may result in epinephrine being given earlier than is possible during OHCA, during which clinicians have to first attend the patient and also obtain intravenous access. One study documented that the mean time of epinephrine administration in human clinical trials was 10 minutes later than in animal models (9.5 min in animal CPR versus 19.4 min in human trials), further questioning the validity of extrapolating animal data to human practice [33].

Dose of Epinephrine

The 1 mg adult bolus dose of epinephrine in CPR was derived from animal experiments (generally on 20–30 kg dogs) in the 1960s [34, 35]. Given that humans are larger than dogs, clinical trials have investigated whether higher doses of epinephrine may be beneficial. In 1995, Australian investigators randomized patients to receive initially either two 10 mg doses of epinephrine or saline placebo, 5 minutes apart [36]. Patients in both groups were then given 1 mg doses of epinephrine according to the prevailing resuscitation guidelines. There were no significant differences between the groups in immediate survival or survival to hospital discharge. A later meta-analysis concluded that there was no evidence of increased survival with high-dose compared with standard-dose epinephrine [37].

The effect of doses less than 1 mg, or of giving epinephrine by infusion rather than as a bolus, has yet to be investigated in humans. Infusion of epinephrine has been compared to bolus doses in animal models. In a pig model, CPR was started after 5 minutes of induced VF, following which the animals (n = 24) were randomized to receive either three boluses of epinephrine (20 mcg/kg) at 3-min intervals or an initial bolus of epinephrine (20 mcg/kg) followed by an infusion of epinephrine (10 mcg/kg/min) [38]. Cortical cerebral blood flow was measured continuously using laser-Doppler flowmetry. Global cerebral oxygenation was measured via jugular bulb oxygen saturation. Defibrillation was attempted after 9 min of CPR. Infusion resulted in a higher and more sustained increase in cortical cerebral blood flow (p = 0.009) compared with that produced with repeated boluses.

Alternative Drugs to Epinephrine for CPR

Given that epinephrine possesses several properties that make it less than ideal when administered during cardiac arrest, there may be other drugs that are equally, or more, effective. It is the vasoconstrictive properties of epinephrine, not the cardiac stimulating effects, which increase the rate of ROSC during CPR. Other vasopressors that have been compared with epinephrine during CPR include vasopressin [39], norepinephrine [40], methoxamine [41–43], and phenylephrine [44].

A 2011 meta-analysis of RCTs comparing vasopressin with epinephrine documented no difference in rates of sustained ROSC, long-term survival or favorable neurological outcome following all-rhythm cardiac arrest [45]. However, in the subset of patients in asystole, vasopressin was associated with a higher rate of long-term survival (OR 1.80, 95 % CI 1.04–3.12, p = 0.04) compared with epinephrine. The authors concluded that use of vasopressin in cardiac arrest was not associated with any net benefit or harm compared with epinephrine, but that there may be some benefit from early administration of vasopressin in patients with asystolic cardiac arrest. This weak evidence is insufficient to be reflected in the recommendations made in existing resuscitation guidelines.

High-dose norepinephrine (11 mg) has been compared to standard (1 mg) and high-dose (15 mg) epinephrine in a RCT of OHCA (n = 816) [40]. Although patients receiving norepinephrine had a numerically higher rate of ROSC compared with standard dose epinephrine (13 % versus 8 %), this was not significant (p = 0.19), and survival to hospital discharge and the CPC score at 7 days were similar in the two groups.

Three RCTs compared methoxamine with epinephrine [41–43]. Wide variations in dose regimens were used, making comparisons difficult; however, no study demonstrated an increase in either ROSC or survival with methoxamine over epinephrine.

Phenylephrine has been compared with epinephrine in a single RCT of OHCA [44]. Similar rates of ROSC were achieved in patients receiving two doses of either phenylephrine 1 mg or epinephrine 0.5 mg, as the initial vasopressor; survival data were not reported.

Epinephrine in Combination with Other Drugs during CPR

Given that the beta effects of epinephrine injected during CPR are thought to be harmful, the possibility of giving beta-blockers to reduce these effects seems attractive. A systematic review found evidence from human trials to be lacking; however, in VF/VT in animals, beta-blockade may reduce myocardial oxygen requirements and the number of shocks required for defibrillation [46]. Post-resuscitation myocardial function may also be improved.

Although the benefits of epinephrine during CPR are the result of its ability to augment coronary perfusion pressure and thus increase the chance of ROSC, the vasoconstriction that occurs to effect this may have adverse consequences. These consequences are particularly apparent in the cerebral and coronary microcirculation, where vasoconstriction may contribute to worsening of energy balance and increase in ischemia. In a porcine model of VF, sodium nitroprusside (SNP), a potent vasodilator, improved carotid blood flow, end tidal CO_2, and arterial pH, when used in conjunction with active compression-decompression CPR, an inspiratory impedance device, and abdominal binding (SNP-enhanced CPR) [47]. The SNP group also had improved rates of ROSC, short-term survival, and neurological recovery. In another porcine model, the addition of SNP to standard CPR improved post-resuscitation left ventricular ejection fraction, but not neurologic injury [48]. There are no clinical data supporting the use of SNP in CPR.

Conclusions

Epinephrine remains in wide use for the treatment of cardiac arrest and is commonly included in ALS algorithms. The origins of epinephrine use in cardiac arrest can be traced to observations on its effects on aortic diastolic pressure and coronary perfusion pressure in animal experiments half a century ago. This effect appears to increase rates of ROSC and is supported by evidence from RCTs and observational studies in humans. There is no convincing evidence of improvement in long-term survival, or survival with good neurological outcome, and there are many mechanisms by which epinephrine could potentially cause harm during resuscitation. The most pressing need is for an adequately powered study comparing epinephrine with placebo; there is enough doubt over the net benefit of epinephrine to justify such a study, i.e., there is clinical equipoise. Subsequently, other vasopressors could be compared with epinephrine and other drugs studied in combination with epinephrine.

References

1. Safar P (1964) Community-wide cardiopulmonary resuscitation. J Iowa Med Soc 54:629–635
2. Oliver G, Schafer EA (1895) The physiological effects of extracts of the suprarenal capsules. J Physiol 18:230–276
3. Crile G, Dolley DH (1906) An experimental research into the resuscitation of dogs killed by anesthetics and asphyxia. J Exp Med 8:713–725
4. Deakin CD, Morrison LJ, Morley PT et al (2010) Part 8: Advanced life support: 2010 International Consensus on cardiopulmonary resuscitation and emergency cardiovascular care science with treatment recommendations. Resuscitation 81:e93–e174
5. Deakin CD, Nolan JP, Soar J et al (2010) European Resuscitation Council Guidelines for Resuscitation 2010 Section 4. Adult advanced life support. Resuscitation 81:1305–1352
6. Paradis NA, Martin GB, Rivers EP et al (1990) Coronary perfusion pressure and the return of spontaneous circulation in human cardiopulmonary resuscitation. JAMA 263:1106–1113
7. Michael JR, Guerci AD, Koehler RC et al (1984) Mechanisms by which epinephrine augments cerebral and myocardial perfusion during cardiopulmonary resuscitation in dogs. Circulation 69:822–835
8. Yakaitis RW, Otto CW, Blitt CD (1979) Relative importance of a and b adrenergic receptors during resuscitation. Crit Care Med 7:293–296
9. Ditchey RV, Lindenfeld J (1988) Failure of epinephrine to improve the balance between myocardial oxygen supply and demand during closed-chest resuscitation in dogs. Circulation 78:382–389
10. Ristagno G, Tang W, Huang L et al (2009) Epinephrine reduces cerebral perfusion during cardiopulmonary resuscitation. Crit Care Med 37:1408–415
11. Burnett AM, Segal N, Salzman JG, McKnite MS, Frascone RJ (2012) Potential negative effects of epinephrine on carotid blood flow and ETCO2 during active compression-decompression CPR utilizing an impedance threshold device. Resuscitation 83:1021–1024
12. Nordseth T, Olasveengen TM, Kvaloy JT, Wik L, Steen PA, Skogvoll E (2012) Dynamic effects of adrenaline (epinephrine) in out-of-hospital cardiac arrest with initial pulseless electrical activity (PEA). Resuscitation 83:946–952
13. Sun S, Tang W, Song F et al (2010) The effects of epinephrine on outcomes of normothermic and therapeutic hypothermic cardiopulmonary resuscitation. Crit Care Med 38:2175–2180
14. Perkins GD, Nathani N, McAuley DF, Gao F, Thickett DR (2007) vitro and in vivo effects of salbutamol on neutrophil function in acute lung injury. Thorax 62:36–42
15. Perkins GD, McAuley DF, Richter A, Thickett DR, Gao F (2004) Bench-to-bedside review: beta2-Agonists and the acute respiratory distress syndrome. Crit Care 8:25–32
16. Maris NA, de Vos AF, Dessing MC et al (2005) Antiinflammatory effects of salmeterol after inhalation of lipopolysaccharide by healthy volunteers. Am J Respir Crit Care Med 172:878–884
17. Perbet S, Mongardon N, Dumas F et al (2011) Early-onset pneumonia after cardiac arrest: characteristics, risk factors and influence on prognosis. Am J Respir Crit Care Med 184:1048–1054
18. Davies KJ, Walters JH, Kerslake IM, Greenwood R, Thomas MJ (2013) Early antibiotics improve survival following out-of hospital cardiac arrest. Resuscitation 84:616–619
19. Myerburg RJ, Junttila MJ (2012) Sudden cardiac death caused by coronary heart disease. Circulation 125:1043–1052
20. Larsson PT, Hjemdahl P, Olsson G, Egberg N, Hornstra G (1989) Altered platelet function during mental stress and adrenaline infusion in humans: evidence for an increased aggregability in vivo as measured by filtragometry. Clin Sci (Lond) 76:369–376
21. Cocchi MN, Miller J, Hunziker S et al (2011) The association of lactate and vasopressor need for mortality prediction in survivors of cardiac arrest. Minerva Anestesiol 77:1063–1071

22. Beiser DG, Carr GE, Edelson DP, Peberdy MA, Hoek TL (2009) Derangements in blood glucose following initial resuscitation from in-hospital cardiac arrest: a report from the national registry of cardiopulmonary resuscitation. Resuscitation 80:624–630
23. Jacobs IG, Finn JC, Jelinek GA, Oxer HF, Thompson PL (2011) Effect of adrenaline on survival in out-of-hospital cardiac arrest: A randomised double-blind placebo-controlled trial. Resuscitation 82:1138–1143
24. Olasveengen TM, Sunde K, Brunborg C, Thowsen J, Steen PA, Wik L (2009) Intravenous drug administration during out-of-hospital cardiac arrest: a randomized trial. JAMA 302:2222–2229
25. Hagihara A, Hasegawa M, Abe T, Nagata T, Wakata Y, Miyazaki S (2012) Prehospital epinephrine use and survival among patients with out-of-hospital cardiac arrest. JAMA 307:1161–1168
26. Olasveengen TM, Wik L, Sunde K, Steen PA (2012) Outcome when adrenaline (epinephrine) was actually given vs. not given – post hoc analysis of a randomized clinical trial. Resuscitation 83:327–332
27. Holmberg M, Holmberg S, Herlitz J (2002) Low chance of survival among patients requiring adrenaline (epinephrine) or intubation after out-of-hospital cardiac arrest in Sweden. Resuscitation 54:37–45
28. Stiell IG, Wells GA, Field B et al (2004) Advanced cardiac life support in out-of-hospital cardiac arrest. N Engl J Med 351:647–656
29. Ong ME, Tan EH, Ng FS et al (2007) Survival outcomes with the introduction of intravenous epinephrine in the management of out-of-hospital cardiac arrest. Ann Emerg Med 50:635–642
30. Mentzelopoulos SD, Zakynthinos SG, Tzoufi M et al (2009) Vasopressin, epinephrine, and corticosteroids for in-hospital cardiac arrest. Arch Intern Med 169:15–24
31. Mentzelopoulos SD, Malachias S, Chamos C et al (2013) Vasopressin, steroids, and epinephrine and neurologically favorable survival after in-hospital cardiac arrest: a randomized clinical trial. JAMA 310:270–279
32. Lemiale V, Dumas F, Mongardon N et al (2013) Intensive care unit mortality after cardiac arrest: the relative contribution of shock and brain injury in a large cohort. Intensive Care Med 39:1972–1980
33. Reynolds JC, Rittenberger JC, Menegazzi JJ (2007) Drug administration in animal studies of cardiac arrest does not reflect human clinical experience. Resuscitation 74:13–26
34. Redding JS, Pearson JW (1968) Resuscitation from ventricular fibrillation: drug therapy. JAMA 203:255–260
35. Redding JS, Pearson JW (1962) Resuscitation from asphyxia. JAMA 182:283–286
36. Woodhouse SP, Cox S, Boyd P, Case C, Weber M (1995) High dose and standard dose adrenaline do not alter survival, compared with placebo, in cardiac arrest. Resuscitation 30:243–249
37. Vandycke C, Martens P (2000) High dose versus standard dose epinephrine in cardiac arrest – a meta-analysis. Resuscitation 45:161–166
38. Johansson J, Gedeborg R, Basu S, Rubertsson S (2003) Increased cortical cerebral blood flow by continuous infusion of adrenaline (epinephrine) during experimental cardiopulmonary resuscitation. Resuscitation 57:299–307
39. Wenzel V, Krismer AC, Arntz HR, Sitter H, Stadlbauer KH, Lindner KH (2004) A comparison of vasopressin and epinephrine for out-of-hospital cardiopulmonary resuscitation. N Engl J Med 350:105–113
40. Callaham M, Madsen CD, Barton CW, Saunders CE, Pointer J (1992) A randomized clinical trial of high-dose epinephrine and norepinephrine vs standard-dose epinephrine in prehospital cardiac arrest. JAMA 268:2667–2672
41. Olson DW, Thakur R, Stueven HA et al (1989) Randomized study of epinephrine versus methoxamine in prehospital ventricular fibrillation. Ann Emerg Med 18:250–253

42. Patrick WD, Freedman J, McEwen T, Light RB, Ludwig L, Roberts D (1995) A randomized, double-blind comparison of methoxamine and epinephrine in human cardiopulmonary arrest. Am J Respir Crit Care Med 152:519–523
43. Turner LM, Parsons M, Luetkemeyer RC, Ruthman JC, Anderson RJ, Aldag JC (1988) A comparison of epinephrine and methoxamine for resuscitation from electromechanical dissociation in human beings. Ann Emerg Med 17:443–449
44. Silfvast T, Saarnivaara L, Kinnunen A et al (1985) Comparison of adrenaline and phenylephrine in out-of-hospital cardiopulmonary resuscitation. A double-blind study. Acta Anaesthesiol Scand 29:610–613
45. Mentzelopoulos SD, Zakynthinos SG, Siempos I, Malachias S, Ulmer H, Wenzel V (2012) Vasopressin for cardiac arrest: meta-analysis of randomized controlled trials. Resuscitation 83:32–39
46. de Oliveira FC, Feitosa-Filho GS, Ritt LE (2012) Use of beta-blockers for the treatment of cardiac arrest due to ventricular fibrillation/pulseless ventricular tachycardia: a systematic review. Resuscitation 83:674–683
47. Yannopoulos D, Matsuura T, Schultz J, Rudser K, Halperin HR, Lurie KG (2011) Sodium nitroprusside enhanced cardiopulmonary resuscitation improves survival with good neurological function in a porcine model of prolonged cardiac arrest. Crit Care Med 39:1269–1274
48. Yannopoulos D, Segal N, Matsuura T et al (2013) Ischemic post-conditioning and vasodilator therapy during standard cardiopulmonary resuscitation to reduce cardiac and brain injury after prolonged untreated ventricular fibrillation. Resuscitation 84:1143–1149

Part XI
Ischemic Brain Damage

Preventing Ischemic Brain Injury after Sudden Cardiac Arrest Using NO Inhalation

K. Kida and F. Ichinose

Introduction

Sudden cardiac arrest is a leading cause of death worldwide [1]. Despite advances in cardiopulmonary resuscitation (CPR) methods, including the introduction of the automatic electrical defibrillator (AED) and therapeutic hypothermia [2, 3], only about 10 % of adult out-of-hospital cardiac arrest (OHCA) victims survive to hospital discharge [4], and the majority of survivors have moderate to severe cognitive deficits 3 months after resuscitation [5]. Resuscitation from cardiac arrest is the ultimate whole body ischemia-reperfusion (I/R) injury affecting multiple organ systems including brain and heart [6]. No pharmacological agent is available to improve outcome from post-cardiac arrest syndrome.

Inhaled nitric oxide (NO) has been widely used for the treatment of neonatal hypoxemia with acute pulmonary hypertension. However, accumulating evidence has demonstrated that inhaled NO exerts beneficial effects on I/R injury in extra-pulmonary organs without causing hypotension. Along these lines, we recently reported that inhaled NO improved outcomes after cardiac arrest/CPR in mice. This chapter provides insights into the potential salutary effects of inhaled NO in ischemic brain injury associated with sudden cardiac arrest.

Importance of Sudden Cardiac Arrest to Public Health

Approximately 360,000 Americans experience OHCA each year [4]. In a recent meta-analysis of more than 140,000 patients with OHCA, survival to hospital admission was 23.8 %, and survival to hospital discharge was only 7.6 % [7]. Densely populated urban areas such as New York, NY, and Chicago, Ill, where a large num-

K. Kida · F. Ichinose ✉
Dept of Anesthesia and Intensive Care, Massachusetts General Hospital, Charlestown, MA USA
e-mail: fichinose@partners.org

J.-L. Vincent (Ed.), *Annual Update in Intensive Care and Emergency Medicine 2014*,
DOI 10.1007/978-3-319-03746-2_34, © Springer International Publishing Switzerland
and BioMed Central Ltd. 2014

ber of cardiac arrests occur, report even lower (1.4 % to 2 %) survival rates [8,9]. Unlike other areas of cardiovascular health, such as myocardial infarction (MI) which has seen a 3-fold decrease in acute mortality [10], improvements in outcome from OHCA have remained modest over the last 25 years [11]. Although OHCA is obviously a life-threatening condition, it is a 'treatable disease' in the sense that medical interventions can improve survival significantly [12–14]. A nearly 500 % difference in survival rates exists across communities in the United States, suggesting that variability in the quality of resuscitation care is driving large differences in community survival rates [15]. Collectively, these data suggest the potential that a major improvement in survival rates could save tens of thousands of lives. Moreover, the financial burden of care of post-arrest patients on society is enormous. A recent estimate suggests that on average it costs $ 102,017 to take care of a patient after OHCA with conventional care (without therapeutic hypothermia) [16]. More than $ 33 billion of health care cost is spent on OHCA annually in US.

Pathophysiology and Current Treatment for Post-cardiac Arrest Syndrome

The greatest proportion of post-cardiac arrest mortality and morbidity is caused by global ischemic brain injury [17]. The mechanisms responsible for post-cardiac arrest brain injury include excitotoxicity, free radical formation, pathological activation of proteases, and cell death signaling [18,19]. Many of the injurious pathways are executed over hours to days following return of spontaneous circulation (ROSC) [20,21]. While the protracted time-course of brain injury suggests a broad therapeutic window for neuroprotective strategies following cardiac arrest [19], no pharmacological agents have been proven to be effective in improving neurological outcomes in post-cardiac arrest patients. Two randomized clinical trials have shown that therapeutic hypothermia confers significant protective effects when applied for 12–24 h after ventricular fibrillation (VF)-induced cardiac arrest in adults [2, 3]. Based on these findings, the American Heart Association 2010 ACLS guidelines gave the highest level of recommendation for the use of hypothermia in comatose patients after OHCA. Currently, mortality at six months after cardiac arrest in patients treated with or without therapeutic hypothermia is 41 % and 55 %, respectively. At six months, 55 % and 39 % of the patients treated with or without therapeutic hypothermia, respectively, have a favorable neurologic outcome. A meta-analysis concluded that the number needed to treat to achieve one additional patient with good neurological outcome was 6 [22]. Although therapeutic hypothermia clearly provides a statistically significant improvement in OHCA patients, the benefit is clinically quite modest [22]. In 40 %–66 % of patients treated with therapeutic hypothermia after cardiac arrest, consciousness never returns [2, 3, 23]. Therefore, additional therapies are urgently needed [6].

Nitric Oxide

NO is synthesized from L-arginine by NO synthases (NOS1, NOS2, and NOS3). One of the primary targets of NO is soluble guanylate cyclase (sGC), which generates the second messenger, cGMP, upon activation. sGC is a heme-containing heterodimeric enzyme composed of one α and one β subunit. In most tissues, including heart, lung, and vascular smooth muscle cells, the sGC$\alpha 1 \beta 1$ heterodimer is the predominant isoform. NO binds to the heme moiety of sGC and stimulates the synthesis of cGMP [24]. cGMP exerts its effects by interacting with cGMP-dependent protein kinase (PKG), cGMP-regulated phosphodiesterases (PDE), and cGMP-regulated ion channels. Although the biological effects of NO are mainly mediated via a cGMP-dependent mechanism, studies have demonstrated that cGMP-independent signaling plays an important role in diverse aspects of NO signaling. For example, a number of effects of NO are mediated by S-nitrosylation, which is the covalent modification of a protein cysteine thiol (-SH) to generate an S-nitrosothiol (-SNO) by NO [25].

NO/sGC and Ischemia-reperfusion Injury

NO exerts a variety of effects that would be expected to be beneficial during I/R injury [26]. For example, NO is a potent vasodilator that inhibits platelet and leukocyte activation and adhesion, inhibits reactive oxygen species (ROS)-producing enzymes, and directly scavenges ROS [27]. Deficiency of NOS3 has been shown to aggravate I/R injury in brain and heart [28, 29]. We reported that deficiency of NOS3 or sGCα1 worsened outcomes of cardiac arrest/CPR, whereas cardiomyocyte-specific overexpression of NOS3 rescued NOS3-deficient mice from myocardial and neurological dysfunction and death after cardiac arrest/CPR [30]. Along these lines, Beiser and colleagues reported that poor cardiovascular outcomes and survival in NOS3-deficient mice after cardiac arrest/CPR were associated with decreased myocardial cGMP levels [31].

The salutary effects of NO in I/R appear to be mediated via multiple mechanisms. Dezfulian and colleagues showed that systemic administration of nitrite, which is converted *in vivo* to NO, improves outcomes in mice 24 h after cardiac arrest/CPR by reducing pathological cardiac mitochondrial oxygen consumption resulting from ROS formation [32]. Systemic administration of nitrite prevented oxidative enzymatic injury via reversible specific inhibition of mitochondrial respiratory chain complex I after cardiac arrest/CPR. cGMP may elicit its cytoprotective effects via protein kinase G (PKG), which, in turn, activates mitochondrial protein kinase Cε via ERK signaling [33]. Recent studies showed that activation of cGMP-PKG-dependent signaling altered the glial inflammatory response and decreased oxidative stress and cell death induced by focal brain injury [34].

Inhaled NO and I/R injury

Inhaled NO is a selective pulmonary vasodilator that does not produce systemic hypotension when inhaled at concentrations up to 80 ppm in multiple species, including man [35]. The absence of systemic vasodilation during NO inhalation is due to the rapid scavenging of NO by hemoglobin in the blood. Inhaled NO has been approved for the treatment of neonatal hypoxemia with acute pulmonary hypertension [36]. However, breathing NO also has systemic effects [37]. Breathing NO was shown to reduce I/R injury of extrapulmonary organs in a variety of animal models [38–42]. For example, Hataishi and colleagues examined the ability of breathing NO to decrease cardiac I/R injury in intact mice [40]. They observed that breathing NO for the final 20 minutes of ischemia and for 24 h after reperfusion decreased the size of MI and improved systolic and diastolic function. Breathing 80 ppm NO decreased MI size similarly after 30, 60, or 120 min of ischemia. Breathing 40 and 80 ppm NO decreased myocardial I/R injury to a similar degree, but 20 ppm was not effective. Breathing NO decreased cardiac neutrophil accumulation, and leukocyte depletion prevented the beneficial effects of NO on MI size. Observations in rodents have been extended to a clinically-relevant porcine model of cardiac I/R injury: Liu and colleagues reported that, in pigs subjected to 50 min of cardiac ischemia and 4 h of reperfusion, breathing 80 ppm NO decreased MI size and improved myocardial perfusion [41]. Taken together, these observations suggest that inhaled NO exerts beneficial effects on I/R and protects extrapulmonary organs from I/R injury in small and large mammals.

The ability of inhaled NO to reduce I/R injury was subsequently reproduced in 'proof-of-concept' human studies [43–45]. Lang and colleagues reported a prospective, blinded, placebo-controlled study that demonstrated that 80 ppm NO inhalation during liver transplantation prevented hepatic I/R injury after transplantation. The investigators observed significantly decreased hospital length of stay, serum transaminases, coagulation times, and hepatic apoptosis after liver transplantation [43]. Gianetti and colleagues reported that breathing 20 ppm NO during and after cardiopulmonary bypass decreased myocardial injury and left ventricular dysfunction in patients undergoing aortic valve replacement via anti-inflammatory properties [44]. Mathru and colleagues reported that breathing 80 ppm NO reduced I/R induced inflammatory injury in patients undergoing knee surgery [45]. Based on these observations, we hypothesized that NO inhalation could improve outcomes after cardiac arrest/CPR.

Inhaled NO Improves Outcomes after Cardiac Arrest and CPR in Mice

To examine the effects of NO inhalation on the outcome of cardiac arrest/CPR in a clinically relevant manner, we developed and thoroughly characterized a murine model of cardiac arrest/CPR, in which mice exhibit poor neurological outcomes and survival rates after successful resuscitation from cardiac arrest [30, 46–48]. Briefly,

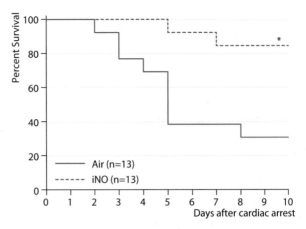

Fig. 1 Survival rate of wild-type mice during the first 10 days after cardiac arrest and CPR. Air: mice breathed air for 23 hours starting 1 hour after CPR; iNO: mice breathed air supplemented with NO for 23 hours starting 1 hour after CPR. * p = 0.003 vs. air

after instrumentation under general anesthesia, cardiac arrest was induced by an intravenous injection of potassium chloride (KCl). After 7.5 min of arrest time, chest compressions were delivered with a finger at a rate of 300–350 per minute with resumption of mechanical ventilation ($FiO_2 = 1.0$) and continuous intravenous infusion of epinephrine. Mice were weaned from mechanical ventilation and extubated at 1 h after CPR. Mice were then randomized to breath air with or without 40 ppm NO for 23 h in custom-made chambers. Whereas only 4 out of 13 mice that breathed air alone survived 10 days after CPR, 11 out of 13 mice that breathed air combined with NO survived for 10 days (p = 0.003, Fig. 1).

It is increasingly recognized that post-cardiac arrest care after ROSC can improve the likelihood of patient survival with good neurological function. Clinical trials showed that therapeutic hypothermia conferred neuroprotective effects when it was applied for 12–24 h starting minutes to hours after successful CPR from cardiac arrest due to ventricular fibrillation [2, 3]. The apparent presence of a temporal therapeutic window after successful CPR is consistent with the observations that many of the pathogenetic mechanisms responsible for post-cardiac arrest brain injury are executed over hours to days following ROSC [18–21]. The protective effects of breathing NO for 23 h beginning 1 h after successful CPR further support the notion that outcomes from sudden cardiac arrest can be improved by implementing innovative therapies in the post-cardiac arrest 'golden hours' after successful CPR.

Mice that breathed air alone exhibited a marked abnormality in water diffusion in the hippocampus, caudoputamen, and cortex 24 h after CPR (Fig. 2). The presence of abnormal diffusion-weighted imaging (DWI) signals in the vulnerable regions of the brain 24 h after cardiac arrest/CPR correlated with worse neurological function and increased apoptosis of hippocampal neurons 4 days after CPR, as well as a poor survival rate. In contrast, NO breathing markedly attenuated the development of abnormality in water diffusion in the brain and improved neurological outcomes and survival rate. These observations are consistent with a recent clinical study that showed that diffuse cortical abnormalities in DWI were associated with poor out-

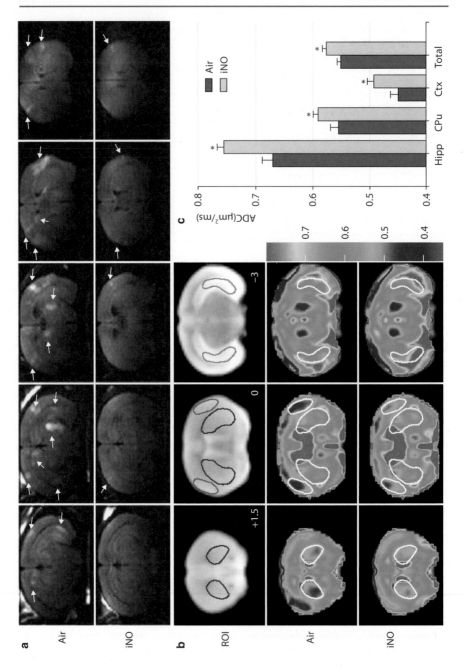

Fig. 2 **a** Representative diffusion weighted image (DWI) of brain in mice that breathed air (Air) or air supplemented with NO (iNO). White arrows indicate areas of hyperintense DWI. **b** Representative magnetic resonance images showing three brain slices containing regions of interest (ROI). Slice positions are identified in millimeters (+1.5, 0, or −3 mm) with respect to bregma in the coordinate space of the Allen Mouse Brain Atlas. Colored outlines indicate portions of ROI (*blue*: caudoputamen; *red*: lateral cortex; *green*: ventral lateral hippocampus) that intersect with these slice planes. Average apparent diffusion coefficient (ADC) values of the slice plane for mice that breathed air (Air) or NO (iNO) after cardiac arrest and cardiopulmonary resuscitation (CPR). The color bar on the right side indicates the color-code for the ADC values (μm^2/ms). **c** Average ADC values of each three-dimensional ROI (Hipp: ventral lateral hippocampus; CPu: caudoputamen; Ctx: lateral cortex; Total: total brain) across all planes in mice that breathed air (Air, n = 6) or NO (iNO, n = 7) after cardiac arrest and CPR. p < 0.05 vs. Air

comes in patients resuscitated from cardiac arrest [49]. Hyperintense DWI signals indicate the presence of brain edema, presumably due to disruption of ion pump function and membrane failure. Therefore, these observations suggest that NO inhalation after successful CPR can preserve ion pump homeostasis and membrane integrity early after cardiac arrest/CPR.

Neuroinflammation induced by the whole body I/R injury associated with cardiac arrest/CPR hinders the neurological recovery from cardiac arrest. We observed that cardiac arrest/CPR markedly upregulated the expression of genes encoding inflammatory cytokines and NADPH oxidase in the brain of mice that breathed air alone, but not in mice that breathed air combined with NO. These observations suggest that NO inhalation prevents neuroinflammation after cardiac arrest/CPR. Furthermore, these results demonstrate a correlation between neuroinflammation, neurological dysfunction, and mortality after resuscitation.

NO elicits biological effects via sGC-dependent and/or independent mechanisms. To examine the role of sGC in the beneficial effects of inhaled NO on outcomes after resuscitation, sGC$\alpha 1^{-/-}$ mice were subjected to cardiac arrest/CPR. We observed that sGCα1-deficiency abolished the ability of inhaled NO to prevent induction of inflammatory cytokines in the brain and to improve neurological function and 10-day survival rate after resuscitation [48]. These observations suggest that beneficial effects of inhaled NO on outcomes after cardiac arrest/CPR are largely mediated via sGC-dependent mechanisms.

Inhaled NO may exert systemic effects via interaction with circulating bone marrow-derived cells (e. g., leukocytes) as they transit lungs. We previously reported that neutrophils are required for inhaled NO to reduce MI size in wild-type (WT) mice subjected to transient left coronary artery occlusion [40]. Along these lines, we recently observed that NO breathing markedly decreased MI size in WT but not in sGC$\alpha 1^{-/-}$ mice [50]. Furthermore, breathing NO decreased MI size in chimeric sGC$\alpha 1^{-/-}$ mice carrying WT bone marrow generated by bone marrow transplantation. These results raise the possibility that the neuroprotective effects of inhaled NO after cardiac arrest/CPR may be mediated by bone marrow-derived cells in a sGC-dependent manner.

From the viewpoint of translating our results into clinical benefit, it is of particular importance that NO inhalation started 1 h after CPR can improve neurological and myocardial function and survival rate after cardiac arrest and CPR. Although the therapeutic window in humans remains to be determined, our observations suggest that inhaled NO can be started after patients are transported to the hospital, and informed consent is obtained. To date, therapeutic hypothermia is the only therapeutic approach that has been proved to improve outcomes after cardiac arrest/CPR when applied hours after successful CPR [2, 3]. Since the body temperature of the mice was allowed to decrease to $\sim 30\,°C$ in the early period after CPR in our recent study, these observations raise the possibility that inhaled NO may confer additional protective effects in the setting of mild hypothermia. Nonetheless, whether inhaled NO combined with therapeutic hypothermia further improves outcomes after cardiac arrest/CPR compared to mice treated with therapeutic hypothermia alone remains to be formally determined in future studies.

Conclusions

Although mounting evidence suggests that NO-dependent signaling exerts multifaceted protection against I/R injury, the vasodilating effects of systemically-administered NO-donor compounds preclude their use in post-cardiac arrest patients with unstable blood pressure. Based upon our prior studies of the beneficial effects of breathing NO on cardiac I/R injury, which were not associated with systemic hypotension [40], we tested the hypothesis that breathing NO could improve outcomes after cardiac arrest/CPR. We observed that breathing NO beginning 1 h after ROSC markedly improved neurological and myocardial function, as well as survival at 10 days without causing hypotension. Of note, the protective effects of inhaled NO in I/R injury of remote organs were first demonstrated in small animals [38, 39] and then later confirmed in patients [43–45], suggesting that the beneficial effects of inhaled NO in mice subjected to cardiac arrest/CPR are likely to be readily translated to benefit patients. Moreover, the established safety profile of NO inhalation (including FDA approval in 1999 for babies with hypoxic respiratory failure and pulmonary hypertension) further enhances the probability that observations in animal models will be rapidly translatable to patients with post-cardiac arrest syndrome.

References

1. Field JM, Hazinski MF, Sayre MR et al (2010) Part 1: Executive Summary: 2010 American Heart Association Guidelines for Cardiopulmonary Resuscitation and Emergency Cardiovascular Care. Circulation 122:S640–S656
2. Bernard SA, Gray TW, Buist MD et al (2002) Treatment of comatose survivors of out-of-hospital cardiac arrest with induced hypothermia. N Engl J Med 346:557–563
3. Hypothermia after Cardiac Arrest Study Group (2002) Mild therapeutic hypothermia to improve the neurologic outcome after cardiac arrest. N Engl J Med 346:549–556
4. Go AS, Mozaffarian D, Roger V et al (2013) Heart Disease and Stroke Statistics-2013 Update: A report from the American Heart Association. Circulation 127:e6–e245

5. Roine RO, Kajaste S, Kaste M (1993) Neuropsychological sequelae of cardiac arrest. JAMA 269:237–242
6. Peberdy MA, Callaway CW, Neumar RW et al (2010) Part 9: Post-Cardiac Arrest Care: 2010 American Heart Association Guidelines for Cardiopulmonary Resuscitation and Emergency Cardiovascular Care. Circulation 122:S768–S786
7. Sasson C, Rogers MAM, Dahl J, Kellermann AL (2010) Predictors of survival from out-of-hospital cardiac arrest: A systematic review and meta-analysis. Circ Cardiovasc Qual Outcomes 3:63–81
8. Lombardi G, Gallagher J, Gennis P (1994) Outcome of out-of-hospital cardiac arrest in New York City. The Pre-Hospital Arrest Survival Evaluation (PHASE) Study. JAMA 271:678–683
9. Becker LB, Ostrander MP, Barrett J, Kondos GT (1991) Outcome of CPR in a large metropolitan area – where are the survivors? Ann Emerg Medicine 20:355–361
10. Heidenreich PA, McClellan M (2001) Trends in treatment and outcomes for acute myocardial infarction: 1975–1995. Am J Med 110:165–174
11. Weil MH, Becker L, Budinger T et al (2001) Workshop Executive Summary Report: Post-Resuscitative and Initial Utility in Life Saving Efforts (PULSE). Circulation 103:1182–1184
12. Cobb LA, Fahrenbruch CE, Walsh TR (1999) Influence of cardiopulmonary resuscitation prior to defibrillation in patients with out-of-hospital ventricular fibrillation. JAMA 281:1182–1188
13. Hallstrom AP, Ornato JP, Weisfeldt M et al (2004) Public-access defibrillation and survival after out-of-hospital cardiac arrest. N Engl J Med 351:637–646
14. Bobrow BJ, Clark LL, Ewy GA (2008) Minimally interrupted cardiac resuscitation by emergency medical services for out-of-hospital cardiac arrest. JAMA 299:1158–1165
15. Nichol G, Thomas E, Callaway CW (2008) Regional variation in out-of-hospital cardiac arrest incidence and outcome. JAMA 300:1423–1431
16. Merchant RM, Becker LB, Abella BS, Asch DA, Groeneveld PW (2009) Cost-effectiveness of therapeutic hypothermia after cardiac arrest. Circ Cardiovasc Qual Outcomes 2:421–428
17. Laver S, Farrow C, Turner D, Nolan J (2004) Mode of death after admission to an intensive care unit following cardiac arrest. Intensive Care Med 30:2126–2128
18. Neumar RW (2000) Molecular mechanisms of ischemic neuronal injury. Ann Emerg Med 36:483–506
19. Neumar RW, Nolan JP, Adrie C et al (2008) Post-cardiac arrest syndrome: Epidemiology, pathophysiology, treatment, and prognostication. A Consensus Statement From the International Liaison Committee on Resuscitation (American Heart Association, Australian and New Zealand Council on Resuscitation, European Resuscitation Council, Heart and Stroke Foundation of Canada, InterAmerican Heart Foundation, Resuscitation Council of Asia, and the Resuscitation Council of Southern Africa); the American Heart Association Emergency Cardiovascular Care Committee; the Council on Cardiovascular Surgery and Anesthesia; the Council on Cardiopulmonary, Perioperative, and Critical Care; the Council on Clinical Cardiology; and the Stroke Council. Circulation 118:2452–2483
20. Sharma H, Miclescu A, Wiklund L (2011) Cardiac arrest-induced regional blood-brain barrier breakdown, edema formation and brain pathology: a light and electron microscopic study on a new model for neurodegeneration and neuroprotection in porcine brain. J Neural Transm 118:87–114
21. Fujioka M, Taoka T, Matsuo Y et al (2003) Magnetic resonance imaging shows delayed ischemic striatal neurodegeneration. Ann Neurol 54:732–747
22. Holzer M, Bernard SA, Hachimi-Idrissi S et al (2005) Hypothermia for neuroprotection after cardiac arrest: Systematic review and individual patient data meta-analysis. Crit Care Med 33:414–418
23. Bouwes A, Binnekade JM, Zandstra DF et al (2009) Somatosensory evoked potentials during mild hypothermia after cardiopulmonary resuscitation. Neurology 73:1457–1461
24. Friebe A, Koesling D (2003) Regulation of nitric oxide-sensitive guanylyl cyclase. Circ Res 93:96–105

25. Lima B, Forrester MT, Hess DT, Stamler JS (2010) S-nitrosylation in cardiovascular signaling. Circ Res 106:633–646
26. Bloch KD, Ichinose F, Roberts JD, Zapol WM (2007) Inhaled NO as a therapeutic agent. Cardiovasc Res 75:339–348
27. Kubes P, Suzuki M, Granger DN (1991) Nitric oxide: an endogenous modulator of leukocyte adhesion. Proc Natl Acad Sci U S A 88:4651–4655
28. Jones SP, Girod WG, Palazzo AJ et al (1999) Myocardial ischemia-reperfusion injury is exacerbated in absence of endothelial cell nitric oxide synthase. Am J Physiol 276:H1567–H1573
29. Huang Z, Huang PL, Ma J et al (1996) Enlarged infarcts in endothelial nitric oxide synthase knockout mice are attenuated by nitro-l-arginine. J Cereb Blood Flow Metab 16:981–987
30. Nishida T, Yu JD, Minamishima S et al (2009) Protective effects of nitric oxide synthase 3 and soluble guanylate cyclase on the outcome of cardiac arrest and cardiopulmonary resuscitation in mice. Crit Care Med 37:256–262
31. Beiser DG, Orbelyan GA, Inouye BT et al (2011) Genetic deletion of NOS3 increases lethal cardiac dysfunction following mouse cardiac arrest. Resuscitation 82:115–121
32. Dezfulian C, Shiva S, Alekseyenko A et al (2009) Nitrite therapy after cardiac arrest reduces reactive oxygen species generation, improves cardiac and neurological function, and enhances survival via reversible inhibition of mitochondrial complex I. Circulation 120:897–905
33. Ping P, Zhang J, Cao X et al (1999) PKC-dependent activation of p44/p42 MAPKs during myocardial ischemia-reperfusion in conscious rabbits. Am J Physiol 276:H1468–H1481
34. Pifarré P, Prado J, Giralt M, Molinero A, Hidalgo J, Garcia A (2010) Cyclic GMP phosphodiesterase inhibition alters the glial inflammatory response, reduces oxidative stress and cell death and increases angiogenesis following focal brain injury. J Neurochem 112:807–817
35. Ichinose F, Roberts JD Jr., Zapol WM (2004) Inhaled nitric oxide: a selective pulmonary vasodilator: current uses and therapeutic potential. Circulation 109:3106–3111
36. Griffiths MJ, Evans TW (2005) Inhaled nitric oxide therapy in adults. N Engl J Med 353:2683–2695
37. Hogman M, Frostell C, Arnberg H, Hedenstierna G (1993) Bleeding time prolongation and NO inhalation. Lancet 341:1664–1665
38. Fox-Robichaud A, Payne D, Hasan SU et al (1998) Inhaled NO as a viable antiadhesive therapy for ischemia/reperfusion injury of distal microvascular beds. J Clin Invest 101:2497–2505
39. Guery B, Neviere R, Viget N et al (1999) Inhaled NO preadministration modulates local and remote ischemia-reperfusion organ injury in a rat model. J Appl Physiol 87:47–53
40. Hataishi R, Rodrigues AC, Neilan TG et al (2006) Inhaled nitric oxide decreases infarction size and improves left ventricular function in a murine model of myocardial ischemia-reperfusion injury. Am J Physiol Heart Circ Physiol 291:H379–H384
41. Liu X, Huang Y, Pokreisz P et al (2007) Nitric oxide inhalation improves microvascular flow and decreases infarction size after myocardial ischemia and reperfusion. J Am Coll Cardiol 50:808–817
42. Nagasaka Y, Fernandez BO, Garcia-Saura MF et al (2008) Brief periods of nitric oxide inhalation protect against myocardial ischemia-reperfusion injury. Anesthesiology 109:675–682
43. Lang JD Jr., Chumley P, Teng X et al (2007) Inhaled NO accelerates restoration of liver function in adults following orthotopic liver transplantation. J Clin Invest 117:2583–2591
44. Gianetti J, Del Sarto P, Bevilacqua S et al (2004) Supplemental nitric oxide and its effect on myocardial injury and function in patients undergoing cardiac surgery with extracorporeal circulation. J Thorac Cardiovasc Surg 127:44–50
45. Mathru M, Huda R, Solanki DR, Hays S, Lang JD (2007) Inhaled nitric oxide attenuates reperfusion inflammatory responses in humans. Anesthesiology 106:275–282
46. Kida K, Minamishima S, Wang H et al (2012) Sodium sulfide prevents water diffusion abnormality in the brain and improves long term outcome after cardiac arrest in mice. Resuscitation 83:1292–1297

47. Minamishima S, Bougaki M, Sips PY et al (2009) Hydrogen sulfide improves survival after cardiac arrest and cardiopulmonary resuscitation via a nitric oxide synthase 3-dependent
mechanism in mice. Circulation 120:888–896
48. Minamishima S, Kida K, Tokuda K et al (2011) Inhaled nitric oxide improves outcomes after
successful cardiopulmonary resuscitation in mice. Circulation 124:1645–1653
49. Wijman cardiac arrest, Mlynash M, Caulfield AF et al (2009) Prognostic value of brain
diffusion-weighted imaging after cardiac arrest. Ann Neurol 65:394–402
50. Nagasaka Y, Buys E, Spagnolli E et al (2011) Soluble guanylate cyclase-α1 is required for the
cardioprotective effects of inhaled nitric oxide. Am J Physiol Heart Circ Physiol 300:H1477–
H1483

Neurological Prognostication After Cardiac Arrest in the Era of Hypothermia

C. Sandroni, S. D'Arrigo, and M. Antonelli

Introduction

Despite recent improvements in resuscitation techniques and post-resuscitation care, cardiac arrest still has a poor prognosis. Mortality exceeds 80 %–90 % and more than one quarter of those who survive to hospital discharge have severe persistent neurological dysfunction [1]. Prediction of poor neurological outcome in comatose survivors of cardiac arrest is important, both to give correct information to their relatives and to avoid futile care. In 2006, the criteria for prediction of poor outcome in those patients were codified in the landmark review from the Quality Standards Subcommittee of the American Academy of Neurology (AAN) [2]. According to that review, myoclonus status epilepticus on day 1 after cardiac arrest, an absent N20 wave of somatosensory evoked potentials (SSEP) or a serum neuron specific enolase (NSE) $> 33 \, \mu g/l$ from day 1 to day 3, and absent pupillary or corneal reflexes or an extensor or absent motor response on day 3 accurately predicted a poor outcome, defined as death or unconsciousness after 1 month, or unconsciousness or severe disability after 6 months. In that review, electroencephalogram (EEG) and imaging techniques, such as magnetic resonance imaging (MRI), were considered promising, but not ready for routine clinical use.

The major limitation of the AAN 2006 review was the fact that it was based on studies conducted before the advent of therapeutic hypothermia, which now represents a standard treatment for comatose patients resuscitated from out-of-hospital cardiac arrest (OHCA) due to shockable rhythms, and is often used also for patients resuscitated from in-hospital cardiac arrest or arrest due to non-shockable rhythms. Studies published after the AAN 2006 review [3, 4] have suggested that therapeutic hypothermia may affect neurological prognostication and that the AAN 2006 crite-

C. Sandroni · S. D'Arrigo · M. Antonelli ✉
Department of Anesthesiology and Intensive Care, Catholic University School of Medicine, Rome, Italy
e-mail: m.antonelli@rm.unicatt.it

J.-L. Vincent (Ed.), *Annual Update in Intensive Care and Emergency Medicine 2014*, 461
DOI 10.1007/978-3-319-03746-2_35, © Springer International Publishing Switzerland 2014

ria may not be applicable to therapeutic hypothermia-treated patients [5]. Moreover, recent clinical studies [6, 7] and systematic reviews [8] have challenged the results of the AAN 2006 paper, suggesting that even in patients not treated with therapeutic hypothermia the criteria for predicting poor outcome may need an update. A critical revision of recommendations on prognostication in comatose resuscitated patients based on latest evidence has recently been advocated [9].

Predictors of Poor Neurological Outcome after Cardiac Arrest

The four main types of predictors on which neurological prognostication after cardiac arrest can be based are clinical examination, electrophysiological studies, biochemical markers, and imaging.

Clinical Examination

Clinical examination represents an immediate, bedside-available, and costless approach for prognostication in comatose resuscitated patients. Bilateral absence of pupillary reflex to light is common and has no predictive value when recorded immediately after the arrest [10, 11], but accurately predicts poor outcome at 72 h in therapeutic hypothermia-treated and in non-therapeutic hypothermia-treated patients [8, 12, 13] (Table 1). Bilateral absence of corneal reflex at 72 h is less accurate than that of pupillary reflex, having a 2 %–5 % false positive rate (FPR) [8, 12, 13]. Both these signs have a low sensitivity, being present in only one third or less of patients with an eventually poor outcome [8, 12]. An extensor or absent motor response to pain (M ≤ 2) at 72 h had been previously recommended as an accurate predictor of poor outcome in non-therapeutic hypothermia-treated patients after cardiac arrest [2], but results of a large multicenter observational study [14] showed that this sign actually has a high FPR. This was confirmed by a recent systematic review in therapeutic hypothermia-treated patients as well [13] (Table 1).

In therapeutic hypothermia-treated patients, results of clinical examination at 72 h can be altered due to a persistent effect of sedatives and muscle relaxants given during the hypothermia phase. Therapeutic hypothermia prolongs the effect of these drugs. Corneal reflexes and motor response are more likely to be affected by muscle relaxants than pupillary reflex, which has the ciliary smooth muscle as an effector.

In patients who have not been treated with therapeutic hypothermia, presence of myoclonus status epilepticus, defined as spontaneous, repetitive, unrelenting, generalized multifocal myoclonus involving the face, limbs, and axial musculature, in comatose patients within 24 h is almost invariably associated with death or vegetative state [2, 8]. In therapeutic hypothermia-treated patients, occurrence of myoclonus status epilepticus within 72 h is also an ominous sign [3, 15]. However, cases of neurological recovery despite early and prolonged myoclonus have been reported in both populations [16–19]. Some of these cases have been identified as Lance-Adams syndrome (LAS), a chronic benign form of posthypoxic myoclonus

Table 1 Accuracy of major predictors of poor outcome at 72 h after cardiac arrest in patients treated with and without therapeutic hypothermia as reported in two recent meta-analyses. Data from [8] and [13]

Index	Not treated with therapeutic hypothermia		Treated with therapeutic hypothermia	
	Sensitivity % [95 % CI]	FPR % [95 % CI]	Sensitivity % [95 % CI]	FPR % [95 % CI]
Absent pupillary light reflex	18 [15–23]	0 [0–8]	22 [18–27]	0.4 [0.1–3]
Absent corneal reflex	29 [23–34]	5 [0–5]	32 [27–39]	2 [0–13]
Extensor or absent motor response to pain	74 [68–79]	27 [12–48]	80 [63–91]	21 [8–43]
Bilaterally absent SSEP N20 wave	46 [40–52]	0 [0–9]	50 [42–57]	0.7 [0.1–4.7]

CI: confidence interval; FPR: false positive rate; SSEP: short-latency somatosensory evoked potentials.

induced by voluntary movements. Patients with LAS are typically aware, but this may not be evident in patients who are intubated and sedated after resuscitation. Misinterpretation of early-onset LAS as a malignant myoclonic status epilepticus could lead to an inappropriate prognostication of poor outcome in patients having good chances of recovery. In patients with post-cardiac arrest myoclonus, an accurate clinical neurological evaluation should be made off sedation. Performing an EEG could be helpful to both assess the level of consciousness and identify the presence of associated epileptiform activity or malignant EEG patterns.

An important limitation to the use of myoclonus status epilepticus for prognostication in postanoxic coma is its inconsistent terminology and definition. Postanoxic myoclonus has a variety of clinical features, none of which *per se* is 100 % specific of poor outcome [8, 12]. In particular, multifocal distribution, long duration or absence of EEG reactivity are still compatible with neurological recovery [18, 20, 21], although the outcome is generally worse with prolonged and continuous myoclonus [3, 7, 15, 18]. Another limitation of early myoclonus status epilepticus is its low sensitivity [8].

Biochemical Markers

During the last 25 years, various biochemical markers of brain damage have been investigated, the most popular of which is NSE, also known as gamma enolase or enolase 2. NSE is released in blood and cerebrospinal fluid (CSF) after neuronal ischemia and its serum concentrations correlate with the extent of brain damage [22]. According to the AAN 2006 review [2], serum levels of NSE > 33 μg/l during the first 72 h after cardiac arrest were a reliable predictor of an invariably poor neurological outcome in patients who had not been treated with therapeutic hypothermia. However, analysis of studies published after that review [6, 7] and a reappraisal of older studies showed that levels up to 80 μg/l are needed to ensure 100 % specificity at 72 h. Similar values have been found in therapeutic hypothermia-treated patients [4, 23].

The major limitation to using NSE for early prognostication after cardiac arrest is the inconsistency of its thresholds for 100 % specificity, which vary largely not only among studies, but also within a single study population according to timing from cardiac arrest. A possible cause for this inconsistency is the use of different analytic techniques. Another cause is the presence of extracerebral sources of NSE, the most common of which are the red blood cells. Neuroendocrine tumors and small-cell lung carcinoma are other less common sources of NSE.

The glial S-100B protein is another biochemical marker that has been investigated as a predictor of poor neurological outcome after cardiac arrest. Unfortunately, similarly to NSE, the S-100B thresholds for 100 % specificity vary largely, ranging from 0.2 to 5.2 µg/l in patients not treated with therapeutic hypothermia and from 0.18 to 0.30 in therapeutic hypothermia-treated patients [8, 12]. S-100B appears to be affected by the same limitations as NSE, and it has been less well documented. S-100B is contained in muscle and adipose tissue, therefore its levels could be increased by thoracic trauma caused by prolonged resuscitation [24].

Electrophysiological Studies

SSEP are the most extensively studied predictors based on electrophysiology. In patients who have not been treated with therapeutic hypothermia, the bilateral absence of a cortical N20 SSEP wave at 24 h–72 h from cardiac arrest almost invariably predicts a poor outcome (FPR 0.7 [0–3.7]) [2, 8]. In therapeutic hypothermia-treated patients, SSEP was confirmed as a robust and early predictor of neurological outcome, being 100 % accurate as early as 24 h from cardiac arrest [12]. In a recent review[13], among 492 patients with absent N20 SSEPs within 72 h after cardiac arrest there was only one false positive result (FPR 0.7 % [0.1–5]) [25]. The sensitivity of SSEP is around 50 %, therefore higher than that of clinical examination (Table 1).

In therapeutic hypothermia-treated patients, SSEPs have the advantage of being resistant to the effects of both low body temperature and sedative drugs [26–28]. SSEP are highly reproducible; however, studies showed that experts may sometimes disagree on the interpretation of a bilaterally absent N20 SSEP wave when the tracing has a low voltage or when there is interference from muscular artifacts or electrical equipment [4, 29, 30]. Although SSEP recording is technically simple, it requires expertise, which is not universally available.

The EEG has long been used for outcome prediction in post-anoxic coma. Several classification systems have been used to grade the EEG changes observed after anoxic injury and find a correlation with patient outcome. Most of these systems include five grades of increasing severity, with Grade I indicating predominant alpha rhythm, Grade II a predominant theta, Grade III a predominant delta, Grade IV the presence of isoelectric intervals, as in burst-suppression, and Grade V an isoelectric or very depressed tracing. However, the classification criteria for these systems are not consistent [8].

In two large cohort studies in patients not treated with therapeutic hypothermia [31, 32], a low-voltage EEG ($\leq$ 20–21 µV) at 24 h–72 h predicted poor outcome with 0 % [0–8] FPR. However, the application of this index for prognostication requires caution, since the amplitude of the EEG signal may depend on a variety of technical conditions, such as skin and scalp impedance, inter-electrode distances, size, type and placement of the exploring electrodes, type of filters adopted [33].

In contrast to SSEP, EEG is a widely available technology. However, it is also prone to the effects of hypothermia, sedative drugs and toxic-metabolic derangements. Barbiturates, opiates and benzodiazepines can induce alpha coma, while propofol and barbiturates at high doses can induce burst-suppression. Interference from therapeutic hypothermia and sedation and the inconsistencies of EEG patterns after cardiac arrest stimulated research towards a reliable and standardized method of EEG analysis for prognostication in therapeutic hypothermia-treated patients. Three cohort studies – two of which were from the same group – [20, 21, 34] showed that absence of EEG reactivity was a sensitive and highly specific predictor of poor outcome both during therapeutic hypothermia and after rewarming. The major limitation of this index is the lack of standardization of techniques to induce EEG reactivity (which include auditory, tactile, or noxious stimulation), and of the EEG reaction to the stimulus.

Presence of a burst-suppression pattern on the EEG within 72 h after cardiac arrest is often associated with poor outcome [8, 12], but may transiently appear in the early recovery phase after cardiac arrest in patients who eventually have a good outcome [35]. Reappearance of a continuous pattern is a reliable predictor of awakening in post-anoxic coma [36].

Presence of prolonged seizures, i. e., status epilepticus, is usually associated with poor outcome, in patients not treated with therapeutic hypothermia [32] and in therapeutic hypothermia-treated patients [21, 34, 37, 38]. However, it is unclear whether the epileptiform activity in these patients is just a marker of irreversible postanoxic brain injury or whether it contributes to poor outcome by causing direct or indirect neuronal damage [39, 40]. In this last case, aggressive seizure detection could improve final patient outcome. Both burst suppression and status epilepticus have inconsistent definitions [12].

Imaging

Evidence supporting the use of brain neuroimaging for outcome prediction in postanoxic coma is still limited. The two most investigated techniques are brain computer tomography (CT) and MRI.

The main CT finding of anoxic-ischemic cerebral insult is brain swelling, which appears as a reduction in ventricle size and sulci and an attenuation of the gray-white matter interface, measured as a reduction in the density ratio in Hounsfield units. A CT density ratio < 1.22 between the caudate and the posterior internal capsula was associated with death or vegetative state in 100 % of cases in both therapeutic hypothermia-treated and non-therapeutic hypothermia-treated patients [41, 42].

MRI has better spatial definition and higher sensitivity for anoxic-ischemic injury than brain CT, but its high costs and limited feasibility in unstable patients have hindered its use in the acute phase after cardiac arrest. The earliest post-anoxic MRI change is hyperintensity on diffuse weighted imaging (DWI) sequences, which reflects a restriction of water diffusion through neuronal membranes caused by ischemic dysfunction of the membrane-bound Na-K-ATPase pump. Presence of extensive DWI changes measured qualitatively at 4 h–32 h predicted poor outcome with 0 % FPR in one study [43] conducted in patients not treated with therapeutic hypothermia. In two studies conducted in therapeutic hypothermia-treated patients, extensive DWI changes in both cortical and deep gray matter nuclei within 5 days from cardiac arrest were 100 % specific for poor outcome [42, 44]. Being a qualitative technique, DWI is prone to interobserver variability, but it can be partly standardized using quantitative methods, such as the absolute diffusion coefficient (ADC). In two studies on therapeutic hypothermia-treated patients [45, 46], ADC reduction on MRI peaked from 3 to 5 days after cardiac arrest and was a highly specific predictor of poor outcome. The spatial distribution of MRI postanoxic changes in the brain is complex, and all the encephalic structures, including brain stem, basal ganglia and various cortical areas, can be affected.

Brain MRI in resuscitated comatose patients has mainly been used as a research rather than a prognostication tool and it has not attained widespread use yet. However, it can be used to improve sensitivity of more conventional predictors [46]. Relatively long measurement times and lack of bedside availability may limit MRI use in the most unstable resuscitated patients.

Self-fulfilling Prophecy

Studies on prediction of poor outcome in comatose patients resuscitated from cardiac arrest are prone to 'self-fulfilling prophecy', a bias which occurs when the treating physicians are not blinded to the results of the outcome predictor under investigation and use it to make a decision to withdraw treatment [47]. In a recent systematic review on prognostication in comatose therapeutic hypothermia-treated patients [12] only four of the 37 included studies reported blinding of the treating team from the results of the investigated predictors. In that review, treatment suspension policy was reported in 20/37 studies (54 %), in half of which it was based, at least in part, on one or more of the investigated predictors.

Prediction of poor outcome that is made too early when the patient may still be under the effect of sedatives/muscle relaxants or in the recovery phase from post-anoxic injury, can also increase the risk of inappropriate withdrawal of life sustaining treatment. At present, several authors agree that in therapeutic hypothermia-treated patients the time to prognostication should be delayed beyond 72 h after rewarming [7, 9, 48] especially with respect to clinical examination.

Another way of limiting the risk of falsely pessimistic predictions would be to use a multimodal approach. Combining predictors of poor outcome seems to be the most logical solution to reduce the risk of false positives, even though this would reduce sensitivity in some cases.

Conclusions

Prediction of poor neurological outcome in comatose resuscitated patients should be made with caution and possibly be based on multiple predictors. The predictive value of both clinical examination and SSEP at 72 h is very similar between therapeutic hypothermia-treated and non-treated patients. Absent pupillary reflex to light is the most specific clinical predictor, while absent corneal reflex is less accurate. A bilaterally absent N20 SSEP wave is highly specific (FPR < 1 %) and is more sensitive than ocular reflexes. In contrast to predictors based on clinical examination, SSEPs are not influenced by hypothermia or sedation, but require expertise and technology that are not yet universally available. Myoclonus status epilepticus is an infrequent but early and highly specific predictor of poor outcome. Its major limitations include an inconsistent definition and the possible confusion with benign forms of intentional myoclonus in patients with preserved brain function whose awareness is masked by sedation or paralysis.

EEG is widely available, but is less standardized than SSEP and is prone to interference from hypothermia and sedative drugs. EEG patterns like burst suppression and status epilepticus are usually associated with a poor outcome but their definition is inconsistent in the literature. EEG reactivity is relatively reproducible and is an accurate predictor in patients undergoing therapeutic hypothermia.

Biochemical markers, such as NSE and S-100B protein, are easy to use and are independent of sedation or paralysis, but there is wide variability in their thresholds for 100 % specificity both in therapeutic hypothermia-treated patients and in those not treated with therapeutic hypothermia.

MRI is a promising adjunctive prognostication tool; however, the evidence supporting its use is still limited and the complex spatial results it provides in post-anoxic comatose patients still need to be fully interpreted and standardized.

References

1. Stiell IG, Nichol G, Leroux BG et al (2011) Early versus later rhythm analysis in patients with out-of-hospital cardiac arrest. N Engl J Med 365:787–797
2. Wijdicks EF, Hijdra A, Young GB, Bassetti CL, Wiebe S (2006) Practice parameter: prediction of outcome in comatose survivors after cardiopulmonary resuscitation (an evidence-based review): report of the Quality Standards Subcommittee of the American Academy of Neurology. Neurology 67:203–210
3. Thenayan AE, Savard M, Sharpe M, Norton L, Young B (2008) Predictors of poor neurologic outcome after induced mild hypothermia following cardiac arrest. Neurology 71:1535–1537
4. Bouwes A, Binnekade JM, Kuiper MA et al (2012) Prognosis of coma after therapeutic hypothermia: a prospective cohort study. Ann Neurol 71:206–212

5. Mayer SA (2011) Outcome prediction after cardiac arrest: new game, new rules. Neurology 77:614–615
6. Reisinger J, Hollinger K, Lang W et al (2007) Prediction of neurological outcome after cardiopulmonary resuscitation by serial determination of serum neuron-specific enolase. Eur Heart J 28:52–58
7. Samaniego EA, Mlynash M, Caulfield AF, Eyngorn I, Wijman CA (2011) Sedation confounds outcome prediction in cardiac arrest survivors treated with hypothermia. Neurocrit Care 15:113–119
8. Sandroni C, Cavallaro F, Callaway CW et al (2013) Predictors of poor neurological outcome in adult comatose survivors of cardiac arrest: A systematic review and meta-analysis. Part 1: Patients not treated with therapeutic hypothermia. Resuscitation 84:1310–1324
9. Cronberg T, Brizzi M, Liedholm LJ et al (2013) Neurological prognostication after cardiac arrest-recommendations from the Swedish Resuscitation Council. Resuscitation 84:867–872
10. Zandbergen EG, de Haan RJ, Stoutenbeek CP, Koelman JH, Hijdra A (1998) Systematic review of early prediction of poor outcome in anoxic-ischaemic coma. Lancet 352:1808–1812
11. Young GB (2009) Clinical practice. Neurologic prognosis after cardiac arrest. N Engl J Med 361:605–611
12. Sandroni C, Cavallaro F, Callaway CW et al (2013) Predictors of poor neurological outcome in adult comatose survivors of cardiac arrest: A systematic review and meta-analysis. Part 2: Patients treated with therapeutic hypothermia. Resuscitation 84:1324–1328
13. Kamps MJ, Horn J, Oddo M et al (2013) Prognostication of neurologic outcome in cardiac arrest patients after mild therapeutic hypothermia: a meta-analysis of the current literature. Intensive Care Med 39:1671–1682
14. Rundgren M, Westhall E, Cronberg T, Rosen I, Friberg H (2010) Continuous amplitude-integrated electroencephalogram predicts outcome in hypothermia-treated cardiac arrest patients. Crit Care Med 38:1838–1844
15. Rittenberger JC, Popescu A, Brenner RP, Guyette FX, Callaway CW (2012) Frequency and timing of nonconvulsive status epilepticus in comatose post-cardiac arrest subjects treated with hypothermia. Neurocrit Care 16:114–122
16. Datta S, Hart GK, Opdam H, Gutteridge G, Archer J (2009) Post-hypoxic myoclonic status: the prognosis is not always hopeless. Crit Care Resusc 11:39–41
17. English WA, Giffin NJ, Nolan JP (2009) Myoclonus after cardiac arrest: pitfalls in diagnosis and prognosis. Anaesthesia 64:908–911
18. Bouwes A, van Poppelen D, Koelman JH et al (2012) Acute posthypoxic myoclonus after cardiopulmonary resuscitation. BMC Neurol 12:63
19. Lucas JM, Cocchi MN, Salciccioli J et al (2012) Neurologic recovery after therapeutic hypothermia in patients with post-cardiac arrest myoclonus. Resuscitation 83:265–269
20. Rossetti AO, Oddo M, Logroscino G, Kaplan PW (2010) Prognostication after cardiac arrest and hypothermia: a prospective study. Ann Neurol 67:301–307
21. Rossetti AO, Carrera E, Oddo M (2012) Early EEG correlates of neuronal injury after brain anoxia. Neurology 78:796–802
22. Fogel W, Krieger D, Veith M et al (1997) Serum neuron-specific enolase as early predictor of outcome after cardiac arrest. Crit Care Med 25:1133–1138
23. Steffen IG, Hasper D, Ploner CJ et al (2010) Mild therapeutic hypothermia alters neuron specific enolase as an outcome predictor after resuscitation: 97 prospective hypothermia patients compared to 133 historical non-hypothermia patients. Crit Care 14:R69
24. Anderson RE, Hansson LO, Nilsson O, Dijlai-Merzoug R, Settergren G (2001) High serum S100B levels for trauma patients without head injuries. Neurosurgery 48:1255–1258
25. Leithner C, Ploner CJ, Hasper D, Storm C (2010) Does hypothermia influence the predictive value of bilateral absent N20 after cardiac arrest? Neurology 74:965–969
26. Tiainen M, Kovala TT, Takkunen OS, Roine RO (2005) Somatosensory and brainstem auditory evoked potentials in cardiac arrest patients treated with hypothermia. Crit Care Med 33:1736–1740

27. Kottenberg-Assenmacher E, Armbruster W, Bornfeld N, Peters J (2003) Hypothermia does not alter somatosensory evoked potential amplitude and global cerebral oxygen extraction during marked sodium nitroprusside-induced arterial hypotension. Anesthesiology 98:1112–1118
28. Stecker MM, Cheung AT, Pochettino A et al (2001) Deep hypothermic circulatory arrest: I. Effects of cooling on electroencephalogram and evoked potentials. Ann Thorac Surg 71:14–21
29. Pfeifer R, Weitzel S, Gunther A et al (2013) Investigation of the inter-observer variability effect on the prognostic value of somatosensory evoked potentials of the median nerve (SSEP) in cardiac arrest survivors using an SSEP classification. Resuscitation 84:1375–1381
30. Zandbergen EG, Hijdra A, de Haan RJ et al (2006) Interobserver variation in the interpretation of SSEPs in anoxic-ischaemic coma. Clin Neurophysiol 117:1529–1535
31. Young GB, Doig G, Ragazzoni A (2005) Anoxic-ischemic encephalopathy: clinical and electrophysiological associations with outcome. Neurocrit Care 2:159–164
32. Zandbergen EG, Hijdra A, Koelman JH et al (2006) Prediction of poor outcome within the first 3 days of postanoxic coma. Neurology 66:62–68
33. Reilly EL (1993) EEG recording and operation of the apparatus. In: Niedermeyer E, Lopes Da Silva F (eds) Electroencephalography. Williams & Wilkins, Baltimore, pp 104–124
34. Crepeau AZ, Rabinstein AA, Fugate JE et al (2013) Continuous EEG in therapeutic hypothermia after cardiac arrest: prognostic and clinical value. Neurology 80:339–344
35. Jorgensen EO, Holm S (1998) The natural course of neurological recovery following cardiopulmonary resuscitation. Resuscitation 36:111–122
36. Kim YM, Yim HW, Jeong SH, Klem ML, Callaway CW (2012) Does therapeutic hypothermia benefit adult cardiac arrest patients presenting with non-shockable initial rhythms?: A systematic review and meta-analysis of randomized and non-randomized studies. Resuscitation 83:188–196
37. Legriel S, Hilly-Ginoux J, Resche-Rigon M et al (2013) Prognostic value of electrographic postanoxic status epilepticus in comatose cardiac-arrest survivors in the therapeutic hypothermia era. Resuscitation 84:343–350
38. Mani R, Schmitt SE, Mazer M, Putt ME, Gaieski DF (2012) The frequency and timing of epileptiform activity on continuous electroencephalogram in comatose post-cardiac arrest syndrome patients treated with therapeutic hypothermia. Resuscitation 83:840–847
39. DeGiorgio CM, Tomiyasu U, Gott PS, Treiman DM (1992) Hippocampal pyramidal cell loss in human status epilepticus. Epilepsia 33:23–27
40. VanLandingham KE, Lothman EW (1991) Self-sustaining limbic status epilepticus. I. Acute and chronic cerebral metabolic studies: limbic hypermetabolism and neocortical hypometabolism. Neurology 41:1942–1949
41. Choi SP, Park HK, Park KN et al (2008) The density ratio of grey to white matter on computed tomography as an early predictor of vegetative state or death after cardiac arrest. Emerg Med J 25:666–669
42. Choi SP, Youn CS, Park KN et al (2012) Therapeutic hypothermia in adult cardiac arrest because of drowning. Acta Anaesthesiol Scand 56:116–123
43. Els T, Kassubek J, Kubalek R, Klisch J (2004) Diffusion-weighted MRI during early global cerebral hypoxia: a predictor for clinical outcome? Acta Neurol Scand 110:361–367
44. Cronberg T, Rundgren M, Westhall E et al (2011) Neuron-specific enolase correlates with other prognostic markers after cardiac arrest. Neurology 77:623–630
45. Mlynash M, Campbell DM, Leproust EM et al (2010) Temporal and spatial profile of brain diffusion-weighted MRI after cardiac arrest. Stroke 41:1665–1672
46. Wijman CA, Mlynash M, Caulfield AF et al (2009) Prognostic value of brain diffusion-weighted imaging after cardiac arrest. Ann Neurol 65:394–402
47. Geocadin RG, Peberdy MA, Lazar RM (2012) Poor survival after cardiac arrest resuscitation: a self-fulfilling prophecy or biologic destiny? Crit Care Med 40:979–980
48. Blondin NA, Greer DM (2011) Neurologic prognosis in cardiac arrest patients treated with therapeutic hypothermia. Neurologist 17:241–248

Part XII
Gastrointestinal Problems

Stress Ulceration: Prevalence, Pathology and Association with Adverse Outcomes

M. P. Plummer, A. Reintam Blaser, and A. M. Deane

Introduction

So-called 'stress-related mucosal damage' (SRMD) is the broad term used to describe the spectrum of pathology attributed to the acute, erosive, inflammatory insult to the upper gastrointestinal tract associated with critical illness [1]. SRMD represents a continuum from asymptomatic superficial lesions found incidentally during endoscopy, occult gastrointestinal bleeding causing anemia, overt gastrointestinal bleeding and clinically significant gastrointestinal bleeding.

Prevalence

Stress ulceration was first described in 1969 when focal lesions in the mucosa of the gastric fundus were reported during post-mortem examinations in 7 (out of 150) critically ill patients [2]. Endoscopic studies have since identified that between 74–100 % of critically ill patients have stress-related mucosal erosions and subepithelial hemorrhage within 24 hours of admission (Fig. 1a) [3]. These lesions are generally superficial and asymptomatic, but can extend into the submucosa and muscularis propria and erode larger vessels causing overt and clinically significant bleeding (Fig. 1b).

The prevalence of overt and clinically significant bleeding depends on how these conditions are defined, with the definitions by Cook and colleagues the most widely accepted [4]. These authors defined overt gastrointestinal bleeding as the presence of hematemesis, bloody gastrointestinal aspirate or melena, while clinically

M. P. Plummer ✉ · A. M. Deane
Discipline of Acute Care Medicine, University of Adelaide, Adelaide, Australia
Department of Critical Care Services, Level 4, Royal Adelaide Hospital, Adelaide, Australia
e-mail: mark.philip.plummer@gmail.com

A. Reintam Blaser
Department of Anaesthesiology and Intensive Care, University of Tartu, Tartu, Estonia

J.-L. Vincent (Ed.), *Annual Update in Intensive Care and Emergency Medicine 2014*,
DOI 10.1007/978-3-319-03746-2_36, © Springer International Publishing Switzerland
and BioMed Central Ltd. 2014

Fig. 1 Stress-related mucosal disease. **a** Gastric antral erosions; **b** Pyloric ulcer with adherent clot

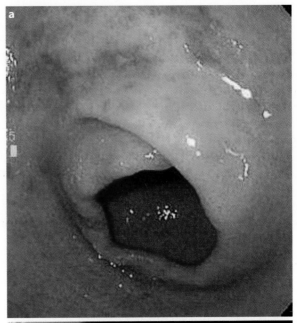

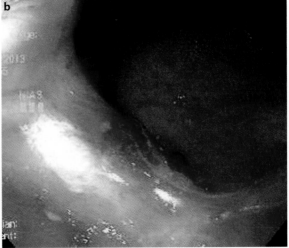

significant bleeding is the association of overt gastrointestinal bleeding and either hemodynamic compromise, or the requirement for blood transfusion, or surgery. It is important to emphasize that SRMD excludes variceal bleeding. However, bleeding *per se* is a clinical endpoint, and some studies may have incorrectly included bleeding attributable to varices, as well as that from the lower gastrointestinal tract, as part of the SRMD spectrum. This distinction is often not clear in the literature, particularly in observational studies of SRMD in which clinically significant bleeding is a primary outcome, which may led to investigators inappropriately including variceal, or non-SRMD bleeding. The importance of this distinction is highlighted in a prospective study by Cook and colleagues, which identified the cause of hemorrhage in 22 (of 33) patients with clinically significant gastrointestinal bleeding by the use of endoscopy or surgery [4]. In this study, stress ulceration was identified as the sole source of bleeding in 14 patients, with evidence of ulceration noted in 4 (of the remaining 8) patients in whom another bleeding site was identified, which included esophageal and gastric varices, vascular anomalies, and an anastomosis bleed [4]. Accordingly, variceal or non-SRMD pathologies, which will not be prevented by stress ulcer prophylactic therapies, are a frequent cause of overt and clinically significant bleeding. This distinction is often not identified in observational studies, whereas randomized controlled studies comparing different therapies for the prevention of SRMD have excluded patients with previous ulcer and variceal disease. For this reason, prevalence data from intervention studies may not be comparable to that from observational studies.

Nevertheless, data from earlier studies suggested that overt gastrointestinal bleeding occurred frequently, and in some studies up to 25 % of critically ill patients developed overt gastrointestinal bleeding [5]. It is now accepted that the condition is far more infrequent, with the prevalence reported as between 0.6 and 4 % of patients [4, 6]. The variation in prevalence is due, at least in part, to the cohort of patients studied and their risk factors for developing SRMD and it has been estimated that episodes of clinically significant stress ulcer bleeding in patients without risk factors is negligible (~0.1 %) [4]. The infrequency of the diagnosis in more recent epidemiological studies probably reflects an improvement in the overall management of the critically ill patient, including a focus on early aggressive resuscitation, attenuating mucosal hypoperfusion, and an awareness of the importance of early enteral nutrition [7].

Importance

Clinically significant gastrointestinal bleeding, as the name suggests, indicates that bleeding is substantive and important. It has been estimated that up to half of all patients with clinically significant upper gastrointestinal bleeding die in the intensive care unit (ICU) and, in survivors, the length of ICU stay increases by approximately 8 days [8]. It is, therefore, intuitive that preventing episodes of clinically significant gastrointestinal bleeding will lead to better patient outcomes. However, interventional studies that have reduced the incidence of stress ulceration have had no effect on either mortality or length of stay [6, 9]. Plausible explanations for this lack of effect following intervention are that:

(i)   a demonstrable proportion of clinically significant bleeding is not attributable to SRMD and will not respond to acid suppressive therapy;
(ii) previous studies were underpowered;
(iii) the interventions studied have adverse effects that negate any benefit from a reduction in stress ulceration; and

(iv) the association between development of clinically significant bleeding and mortality may not be causal, and that clinically significant bleeding may just be heralding a poor outcome.

Mechanisms

Putative mechanisms underlying SRMD include reduced gastric blood flow, mucosal ischemia and reperfusion injury, all of which occur frequently in the critically ill [9]. In a prospective observational study of 2,200 critically ill patients, mechanical ventilation > 48 hours and coagulopathy were identified as substantial risk factors for clinically significant bleeding (odds ratios 15.6 and 4.3, respectively) [4]. Studies of smaller cohorts, which were performed over 30 years ago, also reported associations between clinically significant bleeding and hypotension, sepsis, hepatic failure, renal failure, burns and major trauma [10].

Prevention of Stress Ulceration

Although clinically significant bleeding occurs infrequently, the severity of the associated complications has encouraged preventative approaches. For example, the FAST HUG mnemonic reminds clinicians to consider the need for stress ulcer prophylaxis on a daily basis [11]. Moreover, the recent Surviving Sepsis Campaign guidelines recommend the use of stress ulcer prophylaxis in patients with severe sepsis who have a risk factor, one of which is need for mechanical ventilation > 48 hours [12]. Somewhat surprisingly, the recommendation to prescribe a stress ulcer prophylaxis drug was listed as a 1B recommendation – translating into a 'strong' recommendation. This recommendation was endorsed despite the accompanying discussion acknowledging that there are no data to demonstrate a mortality benefit when prescribing these drugs [12].

Several drugs/techniques have been described to reduce the incidence of SRMD, including sucralfate, histamine-2 receptor blockers (H2RBs) and proton pump inhibitors (PPIs). Sucralfate acts by adhering to epithelial cells forming a physical cytoprotective barrier at the ulcer site, thereby protecting the gastric mucosa from the effects of acid and pepsin. Sucralfate is more effective than placebo in reducing overt bleeding, but has been shown to be inferior to H2RBs to reduce clinically significant bleeding [13]. Furthermore, sucralfate can impair the absorption of enteral feeds and co-administered oral medication [14], and there is a potential risk of bezoar formation (particularly in the setting of impaired gastric motility) when administering sucralfate to patients who are concurrently receiving enteral liquid nutrient [15]. Since intravenous H2RBs and PPIs are now widely available, sucralfate is rarely used as a first-line therapy.

H2RBs competitively inhibit histamine binding to its G-protein coupled receptor on the basolateral membrane of gastric parietal cells, which results in a reduction in acid production and an overall decrease in gastric secretions. H2RBs were used in early studies as first-line stress ulcer prophylaxis therapy, and were shown to significantly reduce the risk of clinically important bleeding when compared to placebo [13]. A limitation of H2RB administration is that tachyphylaxis can occur rapidly. In health, the anti-secretory effect of continuously infused intravenous ranitidine is dramatically reduced within the first day of administration [16]. With intragastric pH monitoring, studies in health have demonstrated that 70 % of patients have an intragastric pH > 4 in the first 24 hours of ranitidine intravenous infusion which falls to 26 % on the third day of continuous infusion [16]. Although similar studies have not been performed in the critically ill, these data raise concerns about the efficacy of H2RBs during longer term use in the critically ill [16].

PPIs inactivate the H^+/K^+ ATPase enzyme at the secretory surface of the parietal cell, inhibiting the secretion of H^+ ions and thereby increasing the pH of the gastric contents. In contrast to H2RBs the use of PPIs is not associated with the development of tolerance, with 100 % of healthy subjects maintaining an intragastric pH > 4 after 72 hours of continuous infusion of omeprazole [16]. In a recent meta-analysis, Alhazzani and colleagues reported that PPIs were more effective than H2RBs at reducing clinically important and overt upper gastrointestinal bleeding, without appearing to increase the risk of nosocomial pneumonia [6]. The Surviving Sepsis Campaign guidelines recommend the use of PPIs rather than H2RBs for stress ulcer prophylaxis citing level 2C evidence [12]. Previous studies of SRMD prophylaxis in the critically ill with PPIs are summarized in Table 1 [17–29]. Although these studies have been subject to meta-analyses by various groups [6, 9], with somewhat divergent results, even when these analyses have shown a reduction in clinically significant bleeding with PPI use, there has been no corresponding reduction in mortality.

Potential Adverse Effects Associated with Stress Ulcer Prophylaxis Therapy

Controversy surrounds the relationship between the use of stress ulcer prophylaxis and the development of infectious complications, particularly infection-related ventilator-associated complications (IVAC) and *Clostridium difficile* infection. Gastric acid plays an important role in natural host defense, with an intragastric pH < 4 being optimal for bactericidal action [30]. Accordingly, suppressing gastric acid production and raising the intragastric pH above this bactericidal threshold has the capacity to increase colonization of the stomach with pathogenic organisms.

Stress Ulcer Prophylaxis and Infection-related Ventilator-associated Complications

For the purpose of this review, the updated term 'infection-related ventilator-associated complication' has been used in preference to the previous term ventilator-associated pneumonia (VAP). In 2013, the Centers for Disease Control and

Table 1 A summary of trials of proton pump inhibitors for stress ulcer prophylaxis

Author (year)	Population	Intervention	UGI bleeding	Pneumonia
Powell et al. (1993) [17]	Post-CABG, surgical ICU. Age: 57; APACHE II: N/R	Omeprazole i.v. 80 mg × 1, then i.v. 40 mg/day (n = 10) Omeprazole i.v. 80 mg × 1, then i.v. 40 mg/8 h (n = 10) Ranitidine i.v. 50 mg/8 h (n = 11)	0 (0%) 0 (0%) 0 (0%)	N/R N/R N/R
Risaliti and Uzzau (1993) [18]	Post-major surgery, surgical ICU. Age: 62; APACHE II: N/R	Omeprazole i.v. 40 mg, then PO 20 mg/day (n = 14) Ranitidine i.v. 150 mg, then PO 300 mg/day (n = 14)	0 (0%) 0 (0%)	N/R N/R
Levy et al. (1997) [19]	Medical and surgical ICU. Age: 57; APACHE II: 19	Omeprazole NG 40 mg/day (n = 32) Ranitidine i.v. 50 mg bolus, then i.v. 50 mg/day (n = 35)	1 (3%)* 11 (35%)	5 (14%) 6 (18%)
Lasky et al. (1998) [10]	Post-trauma, mechanically ventilated. Age: N/A; APACHE II: N/R	Omeprazole NG 40 mg × 2, then NG 20 mg/day (n = 60)	0 (0%)	17 (28%)
Phillips et al. (1998) [21]	General ICU. Age: N/A; APACHE II: N/R	Omeprazole NG 40 mg × 2, then NG 20 mg/day (n = 33) Ranitidine i.v. 50 mg × 1, c.i.v. 150–200 mg/24 h (n = 25)	1 (3%)* 4 (16%)	6 (18%) 4 (16%)
Azvedo et al. (1999) [22]	General ICU. Age: 57; APACHE II: N/R	Omeprazole i.v. 40 mg/12 h (n = 38) Ranitidine c.i.v. 150 mg/24 h (n = 38) Sucralfate NG 1 mg/6 h (n = 32)	0 (0%) 4 (11%) 3 (9%)	5 (13.1%) 4 (11%) 3 (9%)
Kantorova et al. (2004) [23]	Surgical ICU. Age: 47; APACHE II: 18	Omeprazole i.v. 40 mg/day (n = 72) Famotidine i.v. 40 mg/12 h (n = 71) Sucralfate NG 1 mg/6 h (n = 69) Placebo (n = 75)	1 (1%) 2 (3%) 3 (4%) 1 (1%)	8 (11%) 7 (10%) 6 (9%) 5 (7%)
Pan and Li (2004) [24]	Critically ill patients with severe acute pancreatitis. Age: 48; APACHE II: 12	Rabeprazole PO 20 mg/day (n = 20) Famotidine i.v. 40 mg/12 h (n = 10)	0 (0%) 1 (10%)	N/R N/R
Conrad et al. (2005) [25]	General ICU. Age: 55; APACHE II: 23	Omeprazole NG 40 mg × 2, then NG 40 mg/day (n = 178) Cimetidine i.v. 300 mg bolus, then c.i.v. 1200 mg/24 h (n = 181)	7 (4%) 10 (6%)	20 (11%) 17 (9%)
Hata et al. (2005) [26]	Cardiac ICU. Age: 65; APACHE II: N/R	Rabeprazole PO 10 mg/day (n = 70) Ranitidine PO 300 mg/day (n = 70) Teprenone NG 150 mg/day (n = 70)	0 (0%) 4 (6%) 4 (6%)	N/R N/R N/R
Kotlyanskaya et al. (2008) [27]	Medical ICU. Age: 72; APACHE II: 28	Lanzoprazole PO (n = 45), dose not given Ranitidine (n = 21), dose and route not given	0 (0%) 3 (14%)	2 (4%) 4 (19%)

Continuation see next page

Table 1 *Continued*

Author (year)	Population	Intervention	UGI bleeding	Pneumonia
Somberg et al. (2008) [28]	Mixed ICU. Age 42; APACHE II: 15	Pantoprazole i.v. 40 mg/day (n = 32) Pantoprazole i.v. 40 mg/12 h (n = 38) Pantoprazole i.v. 80 mg/day (n = 23) Pantoprazole i.v. 80 mg/12 h (n = 39) Pantoprazole i.v. 80 mg/8 h (n = 35) Cimetidine i.v. 300 mg bolus, then CIV 1200 mg/24 h (n = 35)	0 (0 %) 0 (0 %) 0 (0 %) 0 (0 %) 0 (0 %) 0 (0 %)	3 (9 %) 8 (21 %) 1 (4.3 %) 2 (5.1 %) 2 (5.7 %) 3 (9.1 %)
Solouki and Kouchak (2009) [29]	General ICU. Age 50; APACHE II: N/R	Omeprazole NG 20 mg/12 h (n = 61) Ranitidine i.v. 50 mg/12 h (n = 68)	4 (7 %) 18 (26 %)	8 (13 %) 6 (9 %)

* Study reported clinical significance, age and APACHE data are presented as mean.
APACHE II: Acute Physiological and Chronic Health Evaluation II; CABG: coronary artery by-pass graft; c.i.v.: continuous intravenous infusion; i.v.: intravenous; NG: nasogastric; N/R: not recorded, PO: per oral; UGI: upper gastrointestinal.

Prevention proposed new definitions for patients receiving mechanical ventilation, including IVAC to improve objectivity and facilitate comparability [31]. Although prior studies investigating stress ulcer prophylaxis have exclusively used the term VAP to report data, with the inherent subjectivity associated with this diagnosis, we believe that using the recently proposed definitions for IVAC in future studies will more accurately determine whether stress ulcer prophylaxis increases adverse events during mechanical ventilation. It should be recognized, however, that the previous studies all referred to VAP rather than IVAC.

A mechanism that has been proposed to contribute to IVAC is the contamination of the oropharyngeal area by reflux of gastric fluid, with subsequent aspiration of the oropharyngeal bacteria to the lower airways [32]. Because numerous organisms are unable to live in an acidic environment, the administration of drugs to increase gastric pH could facilitate gastric colonization with pathogenic organisms and pre-dispose to respiratory infections [30]. In ambulant patients, use of PPIs has been associated with an increased risk of community-acquired pneumonia (CAP) [33]. Laheij et al. reported a 1.89 fold increase in the risk of CAP in those taking PPIs versus those who had stopped using PPIs [33], with a correlation between dose of PPI and risk of pneumonia [33].

In the critically ill, however, data relating intragastric pH and pulmonary infections are inconsistent. Some studies have reported a higher occurrence of IVAC in patients who received drugs to increase gastric pH compared to those who received sucralfate [34], supporting the importance of gastric acidity and the role of the entero-pulmonary route. However, Heyland et al. reported that while the delivery of acidified enteral feeds (pH 3.5) preserved gastric acidity and dramatically reduced gastric bacterial growth and lowered the rate of Gram-negative bacterial growth in tracheal suction, there was no reduction in frequency of VAP [35]. In a meta-analysis of data comparing H2RBs and placebo, which did not adjust for enteral nutrition, Cook et al. reported a trend towards increased rates of pneumonia with the routine use of H2RBs [13].

Despite PPI prophylaxis being a key recommendation of the Surviving Sepsis Guidelines, there have been no large-scale prospective randomized trials that have compared PPIs and placebo to determine the efficacy and/or adverse events associated with their use [12]. Nevertheless, the rate of IVAC associated with PPI use is likely to be at least similar to that observed with H2RBs [6]. Furthermore, if tolerance to H2RBs occurs, and increasing pH increases the risk of IVAC, it is plausible that VAP rates will be even greater in patients receiving PPIs. Regardless of whether H2RBs or PPIs are more harmful in creating the ideal environment to alter bacterial colonization of the stomach, this issue is likely to be particularly relevant for enterally fed patients, as enteral feeding *per se* may be a risk factor for IVAC [36].

Stress Ulcer Prophylaxis and *Clostridium difficile* Infection

Symptomatic infection with *C. difficile* occurs relatively frequently in mechanically ventilated critically ill patients. Using data from over 65,000 patients in the United States who required prolonged ventilation, *C. difficile*-associated diseases were present in >5 % of patients [37]. Furthermore *C. difficile* infections are important because infection leads to a substantial increase in hospital length of stay (6.1 days; 95 % confidence interval 4.9–7.4) [37].

There is a plausible biological mechanism that acid-suppression increases the risk of developing *C. difficile* colonization, because host immunity is compromised by a higher pH environment in the stomach [38]. Observational studies have reported an association between iatrogenic acid suppression and *C. difficile*-associated diseases [38]. In a prospective case-control study of 303 patients admitted to a general medical ward, Yearsley et al. reported a two-fold increase in *C. difficile*-associated diseases in patients receiving PPIs [39]. However, to the best of our knowledge, there are no epidemiological data detailing *C. difficile*-associated diseases in critically ill patients receiving stress ulcer prophylaxis.

Complications Associated with Long-term Use of Drug Therapies

Although complications associated with the acute use of H2RBs and PPIs are of more relevance to critically ill patients, it should be recognized that chronic use of PPIs has been associated with osteoporosis and fractures [40]. Adverse effects associated with chronic use may be important, as a recent observational study reported that around a third of patients given PPIs for stress ulcer prophylaxis went home on the drug despite there being no indication on discharge from hospital for their continued use [41].

Enteral Feeds and the Role of Stress Ulcer Prophylaxis

The majority of the studies on which current recommendations are based were performed over 20 years ago. Over that time, there have been changes to the perceived importance of enteral nutrition, with intragastric feeds commenced sooner after admission [42]. Liquid nutrient buffers gastric acid, increases mucosal blood flow and induces the secretion of cytoprotective prostaglandins and mucus [43]. It is uncertain what influence the route of enteral feeding has on the effect of liquid nutrient. Although it is intuitive that only liquid nutrient administered into the stomach could have these potentially beneficial effects, delivery directly into the small intestine may have other advantages that lead to favorable outcomes [42]. Furthermore, because of duodenal-gastric reflux of liquid [32] and increase in mesenteric blood flow due to small intestinal delivery [44], postpyloric delivery may still prevent development of stress ulceration. Nevertheless the so-called 'early' administration of enteral nutrition into the stomach has been suggested to have contributed substantially to the diminishing frequency of stress ulcer-related bleeding that has been observed over the last 30 years [7]. In the critically ill, continuous enteral nutrition has been shown to be more effective at increasing intragastric pH than H2RBs and PPIs [45] and, in rats, enteral nutrition provides better protection against stress ulceration than do intravenous H2RBs [46]. Studies in humans to evaluate the effects of enteral nutrition on gastrointestinal bleeding reduction have primarily been performed in patients post-burn injury. Interpretation of these data are problematic because of inconsistencies around the definitions of SRMD, clinically significant upper gastrointestinal bleeding and enteral nutrition [47]. Marik et al. performed a meta-analysis to evaluate the effects of H2RBs and placebo [9]. In the subgroup of patients who received enteral feeds, stress ulcer prophylaxis did not reduce the risk of bleeding but increased VAP rates and mortality [9]. However, as acknowledged by the authors, subgroup analysis within a systematic review should be interpreted with caution. For this reason we consider the Marik review hypothesis-generating and prospective studies to determine the influence of enteral nutrition on SRMD and stress ulcer prophylaxis-associated IVAC are urgently required.

Cost of Routine Prophylaxis

Models of cost-effectiveness of stress ulcer prophylaxis advocate that prophylactic therapy be limited to patients with established risk factors for clinically significant bleeding [48]. In comparison to routine prophylaxis for all critically ill patients, this strategy has been shown to decrease H2RB drug costs by 80 % without altering the frequency of gastrointestinal bleeding [49]. To our knowledge, a cost analysis has not been performed with PPIs in the critically ill. Based on historical data, however, stress ulcer prophylaxis would need to be routinely administered to 900 hospitalized patients to prevent one episode of clinically significant bleeding [50]. Since clinically significant stress ulcer bleeding occurs infrequently in patients without risk factors, routine stress ulcer prophylaxis is unlikely to be cost-effective and should probably be avoided in this subgroup, particularly given the potential for harm with PPI and H2RB use. As described [41], almost a third of patients have PPIs continued on hospital discharge, which in itself will lead to increases in costs to individual patients and communities, independent of any long-term health concerns.

Conclusions

Using current resuscitation and feeding practices, clinically significant gastrointestinal bleeding, as a consequence of SRMD, appears to occur infrequently. Nevertheless, should clinically significant bleeding occur, it is associated with significant morbidity and at least a 4-fold increase in ICU mortality. Patients with respiratory failure requiring mechanical ventilation for > 48 hours and those with coagulopathy are at the highest risk of clinically significant bleeding. Based on these observations, current guidelines suggest that this group is most likely to benefit from prophylactic therapy. The superior efficacy of PPIs has shaped recommendations that these agents be used as first-line therapy. However, the routine use of stress ulcer prophylaxis in all critically patients may be harmful and is unlikely to be cost-effective. Controversy surrounds pharmacologically increasing gastric pH, but there is mechanistic plausibility that this may increase the rate of IVAC and *C. difficile* infections – both of which are associated with substantial morbidity and increased costs – particularly in those ventilated for > 48 hours. In contrast to recent recommendations from the Surviving Sepsis Campaign, we contend that the issue of stress ulcer prophylaxis is not settled and further prospective randomized trials are required to guide decision-making.

References

1. Peura D (1986) Stress-related mucosal damage. Clin Ther 8(A):14–23
2. Skillman JJ, Bushnell LS, Goldman H, Silen W (1969) Respiratory failure, hypotension, sepsis, and jaundice. A clinical syndrome associated with lethal hemorrhage from acute stress ulceration of the stomach. Am J Surg 117:523–530
3. Mutlu GM, Mutlu EA, Factor P (2001) GI complications in patients receiving mechanical ventilation. Chest 119:1222–1241
4. Cook DJ, Fuller HD, Guyatt GH et al (1994) Risk factors for gastrointestinal bleeding in critically ill patients. Canadian Critical Care Trials Group. N Engl J Med 330:377–381
5. Hastings PR, Skillman JJ, Bushnell LS, Silen W (1978) Antacid titration in the prevention of acute gastrointestinal bleeding. N Engl J Med 298:1041–1045
6. Alhazzani W, Alenezi F, Jaeschke RZ, Moayyedi P, Cook DJ (2013) Proton pump inhibitors versus histamine 2 receptor antagonists for stress ulcer prophylaxis in critically ill patients: a systematic review and meta-analysis. Crit Care Med 41:693–705

7. Faisy C, Guerot E, Diehl JL, Iftimovici E, Fagon JY (2003) Clinically significant gastrointestinal bleeding in critically ill patients with and without stress-ulcer prophylaxis. Intensive Care
Med 29:1306–1313

8. Cook DJ, Griffith LE, Walter SD et al (2001) The attributable mortality and length of intensive
care unit stay of clinically important gastrointestinal bleeding in critically ill patients. Crit Care
5:368–375

9. Marik PE, Vasu T, Hirani A, Pachinburavan M (2010) Stress ulcer prophylaxis in the new
millennium: a systematic review and meta-analysis. Crit Care Med 38:2222–2228

10. Fiddian-Green RG, Mcgough E, Pittenger G, Rothman E (1983) Predictive value of intramu-
ral pH and other risk factors for massive bleeding from stress ulceration. Gastroenterology
85:613–620

11. Vincent JL (2005) Give your patient a fast hug (at least) once a day. Crit Care Med 33:1225–
1229

12. Dellinger RP, Levy MM, Rhodes A et al (2013) Surviving Sepsis Campaign: international
guidelines for management of severe sepsis and septic shock: 2012. Crit Care Med 41:580–
637

13. Cook DJ, Reeve BK, Guyatt GH et al (1996) Stress ulcer prophylaxis in critically ill patients.
Resolving discordant meta-analyses. JAMA 275:308–314

14. Daley RJ, Rebuck JA, Welage LS, Rogers FB (2004) Prevention of stress ulceration: current
trends in critical care. Crit Care Med 32:2008–2013

15. Guy C, Ollagnier M (1999) Sucralfate and bezoars: data from the system of pharmacologic
vigilance and review of the literature. Therapie 54:55–58

16. Netzer P, Gaia C, Sandoz M et al (1999) Effect of repeated injection and continuous infusion of
omeprazole and ranitidine on intragastric pH over 72 hours. Am J Gastroenterol 94:351–357

17. Powell H, Morgan M, Li SK, Baron J (1993) Inhibition of gastric acid secretion in the intensive
care unit after coronary artery bypass graft. A pilot control study of intravenous omeprazole
by bolus and infusion, ranitidine and placebo. Theor Surg 8:125–130

18. Risaliti ATG, Uzzau A (1993) Intravenous omeprazole vs ranitidine in the prophylaxis of stress
ulcers. Acta. Chir Ital 49:397–401

19. Levy MJ, Seelig CB, Robinson NJ, Ranney JE (1997) Comparison of omeprazole and ranitidine for stress ulcer prophylaxis. Dig Dis Sci 42:1255–1259

20. Lasky MR, Metzler MH, Phillips JO (1998) A prospective study of omeprazole suspension
to prevent clinically significant gastrointestinal bleeding from stress ulcers in mechanically
ventilated trauma patients. J Trauma 44:527–533

21. Phillips JO, Metzler MH, Huckfeldt RE, Olsen K (1998) Multicenter prospective randomized
clinical trial of continuous infusion I.V. Ranitidine vs. Omeprazole suspension in the prophylaxis of stress ulcers. Crit Care Med 26:101A (abst)

22. Azevedo SM Jr, Silva G, Palacio G (1999) Prevention of stress ulcer bleeding in high risk
patients. Comparison of three drugs. Crit Care Med 27:A145 (abst)

23. Kantorova I, Svoboda P, Scheer P et al (2004) ulcer prophylaxis in critically ill patients: a
randomized controlled trial. Hepatogastroenterology. Stress 51:757–761

24. Pan XZW, Li Z (2004) The preventive effects of rabeprazole on upper gastrointestinal tract
hemorrhage in patients with severe acute pancreatitis. Chin J Gastroenterol 9:30–32

25. Conrad SA, Gabrielli A, Margolis B et al (2005) Randomized, double-blind comparison of
immediate-release omeprazole oral suspension versus intravenous cimetidine for the prevention of upper gastrointestinal bleeding in critically ill patients. Crit Care Med 33:760–765

26. Hata M, Shiono M, Sekino H et al (2005) Prospective randomized trial for optimal prophylactic
treatment of the upper gastrointestinal complications after open heart surgery. Circ J 69:331–
334

27. Kotlyanskaya A, Luka B, Mukherji R et al (2008) A comparison of lansoprazole disintegrat-
ing tablet, lansoprazole suspension or ranitidine for stress ulcer prophylaxis in critically ill
patients. Crit Care Med 7:A194 (abst)

28. Somberg L, Morris J Jr, Fantus R et al (2008) Intermittent intravenous pantoprazole and continuous cimetidine infusion: effect on gastric pH control in critically ill patients at risk of developing stress-related mucosal disease. J Trauma 64:1202–1210
29. Solouki MMS, Kouchak M (2009) Comparison between the preventive effects of ranitidine and omeprazole on upper gastrointestinal bleeding among ICU patients. Tanaffos 8:37–42
30. Heyland D, Bradley C, Mandell LA (1992) Effect of acidified enteral feedings on gastric colonization in the critically ill patient. Crit Care Med 20:1388–1394
31. Klompas M (2013) Complications of mechanical ventilation – the CDC's new surveillance paradigm. N Engl J Med 368:1472–1475
32. Chapman MJ, Nguyen NQ, Deane AM (2011) Gastrointestinal dysmotility: clinical consequences and management of the critically ill patient. Gastroenterol Clin North Am 40:725–739
33. Laheij RJ, Sturkenboom MC, Hassing RJ, Dieleman J, Stricker BH, Jansen JB (2004) Risk of community-acquired pneumonia and use of gastric acid-suppressive drugs. JAMA 292:1955–1960
34. Prod'hom G, Leuenberger P, Koerfer J et al (1994) Nosocomial pneumonia in mechanically ventilated patients receiving antacid, ranitidine, or sucralfate as prophylaxis for stress ulcer. A randomized controlled trial. Ann Intern Med 120:653–662
35. Heyland DK, Cook DJ, Schoenfeld PS, Frietag A, Varon J, Wood G (1999) The effect of acidified enteral feeds on gastric colonization in critically ill patients: results of a multicenter randomized trial. Canadian Critical Care Trials Group. Crit Care Med 27:2399–2406
36. Jacobs S, Chang RW, Lee B, Bartlett FW (1990) Continuous enteral feeding: a major cause of pneumonia among ventilated intensive care unit patients. JPEN J Parenter Enteral Nutr 14:353–356
37. Zilberberg MD, Nathanson BH, Sadigov S, Higgins TL, Kollef MH, Shorr AF (2009) Epidemiology and outcomes of clostridium difficile-associated disease among patients on prolonged acute mechanical ventilation. Chest 136:752–758
38. Howell MD, Novack V, Grgurich P et al (2010) Iatrogenic gastric acid suppression and the risk of nosocomial Clostridium difficile infection. Arch Intern Med 170:784–790
39. Yearsley KA, Gilby LJ, Ramadas AV, Kubiak EM, Fone DL, Allison MC (2006) Proton pump inhibitor therapy is a risk factor for Clostridium difficile-associated diarrhoea. Aliment Pharmacol Ther 24:613–619
40. Khalili H, Huang ES, Jacobson BC, Camargo CA Jr, Feskanich D, Chan AT (2012) Use of proton pump inhibitors and risk of hip fracture in relation to dietary and lifestyle factors: a prospective cohort study. BMJ 344:e372
41. Farley KJ, Barned KL, Crozier TM (2013) Inappropriate continuation of stress ulcer prophylaxis beyond the intensive care setting. Crit Care Resusc 15:147–151
42. Deane AM, Dhaliwal R, Day AG, Ridley EJ, Davies AR, Heyland DK (2013) Comparisons between intragastric and small intestinal delivery of enteral nutrition in the critically ill: a systematic review and meta-analysis. Crit Care 17:R125
43. Ephgrave KS, Kleiman-Wexler RL, Adair CG (1990) Enteral nutrients prevent stress ulceration and increase intragastric volume. Crit Care Med 18:621–624
44. Sim JA, Horowitz M, Summers MJ et al (2013) Mesenteric blood flow, glucose absorption and blood pressure responses to small intestinal glucose in critically ill patients older than 65 years. Intensive Care Med 39:258–266
45. Bonten MJ, Gaillard CA, Van Tiel FH, Van Der Geest S, Stobberingh EE (1994) Continuous enteral feeding counteracts preventive measures for gastric colonization in intensive care unit patients. Crit Care Med 22:939–944
46. Harju E, Sajanti J (1987) The protective effect of nutrients against stress induced gastric ulcers in the rat. Surg Gynecol Obstet 165:530–534
47. Stollman N, Metz DC (2005) Pathophysiology and prophylaxis of stress ulcer in intensive care unit patients. J Crit Care 20:35–45

48. Ben-Menachem T, Mccarthy BD, Fogel R et al (1996) Prophylaxis for stress-related gastrointestinal hemorrhage: a cost effectiveness analysis. Crit Care Med 24:338–345
49. Devlin JW, Claire KS, Dulchavsky SA, Tyburski JG (1999) Impact of trauma stress ulcer prophylaxis guidelines on drug cost and frequency of major gastrointestinal bleeding. Pharmacotherapy 19:452–460
50. Cash BD (2002) Evidence-based medicine as it applies to acid suppression in the hospitalized patient. Crit Care Med 30:S373–S378

Surgical Complications Following Bariatric Surgery

P. Montravers, P. Fournier, and P. Augustin

Introduction

Bariatric surgery is an increasingly common treatment for morbid obesity [1], because it is the only technique with demonstrated efficacy in terms of long-term, sustained weight loss. Most studies have shown that these operations are safe, with decreased overall mortality and morbidity, and reversal of related comorbidities in obese patients. However, the beneficial effects of bariatric surgery need to be weighed against the risks of perioperative complications and postoperative or short-term adverse outcomes [2].

From the intensive care unit (ICU) physician's perspective, these patients represent new and challenging issues and raise specific concerns. Several medical postoperative complications may require ICU admission, the most common being acute respiratory failure and thromboembolic disease with deep vein thrombosis and pulmonary embolism. Surgical complications are specific to the procedure performed, but anastomotic leaks are probably the most common life-threatening events [3, 4]. The purpose of this chapter is to review the surgical complications most commonly observed during bariatric surgery in order to help surgeons and ICU physicians provide high-quality care for these high-risk patients.

P. Montravers ✉ · P. Augustin
APHP, CHU Bichat-Claude Bernard, Département d'Anesthésie Réanimation, Université Paris Diderot, Paris, France
e-mail: philippe.montravers@bch.aphp.fr

P. Fournier
APHP, CHU Bichat-Claude Bernard, Service de Chirurgie Générale, Université Paris Diderot, Paris, France

J.-L. Vincent (Ed.), *Annual Update in Intensive Care and Emergency Medicine 2014*,   487
DOI 10.1007/978-3-319-03746-2_37, © Springer International Publishing Switzerland 2014

Description of Surgical Procedures

Bariatric surgery, mostly developed in recent decades and usually performed laparo-scopically, can be divided into restrictive and malabsorptive operations [1]. These procedures are designed to reduce caloric intake by modifying the anatomy of the upper mesocolic gastrointestinal tract.

Restrictive Procedures (Fig. 1)

Several restrictive procedures have been described, designed to limit food intake by creating a small gastric reservoir with a narrow outlet resulting in delayed emptying.

Adjustable gastric banding consists of placement of an adjustable silicone ring around the stomach 2 cm below the cardia to create a small pouch with a narrow outlet, combined with insertion of a subcutaneous port to adjust gastric restriction by means of saline injections. The small stomach pouch rapidly becomes filled, causing satiety.

Vertical restrictive (sleeve) gastrectomy was initially proposed as the first step of the duodenal switch procedure, but, more recently, has become an independent treatment option for morbid obesity. This procedure removes the terminal two-thirds of the gastric volume to leave a narrow stomach tube by stapling along the entire length of the greater curvature.

Malabsorptive Procedures (Fig. 2)

Malabsorptive procedures bypass various portions of the small intestine in which nutrient absorption occurs in order to reduce jejunal absorption.

Proximal Roux-en-Y gastric bypass (RYGB), often considered to be a mixed restriction-malabsorption procedure, involves stapling of the stomach to create a small (30–50 ml) upper gastric pouch, while the small intestine is divided at the midjejunum, and the distal portion (called the alimentary, or Roux, limb) is anasto-mosed to the gastric pouch. The longer the Roux limb, the less nutrient absorption will occur. Two types of anastomosis can be performed: Gastrojejunal anastomosis and jejunojejunal anastomosis.

Other malabsorptive procedures, such as duodenal switch, are usually selected for super-obese patients (BMI > 50 kg/m^2) or after failure of previous bariatric pro-cedures. This procedure comprises reduction of the stomach by means of sleeve gastrectomy together with creation of a duodeno-ileal short circuit with two anas-tomoses (duodeno-ileal and ileo-ileal) [5].

a

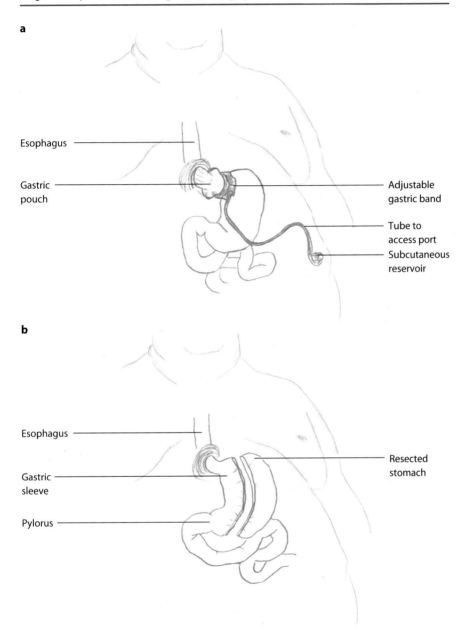

Esophagus

Gastric
pouch

Adjustable
gastric band

Tube to
access port

Subcutaneous
reservoir

b

Esophagus

Gastric
sleeve

Pylorus

Resected
stomach

Fig. 1 Surgical consequences of restrictive procedures: Adjustable gastric banding (**a**); vertical restrictive sleeve gastrectomy (**b**)

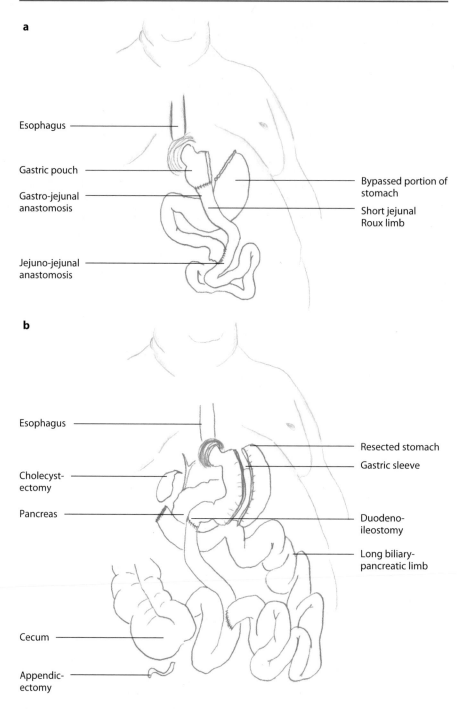

Fig. 2 Surgical consequences of malabsorptive procedures: Proximal Roux-en-Y gastric by-pass (**a**); duodenal switch (**b**)

Epidemiology of Surgical Complications and Clinical Presentation

Surgical complications can occur during the procedure, but more often occur during the early postoperative period (usually the first month) or later. The time to diagnosis usually peaks between day 1 and day 18, as these patients are frequently asymptomatic or have only limited clinical signs [6–8]. Descriptions of surgical postoperative complications are mainly based on analyses of general or surgical site complications [9]. Most of these cases are treated in surgical wards and never require ICU management [10]. Very few data are available concerning patients requiring ICU management, usually limited to case reports [11] or small case series [12, 13]. Most epidemiologic reports are based on large database analyses concerning patients referred to the surgical ward and ICU for these complications and the proportion of patients requiring ICU admission cannot be accurately estimated.

Surgical causes of ICU admission can be classified into two main categories: Intra-abdominal sepsis, mainly due to fistula and anastomotic leaks, and non-septic complications, mainly hemorrhage. Anastomotic leaks may occur in up to 5.6 % of cases, making these events a more common postoperative complication than pulmonary embolism [3, 14]. This issue was confirmed by Goldfeder et al. in an analysis of 107 autopsies following bariatric surgery [15]. They reported 97 deaths linked to complications of surgery, with anastomotic leaks (36 %) as the leading cause of death, whereas pulmonary embolism accounted for only 13 % of deaths [15].

Complications Following Restrictive Procedures

The morbidity rates for adjustable gastric banding range from 11 to 32 % with a short-term mortality rate between 0.05 and 0.09 %, the lowest of all bariatric surgery procedures [16, 17]. However, many early complications have been described and can be potentially life-threatening when the diagnosis is delayed:

- Gastric or esophageal perforation is sometimes diagnosed intraoperatively, constituting a contraindication to ring placement. In other cases, unexplained signs of sepsis with tachycardia are usually observed during the early postoperative period, from day 1–2, leading to delayed diagnosis. Among 22 studies reviewed by the French ANAES (French National Agency for Accreditation and Evaluation in Health) agency, the incidence of gastric perforation was 0.3 % (15/5,237 patients) [18].
- Infection of the ring or port may lead to suppuration at the port site [16, 17], possibly due to initially unrecognized perforation. Port infection is not systematically associated with ring infection, in which case the ring can be left in place.
- Ring malposition is a postoperative complication that can result in complete dysphagia, whereas band slippage is reported as a late complication in 6 to 13 % of cases, requiring reoperation in one half of cases [17].

The most common complications following sleeve gastrectomy are fistulas, reported in 0 to 5 % of cases [19]. In a meta-analysis comprising nearly 10,000 sleeve gastrectomies, Parikh et al. reported a fistula rate of 2.2 % [20]. Tachycardia, abdominal pain, fever and clinical signs are the usual precursor signs of surgical complications, but signs of sepsis can be severe. Bleeding on the stapling line occurs in approximately 3.5 % of cases [19]. Postoperative tachycardia is the main sign suggestive of bleeding [19], which may often be difficult to suspect until a low plasma hemoglobin concentration is observed.

Complications of Malabsorptive Procedures

Malabsorptive procedures are associated with the highest complication rates. Buchwald et al. reported mortality rates of 0.5 % in their meta-analysis analyzing gastric bypass [21]. Podnos and colleagues reported a complication rate of 19 % [22]. The most common complications of RYGB are anastomotic leaks, with an incidence ranging from 0 to 8 % according to various authors [3, 14]. Each segment of the procedure is at risk of fistula: Gastric pouch, excluded part of the stomach, gastrojejunal anastomosis, jejunojejunal anastomosis, and sliced section of the small intestine. The diagnosis of fistula is based on conventional clinical signs (abdominal pain, fever, leukocytosis, tachycardia), fluid drainage, and finally radiological examinations (upper gastrointestinal imaging and computed tomography [CT] scan) [23]. Bleeding in the various segments occurs in 1 % of procedures [24]. The origin of bleeding can be intraluminal or intraperitoneal with the same diagnostic difficulties as those described for restrictive procedures.

Buchwald et al. [21] reported the highest mortality rate of 11 % in duodenal switch procedures. Complications of duodenal switch, which are highly dependent on the surgical technique, are also fairly common, with rates ranging between 2.8 and 34 % depending on the author. The complications observed in these cases comprise those observed with sleeve gastrectomy and gastric bypass.

Clinical Presentation at the Time of ICU Admission

Surgical postoperative complications and especially postoperative intra-abdominal sepsis after bariatric surgery appear to be difficult to detect [25]. One of the most difficult issues is identification of these complications before the onset of organ dysfunction. Bariatric surgery patients represent an atypical group that differs from other 'common' groups with surgical postoperative complications and peritonitis. We recently compared a group of 134 patients admitted to the ICU for postoperative peritonitis not related to bariatric surgery and a group of 49 patients who developed postoperative peritonitis following bariatric surgery [26]. The bariatric surgery patients were younger (45 ± 10 versus 63 ± 16 years; $p < 0.0001$), did not suffer from cancer and presented lower rates of fatal underlying disease (39 vs 64 %; $p = 0.002$). However, the time to diagnosis of surgical complications was similar

Table 1 Clinical presentation at the time of diagnosis of gastric bypass anastomotic leakage

	Ballesta [7]	Thodiyil [8]	Gonzalez [23]
Number of cases	59	46	63
No clinical signs	49 %	11 %	8 %
Abdominal pain	50 %	24 %	54 %
Left shoulder pain	–	8 %	14 %
Nausea/vomiting	18 %	6 %	17 %
Abnormal drainage	49 %	28 %	24 %
Fever > 38 °C	49 %	28 %	63 %
White blood cell count > 12,000/mm^3	–	67 %	51 %
Tachycardia	22 %	17 %	72 %
Polypnea	–	9 %	–
Hypotension	12 %	2 %	17 %
Oliguria	13 %	4 %	21 %

to that reported during non-bariatric surgery both above and below the transverse mesocolon [26].

Clinical signs can be misleading or atypical in obese patients and can make the diagnosis challenging [3, 27]. Hamilton et al. reported that tachycardia > 120 bpm and respiratory distress were the most sensitive indicators of gastrointestinal leakage after RYGB [27]. Several authors analyzed the frequency of clinical signs at the time of diagnosis of anastomotic leaks in cohorts of gastric bypass patients not admitted to the ICU (Table 1). Interestingly, many of these complicated patients did not show any clinical signs, at least at the time of the diagnostic process [7, 8, 23]. This paucity of symptoms was confirmed in 27 ICU bariatric surgery cases reported by Kermarrec et al. suggesting that the diagnosis of postoperative peritonitis is difficult, even in patients with a deteriorating clinical status [28]. Extraabdominal signs were the symptoms most frequently reported (fever, dyspnea and tachycardia in 74, 98 and 100 % of cases, respectively), while abdominal signs were rarely reported (tenderness, pus, ileus in 30 %, 33 % and 37 % of cases, respectively) [28]. The predominance of respiratory signs over abdominal signs guided the initial diagnosis toward pleural or pulmonary diseases, resulting in an incorrect diagnosis in more than 50 % (15/27) of patients. The attending teams more frequently proposed diagnoses of pneumonia (n = 7), pulmonary embolism (n = 4), wound abscess (n = 2), and bowel obstruction (n = 2) [28]. Unfortunately, most of the complicated cases admitted to the ICU already exhibited organ dysfunction. Interestingly, bariatric surgery patients do not differ from patients with common forms of postoperative peritonitis with a similar sequential organ failure assessment (SOFA) score and almost two-thirds of cases require vasoactive support and mechanical ventilation, and one-third present renal failure as assessed by the SOFA score [26]. Overall, the reasons for the poor sensitivity of physical examination in morbidly obese patients remain unclear, but could be related to many issues such as the large mass of abdominal subcutaneous tissue, the subphrenic site of intraperitoneal sepsis, or the postoperative nature of the peritonitis.

Radiologic Studies

Radiographic imaging is highly recommended in the decision-making process for patients with suspected postoperative surgical complications [29]. However, the lack of specificity of imaging studies can make the diagnosis challenging [3, 27]. Madan et al. reported that routine upper gastrointestinal studies after RYGB were more predictive of an early leak diagnosis than clinical signs [30]. In this study, positive and negative predictive values of leak using upper gastrointestinal studies on the first postoperative day were 67 % and 99 %, respectively. Limited data are available concerning the capacity of CT scan to detect surgical complications and anastomotic leaks after bariatric surgery. Lyass et al suggested the advantage of CT scan over upper gastrointestinal studies, because it also allowed detection of complications other than anastomotic leaks [31]. To the best of our knowledge, no study has ever assessed the specificity and sensitivity of CT scan in the diagnosis of complicated bariatric surgery in the ICU setting. This point is of major importance and could be linked to certain limitations in the use of imaging procedures encountered in this population: Patients exceeding the weight limit of CT scan systems, limited use of contrast load due to renal dysfunction, and/or the radiologist's experience.

In complicated bariatric surgery patients admitted to the ICU, Kermarrec et al. reported frequent chest radiograph abnormalities, including basal pulmonary atelectasis and/or left-sided pleural effusion in 37 and 44 % of cases, respectively [28]. In

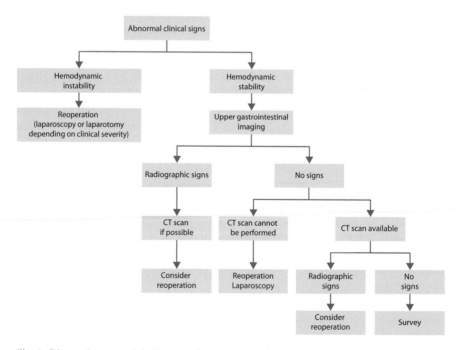

Fig. 3 Diagnostic approach in the case of suspected fistula

this cohort, upper gastrointestinal studies were obtained in only 44 % of patients and were reported as normal in half the cases. CT scan of the abdomen was performed in only one half of patients at a median interval of 8 days after initial surgery and was reported to be normal in 4 patients who suffered from generalized (n = 2) and localized (n = 2) intra-abdominal sepsis. Abnormal CT scan revealed subphrenic collections (n = 7), supramesocolic collections (n = 2), and small bowel obstruction (n = 1) [28].

In summary, the diagnostic process is based on the presence of abnormal clinical signs supported by the presence of signs of poor tolerance such as hemodynamic instability or respiratory failure and abnormal radiographic imaging findings. When in doubt and depending on the patient's tolerance, the medical team may decide on watchful waiting or reoperation. Based on the literature and our local experience, we use the decision tree presented in Fig. 3 as a possible diagnostic approach in the case of suspected fistula.

Therapeutic Management

Management of complicated bariatric surgery patients is based on a combination of surgical or endoscopic procedures, largely influenced by the type of surgical complication, and medical care. Severity at the time of diagnosis is a key issue in the decision-making process.

Surgical Management of Postoperative Complications

The surgical management of intraabdominal sepsis corresponds to the rules of septic surgery, including evacuation of purulent necrotic material, debridement of devitalized tissues, identification and elimination of the source of infection, intraoperative lavage of the abdominal cavity and possibly drainage depending on the severity and the site of the source. In the case of bleeding, surgery is required either for direct hemostasis or for reinforcement of the anastomoses, depending on the site of hemorrhage. Figure 4 proposes a possible therapeutic approach in the case of suspected fistula depending on the clinical presentation.

Restrictive and malabsorptive procedures share some similarities in terms of complications and clinical presentation. However, management of these complications has some specificities, depending on the initial surgery.

Gastric or esophageal perforation complicating gastric banding requires second-look laparoscopy, removal of the ring, abundant lavage-drainage of the peritoneal cavity (supramesocolic peritonitis) and sometimes suture if a perforation is found. Infection of the ring or port of gastric banding requires removal of the device, with delayed insertion of a new prosthesis. Malposition of the band requires urgent removal of the gastric band or repositioning [16, 17].

In complicated sleeve gastrectomy, reoperation is required in the case of fistula, usually by laparoscopy, and includes peritoneal toilet, sometimes suture (either

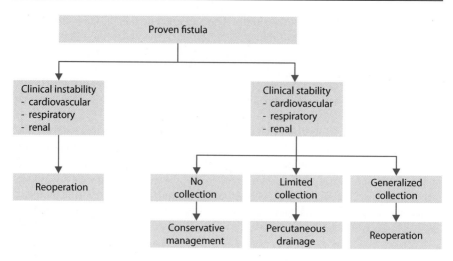

Fig. 4 Therapeutic approach in the case of proven fistula

manual or mechanical), and, in every case, drainage in contact with the fistula. If the fistula is closed properly, the outcome is usually uneventful. In the case of failure to control the contamination, insertion of an endoscopic prosthesis into the fistulous opening is an effective technique. The use of pigtail drains has been recently proposed in this situation [32]. In the case of failure of these options and in the presence of necrosis of the stomach, total gastrectomy with primary reconstruction or delayed esophagojejunal anastomosis has been successfully performed [26, 33] depending on the patient's clinical status and tolerance of sepsis. Similar management is proposed in the case of leaks observed following RYGB with revision of the anastomosis either alone or combined with primary or delayed total gastrectomy.

Based on the literature and our local experience, we use the decision tree presented in Fig. 4 for the treatment of all fistulas observed following bariatric surgery.

Medical Management

Medical management consists of nutritional support, appropriate antibiotics and treatment of associated complications. Although some publications have addressed the medical issues raised by the management of morbidly obese patients in the ICU setting, very few data are available concerning the medical management of postoperative complications, such as nutrition support [34], and the nature and modalities of parenteral or enteral nutrition via the accessible intestinal segment are major sources of concern. However, the overall clinical management does not appear to differ from that applied to other bariatric surgery cases. In addition, supportive ICU care, such as mechanical ventilation, prevention of complications, monitoring or pharmacokinetic issues, remains largely based on extrapolations of medical management in non-obese cases.

Microbiologic and Anti-Infective Issues

A high frequency of Gram-positive cocci and fungi has been previously reported in patients with gastroduodenal or upper mesocolic perforations during non-bariatric surgery. High concentrations of aerobes, anaerobes and fungi have been observed in the stomach flora of patients undergoing bypass for morbid obesity [35]. A high pH reported in these patients can also be considered to be a predisposing factor for yeast growth [35]. Few data are available in complicated postoperative bariatric surgery patients. We recently reported that, compared to patients who developed postoperative peritonitis following nonbariatric surgery, bariatric surgery patients had a 37 % higher rate of Gram-positive cocci, a 33 % lower rate of Gram-negative bacilli, and a 50 % lower rate of anaerobes and multidrug-resistant strains [26]. High rates of fungi, similar to those previously reported in non-bariatric surgery cases [26], were recently confirmed in a cohort of mixed ICU and non-ICU complicated bariatric surgery patients [36]. The microbiological characteristics of patients with complicated RYGB suggest that these cases should be considered to present small bowel perforation rather than upper gastrointestinal perforation [26]. The extensive use of antibiotics between initial surgery and the diagnosis of septic surgical complication contributes to the emergence of multi-drug resistance strains and fungi. These observations justify the use of empiric antibiotic therapy protocols comprising broad-spectrum agents and antifungal agents that ensure a high adequacy rate, targeting all microorganisms in more than 80 % of cases [26]. Interestingly, de-escalation can be performed in more than two-thirds of cases.

No data are available on the appropriate antibiotic dose in these specific cases. Recent data suggest a risk of high variability in serum beta-lactam concentrations in obese patients including insufficient serum concentrations in 32 % of patients and overdose concentrations in 25 % [37]. General recommendations for ICU patients are usually applied, but additional studies are required, especially as diffusion of antibiotics in the peritoneal space is difficult to predict and impossible to monitor.

Prognosis of Surgical Complications

Bariatric surgery has a reputation for being safe and well tolerated. Surgical complications can be analyzed from the perspective of large cohorts or smaller groups, allowing a more accurate description of the outcome.

From the surgical point of view, Buchwald et al. published, in 2007, a meta-analysis of nearly 85,000 patients and reported a postoperative mortality of 0.07 % for laparoscopic restrictive techniques, 0.16 % for gastric bypass and 1.1 % for duodenal switch [21]. In a large database comprising more than 44,000 patients be-

Table 2 Outcome of anastomotic leaks following Roux-en-Y gastric bypass among cases treated conservatively and there who underwent reoperation

	Leaks	Conservative treatment		Reoperation	
	n	n	Death rate (%)	n	Death rate (%)
Ballesta [7]	59	36	0	23	22
Gonzalez [23]	63	23	0	40	10
Marshall [49]	21	10	0	11	18

tween 2007 and 2209, Khan et al. identified independent risk factors of mortality as age greater than 45 years, male sex, BMI greater than or equal to $50\,kg/m^2$, bariatric surgery laparotomy, loss of autonomy before surgery, coronary angioplasty, dyspnea, preoperative intentional weight loss > 10 % and bleeding disorders [38]. Anastomotic leaks are considered to be one of the most life-threatening complications among morbidly obese patients undergoing bariatric surgery [23]. Based on a series of 3,073 RYGB cases, Fernandez et al. identified predictive factors of mortality as male sex, age, weight, and obstructive sleep apnea [39]. The authors advised surgeons to avoid operating on such patients early in their learning curve.

From the intensivist's perspective, the prognosis is more difficult to assess. Contradictory results have been published on the outcome of morbidly obese patients admitted to the ICU, from a decreased risk of in-hospital mortality in surgical patients [40] to increased morbidity in a mixed population [41] and even an increased (33 %) risk of death among surgical patients who required prolonged ICU stays [42]. Some authors have reported obesity to be an independent risk factor for death among critically ill patients [43, 44]. Obese patients undergoing surgery seem to be more susceptible than non-obese patients to postoperative complications, such as wound infections, acute respiratory distress, and multiple organ failure [45]. In a meta-analysis based on a total of 62,045 critically ill subjects, obesity was not associated with excess mortality, but was significantly related to prolonged duration of mechanical ventilation and ICU length of stay [46].

Several publications have reported mortality rates after anastomotic leaks ranging between 6 % and 22 % [3, 6, 47] and up to 66 % in some series [39, 48] of patients who underwent RYGB. No deaths were reported among cases treated conservatively, while patients who underwent reoperation had high mortality rates of up to 18 to 22 % [7, 49], and even 40 % in some specific subpopulations [50] (Table 2). Interstingly, these cases treated conservatively seem to be less severe than those who underwent reoperation. In a small group of patients referred to our unit with a diagnosis of postoperative peritonitis following bariatric surgery, we previously reported that identification of the complication was usually delayed and the prognosis was severe because of delayed source control, frequently at the time of onset of organ dysfunction [28]. Complicated bariatric surgery patients had similar reoperation rates and mortality rates to those of complicated non-bariatric surgery patients [26]. In addition, bariatric surgery did not appear to be a significant risk factor for mortality on multivariate analysis.

Delayed surgery has been largely reported to be associated with increased organ dysfunction and mortality among non-bariatric surgery patients. When a surgical complication is suspected, standard practice based on clinical assessment and radiographic imaging should be the rule, at least before the onset of multiple organ dysfunction syndrome. This issue was recently stressed by Gonzales et al., who reported a mortality rate as low as 6 % for anastomotic leaks after RYGB [23]. In this study, performed in four high-volume academic centers, the vast majority of patients had no organ failure and leaks were detected early (< 48 h) after the index surgery, even before the onset of any clinical symptoms [23].

Conclusions

Morbidly obese patients represent new and challenging issues for intensivists. With the increasing prevalence of overweight in the general population, bariatric surgery may become an increasingly popular approach in the years to come in many countries. Consequently, more intensivists will be required to manage these patients. The technical and logistical problems (beds, tables, CT scans and radiology tables, etc.) will probably be progressively resolved in the near future. On the other hand, expertise in the management of these difficult cases is only at an early stage. Many surgical and medical issues need to be resolved that will require collaborative and multidisciplinary approaches to improve the quality of care of these high-risk patients.

References

1. DeMaria EJ (2007) Bariatric surgery for morbid obesity. N Engl J Med 356:2176–2183
2. Buchwald H, Avidor Y, Braunwald E et al (2004) Bariatric surgery: a systematic review and meta-analysis. JAMA 292:1724–1737
3. Fernandez AZ Jr., Tichansky DS, Demaria EJ et al (2004) Multivariate analysis of risk factors for death following gastric bypass for treatment of morbid obesity. Ann Surg 239:698–702
4. Morino M, Toppino M, Forestieri P et al (2007) Mortality after bariatric surgery: analysis of 13,871 morbidly obese patients from a national registry. Ann Surg 246:1002–1007
5. Gagner M, Boza C (2006) Laparoscopic duodenal switch for morbid obesity. Exp Rev Med Devices 3:105–112
6. Al-Sabah S, Ladouceur M, Christou N (2008) Anastomotic leaks after bariatric surgery: it is the host response that matters. Surg Obes Relat Dis 4:152–157
7. Ballesta C, Berindoague R, Cabrera M, Palau M, Gonzales M (2008) Management of anastomotic leaks after laparoscopic Roux-en-Y gastric bypass. Obes Surg 18:623–630
8. Thodiyil PA, Yenumula P, Rogula T et al (2008) Selective nonoperative management of leaks after gastric bypass: lessons learned from 2,675 consecutive patients. Ann Surg 248:782–792
9. Flum DR, Belle SH, King WC et al (2009) Perioperative safety in the longitudinal assessment of bariatric surgery. N Engl J Med 361:445–454
10. Dillemans B, Sakran N, Van Cauwenberge S et al (2009) Standardization of the fully stapled laparoscopic Roux-en-Y gastric bypass for obesity reduces early immediate postoperative morbidity and mortality: a single center study on 2,606 patients. Obes Surg 19:1355–1364

11. Chen CC, Huang MT, Wei PL et al (2010) Severe peritonitis due to Streptococcus viridans following adjustable gastric banding. Obes Surg 20:1603–1605
12. Benotti PN, Wood GC, Rodriguez H, Carnevale N, Liriano E (2006) Perioperative outcomes and risk factors in gastric surgery for morbid obesity: a 9-year experience. Surgery 139:340–346
13. van den Broek RJ, Buise MP, van Dielen FM et al (2009) Characteristics and outcome of patients admitted to the ICU following bariatric surgery. Obes Surg 19:560–564
14. Gonzalez R, Nelson LG, Gallagher SF, Murr MM (2004) Anastomotic leaks after laparoscopic gastric bypass. Obes Surg 14:1299–1307
15. Goldfeder LB, Ren CJ, Gill JR (2006) Fatal complications of bariatric surgery. Obes Surg 16:1050–1056
16. Chapman AE, Kiroff G, Game P et al (2004) Laparoscopic adjustable gastric banding in the treatment of obesity: a systematic literature review. Surgery 135:326–351
17. Owers C, Ackroyd R (2013) A study examining the complications associated with gastric banding. Obes Surg 23:56–59
18. Agence Nationale d'Accréditation et d'Evaluation en Santé. Service évaluation des technologies (2001) Chirurgie de l'obésité morbide de l'adulte. Available at: http://prod1-has-portail.integra.fr/portail/upload/docs/application/pdf/chirurgie_obesite_rap.pdf. Accessed September 2013
19. Shi X, Karmali S, Sharma AM, Birch DW (2010) A review of laparoscopic sleeve gastrectomy for morbid obesity. Obes Surg 20:1171–1177
20. Parikh M, Issa R, McCrillis A et al (2013) Surgical strategies that may decrease leak after laparoscopic sleeve gastrectomy: a systematic review and meta-analysis of 9,991 cases. Ann Surg 257:231–237
21. Buchwald H, Estok R, Fahrbach K, Banel D, Sledge I (2007) Trends in mortality in bariatric surgery: a systematic review and meta-analysis. Surgery 142:621–632
22. Podnos YD, Jimenez JC, Wilson SE, Stevens CM, Nguyen NT (2003) Complications after laparoscopic gastric bypass: a review of 3,464 cases. Arch Surg 138:957–961
23. Gonzalez R, Sarr MG, Smith CD et al (2007) Diagnosis and contemporary management of anastomotic leaks after gastric bypass for obesity. J Am Coll Surg 204:47–55
24. Heneghan HM, Meron-Eldar S, Yenumula P et al (2012) Incidence and management of bleeding complications after gastric bypass surgery in the morbidly obese. Surg Obes Relat Dis 8:729–735
25. Mehran A, Liberman M, Rosenthal R, Szomstein S (2003) Ruptured appendicitis after laparoscopic Roux-enY gastric bypass: pitfalls in diagnosing a surgical abdomen in the morbidly obese. Obes Surg 13:938–940
26. Montravers P, Guglielminotti J, Zappella N et al (2013) Clinical features and outcome of postoperative peritonitis following bariatric surgery. Obes Surg 23:1536–1544
27. Hamilton EC, Sims TL, Hamilton TT et al (2003) Clinical predictors of leak after laparoscopic Roux-en-Y gastric bypass for morbid obesity. Surg Endosc 17:679–684
28. Kermarrec N, Marmuse JP, Faivre J et al (2008) High mortality rate for patients requiring intensive care after surgical revision following bariatric surgery. Obes Surg 18:171–178
29. Merkle EM, Hallowell PT, Crouse C et al (2005) Roux-en-Y gastric bypass for clinically severe obesity: normal appearance and spectrum of complications at imaging. Radiology 234:674–683
30. Madan AK, Stoecklein HH, Ternovits CA et al (2007) Predictive value of upper gastrointestinal studies versus clinical signs for gastrointestinal leaks after laparoscopic gastric bypass. Surg Endosc 21:194–196
31. Lyass S, Khalili TM, Cunneen S et al (2004) Radiological studies after laparoscopic Roux-en-Y gastric bypass: routine or selective? American Surg 70:918–921
32. Pequignot A, Fuks D, Verhaeghe P et al (2012) Is there a place for pigtail drains in the management of gastric leaks after laparoscopic sleeve gastrectomy? Obes Surg 22:712–720

33. Moszkowicz D, Arienzo R, Khettab I et al (2013) Sleeve gastrectomy severe complications: is it always a reasonable surgical option? Obes Surg 23:676–686
34. Choban PS, Dickerson RN (2005) Morbid obesity and nutrition support: is bigger different? Nutr Clin Pract 20:480–487
35. Ishida RK, Faintuch J, Paula AM et al (2007) Microbial flora of the stomach after gastric bypass for morbid obesity. Obes Surg 17:752–758
36. Rebibo L, Dupont H, Levrard M et al (2013) Letter to Editor: "Gastric fistula after laparoscopic sleeve gastrectomy: Don't forget to treat for candida". Obes Surg 23:2106–2108
37. Hites M, Taccone FS, Wolff F et al (2013) Case-control study of drug monitoring of beta-lactams in obese critically ill patients. Antimicrob Agents Chemother 57:708–715
38. Khan MA, Grinberg R, Johnson S, Afthinos JN, Gibbs KE (2013) Perioperative risk factors for 30-day mortality after bariatric surgery: is functional status important? Surg Endosc 27:1772–1777
39. Fernandez AZ Jr, DeMaria EJ, Tichansky DS et al (2004) Experience with over 3,000 open and laparoscopic bariatric procedures: multivariate analysis of factors related to leak and resultant mortality. Surg Endosc 18:193–197
40. Hutagalung R, Marques J, Kobylka K et al (2011) The obesity paradox in surgical intensive care unit patients. Intensive Care Med 37:1793–1799
41. Sakr Y, Madl C, Filipescu D et al (2008) Obesity is associated with increased morbidity but not mortality in critically ill patients. Intensive Care Med 34:1999–2009
42. Nasraway SA Jr, Albert M, Donnelly AM et al (2006) Morbid obesity is an independent determinant of death among surgical critically ill patients. Crit Care Med 34:964–970
43. Bercault N, Boulain T, Kuteifan K et al (2004) Obesity-related excess mortality rate in an adult intensive care unit: a risk-adjusted matched cohort study. Crit Care Med 32:998–1003
44. Ray DE, Matchett SC, Baker K et al (2005) The effect of body mass index on patient outcomes in a medical ICU. Chest 127:2125–2131
45. Pasulka PS, Bistrian BR, Benotti PN, Blackburn GL (1986) The risks of surgery in obese patients. Ann Intern Med 104:540–546
46. Akinnusi ME, Pineda LA, El Solh AA (2008) Effect of obesity on intensive care morbidity and mortality: a meta-analysis. Crit Care Med 36:151–158
47. Csendes A, Burdiles P, Burgos AM, Maluenda F, Diaz JC (2005) Conservative management of anastomotic leaks after 557 open gastric bypasses. Obes Surg 15:1252–1256
48. Papasavas PK, Caushaj PF, McCormick JT et al (2003) Laparoscopic management of complications following laparoscopic Roux-en-Y gastric bypass for morbid obesity. Surg Endosc 17:610–614
49. Marshall JS, Srivastava A, Gupta SK, Rossi TR, DeBord JR (2003) Roux-en-Y gastric bypass leak complications. Arch Surg 138:520–523
50. Lee S, Carmody B, Wolfe L et al (2007) Effect of location and speed of diagnosis on anastomotic leak outcomes in 3,828 gastric bypass cases. J Gastrointest Surg 11:708–713

Acute Liver Failure

L. A. Possamai and J. A. Wendon

Introduction and Definition

Acute liver failure is a complex clinical syndrome that develops when a sudden and critical loss of hepatocellular function occurs in the context of a previously normal liver. The most prominent clinical consequences of this loss in hepatic function are jaundice, coagulopathy and encephalopathy with a clinical course that may rapidly progress to multi-organ failure and death. A number of different definitions of acute liver failure have been proposed, as highlighted by a recent systematic review that found over 40 definitions used in published literature [1]. One widely accepted and inclusive definition, referenced in the current American Association for the Study of Liver Diseases (AASLD) guidelines is 'evidence of a coagulation abnormality (INR > 1.5) and mental alteration (encephalopathy) in a patient without pre-existing cirrhosis and with an illness of < 26 weeks duration' [2]. A number of sub-classifications of acute liver failure according to the duration from onset of jaundice to the development of encephalopathy have been described [3–5] and are summarized in Table 1. The rationale for these divisions is the different clinical features and prognosis seen in patients with a rapid onset (hyperacute/fulminant) illness in whom brain edema is prominent but who paradoxically stand the best chance of survival with medical therapy alone, to those with a more protracted (subacute/subfulminant) illness who less frequently exhibit cerebral edema but have a worse prognosis without liver transplant. The differences between these groups is largely due to differing etiologies, with acetaminophen and hepatitis A and E associated with hyperacute presentations and non-acetaminophen drug-induced liver

L. A. Possamai
Department of Hepatology, Imperial College London, London, UK

J. A. Wendon ✉
Institute of Liver Studies at King's College School of Medicine, King's College Hospital, London, UK
e-mail: julia.wendon@kcl.ac.uk

J.-L. Vincent (Ed.), *Annual Update in Intensive Care and Emergency Medicine 2014*,   503
DOI 10.1007/978-3-319-03746-2_38, © Springer International Publishing Switzerland
2014

Table 1 A summary of sub-classifications of acute liver failure

Classification	Bernuau et al. 1986 [5]	Fulminant < 2 weeks		Subfulminant 2–12 weeks
	O'Grady et al. 1993 [3]	Hyperacute < 7 days	Acute 8–28 days	Subacute 5–12 weeks
	Tandon et al. 1999 IASL sub-committee statement [4]	Acute hepatic failure		Subacute hepatic failure
		Hyperacute < 10 days	Fulminant 10–30 days	5–24 weeks
Clinical features	Etiology	Acetominophen toxicity Hepatitis A & E	Hepatitis B	Drug-induced liver injury Autoimmune
	Cerebral edema and intercranial hypertension	Prominent feature		Rare
	Survival with medical therapy alone	More common		Unlikely

IASL: International Association for the Study of the Liver

injury, hepatitis B and sero-negative disease typically running a slower clinical course. For the purposes of this chapter, we will refer to acute liver failure according to the inclusive definition above, but aim to clarify how the clinical presentation and management might differ according to the particular manifestation of disease.

Epidemiology

Acute liver failure is a rare disorder, with approximately 1600–2000 cases per year reported in the USA [2, 6]. In the developed world, acetaminophen hepatotoxicity due to either deliberate or unintentional overdose is the commonest cause of acute liver failure accounting for 39–57 % of cases [7–9]. Acetaminophen-induced acute liver failure is becoming increasingly common in the USA. In the United Kingdom, where legislation to reduce acetaminophen pack size was introduced in 1998, both the number and severity of cases of acetaminophen-induced acute liver failure has fallen dramatically [10].

Non-acetaminophen drug-induced liver injury is also a notable cause of acute liver failure, being responsible for 12 % of cases in the USA [8]. These cases are usually severe idiosyncratic reactions to a wide range of drugs, including, but not limited to antibiotics, antiepileptics and antituberculosis medications [11]. Recent epidemiological data from the USA Acute Liver Failure Study Group showing the commonest causes of acute liver failure are summarized in Table 2.

There is great geographical variation in the causes of acute liver failure, with viral hepatitis being the predominant cause in Asia and Africa and acetaminophen-

Table 2 The most common causes of acute liver failure in the USA (adapted from [8])

Cause	
Acetaminophen	46 %
Indeterminate/including seronegative	15 %
Drug induced liver injury (non-acetominophen)	12 %
Hepatitis B	7 %
Autoimmune	6 %
Ischemia	5 %
Hepatitis A	2 %
Wilson Disease	1 %
Pregnancy	< 1 %
Budd-Chiari	< 1 %
Other	5 %

toxicity rarely seen. In South-East Asia, hepatitis E infection causes 44–60 % of cases and hepatitis B 15–20 % of cases [12, 13].

Mortality from acute liver failure has improved markedly in recent decades thanks to the use of emergent orthotopic liver transplant (OLT) and improved supportive critical care. A recent retrospective review of cases from the United Kingdom showed an improvement in hospital survival in acute liver failure patients from just 17 % in the mid-1970s to 62 % in the mid-2000s [14]. This impressive improvement in patient outcomes from acute liver failure has been achieved despite significant barriers to quality clinical research in this area. As acute liver failure is a rare and heterogeneous syndrome, characterized by a rapidly progressive clinical course, recruitment to controlled trials is challenging. Much of the progress in this field has, therefore, been the result of the application of research from other conditions, for example the management of cerebral edema in traumatic brain injury, or through the development of clinical expertise in specialist centers. What follows is, therefore, a synthesis of evidence-based recommendations, current practice guidelines and clinical experience.

Pathophysiology

The common and crucial pathophysiological event in the development of acute liver failure of all etiologies is the death of a mass of hepatocytes, such that vital synthetic and metabolic hepatic functions are critically impaired. The mode and rate of hepatocyte death varies between etiologies, from sudden toxin-mediated necrosis in acetaminophen poisoning to more indolent immune-regulated injury and apoptosis in autoimmune hepatitis. What starts as a local, single-organ condition rapidly progresses to multi-system involvement with numerous clinical manifestations (Fig. 1).

This amplification is due to the systemic effects of toxins, such as ammonia, that would normally be cleared by the liver, hemodynamic disturbances and spill-over of inflammatory mediators produced in response to intra-hepatic events. Acute liver

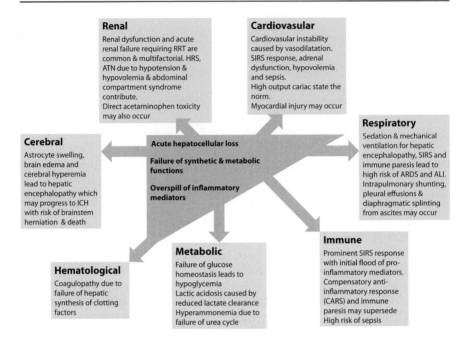

Fig. 1 Summary of the multisystem manifestations of acute liver failure (RRT: renal replacement therapy; HRS: hepatorenal syndrome; ARDS: acute respiratory distress syndrome; ALI: acute lung injury; SIRS: systemic inflammatory response syndrome)

failure is a classic example of a sterile inflammatory condition, in which the presence of uncontrolled cell death provides potent stimuli to the innate immune system and provokes a massive pro-inflammatory response. The systemic consequences of immune activation are similar to sepsis and involve a marked systemic inflammatory response syndrome (SIRS) response. The SIRS response and hemodynamic instability contribute to renal dysfunction, whereas sedation and ventilation to manage hepatic encephalopathy increase the risk of acute respiratory distress syndrome (ARDS) and pulmonary infections. Predicting and acting to halt this apparently inexorable progression from hepatic impairment to multi-system dysfunction and organ failure is the main focus of intensive care management.

Initial Assessment

The initial assessment of the patient presenting with suspected acute liver failure should be aimed at determining the cause and severity of their liver dysfunction and detecting the early presence of complications. As with many areas of clinical medicine the history is of primary importance. There may be a clear precipitant of liver failure, such as in deliberate acetaminophen overdose, however in many cases the cause for acute liver dysfunction is not initially clear.

A thorough enquiry into the history of the presenting problem and its duration should be made. The rate of evolution of symptoms can give important clues to etiology and may also inform prognosis. A detailed medication history should be taken, paying particular attention to the use of 'over-the-counter' medication, illicit drugs or herbal remedies that patients may not initially think to disclose or may deliberately conceal. A recent history of travel to areas with endemic hepatitis A, B and E may suggest a viral etiology. Family history may be significant in Wilson disease.

The clinical examination should be thorough to identify developing multi-system involvement and in particular any evidence of sepsis. Clinical signs of chronic liver disease should be sought to determine whether the presentation is in fact an episode of decompensated chronic liver disease rather than acute liver failure. Bed-side cognitive assessments should be made and documented to detect evidence of early encephalopathy and to provide a baseline against which later assessments can be compared.

Prognosis and Decision to Refer

An important part of the management of acute liver failure is the dynamic assessment of patient prognosis to inform optimal treatment. Early consideration should be given to the decision to refer and possibly transfer to a specialist liver transplant center. Referral criteria for acetaminophen and non-acetaminophen etiologies have been published and offer useful guidance [15] (Table 3). However as a rule, early communication with a local specialist center is advised as each unit may have its own admission criteria. Acute liver failure can progress rapidly and patient transfer becomes increasingly difficult once complications such as cerebral edema occur.

Assessment of a patient's prognosis is also vital when making the decision to list for liver transplantation. The aim of this process is to accurately discriminate between those patients who will survive with supportive care alone and those who would die without liver transplant. This is important not only to prevent patient deaths, but to avoid transplantation in those whose liver would regenerate spontaneously, which needlessly exposes a patient to operative risk and complications, commits them to lifelong immunosuppression and wastes the valuable resource of a transplantable organ.

A number of prognostic scoring systems have been proposed to assist in this difficult clinical decision. Liver-specific scores, such as the Model for End-Stage Liver Disease (MELD), Clichy and King's College Criteria, and general intensive care scores like APACHE II and sequential organ failure assessment (SOFA) have been validated [16–18]. Additionally, numerous serological markers including alpha-fetoprotein and phosphorus have shown prognostic value [19, 20]. Perhaps the most widely used score is the King's College Criteria (KCC), initially described in 1989 [21] and later modified to include arterial lactate [22]. The KCC describe different clinical and laboratory parameters for acetaminophen and non-acetaminophen-induced acute liver failure and are summarized in Table 4. The

Table 3 Guidelines on when to refer to specialist liver transplant centers (from [15])

Acetaminophen toxicity		
Day 2	Day 3	Day 4
Arterial pH < 7.3	Arterial pH < 7.3	PT > 100s (INR > 6.0)
PT > 50s (INR > 3.0)	PT > 75s (INR > 4.4)	Progressive rise in PT
Oliguria	Oliguria	Creatinine > 300 µmol/l
Creatinine > 200 µmol/l	Creatinine > 200 µmol/l	(3.4 mg/dl)
(2.26 mg/dl)	(2.26 mg/dl)	Encephalopathy
Hypoglycemia	Encephalopathy	Severe thrombocytopenia
	Severe thrombocytopenia	
All other etiologies		
Hyperacute	Acute	Subacute
Encephalopathy	Encephalopathy	Encephalopathy
Hypoglycemia	Hypoglycemia	Hypoglycemia
PT > 30s (INR > 2.0)	PT > 30s (INR > 2.0)	PT > 20s (INR > 1.5)
Renal failure	Renal failure	Renal failure
Hyperpyrexia		Hponatremia
		Shrinking liver volume on CT

INR: international normalized ratio; PT: prothrombin time; CT: computed tomography

Table 4 The King's College Hospital criteria for poor prognosis in acute liver failure, including the lactate modification

Acetaminophen-induced acute liver failure	All other etiologies
pH < 7.3 after fluid resuscitation	PT > 100 (INR > 6.5)
OR all of the following:	OR any three of the following:
PT > 100 or INR > 6.5	Seronegative hepatitis or DILI
Serum creatinine > 300 µmol/l (3.4 mg/dL)	Age < 10 or > 40
Grade III or IV encephalopathy	Jaundice to encephalopathy time > 7 days
OR	Bilirubin > 300 µmol/l (17.5 mg/dL)
Serum lactate > 3.5 mmol/l at 4 hours	PT > 50 (INR > 3.5)
or > 3.0 mmol/l at 12 hours	

INR: international normalized ratio; PT: prothrombin time; DILI: drug-induced liver injury

KCC, though widely used have been criticized for a low sensitivity and negative predictive value. A recent systematic review found the pooled specificity of KCC to be excellent at 94 %, but sensitivity poor at 58.2 % [23].

The USA Acute Liver Failure Study Group has recently proposed a new prognostic score the 'ALFSG Index' comprising the patient coma grade, bilirubin, International normalized ratio (INR), phosphorus and serum M30, (an ELISA-based surrogate marker of apoptosis) [24]. This index demonstrated improved prognostic accuracy over the KCC; however the limited availability of serum M30 measurement may limit its clinical applicability.

In the absence of an ideal prognostic test, these scoring systems should be used as guides, with clinical expertise ultimately informing the decision to proceed with transplantation. Consideration of wider factors beyond patient prognosis must also be undertaken, with psychosocial factors impacting on the outcome of a potential liver transplant. One series from Scotland described over 30 % of patients with acetaminophen-induced acute liver failure being unsuitable for transplantation on the basis of pyschosocial problems, largely chronic alcohol abuse [25]. Psychiatric conditions should not, however, be considered a contraindication to transplantation *per se*. A recent case-control study in which over half the patients transplanted for acetaminophen-induced acute liver failure had a pre-existing psychiatric diagnosis and 25 % had previous suicide attempts, showed comparable outcomes in terms of graft failure, compliance and overall survival between acetaminophen and non-acetaminophen etiologies [26].

Intensive Care Management

The intensive care management of acute liver failure is aimed at preventing, if possible, the predictable consequences of acute liver failure, timely and aggressive treatment of those complications that do arise and supportive care to allow hepatic regeneration to occur. Recognition of those patients in whom spontaneous liver regeneration will not occur and who, therefore, require emergent liver transplantation is another vital aspect of patient management.

N-acetylcysteine

The clinical utility of N-acetylcysteine (NAC) in acute liver failure has evolved over the last two decades from limited use as an 'antidote' in early acetaminophen toxicity to a valuable, proven treatment in all etiologies of acute liver failure.

In acetaminophen overdose, NAC may prevent hepatocellular necrosis if given early enough in the evolution of liver injury by replenishing hepatic glutathione and allowing effective detoxification of *N*-acetyl-*p*-benzoquinone imine (NAPQI), the highly reactive, toxic metabolite of acetaminophen. An oral or intravenous regimen of NAC is, therefore, the mainstay of treatment in patients presenting to emergency departments with a history of acetaminophen overdose. Therapeutic nomograms that guide treatment based on the time from ingestion and plasma acetaminophen levels are widely used. These should be interpreted generously, with a tendency to over-treat where there is doubt over the timing of overdose, a history of staggered overdose or risk factors for enhanced response, such as poor nutritional status, chronic alcoholism or the use of enzyme inducing medication. Mild anaphylactoid reactions to NAC are common, but are easily treated and severe side effects are rare [27].

NAC has also proven efficacy in the later stages of acetaminophen overdose, reducing the progression of encephalopathy and improving survival [28]. Given the benefits of this relatively innocuous treatment in established acetaminophen-induced acute liver failure, its use has been extended to the treatment of all forms of acute liver failure and in one of the few randomized controlled trials in acute liver failure management, NAC therapy in non-acetaminophen acute liver failure was shown to improve transplant-free survival in patients with grade I and II hepatic encephalopathy [29]. The mechanism by which NAC exerts its beneficial effects in established acute liver failure are unclear; however, it has been shown to improve oxygen transport and systemic hemodynamics in the late stages of acetaminophen toxicity and may reduce interleukin (IL)-17 production in non-acetaminophen acute liver failure [30, 31].

Sepsis/SIRS

Pathophysiology

Features of SIRS are commonly seen in acute liver failure, with or without the presence of infection and are associated with progressive encephalopathy and increased mortality [32, 33]. In non-acetaminophen-induced acute liver failure, SIRS also correlates with the degree of renal dysfunction [25].

Defects in the immune systems of patients with acute liver failure render them particularly susceptible to infections [34]. Complement deficiency due to failure of hepatic production has been described in acute liver failure along with impaired neutrophil function and phagocytosis [35–37]. The circulating monocytes of patients with acute liver failure have been demonstrated to have a de-activated, endotoxin-tolerant phenotype, similar to those in patients with septic shock. This monocyte defect correlates with patient outcome in acute liver failure [38].

The clinical consequence of immune paresis is a high risk of sepsis and infection-related mortality in this patient population. A number of case series have shown bacterial infection rates of approximately 80 % in acute liver failure [39, 40]. The commonest infections are of the respiratory tract, accounting for approximately 50 % of cases, and urinary tract, causing 25 % of infections [39, 40]. Bacteremia is also common, documented in between 20–35 % of cases [39, 41, 42] and associated with worse hepatic encephalopathy, increased renal replacement therapy (RRT) and ventilation requirements and a longer ICU stay [42]. The causative organisms in acute liver failure-associated blood stream infections are fairly evenly split between Gram-positive (44 %) and Gram-negative bacteria (52 %), with a small but notable percentage of cases caused by candidal fungemia (4 %). A wide range of bacterial species are seen in this population, with a recent series reporting the commonest as *Enterococcus faecium*, *Klebsiella* spp. and vancomycin-resistant *Enterococcus* spp., though these patterns are likely to vary according to geographical location [42]. In up to 30 % of cases of infection in acute liver failure, classical clinical features of sepsis are absent [40].

Management

Sepsis has a devastating effect on the patient with acute liver failure, in terms of their chances of spontaneous survival or successful liver transplantation. Care should be taken to avoid infective complications by the application of good clinical practice with respect to hand hygiene, the avoidance of indwelling lines if possible and routine surveillance and cultures. Any deterioration in clinical condition, whether or not it is associated with a fever or classical signs of infection, should be assumed to be sepsis until proven otherwise. Comprehensive cultures should be sent and the application of early goal-directed therapy instigated to aggressively treat hemodynamic instability [43]. Antibiotic choice will vary depending on local resistant patterns and the clinical situation; however, the guiding principle should be the prompt administration of broad-spectrum antibiotics, with an aim to narrow the spectrum once culture results are available.

There is a strong argument for antibiotic prophylaxis in acute liver failure, given the preponderance of bacterial infections, difficulties in clinical assessment and devastating impact of sepsis; however there is currently no evidence to support routine prophylaxis [44]. A pragmatic approach is to recommend prophylactic antibiotic use in patients in whom infections are known to be common, namely those with grade III–IV encephalopathy, requiring RRT or demonstrating SIRS features [45]. Antibiotics should also be used routinely once the decision to list for liver transplantation is made [45].

Hepatic Encephalopathy, Cerebral Edema and Intracranial Hypertension

Pathophysiology

Hepatic encephalopathy causes a spectrum of neuropsychiatric symptoms that encompass alterations in behavior, cognition and consciousness and range from subtle confusion and personality change in mildest cases, through to coma in more severe cases. This spectrum of disease is generally classified into four grades according to the West-Haven criteria summarized in Table 5 [46]. In acute liver failure, particularly those patients with a fulminant/hyperacute presentation, hepatic encephalopathy progresses rapidly and is frequently complicated by cerebral edema and intracranial hypertension. Intracranial hypertension with brainstem herniation accounts for 20–25 % of deaths in acute liver failure and its treatment is one of the most challenging aspects of patient management. In individuals with a sub-acute presentation of acute liver failure, the occurrence of cerebral edema and intracranial hypertension is less common; however any progression of encephalopathy reflects critical hepatic failure and is associated with a very poor prognosis [15].

The pathogenesis of hepatic encephalopathy and cerebral edema in acute liver failure are incompletely understood. A complex and dynamic interplay occurs between a number of factors, with the best characterized being defects in ammonia metabolism by the failing liver, accumulation of glutamine in astrocytes leading to swelling and a contribution from pro-inflammatory cytokines produced as part of the SIRS response.

There is a clear relationship between arterial ammonia levels in acute liver failure and the progression of hepatic encephalopathy to intracranial hypertension [47–49]. In health, ammonia and glutamate are produced by the action of small intestinal glutaminase on glutamine. The absorbed ammonia is converted in the liver to urea and excreted [50]. When this vital detoxification function of the liver fails, increased

Table 5 The West Haven classification of the grades of hepatic encephalopathy

Grade	Clinical Features
I	Trivial lack of awareness Euphoria or anxiety Shortened attention span Impaired performance of addition
II	Lethargy or apathy Minimal disorientation for time or place Subtle personality change Inappropriate behavior Impaired performance of subtraction
III	Somnolence to semistupor, but responsive to verbal stimuli
IV	Comatose, unresponsive to verbal stimuli or pain

systemic ammonia results. Once hyperammonemia develops, an alternative detoxification pathway is utilized with excess ammonia being converted to glutamine by glutamine synthetase in skeletal muscle and brain astrocytes [51, 52]. Consequently the glutamine content of astrocytes increases, leading to osmotic swelling and alterations in mitochondrial function that affect cellular oxidative metabolism and cause increases in brain lactate [53, 52]. Oxidative stress leads to local vasodilatation and increased cerebral perfusion [54].

SIRS is increasingly recognized as an important factor in the development of hepatic encephalopathy and cerebral edema through the clear clinical association of SIRS with worsening encephalopathy [32, 33, 55, 56]. The initiation of endothelial inflammatory responses, exacerbation of cerebral vasodilatation and contribution to oxidative and nitrosative stress have all been postulated as mechanisms by which the pro-inflammatory cytokines and mediators of SIRS contribute to the pathogenesis of encephalopathy; however clear evidence is lacking [57].

The ultimate clinical consequences of acute astrocyte swelling and brain edema with increased cerebral perfusion within the rigid confines of the skull, is the development of intracranial hypertension, which, if uncontrolled, can result in brainstem herniation and death. The sudden loss of hepatocyte function, with very rapid accumulation of ammonia in acute liver failure overwhelms the adaptive mechanisms that can act to attenuate brain swelling in sub-acute and acute-on-chronic liver failure, thus explaining the inverse relationship between the speed of onset of liver failure and severity of cerebral edema.

Monitoring

The use of invasive intracranial pressure (ICP) monitors remains a controversial area in the management of acute liver failure. There is no randomized controlled-trial level evidence to guide management and so the use of ICP monitors often comes down to local expertise and preference. A 2005 review of practice in the USA suggested ICP monitors are used in the management of acute liver failure in approximately half the transplant centers surveyed [58]. Current pragmatic recommendations in the AALSD treatment guidelines suggest the use of ICP monitoring in patients with high-grade encephalopathy who are awaiting or undergoing liver transplantation, and then only in those centers with expertise [2].

Invasive ICP monitoring gives continuous information, allowing for contemporaneous, reactive management to changes in intracranial pressure. The non-invasive techniques, such as computed tomography (CT), magnetic resonance imaging (MRI) or transcranial Doppler ultrasound, only give intermittent readings, are less accurate than invasive monitors and can be impractical in patients with advanced disease who cannot be transferred for imaging. Evidence suggests patients with invasive monitoring *in situ* are managed more aggressively, with increased use of vasopressors and ICP-related therapeutic interventions [58].

Opponents of invasive ICP monitoring cite the high complication rate, with a 10 % risk of hemorrhage and absence of convincing evidence of survival benefit in available trials [58]. Many of these bleeding complications were, however, incidental findings on imaging and unlikely to be of clinical significance. The use of fresh frozen plasma (FFP) and/or recombinant factor VII to transiently reverse coagulopathy prior to insertion of ICP may be beneficial [59].

Management

The aims of managing intracranial hypertension in acute liver failure are to normalize ICP, preventing permanent neurological damage or death from herniation, while awaiting liver recovery or transplantation. Case reports exist that describe patients making a full neurological recovery following prolonged periods of intracranial hypertension with ICP > 35 mmHg [60] or short-lived spikes > 80 mmHg [61]. However, therapy should be aimed at maintaining ICP below 20 mmHg if possible, while the cerebral perfusion pressure (CPP) should be kept > 60 mmHg [62].

General measures include positioning patients with a 20–30° head up tilt and avoiding maneuvers or interventions that may transiently increase ICP, such as endobronchial suctioning. Adequate sedation and analgesia should be maintained and the combination of propofol and fentanyl is generally recommended [45, 62]. Hyperthermia should be corrected with antipyretics and active cooling and aggressive treatment of sepsis as described above is essential.

The maintenance of CPP is vital to good neurological outcome. Mean arterial pressure (MAP) should, therefore, be measured invasively and maintained with vasoconstrictors, of which norepinephrine is the first choice agent. Seizures may occur in hepatic encephalopathy and should be managed with intravenous (i.v.) phenytoin if they develop; however there is no benefit of prophylactic phenytoin [63].

Liver support devices and RRT may be of some benefit in reducing the systemic ammonia load and improving hepatic encephalopathy. These are discussed in more detail below.

Mannitol

Mannitol is an osmotic agent that can help to treat the astrocyte swelling and brain edema that complicates acute liver failure and gives rise to intracranial hypertension [64]. It is given in boluses of 0.25–0.5 g/kg and will often need to be administered repeatedly as its effects are transient. Serum osmolality should be monitored and repeated boluses can be given providing the osmolality remains < 320 mOsm/l.

Hypertonic Saline

The prophylactic use of hypertonic saline to induce hypernatremia to a target level of 145–155 mmol/l has been shown to reduce the incidence of intracranial hypertension in patients with acute liver failure [65]. No studies have evaluated the use of hypertonic saline boluses in the treatment of elevated ICP in acute liver failure; however, it is widely used and recommended as an alternative osmotic agent to mannitol.

Hypothermia

Therapeutic hypothermia has proven clinical efficacy in other conditions associated with cerebral edema, including traumatic brain injury and post-cardiac arrest [66, 67]. The rationale for its use in acute liver failure is to reduce brain metabolism, blood flow and ammonia uptake and consequently ameliorate the development of brain edema and intracranial hypertension. In experimental models of acute liver failure, the induction of hypothermia has shown great promise. In rodent models, hypothermia reduced ammonia production and uptake, cerebral hyperperfusion and even increased survival in a murine acetaminophen model of acute liver failure [54, 68]. A number of uncontrolled trials of hypothermia in acute liver failure patient groups have been reported [69, 70]. These have shown a range of benefits, including reduction in ICP, cerebral blood flow (CBF), arterial ammonia, brain cytokine production and markers of oxidative stress; however, due to study design these trials were unable to determine whether hypothermia treatment conferred a survival benefit. Concern exists regarding the side effects of prolonged hypothermia, which include bleeding disorders, infection, cardiovascular instability and insulin resistance [71]. These complications tend to be more pronounced at lower temperatures and, therefore, current guidance suggests that if hypothermia is to be used in refractory intracranial hypertension, a moderate temperature of 34–35°C should be the target [2].

Other

A number of other treatment strategies for ICP associated with acute liver failure have been proposed but, with limited evidence for their use or very short-term benefits, their application should be considered a 'last resort' to prevent brainstem herniation if a liver transplantation is pending.

Hyperventilation to induce hypocapnia to a $PaCO_2$ of 25–20 mmHg has been shown to transiently reduce ICP in acute liver failure by restoring cerebral autoregulation [72]. A controlled trial of its use showed no benefits to ICP or survival beyond a slight delay in brainstem herniation [73]. Concerns have also been raised about the possibility of cerebral edema being worsened following hyperventilation due to impaired CBF [74].

Barbiturates have been used in the management of intracranial hypertension and act by reducing cerebral oxygen demand; however their use is complicated by systemic hypotension and their metabolism may be very prolonged due to hepatic impairment, leading to problems with later neurological assessments. Indomethacin may also have some therapeutic benefit in management of intracranial hypertension by inducing cerebral vasoconstriction [75].

One final intervention that may be considered as a short-term bridge to liver transplant is a total hepatectomy and portocaval shunt formation [76]. Removal of the source of pro-inflammatory cytokine formation that drives hepatic encephalopathy can temporarily improve intracranial hypertension allowing time for transplantation to be arranged.

Renal Impairment

Renal impairment commonly accompanies acute liver failure and is a marker of poor prognosis. The causes of renal impairment in acute liver failure are multifactorial and commonly include an element of acute tubular necrosis from hypovolemia. Hepato-renal syndrome can develop due to hemodynamic changes associated with acute liver failure, including decreased systemic vascular resistance reducing the effective circulating volume. The development of ascites in acute liver failure can compromise renal perfusion by increasing intra-abdominal pressure (IAP). Direct renal toxicity from acetaminophen or non-steroidal anti-inflammatory drug overdoses may also contribute to renal impairment in some cases.

Irrespective of the cause of renal impairment, management is aimed at normalizing renal blood flow through the correction of hypovolemia with adequate fluid resuscitation and maintenance of MAP with vasoconstrictors, such as norepinephrine. If abdominal pressure is elevated > 20 mmHg due to ascites, as measured by an intravesical pressure monitor, then paracentesis should be performed for decompression.

When RRT is required in acute liver failure, continuous forms of filtration or dialysis have been shown to be preferable as they reduce hemodynamic instability and do not compromise CPP and ICP, unlike intermittent dialysis [77, 78].

Cardiovascular and Hemodynamic Compromise

Hemodynamic instability in acute liver failure is caused by systemic vasodilatation and exacerbated by hypovolemia. Uncontrolled cell death in the failing liver stimulates a marked pro-inflammatory response with production of cytokines and vasoactive substances that spill over into the systemic circulation and cause profound vasodilatation. A low effective arterial volume results, which, despite a high cardiac output state, causes impaired tissue perfusion and oxygen utilization.

The first line treatment of acute liver failure is adequate fluid resuscitation, and normal saline is the recommended choice for volume resuscitation [2]. Vasoconstrictor therapy should only be considered once the patient is adequately fluid resuscitated, but is commonly required in refractory hypotension to support MAP and

CPP. Norepinephrine is generally recommended as a first line agent, having the benefit of preserved splanchnic blood flow compared to epinephrine [2, 45].

Elevated troponin I levels have been demonstrated in 60–74 % of patients with acute liver failure suggesting that sub-clinical myocardial damage may occur as part of the acute liver failure syndrome [79, 80]. Although troponin levels correlate with the severity of organ failure, they performs poorly as an independent prognostic marker, suggesting myocardial injury may not have a significant clinical impact [79].

Adrenal insufficiency is seen in over 60 % of patients with acute hepatic dysfunction and may contribute to refractory hypotension [81]. A short synacthen test is recommended in all patients with acute liver failure who require vasoconstrictor therapy. If the response to synacthen is inadequate, a trial of hydrocortisone (200–300 mg/day for 7–10 days) may be given as it has been shown to improve vasopressor responsiveness [82].

Respiratory Support

Intubation and controlled mechanical ventilation in acute liver failure is usually indicated for the patient's airway protection due to progressive encephalopathy. As the acute liver failure progresses, a significant proportion (> 30 %) of patients will develop the pulmonary complications of ARDS or acute lung injury (ALI) [83]. As described above, lung infections are also a frequent occurrence in acute liver failure and confer a worse prognosis.

Ventilation strategies in ALI associated with acute liver failure are similar to those in the general intensive care population; however the avoidance of hypercapnia, which can exacerbate intracranial hypertension, should be particularly rigorous. This means that if low tidal volumes are used to guard against ALI, the respiratory rate may need to be increased to maintain normocapnia [45]. Moderate levels of positive end-expiratory pressure (PEEP) can be tolerated without detriment to the ICP and should be used to ensure alveolar recruitment and adequate oxygenation [62].

A further challenge in the ventilation of patients with acute liver failure is the increased respiratory compliance due to fluid overload causing chest wall edema, pleural effusions and ascites, which gives rise to diaphragmatic splinting from raised IAP. IAP monitoring via an intravesical probe should be routine and paracentesis used to decompress the abdominal compartment if pressure rises > 20 mmHg.

Coagulopathy

The coagulopathy of acute liver failure is complex, caused by both a failure in hepatic production of fibrinogen and clotting factors and increased consumption. Thrombocytopenia is common, with platelet counts of $< 150 \times 10^9$ cells/l seen in over 70 % of cases, though the cause for declining platelet counts are not well understood [84]. The marked abnormalities in laboratory indices of clotting may be misleading as hepatic impairment also causes defects in the anti-coagulant system, which can compensate for the bleeding tendency, the so called 'rebalanced hemostasis'. This probably explains why, despite significant prolongation of the INR, spontaneous bleeding in acute liver failure is a rare event. A recent study utilizing thromboelastography (TEG) to assess clotting in patients with acute liver failure, showed that the dynamics of clot formation are well preserved despite an INR range of 1.5–9.6 [85]. The same study also demonstrated that pro- and anti-coagulant factors, except for factor VIII, decreased in direct proportion to one another in acute liver failure.

As significant spontaneous bleeding is rare in acute liver failure there is no requirement for prophylactic correction of clotting indices [2, 86]. Although this advice has been consistent for many years, over-transfusion is common. A recent series showed 92 % of acute liver failure patients received an average of 14 units of FFP within their first week in hospital despite few incidents of spontaneous bleeding or invasive procedures requiring correcting of coagulopathy [86]. The volume associated with transfusion of FFP may cause fluid overload and worsen cerebral edema and this practice also places patients at risk of transfusion-related ALI (TRALI).

If an invasive procedure, such as placement of an ICP monitor is planned, clotting should be corrected. The targets for transfusion have not been clearly set, though an INR of < 1.5 [45] and platelet count of 50,000–70,000/mm^3 has been proposed [86]. The use of recombinant factor VII in addition to or instead of FFP has been recommended by some as it may more efficiently improve clotting indices and reduces the risk of fluid overload [59]. There are, however, significant cost implications to this strategy.

Intravenous vitamin K should be administered to all patients as there is a high prevalence of vitamin K deficiency in acute liver failure [87].

Overall, this is an area where further research is clearly needed. It is recognized that standard laboratory indices poorly reflect *in vivo* coagulopathy and yet no better methods of assessment are available. The optimal targets for transfusion and best strategies to correct coagulopathy currently lack a convincing evidence base.

Nutrition and Electrolyte Homeostasis

Acute liver failure is a catabolic state, with high energy expenditure leading to muscle wasting and nutritional deficiencies. Disorders of glucose, potassium, phosphate and magnesium homeostasis are common and should be monitored and promptly corrected. Hypoglycemia is one of the metabolic hallmarks of acute liver failure and is caused by failure of gluconeogenesis and destruction of hepatic glycogen stores. Treatment with continuous glucose infusions or feed is commonly required to maintain normoglycemia. Hyperglycemia should also be avoided as there is evidence that it may exacerbate intracranial hypertension [62].

Disorders of phosphate handling are also commonly seen in acute liver failure and phosphate levels have been shown to be an accurate predictor of prognosis in acetaminophen-induced acute liver failure, with hyperphosphatemia being seen in non-survivors and hypophosphatemia in survivors [88]. This is thought to be a proxy measure of the absence or presence of hepatic regeneration, which utilizes phosphate in the generation of ATP.

Feeding should be established early and the enteral route is preferred if possible. Acute liver failure is not however a contraindication to parenteral feeding. Protein restriction is not required, so a normal intake of 60 g/day or 1 g/kg/day can be provided. Glutamine-containing feed should be avoided to avoid the theoretical risk of exacerbating hepatic encephalopathy [62].

Liver Support Devices

The potential for hepatic regeneration in acute liver failure if a patient can be supported through their acute illness has led to the development of a number of liver support devices which aim to temporarily take over vital hepatic functions in much the same way a dialysis machine may be used to transiently support kidney function in acute renal failure. Unfortunately the dream of a mechanical 'proxy liver' is a long way from being realized. Systems have been created that use biological components, usually cells from hepatoma lines, or purely artificial components, or a combination of the two in 'bio-artificial' devices. The artificial devices are the only ones to have been used extensively in clinical trials and all work on an albumin dialysis principle, whereby high concentrations of albumin in a dialysate are used to extract albumin-bound toxins from patient blood as it circulates through the device. The two most commonly used devices are the molecular absorbance recirculation system (MARS) and the Prometheus albumin dialysis system. A recent meta-analysis of MARS treatment in acute liver failure demonstrated that it could improve hepatic encephalopathy grade and biochemical indices, but had no overall impact on survival [89]. Further trials on both artificial and the new bioartificial systems are required before they are considered as routine care for acute liver failure [2].

Liver Transplantation

The use of liver transplantation has been the most significant development in the treatment of acute liver failure in the last 40 years and has significantly improved survival [14]. One year survival following an emergent liver transplant is slightly worse than for routine transplants, but stands at an impressive 80 %. The selection for liver transplant depends upon accurate prediction of survival without transplant as discussed above.

A discussion of graft selection and transplantation ethics is beyond the scope of this chapter.

Table 6 A summary of recommendations for management of the multi-system manifestations of acute liver failure

Clinical Manifestation	Recommendation	Rationale
Cerebral edema and ICH	CT scan	Rule out other intracranial pathology or hemorrhage May demonstrate cerebral edema but low sensitivity for ICH
	Invasive ICP monitoring in grade III/IV hepatic encephalopathy	Guide treatment to maintain ICP < 20 mmHg and CPP > 60 mmHg
	Position patient head up 30°	Reduce ICP without compromising CPP
	Sedation with propofol and fentanyl and decreased stimulation	Reduce spikes in ICP associated with movement, agitation and valsalva effects from coughing/gag
	Control seizures with i.v. phenytoin	Seizures can increase ICP
	Aggressive treatment of SIRS	SIRS associated with poor prognosis and progression of hepatic encephalopathy
	Bolus mannitol (0.25–0.5 g/kg). Repeat administration if serum osmolality < 320 mOsm/L	Osmotic reduction in brain water and improved blood rheology
	Hypertonic saline to induce hypernatremia (145–155 mmol/l)	Osmotic reduction in brain swelling. Prevents the development of ICH and may be used in the place of mannitol as treatment
	'Last resort' rescue therapies include: Moderate hypothermia Barbiturates Hyperventilation Total hepatectomy and portocaval shunt	These may transiently lower ICP
Coagulopathy	i.v. proton pump inhibitor	Reduce risk of GI bleeding
	Parenteral vitamin K	Correct vitamin K deficiency
	Do not correct coagulopathy unless significant bleeding or prior to invasive procedure	Transfusion can contribute to volume overload and cerebral edema and cause TRALI
	Correction of coagulopathy prior to invasive procedures with FFP, platelets and rFVII	
Renal impairment	Correct hypovolemia	Improve renal perfusion and GFR
	Avoidance of nephrotoxic drugs	Prevent direct renal toxicity
	Maintain MAP > 75 mmHg with norepinephrine	Improve renal perfusion and GFR
	In presence of ascites monitor intra-abdominal pressure and perform paracentesis if pressure > 20 mmHg	Improve renal perfusion

Continuation see next page

Table 6 *Continued*

Clinical Manifestation	Recommendation	Rationale
	Continuous method of RRT if required.	RRT supports renal function and has added benefit of some systemic ammonia clearance. Continuous methods prevent hemodynamic instability and rises in ICP.
Respiratory compromise	Prompt treatment of pulmonary infections	
	Adjustment of CMV to maintain normocapnia	
	Monitoring of IAP and decompression by paracentesis.	Improves respiratory compliance and facilitates ventilation.
Hemodynamic instability	Fluid resuscitation with normal saline	Correct hypovolemia
	Vasoconstrictor therapy. Norepinephrine preferred.	Maintenance of MAP and CPP, to ensure adequate tissue perfusion
	Short synacthen test on all requiring vasoconstrictors. Hydrocortisone for those with impaired short synacthen test.	Adrenal insufficiency common and may contribute to refractory hypotension
Impaired glucose homeostasis	Continuous glucose infusion or feed to maintain normoglycemia. Avoidance of hyperglycemia	Hyperglycemia may exacerbate ICH
Nutritional deficiency	Enteral feeding if possible aiming for 25–30 kcal/kg/day. Parenteral route if enteral not possible. Normal protein content	
	Frequent monitoring of electrolytes with correction if required	Hypokalemia, hypophosphatemia and hypomagnesemia common.

ICH: intracranial hypertension; CPP: cerebral perfusion pressure; ICP: intracranial pressure; CT: computed tomography; SIRS: systemic inflammatory response syndrome; i.v.: intravenous; TRALI: transfusion-related acute lung injury; FFP: fresh frozen plasma; GFR: glomerular filtration rate; MAP: mean arterial pressure; RRT: renal replacement therapy; IAP: intra-abdominal pressure

Conclusions

The optimal management of acute liver failure requires consideration of the diagnosis and etiological factors (Table 6). The hepatic and extra hepatic manifestations require recognition and management to support end-organ function and increase opportunities for liver repair and regeneration. The time course of deterioration needs to be considered depending on sub-acute, acute or hyperacute etiologies, the latter being associated with rapid changes particularly in regard cardiovascular, metabolic and neurological status. The decision as to whether transplantation is a therapeutic option should be based upon validated prognostic scoring systems and underlying etiology of the acute liver failure.

References

1. Wlodzimirow KA, Eslami S, Abu-Hanna A, Nieuwoudt M, Chamuleau RA (2012) Systematic review: acute liver failure – one disease, more than 40 definitions. Aliment Pharmacol Ther 35:1245–1256
2. Lee WML, Stravitz RT, Larson AM (2011) AASLD Position Paper: The Management of Acute Liver Failure: Update 2011. Available at: http://www.aasld.org/practiceguidelines/Documents/ACuteLiverFailureUpdate2011.pdf. Accessed Nov 2013
3. O'Grady JG, Schalm SW, Williams R (1993) Acute liver failure: redefining the syndromes. Lancet 342:273–275
4. Tandon BN, Bernauau J, O'Grady J et al (1999) Recommendations of the International Association for the Study of the Liver Subcommittee on nomenclature of acute and subacute liver failure. J Gastroenterol Hepatol 14:403–404
5. Bernuau J, Rueff B, Benhamou JP (1986) Fulminant and subfulminant liver failure: definitions and causes. Semin Liver Dis 6:97–106
6. Bower WA, Johns M, Margolis HS, Williams IT, Bell BP (2007) Population-based surveillance for acute liver failure. Am J Gastroenterol 102:2459–2463
7. Ostapowicz G, Fontana RJ, Schiodt FV et al (2002) Results of a prospective study of acute liver failure at 17 tertiary care centers in the United States. Ann Intern Med 137:947–954
8. Lee WM (2012) Recent developments in acute liver failure. Best practice & research. Clin Gastroenterol 26:3–16
9. Bernal W, Auzinger G, Wendon J (2009) Prognostic utility of the bilirubin lactate and etiology score. Clin Gastroenterol Hepatol 7:249
10. Hawton K, Simkin S, Deeks J et al (2004) UK legislation on analgesic packs: before and after study of long term effect on poisonings. BMJ 329:1076
11. Mindikoglu AL, Magder LS, Regev A (2009) Outcome of liver transplantation for drug-induced acute liver failure in the United States: analysis of the United Network for Organ Sharing database. Liver Transpl 15:719–729
12. Sarwar S, Khan AA, Alam A et al (2006) Predictors of fatal outcome in fulminant hepatic failure. J Coll Physicians Surg Pak 16:112–116
13. Khuroo MS, Kamili S (2003) Aetiology and prognostic factors in acute liver failure in India. J Viral Hepat 10:224–231
14. Bernal W, Hyyrylainen A, Gera A et al (2013) Lessons from look-back in acute liver failure? A single centre experience of 3300 patients. J Hepatol 59:74–80
15. Bernal W, Auzinger G, Dhawan A, Wendon J (2010) Acute liver failure. Lancet 376:190–201
16. Cholongitas EB, Betrossian A, Leandro G, Shaw S, Patch D, Burroughs AK (2006) King's criteria, APACHE II, and SOFA scores in acute liver failure. Hepatology 43:881

17. Schmidt LE, Larsen FS (2006) Prognostic implications of hyperlactatemia, multiple organ failure, and systemic inflammatory response syndrome in patients with acetaminophen-induced acute liver failure. Crit Care Med 34:337–343

18. Zaman MB, Hoti E, Qasim A et al (2006) MELD score as a prognostic model for listing acute liver failure patients for liver transplantation. Transplant Proc 38:2097–2098

19. Schmidt LE, Dalhoff K (2005) Alpha-fetoprotein is a predictor of outcome in acetaminophen-induced liver injury. Hepatology 41:26–31

20. Chung PY, Sitrin MD, Te HS (2003) Serum phosphorus levels predict clinical outcome in fulminant hepatic failure. Liver Transpl 9:248–253

21. O'Grady JG, Alexander GJ, Hayllar KM, Williams R (1989) Early indicators of prognosis in fulminant hepatic failure. Gastroenterology 97:439–445

22. Bernal W, Donaldson N, Wyncoll D, Wendon J (2002) Blood lactate as an early predictor of outcome in paracetamol-induced acute liver failure: a cohort study. Lancet 359:558–563

23. Craig DG, Ford AC, Hayes PC, Simpson KJ (2010) Systematic review: prognostic tests of paracetamol-induced acute liver failure. Aliment Pharmacol Ther 31:1064–1076

24. Rutherford A, King LY, Hynan LS et al (2012) Development of an accurate index for predicting outcomes of patients with acute liver failure. Gastroenterology 143:1237–1243

25. Leithead JA, Ferguson JW, Bates CM et al (2009) The systemic inflammatory response syndrome is predictive of renal dysfunction in patients with non-paracetamol-induced acute liver failure. Gut 58:443–449

26. Karvellas CJ, Safinia N, Auzinger G et al (2010) Medical and psychiatric outcomes for patients transplanted for acetaminophen-induced acute liver failure: a case-control study. Liver Int 30:826–833

27. Sandilands EA, Bateman DN (2009) Adverse reactions associated with acetylcysteine. Clin Toxicol 47:81–88

28. Harrison PM, Keays R, Bray GP, Alexander GJ, Williams R (1990) Improved outcome of paracetamol-induced fulminant hepatic failure by late administration of acetylcysteine. Lancet 335:1572–1573

29. Lee WM, Hynan LS, Rossaro L et al (2009) Intravenous N-acetylcysteine improves transplant-free survival in early stage non-acetaminophen acute liver failure. Gastroenterology 137:856–864

30. Harrison PM, Wendon JA, Gimson AE, Alexander GJ, Williams R (1991) Improvement by acetylcysteine of hemodynamics and oxygen transport in fulminant hepatic failure. N Engl J Med 324:1852–1857

31. Stravitz RT, Sanyal AJ, Reisch J et al (2013) Effects of N-acetylcysteine on cytokines in non-acetaminophen acute liver failure: potential mechanism of improvement in transplant-free survival. Liver Int 33:1324–1331

32. Rolando N, Wade J, Davalos M, Wendon J, Philpott-Howard J, Williams R (2000) The systemic inflammatory response syndrome in acute liver failure. Hepatology 32:734–739

33. Vaquero J, Polson J, Chung C et al (2003) Infection and the progression of hepatic encephalopathy in acute liver failure. Gastroenterology 125:755–764

34. Antoniades CG, Berry PA, Wendon JA, Vergani D (2008) The importance of immune dysfunction in determining outcome in acute liver failure. J Hepatol 49:845–861

35. Wyke RJ, Rajkovic IA, Eddleston AL, Williams R (1980) Defective opsonisation and complement deficiency in serum from patients with fulminant hepatic failure. Gut 21:643–649

36. Wyke RJ, Yousif-Kadaru AG, Rajkovic IA, Eddleston AL, Williams R (1982) Serum stimulatory activity and polymorphonuclear leucocyte movement in patients with fulminant hepatic failure. Clin Exp Immunol 50:442–449

37. Clapperton M, Rolando N, Sandoval L, Davies E, Williams R (1997) Neutrophil superoxide and hydrogen peroxide production in patients with acute liver failure. Eur J Clin Invest 27:164–168

38. Antoniades CG, Berry PA, Davies ET et al (2006) Reduced monocyte HLA-DR expression: a novel biomarker of disease severity and outcome in acetaminophen-induced acute liver failure. Hepatology 44:34–43
39. Rolando N, Philpott-Howard J, Williams R (1996) Bacterial and fungal infection in acute liver failure. Sem Liver Dis 16:389–402
40. Rolando N, Harvey F, Brahm J et al (1990) Prospective study of bacterial infection in acute liver failure: an analysis of fifty patients. Hepatology 11:49–53
41. Wyke RJ, Canalese JC, Gimson AE, Williams R (1982) Bacteraemia in patients with fulminant hepatic failure. Liver 2:45–52
42. Karvellas CJ, Pink F, McPhail M et al (2009) Predictors of bacteraemia and mortality in patients with acute liver failure. Intensive Care Med 35:1390–1396
43. Rivers E, Nguyen B, Havstad S et al (2001) Early goal-directed therapy in the treatment of severe sepsis and septic shock. N Engl J Med 345:1368–1377
44. Rolando N, Gimson A, Wade J, Philpott-Howard J, Casewell M, Williams R (1993) Prospective controlled trial of selective parenteral and enteral antimicrobial regimen in fulminant liver failure. Hepatology 17:196–201
45. Stravitz RT, Kramer DJ (2009) Management of acute liver failure. Nat Rev. Gastroenterol Hepatol 6:542–553
46. Atterbury CE, Maddrey WC, Conn HO (1978) Neomycin-sorbitol and lactulose in the treatment of acute portal-systemic encephalopathy. A controlled, double-blind clinical trial. Am J Dig Dis 23:398–406
47. Bernal W, Hall C, Karvellas CJ, Auzinger G, Sizer E, Wendon J (2007) Arterial ammonia and clinical risk factors for encephalopathy and intracranial hypertension in acute liver failure. Hepatology 46:1844–1852
48. Bhatia V, Singh R, Acharya SK (2006) Predictive value of arterial ammonia for complications and outcome in acute liver failure. Gut 55:98–104
49. Clemmesen JO, Larsen FS, Kondrup J, Hansen BA, Ott P (1999) Cerebral herniation in patients with acute liver failure is correlated with arterial ammonia concentration. Hepatology 29:648–653
50. Romero-Gomez M, Jover M, Galan JJ, Ruiz A (2009) Gut ammonia production and its modulation. Metab Brain Dis 24:147–157
51. Chatauret N, Desjardins P, Zwingmann C, Rose C, Rao KV, Butterworth RF (2006) Direct molecular and spectroscopic evidence for increased ammonia removal capacity of skeletal muscle in acute liver failure. J Hepatol 44:1083–1088
52. Cooper AJ, Lai JC (1987) Cerebral ammonia metabolism in normal and hyperammonemic rats. Neurochem Pathol 6:67–95
53. Norenberg MD (2003) Oxidative and nitrosative stress in ammonia neurotoxicity. Hepatology 37:245–248
54. Stravitz RT, Larsen FS (2009) Therapeutic hypothermia for acute liver failure. Crit Care Med 37(7 Suppl):S258–264
55. Wright G, Shawcross D, Olde Damink SW, Jalan R (2007) Brain cytokine flux in acute liver failure and its relationship with intracranial hypertension. Metab Brain Dis 22:375–388
56. Jalan R, Olde Damink SW, Hayes PC, Deutz NE, Lee A (2004) Pathogenesis of intracranial hypertension in acute liver failure: inflammation, ammonia and cerebral blood flow. J Hepatol 41:613–620
57. Bjerring PN, Eefsen M, Hansen BA, Larsen FS (2009) The brain in acute liver failure. A tortuous path from hyperammonemia to cerebral edema. Metab Brain Dis 24:5–14
58. Vaquero J, Fontana RJ, Larson AM et al (2005) Complications and use of intracranial pressure monitoring in patients with acute liver failure and severe encephalopathy. Liver Transpl 11:1581–1589
59. Shami VM, Caldwell SH, Hespenheide EE, Arseneau KO, Bickston SJ, Macik BG (2003) Recombinant activated factor VII for coagulopathy in fulminant hepatic failure compared with conventional therapy. Liver Transpl 9:138–143

60. Davies MH, Mutimer D, Lowes J, Elias E, Neuberger J (1994) Recovery despite impaired cerebral perfusion in fulminant hepatic failure. Lancet 343:1329–1330
61. Tsoulfas G, Elias N, Sandberg WS et al (2012) Liver transplantation results in complete neurologic recovery from malignant hypertension secondary to fulminant hepatic failure: a case report. Ann Transpl 17:117–121
62. Auzinger G, Wendon J (2008) Intensive care management of acute liver failure. Current Opin Crit Care 14:179–188
63. Bhatia V, Batra Y, Acharya SK (2004) Prophylactic phenytoin does not improve cerebral edema or survival in acute liver failure – a controlled clinical trial. J Hepatol 41:89–96
64. Canalese J, Gimson AE, Davis C, Mellon PJ, Davis M, Williams R (1982) Controlled trial of dexamethasone and mannitol for the cerebral oedema of fulminant hepatic failure. Gut 23:625–629
65. Murphy N, Auzinger G, Bernel W, Wendon J (2004) The effect of hypertonic sodium chloride on intracranial pressure in patients with acute liver failure. Hepatology 39:464–470
66. Marion DW, Penrod LE, Kelsey SF et al (1997) Treatment of traumatic brain injury with moderate hypothermia. N Engl J Med 336:540–546
67. Bernard SA, Gray TW, Buist MD et al (2002) Treatment of comatose survivors of out-of-hospital cardiac arrest with induced hypothermia. N Engl J Med 346:557–563
68. Vaquero J, Belanger M, James L et al (2007) Mild hypothermia attenuates liver injury and improves survival in mice with acetaminophen toxicity. Gastroenterology 132:372–383
69. Jalan R, Olde Damink SW, Deutz NE, Hayes PC, Lee A (2004) Moderate hypothermia in patients with acute liver failure and uncontrolled intracranial hypertension. Gastroenterology 127:1338–1346
70. Jalan R, Olde Damink SW, Deutz NE, Lee A, Hayes PC (1999) Moderate hypothermia for uncontrolled intracranial hypertension in acute liver failure. Lancet 354:1164–1168
71. Polderman KH (2004) Application of therapeutic hypothermia in the intensive care unit. Opportunities and pitfalls of a promising treatment modality – Part 2: Practical aspects and side effects. Intensive Care Med 30:757–769
72. Strauss G, Hansen BA, Knudsen GM, Larsen FS (1998) Hyperventilation restores cerebral blood flow autoregulation in patients with acute liver failure. J Hepatol 28:199–203
73. Ede RJ, Gimson AE, Bihari D, Williams R (1986) Controlled hyperventilation in the prevention of cerebral oedema in fulminant hepatic failure. J Hepatol 2:43–51
74. Wendon JA, Harrison PM, Keays R, Williams R (1994) Cerebral blood flow and metabolism in fulminant liver failure. Hepatology 19:1407–1413
75. Tofteng F, Larsen FS (2004) The effect of indomethacin on intracranial pressure, cerebral perfusion and extracellular lactate and glutamate concentrations in patients with fulminant hepatic failure. J Cereb Blood Flow Metab 24:798–804
76. Rozga J, Podesta L, LePage E et al (1993) Control of cerebral oedema by total hepatectomy and extracorporeal liver support in fulminant hepatic failure. Lancet 342:898–899
77. Davenport A, Will EJ, Davidson AM (1993) Improved cardiovascular stability during continuous modes of renal replacement therapy in critically ill patients with acute hepatic and renal failure. Crit Care Med 21:328–338
78. Davenport A, Will EJ, Davison AM (1993) Effect of renal replacement therapy on patients with combined acute renal and fulminant hepatic failure. Kidney Int Suppl 41:S245–251
79. Audimooolam VK, McPhail MJ, Sherwood R et al (2012) Elevated troponin I and its prognostic significance in acute liver failure. Crit Care 16:R228
80. Parekh NK, Hynan LS, De Lemos J, Lee WM (2007) Elevated troponin I levels in acute liver failure: is myocardial injury an integral part of acute liver failure? Hepatology 45:1489–1495
81. Harry R, Auzinger G, Wendon J (2002) The clinical importance of adrenal insufficiency in acute hepatic dysfunction. Hepatology 36:395–402
82. Harry R, Auzinger G, Wendon J (2003) The effects of supraphysiological doses of corticosteroids in hypotensive liver failure. Liver Int 23:71–77

83. Baudouin SV, Howdle P, O'Grady JG, Webster NR (1995) Acute lung injury in fulminant hepatic failure following paracetamol poisoning. Thorax 50:399–402
84. Schiodt FV, Balko J, Schilsky M, Harrison ME, Thornton A, Lee WM (2003) Thrombopoietin in acute liver failure. Hepatology 37:558–561
85. Stravitz RT, Lisman T, Luketic VA et al (2012) Minimal effects of acute liver injury/acute liver failure on hemostasis as assessed by thromboelastography. J Hepatol 56:129–136
86. Munoz SJ, Rajender Reddy K, Lee W (2008) The coagulopathy of acute liver failure and implications for intracranial pressure monitoring. Neurocrit Care 9:103–107
87. Pereira SP, Rowbotham D, Fitt S, Shearer MJ, Wendon J, Williams R (2005) Pharmacokinetics and efficacy of oral versus intravenous mixed-micellar phylloquinone (vitamin K1) in severe acute liver disease. J Hepatol 42:365–370
88. Schmidt LE, Dalhoff K (2002) Serum phosphate is an early predictor of outcome in severe acetaminophen-induced hepatotoxicity. Hepatology 36:659–665
89. Vaid A, Chweich H, Balk EM, Jaber BL (2012) Molecular adsorbent recirculating system as artificial support therapy for liver failure: a meta-analysis. ASAIO J 58:51–59

Part XIII
Renal Issues

Lung/Kidney Interactions: From Experimental Evidence to Clinical Uncertainty

D. Schnell, F. Vincent, and M. Darmon

Introduction

Despite improvements in dialysis technology and supportive care, the morbidity and mortality rates associated with acute kidney injury (AKI) have remained unchanged for several decades [1–6]. Whether this poor prognosis of AKI is ascribable to the severity of underlying disease or to renal dysfunction *per se* has long been debated. Several recent studies suggest that AKI itself might influence patient outcomes, independent of the nature and severity of underlying disease and the metabolic consequences of renal dysfunction. In several studies, AKI was consistently associated with a high relative risk of death even after adjustment for co-morbid conditions and severity of illness [1, 3]. In addition, several studies found that moderate AKI adversely affected patient outcomes [7–9]. Thus, moderate serum creatinine elevation ($> 26 \, \mu mol/l$) was associated with a 6.5-fold increase in the risk of in-hospital death [9]. Based on these data, renal dysfunction is no longer viewed as merely a manifestation of multiple organ failure, but is instead seen as a possible contributor to the development of other organ dysfunctions [3, 9, 10]. Hence, an increasing body of evidence suggests that deleterious interactions might exist between the kidney and distant organs. These interactions may help in understanding the natural history of multiple organ dysfunction and emphasize the central role of AKI in this syndrome. Cardiorenal syndromes [11] and neurological or hepatic consequences of AKI [12] are among the reported interactions. However, lung/kidney interactions are among the most carefully described interactions. This review reports the evidence and mechanisms of these interactions, and delineates a research agenda

D. Schnell
Réanimation médicale, Nouvel Hôpital Civil, Hôpitaux Universitaires de Strasbourg, 67091 Strasbourg Cedex, France

F. Vincent · M. Darmon ✉
Medical ICU, Saint-Etienne University Hospital, 42270 Saint-Priest-en-Jarrez, France
e-mail: michael.darmon@chu-st-etienne.fr

J.-L. Vincent (Ed.), *Annual Update in Intensive Care and Emergency Medicine 2014*, DOI 10.1007/978-3-319-03746-2_39, © Springer International Publishing Switzerland 2014

that may aid in a finer understanding of the clinical consequences of the reported experimental mechanisms.

Pulmonary Consequences of AKI

The primary mechanisms of respiratory failure during AKI have long been debated. The most obvious mechanism is extracellular space overload, which may translate into hydrostatic pulmonary edema [13, 14]. However, more complex mechanisms of lung injury exist in addition to this mechanism. Experimental evidence suggests that pulmonary injury might occur after renal injury [15–17]. Experimental models have demonstrated that renal ischemia-reperfusion and bilateral nephrectomy are associated with increased pulmonary vascular permeability and reduced alveolar fluid clearance, leading to increased pulmonary wet lung and increased bronchoalveolar lavage (BAL) protein concentration [15–17]. All of these findings suggest that pulmonary injury is induced, or at least exacerbated, by renal injury. Pulmonary histology performed after renal injury also revealed interstitial edema, intra-alveolar hemorrhage, and red blood cell (RBC) sludging after renal injury [18]. Additionally, these findings were associated with downregulation of the epithelial sodium channel, the Na^+-K^+-ATPase transporter, and aquaporin 5 in the rodent lung [15]. Finally, genomic analyses revealed the activation of pro-inflammatory and pro-apoptotic pathways after ischemia-reperfusion [17]. The respective influences of uremia (indirectly caused by AKI as a result of the accumulation of urea or other potentially toxic agents) and renal injury *per se* (a direct result of AKI, separate from its metabolic consequences) remain uncertain, and may vary for each of the suspected mechanisms. The effects of renal injury on epithelial sodium and water transporters were observed after bilateral renal ischemia-reperfusion, as well as after bilateral nephrectomy [15]. Similarly, several studies have reported evidence of lung inflammation and injury after bilateral nephrectomy, suggesting that indirect toxicity related to uremia might have occurred [18, 19]. Conversely, transcriptional changes observed after renal ischemia were distinct from changes observed after bilateral nephrectomy, suggesting that at least some of the observed pulmonary consequences were specific to renal ischemia and distinct from hypothetical accumulation of uremic toxicity after AKI [17].

Three mechanisms have been proposed to be involved in the initiation and progression of respiratory response to AKI: A systemic inflammatory response mediated by cytokines; a cellular response involving both neutrophils and macrophages; and a role for reactive oxygen species (ROS). Cellular and humoral inflammatory responses appear to play a major role in the initiation and progression of the respiratory response to AKI [19, 21–23]. Hence, an experimental study conducted in wild type mice reported that both ischemic renal injury and bilateral nephrectomy were followed within 4 hours by lung neutrophil infiltration with increased myeloperoxidase activity, neutrophil chemokines, and capillary leakage [21]. The critical role of interleukin (IL)-6 was demonstrated in IL-6-deficient mice or following the administration of anti-IL-6 antibodies [21]. IL-6-deficient mice and animals treated with anti-IL-6 antibodies exhibited decreased myeloperoxidase levels, capillary leakage, or neutrophil levels of chemokines after both renal interventions [21]. Additional models emphasized the influence of several chemokines and cytokines. Hence, keratinocyte-derived chemokine (or its murine equivalent, Gro-α), macrophage inflammatory protein (MIP)-2 or IL-1β and tumor necrosis factor (TNF)-α have been found to increase during the first 3 hours after AKI [22–24]. Interestingly, the administration of anti-inflammatory IL-10 was associated with decreased lung inflammation and injury in these experimental models [19]. However, beyond cytokines, several studies reported lung leukocyte activation or infiltration after experimental AKI [19, 20]. Therefore, AKI was reportedly associated with pulmonary infiltration independent of the AKI mechanism in animals [19, 20]. Macrophages have also been discussed as potent effectors of lung injury after experimental AKI. Studies have observed that AKI is associated with macrophage infiltration of distant organs [25] and that lung injury is reduced by the administration of macrophage inhibitors [18]. Finally, the influence of ROS has been suggested. Although less thoroughly investigated, experimental studies have suggested that oxidative stress influences systemic organ dysfunction after renal injury. Hence, ischemic renal injury can reportedly decrease hepatic levels of antioxidant compounds (glutathione or superoxide dismutase [SOD]) [26]. Additionally, knockout mice for heme oxygenase 1, a potent antioxidant enzyme, were found to be more sensitive to renal ischemia, with increased IL-6 levels in systemic organs [27].

Despite consistent findings in experimental studies and a high biological plausibility, the respiratory consequences of renal dysfunction remain to be assessed in the clinical setting. Whether these pathophysiological mechanisms translate into meaningful clinical consequences has yet to be demonstrated.

Renal Consequences of Acute Respiratory Failure

In contrast to the previously mentioned interactions, acute lung injury (ALI) adversely affected renal function in experimental studies in animals and healthy volunteers, as well as in critically ill patients. Positive pressure ventilation, hypoxemia and hypercapnia, and systemic inflammation have been involved in this renal response to acute respiratory failure.

Renal Consequences of Positive Pressure Ventilation

Positive pressure ventilation may modify the cardiac preload and has been associated with systemic hemodynamic changes. It has also been associated with changes in renal function, including decreases in glomerular filtration rate (GFR), renal blood flow, and free water clearance [28–34]. An experimental study performed 60 years ago in healthy volunteers reported that high levels of continuous positive airway pressure (24 to 26 mmHg) were associated with decreases in renal plasma flow (as assessed by para-aminohippurate clearance), free water and sodium clearance, and GFR (as assessed by inulin clearance) [29]. Additional studies confirmed these findings with lower levels of positive pressure [30–33, 35] and provided additional insight regarding the pathophysiological mechanisms involved. These studies observed the systematic activation of both sympathetic and renin-angiotensin systems, together with the suppression of atrial natriuretic peptide release [30–33, 35]. Interestingly, no changes in anti-diuretic hormone concentration were observed [35]. Additionally, renal effects of positive pressure were observed in renal transplant recipients, which suggests that renal nerves have little role in altering renal vascular resistance in this setting [32, 34].

Renal Consequences of Hypoxemia and Hypercapnia

Beyond the direct effects of positive pressure ventilation, both hypoxemia and hypercapnia were shown to influence renal perfusion and sodium and water clearance. Oxygen effects are closely related to the relative medullar hypoxemia observed in mammals. This relative medullar hypoxemia is well documented and is closely correlated to the ability of mammals to concentrate urine [36]. However, several regulatory mechanisms enable the maintenance of adequate medullar oxygenation and, therefore, the maintenance of renal function until a critical oxygen concentration is reached [36]. This critical oxygen concentration appears to be reached when the fraction of inspired oxygen (FiO$_2$) is approximately 9 % [36]. Further impairment in medullary oxygenation may lead to medullary hypoxic injury and, therefore, to acute tubular necrosis. However, the effect of milder hypoxemia on kidney function was recognized several decades ago, and includes increases in diuresis, natriuresis, and maintained GFR [37]. The hypoxic diuretic response has secondarily been demonstrated to occur during either normobaric hypoxemia or hypobaric equivalence [38–43]. This effect has been extensively studied in humans and animals at rest and during exercise, as well as in poïkilocapnic and isocapnic conditions [38, 41–43]. This response is believed to be an adaptive phenomenon that allows hemoconcentration (and therefore increased oxygen transportation) in this setting [44]. However, pathophysiological mechanisms of this response are complex and remain poorly understood. Two main mechanisms have been involved. First, hypoxemia may be responsible for stimulation of the respiratory drive, which results in increased minute ventilation, along with the variation of intra-thoracic pressure in a mechanism known as the hypoxic ventilatory response. The hypoxic ventilatory response may participate in the hypoxic diuretic response through several mechanisms. Hence, respiratory alkalosis induced by the hypoxic ventilatory response might enhance sodium bicarbonate excretion [39, 45]. Additionally, intrathoracic pressure changes in response to hyperpnea have been associated with increased diuresis and natriuresis [29].

However, additional mechanisms have been shown to be involved, and the diuretic renal response to hypoxemia has been observed in isocapnic hypoxemia and in animals receiving neuromuscular blockers [44]. Several humoral factors have been involved aside from the hypoxic ventilatory response, including decreased

Fig. 1 Changes in resistive index (RI) in individuals (*light blue lines*) and median (*dark blue line*) following exposure to moderate hypoxemia (SpO$_2$ 88–90 %) in critically ill patients with refractory hypoxemia. Reproduced from [43] (with permission)

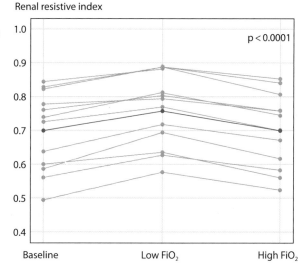

Renal resistive index

p < 0.0001

activity of the renin-angiotensin-aldosterone system [39, 46–48], the role of atrial-natriuretic peptide [49, 50], and the influence of endothelin [39, 51].

Several studies have also emphasized the influence of hypoxemia or hypercapnia on renal perfusion. Although findings have been controversial [52, 53], several studies have reported decreased renal perfusion or increased renal resistance as consequences of hypoxemia [43, 54–58]. Some studies found that both hypoxemia and hypercapnia were associated with increased renal resistance, with synergistic effects when these mechanisms were associated [52, 55, 56]. This effect was reduced but not abolished in renal transplant recipients [57]. This finding suggests an effect, at least partly independent of renal innervation, that could be derived from a humoral mechanism [57]. Suggested mechanisms are numerous, and include chemoreceptor-mediated sympathetic reflexes [57, 59], as well as vasoactive mediators such as bradykinins, angiotensin II, and nitric oxide (NO) [54, 57].

Short-term exposure to moderate hypoxemia appears to have limited consequences on GFR in healthy humans and animals [37, 40, 42, 51–53]. In a recent study performed in critically ill patients with refractory hypoxemia, we found that moderate hypoxemia was associated with an increase in short-term creatinine clearance [43]. This finding, along with an increase in the renal resistive index, might suggest an efferent arteriolar vasoconstriction in response to hypoxemia (Fig. 1) [43]. In contrast, longer duration of exposure to hypobaric hypoxemia in healthy subjects was associated with decreased creatinine clearance [60]. However, the specific role of hypoxemia in this study was difficult to delineate; several confounding factors may have contributed to this finding [60].

Inflammatory Response

Finally, biotrauma and the systemic inflammatory response have been implicated in distant organ dysfunction and renal injury in critically ill patients. Several studies have indicated that the systemic inflammatory response not only affects the lungs, but also leads to further systemic inflammation and organ dysfunction through the release of inflammatory cytokines [61–64]. In these studies, the use of higher tidal volumes was associated with higher levels of cytokines (TNF-α, IL-1β, IL-6, and IL-8), as well as with higher rates of AKI in animals and higher numbers of days with AKI in critically ill patients [61–64]. In an experimental study, ventilation using a higher tidal volume was associated with a higher rate of epithelial cell apoptosis in kidney and intestinal villi [65]. In this study, the contribution of Fas ligand to the observed results was suggested by the correlation between Fas ligand changes and serum creatinine changes, as well as by the attenuated apoptosis that resulted *in vitro* after the inhibition of Fas ligand [65].

Clinical Consequences

Despite the experimental evidence, few studies have evaluated the clinical impact of respiratory failure on renal function by clearly assessing the time of mechanical ventilation initiation relative to the onset of AKI [66–72]. A recent meta-analysis of these studies suggested that both acute respiratory distress syndrome (ARDS) and

Study	Weight	Odds Ratio IV, Random, 95% CI	Odds Ratio IV, Random, 95% CI
Vivino 1998 [66] (PEEP <6)	9.9%	2.89 [0.63, 13.20]	
Vivino 1998 [66] (PEEP <6)	6.7%	20.70 [2.53, 169.35]	
Schortgen 2001 [67]	13.5%	4.02 [1.37, 11.80]	
Rocha 2005 [68]	11.7%	6.16 [1.71, 22.24]	
Brito 2009 [72]	12.7%	0.68 [0.21, 2.17]	
Lahoti 2010 [69]	9.8%	16.00 [3.41, 75.00]	
Jung 2011 [70]	14.7%	1.12 [0.44, 2.87]	
O'Riordan 2011 [71]	20.9%	4.78 [4.19, 5.45]	
Total (95% CI)	**100%**	**3.58 [1.85, 6.92]**	

Heterogeneity: Tau^2 = 0.54; Chi^2 = 24.50, df = 7 (p < 0.001); I^2 = 71%
Test for overall effect: Z = 3.79 (p < 0.001)

0.01 0.1 1 10 100
Favors MV+   Favors MV–

Fig. 2 Forest plot of the studies reporting on mechanical ventilation as a risk factor for AKI in multivariate analysis. MV+: with mechanical ventilation; MV–: without mechanical ventilation; IV: inverse variance; CI: confidence interval; PEEP: positive end-expiratory pressure. Modified from [73]

mechanical ventilation were associated with a 3-fold increase in the risk of AKI (Fig. 2) [73]. However, most of the studies included in this analysis were observational studies that focused on specific populations, such as trauma patients [66], lung transplant recipients [68], cancer patients [69], or patients with hepatic failure [71]. Thus, the general applicability of the findings is unclear. Furthermore, these studies were not specifically designed to assess the influence of respiratory failure on AKI, and the respective influences of mechanical ventilation and ARDS were difficult to delineate [73]. Therefore, and despite the biological plausibility of such an association, these findings do not allow any conclusion regarding the causal relationship between AKI and respiratory failure.

Research Agenda

The large amount of experimental evidence supporting the existence of a lung/kidney interaction contrasts with the limited data regarding the clinical relevance of these interactions. There is a need for confirmatory studies that address the clinical consequences of these interactions. First, epidemiological studies are needed to confirm the association of AKI with respiratory dysfunction or the deterioration of lung function after AKI. Although several studies have suggested such an association during mechanical ventilation, these findings were ancillary results, and the adequacy of adjustment for relevant confounders might be questioned [66–73]. In addition, most of these studies were performed in subgroups of critically ill patients [66, 68–72]. Finally, none of these studies were specifically designed to address this association. Therefore, questions regarding the relevance and generalizability of these findings to an unselected population of critically ill patients remain unanswered. Large cohort studies involving unselected patient populations are needed before any definite conclusion can be drawn regarding this association.

Similarly, addressing the unevaluated question of the influence of ARDS on renal function compared with mechanical ventilation alone might add plausibility to the causal relationship between acute respiratory failure and secondary AKI. In this setting, several physiological studies are needed to assess the influence of mechanical ventilation setting, changes in oxygen or CO_2 level, and biotrauma. Although a previous study demonstrated that short-term changes in FiO_2 setting influenced renal perfusion and free water clearance, as well as GFR [43], this study failed to address the long-term consequences of these changes or the primary mechanisms involved in these associations. Additional observational studies of critically ill patients or randomized studies that focus on these issues are needed to more clearly apprehend the influence of daily changes in ventilator settings on extra-pulmonary function. Whether changes in plateau pressure, positive end-expiratory pressure (PEEP), or oxygen or CO_2 levels translate into clinically relevant changes in fluid balance or renal function in the general intensive care population, in patients with chronic obstructive pulmonary disease (COPD), or in patients with refractory hypoxemia remains to be evaluated.

Finally, assessing the clinical relevance of renal dysfunction to the severity of respiratory failure may be in order, although it would also be more difficult. Large cohort studies may help to address the statistical association between these two events. However, such a study is ultimately likely to fail to discriminate relative consequences of renal injury, uremic state, and fluid balance changes related to renal dysfunction on respiratory failure. A systematic assessment of whether management or preventive measures for AKI might influence the degree of respiratory dysfunction beyond fluid balance may help to highlight such an association more specifically.

Conclusions

Based on existing data regarding the association between renal dysfunction and outcomes, AKI is no longer viewed as merely a manifestation of multiple organ failure. Instead, it is seen as a possible contributor to the development of dysfunction in other organs [12, 18, 74]. Knowledge of the influence of AKI on a distant organ, and conversely, the sensitivity of the kidney to dysfunction in a distant organ, provides insight into the pathophysiology of multiple organ failure [11, 12, 18, 73]. The high prevalence of both AKI and respiratory failure in critically ill patients, along with a growing body of evidence suggesting a lung/kidney interaction, have made this association the perfect experimental example of cross-talk between dysfunctioning organs. Experimental models have demonstrated that renal injury is associated with increased pulmonary vascular permeability and decreased alveolar fluid clearance, leading to increased incidence of pulmonary wet lung and increased BAL protein concentration [15–17]. Pathophysiological mechanisms usually involved in the initiation and progression of the respiratory response to AKI include both cellular and humoral inflammatory responses [19, 21–23]. However, the clinical relevance of these findings remains limited.

ALI has adversely affected renal function in experimental studies in animals, healthy volunteers, and critically ill patients [29, 38, 39, 65]. The consequences of positive pressure ventilation, hypoxemia/hypercapnia, and systemic inflammation are the main mechanisms involved in this renal response to respiratory failure [33, 35, 43, 57, 65]. The relevance of these interactions in a clinical setting has been studied more carefully regarding intermediate outcome variables [31, 35, 43, 56, 57], and also, in some cases, regarding long-term clinical implications [73, 75]. However, there is a lack of studies specifically designed to address long-term clinical consequences.

Studies are needed to more carefully assess the clinical relevance of the experimental mechanisms discussed above. Until such studies are conducted, the previously discussed interactions remain an interesting example of cross-talk between organs, a likely mechanism that may contribute to the puzzle of multiple organ failure, which itself remains a theoretical risk factor for organ dysfunction and a seductive but as-yet-unproven therapeutic target.

References

1. Bagshaw SM, Laupland KB, Doig CJ et al (2005) Prognosis for long-term survival and renal recovery in critically ill patients with severe acute renal failure: a population-based study. Crit Care 9:R700–R709
2. Bagshaw SM, Uchino S, Bellomo R et al (2007) Septic acute kidney injury in critically ill patients: clinical characteristics and outcomes. Clin J Am Soc Nephrol 2:431–439
3. Metnitz PGH, Krenn CG, Steltzer H et al (2002) Effect of acute renal failure requiring renal replacement therapy on outcome in critically ill patients. Crit Care Med 30:2051–2058
4. Joannidis M, Metnitz B, Bauer P et al (2009) Acute kidney injury in critically ill patients classified by AKIN versus RIFLE using the SAPS 3 database. Intensive Care Med 35:1692–1702
5. Palevsky PM, Zhang JH, O'Connor TZ et al (2008) Intensity of renal support in critically ill patients with acute kidney injury. N Engl J Med 359:7–20
6. Brivet FG, Kleinknecht DJ, Loirat P, Landais PJ (1996) Acute renal failure in intensive care units causes, outcome, and prognostic factors of hospital mortality; a prospective, multicenter study. French Study Group on Acute Renal Failure. Crit Care Med 24:192–198
7. Lassnigg A, Schmidlin D, Mouhieddine M et al (2004) Minimal changes of serum creatinine predict prognosis in patients after cardiothoracic surgery: a prospective cohort study. J Am Soc Nephrol 15:1597–1605
8. Loef BG, Epema AH, Smilde TD et al (2005) Immediate postoperative renal function deterioration in cardiac surgical patients predicts in-hospital mortality and long-term survival. J Am Soc Nephrol 16:195–200
9. Chertow GM, Burdick E, Honour M et al (2005) Acute kidney injury, mortality, length of stay, and costs in hospitalized patients. J Am Soc Nephrol 16:3365–3370
10. Khwaja A (2012) KDIGO Clinical Practice Guidelines for Acute Kidney Injury. Nephron Clin Pract 120:179–184
11. Sarraf M, Masoumi A, Schrier RW (2009) Cardiorenal syndrome in acute decompensated heart failure. Clin J Am Soc Nephrol CJASN 4:2013–2026
12. Liu M, Liang Y, Chigurupati S et al (2008) Acute kidney injury leads to inflammation and functional changes in the brain. J Am Soc Nephrol JASN 19:1360–1370
13. National Heart, Lung and Blood Institute Acute Respiratory Distress Syndrome (ARDS), Clinical Trials Network (2006) Comparison of two fluid-management strategies in acute lung injury. N Engl J Med 354:2564–2575
14. Prowle JR, Echeverri JE, Ligabo EV et al (2010) Fluid balance and acute kidney injury. Nat Rev Nephrol 6:107–115
15. Rabb H, Wang Z, Nemoto T et al (2003) Acute renal failure leads to dysregulation of lung salt and water channels. Kidney Int 63:600–606
16. Deng J, Hu X, Yuen PST, Star RA (2004) Alpha-melanocyte-stimulating hormone inhibits lung injury after renal ischemia/reperfusion. Am J Respir Crit Care Med 169:749–756
17. Hassoun HT, Grigoryev DN, Lie ML et al (2007) Ischemic acute kidney injury induces a distant organ functional and genomic response distinguishable from bilateral nephrectomy. Am J Physiol Renal Physiol 293:F30–F40
18. Kramer AA, Postler G, Salhab KF et al (1999) Renal ischemia/reperfusion leads to macrophage-mediated increase in pulmonary vascular permeability. Kidney Int 55:2362–2367
19. Hoke TS, Douglas IS, Klein CL et al (2007) Acute renal failure after bilateral nephrectomy is associated with cytokine-mediated pulmonary injury. J Am Soc Nephrol JASN 18:155–164
20. Kim DJ, Park SH, Sheen MR et al (2006) Comparison of experimental lung injury from acute renal failure with injury due to sepsis. Respir Int Rev Thorac Dis 73:815–824
21. Klein CL, Hoke TS, Fang W-F et al (2008) Interleukin-6 mediates lung injury following ischemic acute kidney injury or bilateral nephrectomy. Kidney Int 74:901–909
22. Feltes CM, Van Eyk J, Rabb H (2008) Distant-organ changes after acute kidney injury. Nephron Physiol 109:80–84

23. Kelly KJ (2003) Distant effects of experimental renal ischemia/reperfusion injury. J Am Soc Nephrol JASN 14:1549–1558
24. Molls RR, Savransky V, Liu M et al (2006) Keratinocyte-derived chemokine is an early biomarker of ischemic acute kidney injury. Am J Physiol Renal Physiol 290:F1187–F1193
25. Tokuyama H, Kelly DJ, Zhang Y et al (2007) Macrophage infiltration and cellular proliferation in the non-ischemic kidney and heart following prolonged unilateral renal ischemia. Nephron Physiol 106:54–62
26. Serteser M, Koken T, Kahraman A, et al (2002) Changes in hepatic TNF-alpha levels, antioxidant status, and oxidation products after renal ischemia/reperfusion injury in mice. J Surg Res
27. Tracz MJ, Juncos JP, Croatt AJ et al (2007) Deficiency of heme oxygenase-1 impairs renal hemodynamics and exaggerates systemic inflammatory responses to renal ischemia. Kidney Int 72:1073–1080
28. Hall SV, Johnson EE, Hedley-Whyte J (1974) Renal hemodynamics and function with continuous positive-pressure ventilation in dogs. Anesthesiology 41:452–461
29. Murdaugh HV Jr, Sieker HO, Manfredi F (1959) Effect of altered intrathoracic pressure on renal hemodynamics, electrolyte excretion and water clearance. J Clin Invest 38:834–842
30. Annat G, Viale JP, Bui Xuan B et al (1983) Effect of PEEP ventilation on renal function, plasma renin, aldosterone, neurophysins and urinary ADH, and prostaglandins. Anesthesiology 58:136–141
31. Lefrant J-Y, Juan J-M, Bruelle P et al (2002) Regional blood flows are affected differently by PEEP when the abdomen is open or closed: an experimental rabbit model. Can J Anaesth J Can Anesth 49:302–308
32. Jacob LP, Chazalet JJ, Payen DM et al (1995) Renal hemodynamic and functional effect of PEEP ventilation in human renal transplantations. Am J Respir Crit Care Med 152:103–107
33. Farge D, De la Coussaye JE, Beloucif S et al (1995) Interactions between hemodynamic and hormonal modifications during PEEP-induced antidiuresis and antinatriuresis. Chest 107:1095–1100
34. Sharkey, Mulloy, Long, O'Neill (1999) The effect of continuous positive airway pressure (CPAP) on renal vascular resistance: the influence of renal denervation. Crit Care 3:33–37
35. Payen DM, Farge D, Beloucif S et al (1987) No involvement of antidiuretic hormone in acute antidiuresis during PEEP ventilation in humans. Anesthesiology 66:17–23
36. Brezis M, Rosen S (1995) Hypoxia of the renal medulla – its implications for disease. N Engl J Med 332:647–655
37. Berger EY, Galdston M, Horwitz SA et al (1949) The effect of anoxic anoxia on the human kidney. J Clin Invest 28:648–652
38. Hildebrandt W, Ottenbacher A, Schuster M et al (2000) Diuretic effect of hypoxia, hypocapnia, and hyperpnea in humans: relation to hormones and O(2) chemosensitivity. J Appl Physiol (1985) 88(2):599–610
39. Höhne C, Boemke W, Schleyer N et al (2002) Low sodium intake does not impair renal compensation of hypoxia-induced respiratory alkalosis. J Appl Physiol (1985) 92:2097–2104
40. Höhne C, Krebs MO, Boemke W et al (2001) Evidence that the renin decrease during hypoxia is adenosine mediated in conscious dogs. J Appl Physiol (1985) 90:1842–1848
41. Swenson ER, Duncan TB, Goldberg SV et al (1985) Diuretic effect of acute hypoxia in humans: relationship to hypoxic ventilatory responsiveness and renal hormones. J Appl Physiol 78:377–383
42. Heyes MP, Farber MO, Manfredi F et al (1982) Acute effects of hypoxia on renal and endocrine function in normal humans. Am J Physiol 243:R265–R270
43. Darmon M, Schortgen F, Leon R et al (2009) Impact of mild hypoxemia on renal function and renal resistive index during mechanical ventilation. Intensive Care Med 35:1031–1038
44. Honig A (1989) Peripheral arterial chemoreceptors and reflex control of sodium and water homeostasis. Am J Physiol 257:R1282–R1302

45. Eiam-ong S, Laski ME, Kurtzman NA, Sabatini S (1994) Effect of respiratory acidosis and respiratory alkalosis on renal transport enzymes. Am J Physiol 267:F390–F399
46. Raff H, Ball DL, Goodfriend TL (1989) Low oxygen selectively inhibits aldosterone secretion from bovine adrenocortical cells in vitro. Am J Physiol 256:E640–E644
47. Milledge JS, Catley DM (1984) Angiotensin converting enzyme response to hypoxia in man: its role in altitude acclimatization. Clin Sci 67:453–456
48. Shigeoka JW, Colice GL, Ramirez G (1985) Effect of normoxemic and hypoxemic exercise on renin and aldosterone. J Appl Physiol 59:142–148
49. Bärtsch P, Shaw S, Franciolli M et al (1988) Atrial natriuretic peptide in acute mountain sickness. J Appl Physiol (1985) 65:1929–1937
50. Kawashima A, Kubo K, Matsuzawa Y et al (1992) Hypoxia-induced ANP secretion in subjects susceptible to high-altitude pulmonary edema. Respir Physiol 89:309–317
51. Nir A, Clavell AL, Heublein D et al (1994) Acute hypoxia and endogenous renal endothelin. J Am Soc Nephrol 4:1920–1924
52. Zillig B, Schuler G, Truniger B (1978) Renal function and intrarenal hemodynamics in acutely hypoxic and hypercapnic rats. Kidney Int 14:58–67
53. Vidiendal Olsen N, Christensen H, Klausen T et al (1998) Effects of hyperventilation and hypocapnic/normocapnic hypoxemia on renal function and lithium clearance in humans. Anesthesiology 89:1389–1400
54. Rose CE Jr, Vance JE, Dacus WS et al (1991) Role of intrarenal angiotensin II and alpha-adrenoceptors in renal vasoconstriction with acute hypoxemia and hypercapnic acidosis in conscious dogs. Circ Res 69:142–156
55. Rose CE Jr, Kimmel DP, Godine RL Jr et al (1983) Synergistic effects of acute hypoxemia and hypercapnic acidosis in conscious dogs. Renal dysfunction and activation of the renin-angiotensin system. Circ Res 53:202–213
56. Sharkey RA, Mulloy EM, O'Neill SJ (1999) The acute effects of oxygen and carbon dioxide on renal vascular resistance in patients with an acute exacerbation of COPD. Chest 115:1588–1592
57. Sharkey RA, Mulloy EM, O'Neill SJ (1998) Acute effects of hypoxaemia, hyperoxaemia and hypercapnia on renal blood flow in normal and renal transplant subjects. Eur Respir J 12:653–657
58. Baudouin SV, Bott J, Ward A et al (1992) Short term effect of oxygen on renal haemodynamics in patients with hypoxaemic chronic obstructive airways disease. Thorax 47:550–554
59. Honig A, Wedler B, Zingler C et al (1985) Kidney function during arterial chemoreceptor stimulation. III. Long-lasting inhibition of renal tubular sodium reabsorption due to pharmacologic stimulation of the peripheral arterial chemoreceptors with almitrine bismesylate. Biomed Biochim Acta 44:1659–1672
60. Richalet JP, Souberbielle JC, Antezana AM et al (1994) Control of erythropoiesis in humans during prolonged exposure to the altitude of 6,542 m. Am J Physiol 266:R756–R764
61. The Acute Respiratory Distress Syndrome Network (2000) Ventilation with lower tidal volumes as compared with traditional tidal volumes for acute lung injury and the acute respiratory distress syndrome. N Engl J Med 342:1301–1308
62. Ranieri VM, Giunta F, Suter PM, Slutsky AS (2000) Mechanical ventilation as a mediator of multisystem organ failure in acute respiratory distress syndrome. JAMA 284:43–44
63. Ranieri VM, Suter PM, Tortorella C et al (1999) Effect of mechanical ventilation on inflammatory mediators in patients with acute respiratory distress syndrome: a randomized controlled trial. JAMA 282:54–61
64. Liu KD, Glidden DV, Eisner MD et al (2007) Predictive and pathogenetic value of plasma biomarkers for acute kidney injury in patients with acute lung injury. Crit Care Med 35:2755–2761
65. Imai Y, Parodo J, Kajikawa O et al (2003) Injurious mechanical ventilation and end-organ epithelial cell apoptosis and organ dysfunction in an experimental model of acute respiratory distress syndrome. JAMA 289:2104–2112

66. Vivino G, Antonelli M, Moro ML et al (1998) Risk factors for acute renal failure in trauma patients. Intensive Care Med 24:808–814
67. Schortgen F, Lacherade JC, Bruneel F et al (2001) Effects of hydroxyethylstarch and gelatin on renal function in severe sepsis: a multicentre randomised study. Lancet 357:911–916
68. Rocha PN, Rocha AT, Palmer SM et al (2005) Acute renal failure after lung transplantation: incidence, predictors and impact on perioperative morbidity and mortality. Am J Transplant 5:1469–1476
69. Lahoti A, Kantarjian H, Salahudeen AK et al (2010) Predictors and outcome of acute kidney injury in patients with acute myelogenous leukemia or high-risk myelodysplastic syndrome. Cancer 116:4063–4068
70. Jung JY, Park BH, Hong S-B et al (2011) Acute kidney injury in critically ill patients with pandemic influenza A pneumonia 2009 in Korea: a multicenter study. J Crit Care 26:577–585
71. O'Riordan A, Brummell Z, Sizer E et al (2011) Acute kidney injury in patients admitted to a liver intensive therapy unit with paracetamol-induced hepatotoxicity. Nephrol Dial Transplant 26:3501–3508
72. Brito DJ, Nina VJ, Nina RV et al (2009) Prevalence and risk factors for acute renal failure in the postoperative of coronary artery bypass grafting. Rev Bras Cir Cardiovasc 17:297–304
73. van den Akker JP, Egal M, Groeneveld ABJ (2013) Invasive mechanical ventilation as a risk factor for acute kidney injury in the critically ill: a systematic review and meta-analysis. Crit Care 17:R98
74. Li X, Hassoun HT, Santora R, Rabb H (2009) Organ crosstalk: the role of the kidney. Curr Opin Crit Care 15:481–487
75. Oba Y, Salzman GA (2000) Ventilation with lower tidal volumes as compared with traditional tidal volumes for acute lung injury. N Engl J Med 343:813

Shifting Paradigms in Acute Kidney Injury

W. De Corte, I. De Laet, and E.A.J. Hoste

Introduction

Acute kidney injury (AKI) is a frequent finding in critically ill patients and associated with adverse outcomes, such as increased length of stay, end-stage-renal disease (ESRD) and mortality [1, 2]. Approximately 50 % of ICU patients have AKI as defined by the sensitive RIFLE definition, and 5–15 % of ICU patients are treated with renal replacement therapy (RRT). Several new concepts, encompassing practically all aspects of AKI from diagnosis to treatment and outcome, have evolved over the last few years. This overview describes the most important new insights on AKI, based on recent research and consensus reports.

Expanding the Scope of AKI

Towards a Consensus Definition

Over the last years, the emphasis in 'acute kidney disease' has shifted from total failure of kidney function, to less severely impaired kidney function, leading to the concept of 'AKI', a grading system describing different levels of acute kidney dysfunction. More recently, a new entity, "subclinical AKI", has been introduced [3].

W. De Corte ✉
Department of Intensive Care Medicine, Ghent University Hospital, Ghent, Belgium
Department of Intensive Care Medicine, Department of Intensive Care, Ziekenhuis Netwerk
Antwerpen, ZNA Stuivenberg, Antwerp, Belgium
e-mail: wouter.decorte@azgroeninge.be

I. De Laet
Department of Intensive Care Medicine, AZ Groeninge Hospital, Kortrijk, Belgium

E.A.J. Hoste
Department of Intensive Care Medicine, Ghent University Hospital, Ghent, Belgium
Research Foundation Flanders, Brussel, Belgium

J.-L. Vincent (Ed.), *Annual Update in Intensive Care and Emergency Medicine 2014*,
DOI 10.1007/978-3-319-03746-2_40, © Springer International Publishing Switzerland
2014

The term 'acute renal failure' was introduced in the 1950s by Homer W. Smith [1]. This terminology was widely used and resulted in over 35 different definitions of acute renal failure in the medical literature [4]. The Acute Dialysis Quality Initiative (ADQI), a group of experts in the field of nephrology and intensive care, recognized the need for a standard definition of kidney failure. They introduced the Risk, Injury, Failure, Loss and End stage renal failure (RIFLE) classification, a grading system for increasing degrees of severity of AKI [4], emphasizing the importance of a small decline in kidney function. This RIFLE classification was later modified by the Acute Kidney Injury Network (AKIN) and the Kidney Disease: Improving Global Outcomes (KDIGO) groups [5, 6]. This allowed for the terminology 'AKI' to cover the whole range from mild impairment of renal function to the need for RRT [5].

Using these new definitions, it became clear that the incidence of AKI is high in critically ill patients, ranging from 16 % to 67 % depending on the baseline characteristics of the study population [7–9]. The increased sensitivity of the AKI definition is related to relevant clinical outcomes. Other, less sensitive definitions, such as the American Society of Surgeons National Surgical Quality Improvement Program (ACS-NSQIP) definition (rise in serum creatinine greater than 2 mg/dl or the acute need for RRT) cannot take into account the risk associated with mild AKI. Bihorac et al. showed, in a large study including over 27,000 patients, that the ACS-NSIQIP definition of postoperative AKI does not detect 93 % of RIFLE-AKI patients. Nevertheless, these patients account for 80 % of the 90-day mortality [10]. The new definitions of AKI have allowed and will continue to allow a much more realistic evaluation of the true incidence, risks and costs of AKI in different patient populations.

The Changing Face of AKI

Change in ICU case-mix and the concept of frailty

The aging society in developed countries is resulting in a change in case-mix of ICU admissions. Patients > 65 years of age now account for approximately 50 % of all ICU admissions and for 60 % of all ICU days [11]. Elderly patients often have impaired cardiac, pulmonary, metabolic and renal function prior to their ICU admission. Increasing age and comorbidity are associated with adverse outcomes. Single point serum creatinine measurement on admission in these patients may underestimate the degree of kidney dysfunction, as decreased muscle mass in these patients leads to decreased creatinine generation and lower serum concentrations.

Together with the admission of this geriatric population came the concept of frailty, initially introduced by the geriatricians. Frailty describes a multidimensional syndrome of loss of physiological reserve that gives rise to the accumulation of deficits and increased risk of vulnerability to adverse events. Frailty has been associated with worse outcomes. In ICU patients, the concept of frailty is quite new and was only recently described [12]. To date, there is no consensus definition of frailty. One of the most widely used descriptions to measure frailty is the definition proposed by Fried et al. [13]. The Clinical Frailty Scale (CFS) a simple and validated seven-point judgment-based tool may be applicable in ICU patients [14]. These frail patients with moderate organ function requiring ICU care for extended periods of time form a new challenge for modern ICU care. As a consequence, the concept of frailty should be considered when studying outcomes in the critically ill population suffering from AKI.

Increasing Incidence of AKI

Interestingly, AKI has been increasingly diagnosed in ICU patients over the past decades. Data from the Australian and New Zealand Intensive Care Society (ANZ-ICS) showed an annual increase of 2.8 % from 1996 to 2005 [15]. Similarly, in the USA, a > 20-fold increase in the incidence of AKI has been observed over the past 30 years [16]. It remains uncertain whether this last finding is the reflection of a true increase in the incidence of AKI or if this is the result of more adequate recording of AKI diagnoses. AKI defined by the need for RRT is diagnosed in approximately 5–10 % of critically ill patients [17, 18].

Organ Crosstalk

Patients with severe AKI mostly suffer from multiple organ dysfunction. Extra-renal organ dysfunction most probably contributes to the high mortality rates in these patients.

In AKI patients there is strong evidence of an 'adverse organ crosstalk' between damaged kidneys and other organ systems such as heart, lung, liver, intestinal tract and brain [19].

Ischemic AKI activates several inflammatory cascades initiating distant organ dysfunction. Of special interest is the crosstalk between the kidney and the heart. Several studies have demonstrated the bidirectional communication and feedback between these organs. Recently the ADQI proposed a consensus definition of car-diorenal syndromes (CRS) [20]. CRS were classified into five subtypes based on the original organ dysfunction. Three subtypes are most interesting to the intensivist. CRS type 1, the acute cardiorenal syndrome, is characterized by an acute deteri-oration in cardiac function leading to AKI. CRS type 3, also known as the acute renocardiac syndrome, is characterized by AKI leading to cardiac injury and/or failure. Both syndromes are associated with adverse outcomes. Finally, type 5 CRS occurs when a systemic disease, such as sepsis, leads to both kidney and heart dysfunction. Preventive and therapeutic strategies in CRS are derived from the management of the individual cardiac and renal dysfunctions. Therefore, the ADQI workgroup advises a multidisciplinary approach combining cardiology, nephrology and critical care medicine. Combining the knowledge from these competencies may contribute to new insights in a better understanding of this complex pathology and better research, but may also facilitate well-designed studies in the field of CRS and organ crosstalk. Future studies should not only focus on the complex pathophysio-logic mechanisms of the complex entity of organ crosstalk in AKI, but should also evaluate possible preventive and therapeutic strategies.

Patients are dying of AKI

In the past, AKI was often considered a surrogate marker for severity of illness. In critically ill patients, AKI often develops in the course of another disease, e. g., sepsis or trauma. Patient mortality was considered a consequence of this underlying disease. In other words, the statement that patients died with AKI and not from AKI was widely accepted. However, epidemiologic data have made it clear that AKI is an independent risk factor for mortality. A whole range of clinical complications of AKI, such as volume overload, electrolyte abnormalities, acidosis, and inadequate drug dosing, may help explain the increased morbidity and mortality in AKI. This facet was already realized for patients treated with RRT, but several more recent studies have demonstrated a correlation between small decreases in kidney function and short-term mortality [2, 21]. These findings suggest that AKI is not a benign syndrome and that patients actually die from AKI, rather than with AKI [22].

Diagnosis and Prevention of AKI

Novel renal biomarkers and the concept of subclinical AKI

The above mentioned paradigm shifts emphasize the need for early recognition of AKI and highlight the importance of early interventions to prevent AKI or to halt the evolution towards severe kidney dysfunction.

Measurements of serum creatinine and its derived calculations of glomerular filtration rate (GFR) have served as the gold standard for the diagnosis of AKI for decades. Even small increases in serum creatinine of ≥ 0.3 mg/dl in hospitalized patients have been associated with an increased risk of death [23]. However, measurement of serum creatinine carries some important limitations. Most importantly, it is a late marker of kidney injury. Changes in serum creatinine reflect alterations in kidney *function* [3]. They do not provide any information concerning kidney *damage*. Unfortunately, functional changes only present after significant kidney damage has taken place. This is in stark contrast to, for example, the management of myocardial ischemia. Patients with myocardial ischemia suffer from chest pain and sensitive and early biomarkers of myocardial ischemia, such as troponin I, are available allowing physicians to intervene early in the course of the disease. The lack of sensitive and specific renal biomarkers has hampered the development of specific interventions to prevent or treat AKI [24].

Until very recently, diagnosis of AKI was based on alterations in GFR, reflected by changes in serum creatinine or urine output, but the absence of clinically manifest AKI does not necessarily mean that the kidney is undamaged. Given the important functional reserve, renal impairment becomes evident only when more than 50 % of the renal mass is compromised. So, the diagnosis of AKI was usually made when GFR had been impaired for at least 24–48 hours after the initial damage had occurred [3].

Very recently, new renal biomarkers, such as neutrophil gelatinase-associated lipocalin (NGAL), urinary interleukin (IL)-18, kidney injury molecule 1 (KIM 1), and the combination of insulin-like growth factor-binding protein 7 (IGFBP-7) and tissue inhibitor of metalloproteinases-2 (TIMP-2) have been introduced [25]. These biomarkers are produced in the kidney itself, making them 'early' indicators of kidney damage. As they are produced even before a decrease in GMR is noticed, an early diagnosis of AKI is made possible [26].

This development has led to concepts like 'subclinical AKI' and 'renal angina', which are biomarker-guided and describe the clinical condition characterized by positive biomarker and negative creatinine findings. Goldstein and Chawla recently suggested that these biomarkers could therefore act as the "renal troponin I" and proposed a framework of AKI based on risk factor assessment, in analogy with the cardiovascular literature [24]. In this framework, intensivists should be aware of the possibility of renal angina in patients at risk for AKI (advanced age, diabetes, liver failure, congestive heart failure, chronic kidney disease [CKD] and cardiopulmonary bypass [CPB]). Further extensive investigation for early signs of AKI should be performed in these patients if signs of oliguria, volume overload or small increases in serum creatinine develop [26]. Measurement of renal biomarkers, urine microscopy and more frequent serum creatinine measurements are advised in this very specific population. This concept has a high negative predictive value. Patients without renal angina have a very low risk of developing AKI (Fig. 1). However, when renal angina is suspected, interventions to prevent further kidney damage are applied earlier in the course of the disease and may, therefore, be more successful. In this respect, modern technologies, such as the use of a real-time electronic alert device, can be of additional help [27].

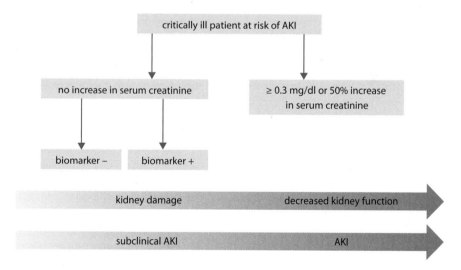

Fig. 1 Biomarker-guided AKI continuum. Serum creatinine is assessed in patients at risk of acute kidney injury (AKI). If there is no significant increase in serum creatinine, renal biomarkers are assessed. A positive biomarker without a significant increase in serum creatinine is suggestive of kidney damage, depicting a subclinical form of AKI. Subclinical AKI can lead to AKI, which is associated with decreased kidney function and, therefore, a significant increase in serum creatinine

At present, the exact role of AKI biomarkers is uncertain. Initial data suggesting high sensitivity and specificity of NGAL for early diagnosis of AKI could not be replicated in other settings. Recently the KDIGO group formulated clinical practice guidelines for prevention and treatment of AKI, advising the maintenance of renal perfusion, the avoidance of nephrotoxic drugs and correction of underlying processes or diseases [6]. Several observational but also interventional studies have demonstrated that early intervention indeed results in a lower incidence of severe AKI [28], but it is uncertain whether earlier diagnosis of AKI using new renal biomarkers can impact on the timing and results of AKI prevention.

Pathophysiology

AKI in critically ill patients is a syndrome with a multifactorial etiology, typically occurring with multiple hits. It is, therefore, probably also a very heterogeneous disease. This concept is not new, but we are now more aware of this. A few decades ago, AKI was considered the consequence of decreased kidney perfusion and ischemia with resulting acute tubular necrosis. However, acute tubular necrosis is seldom found, and markedly decreased renal perfusion could not be demonstrated in animal models of sepsis [29]. On the other hand, decreased microvascular perfusion secondary to inflammation, diffuse intravascular coagulation, tissue edema, vascular shunts in the kidney, and also glomerular changes are probably responsible for decreased kidney function in sepsis. In addition, other pathophysiologic mechanisms, such as increased intra-abdominal pressure (resulting in abdominal hypertension and abdominal compartment syndrome), drug toxicity, and increased venous pressure may contribute to damage and decreased kidney function [30]. Finally, other causes of AKI such as tubulo-interstitial nephritis or glomerulonephritis may play a bigger role than previously thought.

Timing of initiation of RRT

Although RRT has been in use for more than half a decade, many aspects of this therapy remain controversial. The timing of initiation of RRT is a very contentious issue. Over time, there has been a trend towards earlier initiation of RRT. Historically, AKI was considered a problem of uremia and RRT a means of treating uremic symptoms. The world's first successful artificial kidney was presented in 1942 by Willem Johan Kolff as "a new way of treating uremia". As uremic symptoms occur only late in the course of AKI, RRT was also initiated very late and basically considered a life-saving rescue treatment.

This urea-driven approach stood for several decades. Over time, helped by technological advances and more widely available dialysis equipment, early initiation of RRT and its possible positive impact on outcome started to appeal to many. Several – mostly retrospective – studies were published searching for the optimal serum urea threshold for initiation of RRT. Even recently, during the Vancouver meeting in 2006, the AKIN working group considered a blood urea nitrogen (BUN) concentration > 76 mg/dl as a relative indication and a BUN > 100 mg/dl an absolute indication for the initiation of RRT. However, recent retrospective studies showed that serum urea cut-offs at time of initiation of RRT have no predictive value for mortality in ICU patients with AKI [31]. Since the introduction of the AKI definitions that emphasize the importance of less severe stages of AKI and their impact on mortality [4–6, 21], the idea of early initiation of RRT has remained intact, even though the notion of urea-guided initiation of RRT should probably be abandoned.

Based on a meta-analysis of 23 heterogeneous and mostly retrospective studies, Seabra et al. suggested that early initiation of RRT was associated with better outcome [32]. More recently, Karvellas and colleagues updated these findings in a meta-analysis. They made no firm conclusions on the concept of timing of RRT because of absence of a consensus definition of 'early RRT' and the lack of well-designed studies [33].

However, we can make several comments related to this topic of 'early initiation of RRT'. In today's ICU, there is not only a change in case-mix with older patients with more comorbidities, but there is also a change in attitude towards initiation of RRT that leads to a possible 'inclusion bias' in studies on RRT. Patients, who were previously excluded from RRT because of advanced age and severe comorbidity, have more often been included in more recent studies. The general lack of established criteria for the initiation of RRT further complicates the issue. Hopefully, the recently introduced AKI biomarkers could be used in future guidelines for timing of RRT. For now, we argue that there is an urgent need for a consensus definition on what 'early' and 'late' timing of initiation of RRT mean in order to improve study comparability.

Outcomes in AKI: Shift of Focus

Mortality as an Endpoint

Until recently, studies of AKI in ICU patients focused on conventionally accepted short-term outcomes, such as mortality at day 30, or at ICU and hospital discharge. However, these endpoints may underestimate the true burden of kidney disease. In modern-day ICU care, we should aim for more relevant endpoints, such as long-term mortality (90 days, 6 months, one-year).

Initially, studies focused on long-term mortality were mostly performed in patients with AKI defined by treatment with RRT. The RENAL study reported a 44.7 % mortality rate three months after initiation of RRT [34]. Bagshaw and co-workers described a 1-year mortality of 63.8 % in a population-based study [35]. Korkeila et al. reported 65 % mortality at 5 years in a mixed Finnish ICU population with AKI without pre-existing renal failure [36]. Ahlström and colleagues confirmed these findings in a cross-sectional cohort study on patients from a mixed ICU and dialysis unit with a 5 years mortality of 70 % [37].

However, assessing long-term mortality based on 'AKI defined by RIFLE criteria' highlights the stepwise adverse long-term mortality associated with different stages of AKI. Coca et al. demonstrated in a systematic review and meta-analysis of 49 studies that even mild and rapidly reversible forms of AKI are associated with worse short and long-term outcomes [38]. Very recently, in a large retrospective study including more than 15,000 ICU patients with no history of end-stage renal disease (ESRD), Fuchs and co-workers described the strong relationship between AKI and mortality. Patients with AKIN 3 had 61 % higher mortality risk 2 years from ICU discharge compared with patients without AKI [39].

Composite Endpoints

In the cardiovascular literature, composite endpoints, such as major adverse cardiac events (MACE) are widely used. Ideally, these 'pooled' endpoints have a higher incidence than each of their components, reducing required sample size and increasing statistical efficiency. However, the use of composite endpoints in clinical trials can easily be biased, because component endpoints may be selected to ensure statistic significance [40]. Therefore, pooled endpoints have to be well defined and meticulously constructed.

A renal composite endpoint, major adverse kidney events (MAKE), was recently introduced as a concept. However, there is no standard definition for MAKE. This composite endpoint might include death, need for RRT, renal hospitalization within 90 days, persistent decline in kidney function and progression of underlying chronic kidney disease [41].

Renal Recovery

Until recently, it was widely accepted that most patients surviving AKI fully recover renal function [42]. However, because of the increasing focus on long-term outcomes, several studies have investigated the link between AKI, CKD and ESRD [43, 44]. Incomplete recovery after AKI is associated with tubulo-interstitial fibrosis and inflammation. These processes give rise to irreversible loss of functional kidney mass and may eventually lead to ESRD. Despite the lack of a standard definition, the term 'renal recovery' is widely used and is usually interpreted as independency of RRT [45]. Chertow et al. nicely demonstrated that 33 % of patients surviving AKI treated with RRT were still on RRT after one year [46]. Schiffl and Fischer reported that maximal improvement or normalization of renal function took place within the first year [47]. Bell et al. reported, in a 7-year follow-up trial, that 14 % of patients surviving AKI treated with continuous RRT remained on chronic dialysis indefinitely [48]. Interestingly, these and other observational studies suggest that renal recovery is less marked in patients treated with intermittent RRT compared to continuous RRT.

One can argue that 'renal recovery' should encompass more than just independence from RRT. It is well known that patients suffering from an episode of acute-on-chronic kidney disease have an increased risk of progression towards ESRD [43]. Given the fact that CKD stage is associated with a proportionally higher risk of developing new episodes of AKI [49], these patients may eventually be trapped in a downward spiral as their renal functional reserve progressively reduces. Moreover, AKI in patients without preexisting CKD can also cause ESRD directly, depicting the mutual relationship between AKI and CKD. Interestingly, the progression to CKD is facilitated by the frequency of AKI episodes and the severity of AKI [44]. Very recently, Pannu et al. demonstrated, in a retrospective analysis on more than 190,000 patients, that incomplete renal recovery within 90 days of AKI was associated with a higher risk for ESRD [50]. In addition, there is growing evidence that lesser forms of AKI (not requiring RRT) are associated with worse long-term renal outcomes. Even subclinical AKI may result in worse long-term outcomes. With regard to these data and taking into account the social and economic impact of chronic dialysis, some investigators suggest that hospital survivors of severe AKI should be followed by a nephrologist after discharge to prevent undiagnosed CKD in these patients [42].

Quality of Life

The importance of long-term outcomes cannot be overestimated and were recently highlighted in a systematic review on the topic of renal recovery by Bell [51]. This author demonstrated that patients surviving AKI but in need of chronic dialysis have worse quality of life compared to patients without the need for chronic dialysis. Naturally, mortality remains a decisive endpoint, but it is not the only relevant clinical endpoint beyond hospital discharge. For example, failure of renal recovery leading to dialysis dependency is associated with substantial health care costs, but also affects quality of life [52]. Several studies describe health-related quality of life (HRQOL) in patients recovering from AKI. Commonly used HRQOL assessments in critically ill patients include the Short Form-36 (SF-36), the Nottingham Health Profile (NHP) and the European Quality of Life score (EQ-5D). Although most patients who recovered from AKI reported a lower HRQOL than the general population, for the greater part they felt satisfied with their health status; in most patients, quality-of-life after AKI is perceived as acceptable and good [36, 37].

Future Perspectives and Conclusions

The incidence of AKI has increased over the past decades and this condition is becoming a major public health problem. The introduction of a standardized consensus definition for kidney dysfunction and the awareness that even small increases in serum creatinine are associated with adverse outcomes have expanded the scope of AKI and broadened its horizons with the inclusion of less-severely ill AKI patients. At the same time, the concept of organ crosstalk and the increasing numbers of frail elderly patients with co-existing comorbidities have complicated the issue.

At present, we can only speculate as to why even small increases in serum creatinine lead to adverse outcomes. Plausible causes are volume overload, inflammation, adverse effects on other organs and inadequate clearance of potentially toxic waste products of metabolism [1]. The recent introduction of AKI biomarkers may clarify these processes; however, they have limitations. There is currently no single ideal AKI biomarker available, but it is probably naïve to aim for this 'ideal' AKI biomarker that would be suitable in all types of AKI. The question rises whether all AKI is equal? Perhaps we should differentiate several types of AKI, each with their specific AKI biomarker, according to specific populations (e. g., cardiac surgery patients, general ICU patients). These AKI biomarkers may reveal AKI at an early stage, so specific preventive and therapeutic interventions may be implemented halting further decline in kidney function.

Ideally, biomarkers will also help us predict need for RRT, renal recovery, and long-term outcome. New concepts of subclinical AKI and renal angina have been introduced through the use of novel renal biomarkers. These new discoveries may offer new targeting points for preventive interventions and therapeutic strategies. In this way, intensivists may be able to act earlier in the course of AKI, preventing further kidney damage and halting the downward spiral of AKI, thereby preventing the progression to ESRD. Given the increasing incidence of AKI and the burden on health economics, future studies will have to address the most appropriate implementation of strategies preventing and eventually treating AKI. These future interventions can only be successfully studied and implemented if endpoints are optimized with focus on composite endpoints or long-term outcomes.

References

1. Hoste EA, De Corte W (2007) Epidemiology of AKI in the ICU. Acta Clin Belg Suppl 2:314–317
2. Hoste EA, Schurgers M (2008) Epidemiology of acute kidney injury: how big is the problem? Crit Care Med 36:S146–S151
3. Ronco C, Kellum JA, Haase M (2012) Subclinical AKI is still AKI. Crit Care 16:313
4. Bellomo R, Ronco C, Kellum JA, Mehta RL, Palevsky P, Workgroup A (2004) Acute renal failure – definition, outcome measures, animal models, fluid therapy and information technology needs: the Second International Consensus Conference of the Acute Dialysis Quality Initiative (ADQI) Group. Crit Care 8:R204–R212
5. Mehta RL, Kellum JA, Shah SV et al (2007) Acute Kidney Injury Network: report of an initiative to improve outcomes in acute kidney injury. Crit Care 11:R31
6. KDIGO Clinical Practice Guideline for Acute Kidney Injury (2012) Kid Int Suppl 2:16–39
7. Hoste EA, Clermont G, Kersten A et al (2006) RIFLE criteria for acute kidney injury are associated with hospital mortality in critically ill patients: a cohort analysis. Crit Care 10:R73
8. Ostermann M, Chang R, Riyadh ICUPUG (2008) Correlation between the AKI classification and outcome. Crit Care 12:R144
9. Mandelbaum T, Scott DJ, Lee J et al (2011) Outcome of critically ill patients with acute kidney injury using the Acute Kidney Injury Network criteria. Crit Care Med 39:2659–2664
10. Bihorac A, Brennan M, Ozrazgat-Baslanti T et al (2013) National surgical quality improvement program underestimates the risk associated with mild and moderate postoperative acute kidney injury. Crit Care Med 41:2570–2583
11. Marik PE (2006) Management of the critically ill geriatric patient. Crit Care Med 34:176–182
12. McDermid RC, Stelfox HT, Bagshaw SM (2011) Frailty in the critically ill: a novel concept. Crit Care 15:301

13. Fried LP, Tangen CM, Walston J et al (2001) Frailty in older adults: evidence for a phenotype. Gerontol A Biol Sci Med Sci 56:M146–M156
14. Cook WL (2009) The intersection of geriatrics and chronic kidney disease: frailty and disability among older adults with kidney disease. Adv Chronic Kidney Dis 16:420–429
15. Bagshaw SM, George C, Bellomo R, Committee ADM (2007) Changes in the incidence and outcome for early acute kidney injury in a cohort of Australian intensive care units. Crit Care 11:R68
16. Waikar SS, Wald R, Chertow GM et al (2006) Validity of International Classification of Diseases, Ninth Revision, Clinical Modification Codes for acute renal failure. J Am Soc Nephrol 17:1688–1694
17. Uchino S, Kellum JA, Bellomo R et al (2005) Acute renal failure in critically ill patients: a multinational, multicenter study. JAMA 294:813–818
18. Nisula S, Kaukonen KM, Vaara ST et al (2013) Incidence, risk factors and 90-day mortality of patients with acute kidney injury in Finnish intensive care units: the FINNAKI study. Intensive Care Med 39:420–428
19. Rosner MH, Ronco C, Okusa MD (2012) The role of inflammation in the cardio-renal syndrome: a focus on cytokines and inflammatory mediators. Semin Nephrol 32:70–78
20. McCullough PA, Kellum JA, Haase M et al (2013) Pathophysiology of the cardiorenal syndromes: executive summary from the eleventh consensus conference of the Acute Dialysis Quality Initiative (ADQI). Contrib Nephrol 182:82–98
21. Levy EM, Viscoli CM, Horwitz RI (1996) The effect of acute renal failure on mortality. A cohort analysis. JAMA 275:1489–1494
22. Kellum JA, Bellomo R, Ronco C (2012) Kidney attack. JAMA 307:2265–2266
23. Chertow GM, Burdick E, Honour M, Bonventre JV, Bates DW (2005) Acute kidney injury, mortality, length of stay, and costs in hospitalized patients. J Am Soc Nephrol 16:3365–3370
24. Goldstein SL, Chawla LS (2010) Renal angina. Clin. J Am Soc Nephrol 5:943–949
25. Kashani K, Al-Khafaji A, Ardiles T et al (2013) Discovery and validation of cell cycle arrest biomarkers in human acute kidney injury. Crit Care 17:R25
26. Arthur JM, Hill EG, Alge JL et al (2014) Evaluation of 32 urine biomarkers to predict the progression of acute kidney injury after cardiac surgery. Kidney Int (in press)
27. Colpaert K, Hoste EA, Steurbaut K et al (2012) Impact of real-time electronic alerting of acute kidney injury on therapeutic intervention and progression of RIFLE class. Crit Care Med 40:1164–1170
28. Lin SM, Huang CD, Lin HC, Liu CY, Wang CH, Kuo HP (2006) A modified goal-directed protocol improves clinical outcomes in intensive care unit patients with septic shock: a randomized controlled trial. Shock 26:551–557
29. Wan L, Bagshaw SM, Langenberg C, Saotome T, May C, Bellomo R (2008) Pathophysiology of septic acute kidney injury: what do we really know? Crit Care Med 36:198–203
30. De Waele JJ, De Laet I, Kirkpatrick AW, Hoste E (2011) Intra-abdominal Hypertension and Abdominal Compartment Syndrome. Am J Kidney Dis 57:159–169
31. De Corte W, Vanholder R, Dhondt AW et al (2011) Serum urea concentration is probably not related to outcome in ICU patients with AKI and renal replacement therapy. Nephrol Dial Transplant 26:3211–3218
32. Seabra VF, Balk EM, Liangos O, Sosa MA, Cendoroglo M, Jaber BL (2008) Timing of renal replacement therapy initiation in acute renal failure: a meta-analysis. Am J Kidney Dis 52:272–284
33. Karvellas CJ, Farhat MR, Sajjad I et al (2011) A comparison of early versus late initiation of renal replacement therapy in critically ill patients with acute kidney injury: a systematic review and meta-analysis. Crit Care 15:R72
34. Bellomo R, Cass A, Norton R et al (2009) Intensity of continuous renal-replacement therapy in critically ill patients. N Engl J Med 361:1627–1638

35. Bagshaw SM, Laupland KB, Doig CJ et al (2005) Prognosis for long-term survival and renal recovery in critically ill patients with severe acute renal failure: a population-based study. Crit Care 9:R700–R709
36. Korkeila M, Ruokonen E, Takala J (2000) Costs of care, long-term prognosis and quality of life in patients requiring renal replacement therapy during intensive care. Intensive Care Med 26:1824–1831
37. Ahlstrom A, Tallgren M, Peltonen S, Rasanen P, Pettila V (2005) Survival and quality of life of patients requiring acute renal replacement therapy. Intensive Care Med 31:1222–1228
38. Coca SG, Yusuf B, Shlipak MG, Garg AX, Parikh CR (2009) Long-term risk of mortality and other adverse outcomes after acute kidney injury: a systematic review and meta-analysis. Am J Kidney Dis 53:961–973
39. Fuchs L, Lee J, Baumfeld Y, Novack V et al (2013) Severity of acute kidney injury and two-year outcomes in critically ill patients. Chest 144:866–875
40. Cordoba G, Schwartz L, Woloshin S, Bae H, Gotzsche PC (2010) Definition, reporting, and interpretation of composite outcomes in clinical trials: systematic review. BMJ 341:c3920
41. Palevsky PM, Molitoris BA, Okusa MD et al (2012) Design of clinical trials in acute kidney injury: report from an NIDDK workshop on trial methodology. Clin. J Am Soc Nephrol 7:844–850
42. Chawla LS, Kimmel PL (2012) Acute kidney injury and chronic kidney disease: an integrated clinical syndrome. Kidney Int 82:516–524
43. Amdur RL, Chawla LS, Amodeo S, Kimmel PL, Palant CE (2009) Outcomes following diagnosis of acute renal failure in U.S. veterans: focus on acute tubular necrosis. Kidney Int 76:1089–1097
44. Ishani A, Xue JL, Himmelfarb J et al (2009) Acute kidney injury increases risk of ESRD among elderly. J Am Soc Nephrol 20:223–228
45. Rimes-Stigare C, Awad A, Martensson J, Martling CR, Bell M (2012) Long-term outcome after acute renal replacement therapy: a narrative review. Acta Anaesthesiol Scand 56:138–146
46. Chertow GM, Christiansen CL, Cleary PD, Munro C, Lazarus JM (1995) Prognostic stratification in critically ill patients with acute renal failure requiring dialysis. Arch Intern Med 155:1505–1511
47. Schiffl H, Fischer R (2008) Five-year outcomes of severe acute kidney injury requiring renal replacement therapy. Nephrol Dial Transpl 23:2235–2241
48. Bell M, Swing, Granath F, Schon S, Ekbom A, Martling CR (2007) Continuous renal replacement therapy is associated with less chronic renal failure than intermittent haemodialysis after acute renal failure. Intensive Care Med 33:773–780
49. Singbartl K, Kellum JA (2012) AKI in the ICU: definition, epidemiology, risk stratification, and outcomes. Kidney Int 81:819–825
50. Pannu N, James M, Hemmelgarn B, Klarenbach S, Kidney Disease AN (2013) Association between AKI, recovery of renal function, and long-term outcomes after hospital discharge. Clin J Am Soc Nephrol 8:194–202
51. Bell M (2008) Acute kidney injury: new concepts, renal recovery. Nephron Clin Pract 109:c224–c228
52. Oeyen S, Vandijck D, Benoit D, Decruyenaere J, Annemans L, Hoste E (2007) Long-term outcome after acute kidney injury in critically-ill patients. Acta Clin Belg Suppl 2:337–340

Part XIV
Coagulation and Bleeding

Early Identification of Occult Bleeding Through Hypovolemia Detection

A. L. Holder, G. Clermont, and M. R. Pinsky

Introduction

Clinically occult hypovolemia is a significant problem facing hospitalized patients. Tachycardia may occur before hypotension or signs of end-organ injury are apparent, but it is non-specific, often overlooked and may be attributed to other less serious causes. Unless clinicians have a high index of suspicion for subclinical hypovolemia, at-risk patients may progress to overt tissue hypoperfusion, displaying hyperlactatemia and hypotension. Delaying definitive care to reverse both hypovolemia and its causes may have a negative impact on patient outcome. Clinicians need tools to accurately diagnose patients with occult hypovolemia so that these patients receive appropriate resuscitation and definitive care in a timely fashion. We believe that any instrument used to detect clinically occult hypovolemia must use dynamic changes in physiologic parameters. We will review the merit of commonly and less commonly used hemodynamic parameters, measures of global and tissue blood flow and metabolic function, and features embedded within waveform data to identify occult hypovolemia. We will also provide an overview of new approaches to parsimoniously select parameters most predictive of early hypovolemia. All of these parameters and features can be applied to identify any disease process causing occult hypovolemia, e. g., sepsis, bleeding; we will focus on the early identification of occult bleeding.

Subclinical Bleeding from any Cause is a Significant Clinical Problem

There are many causes of hypovolemia in hospitalized patients, all of which could have an adverse impact on patient outcome if they go unrecognized. Occult bleed-

A. L. Holder · G. Clermont · M. R. Pinsky ✉
Department of Critical Care Medicine, University of Pittsburgh, Pittsburgh, PA 15261, USA
e-mail: pinskymr@upmc.edu

J.-L. Vincent (Ed.), *Annual Update in Intensive Care and Emergency Medicine 2014*,
DOI 10.1007/978-3-319-03746-2_41, © Springer International Publishing Switzerland
2014

ing is one cause of hypovolemia and accounts for 50 % of deaths within the first 24 hours of hospitalization for a traumatic injury [1]. Some of these deaths could be related to occult bleeding at initial presentation that went undetected, or from iatrogenic or missed injury among trauma patients taken to the operating room for exploratory surgery. Acute non-variceal upper gastrointestinal bleeding can also go undetected for some time. Urgent definitive endoscopy may improve outcomes by arresting the initial source of bleeding, prevent and predict rebleeding, decrease transfusion requirements and shorten hospital length of stay [2]. One study showed that delayed endoscopy was independently associated with increased in-patient mortality [3].

If the site of bleeding is not readily apparent, health-care practitioners often do not recognize hemorrhage until patients have lost enough blood to cause hemodynamic instability or tissue hypoperfusion as indicated by hypotension, hyperlactatemia and an elevated anion gap. Trauma patients may have lost 30 % of their blood volume before they develop signs of end-organ hypoperfusion or hypotension [4]. Even tachycardia, the most sensitive of the readily-available vital signs, is not present until 15 % of blood volume is lost [4]. Rather large quantities of blood can accumulate in the chest, abdomen, pelvis, and other compartments of the body prior to any clinically detectable signs of hypovolemia. If tissue hypoperfusion persists, subsequent ischemic damage will become irreversible; one indication of irreversible injury is sudden cardiovascular collapse caused by loss of vascular tone [5]. Clearly, waiting for late signs of hypovolemia such as hypotension could be detrimental to patient outcome.

Clinicians Need Better Screening Tools to Identify Subclinical Hemorrhage Early

If clinicians could identify patients with occult hypovolemia earlier in their course, and ultimately predict those at highest risk, then we could initiate resuscitation therapies sooner, minimize tissue hypoperfusion and hopefully avoid the associated increased morbidity and mortality. There are many prognostic tools in the critical care, trauma, and gastrointestinal literature that use mortality as the outcome of interest [6–8]. None of these tools are routinely used in clinical practice. More importantly, one study showed that physician judgment was more accurate at distinguishing survivors from non-survivors than standard prognostic tools in critical illness [9].

It may be more useful to have models to predict the need for targeted clinical interventions that could improve overall patient outcomes. Unfortunately, most of the clinical scoring systems for acute non-variceal upper gastrointestinal hemorrhage are not sensitive enough to identify the need for clinical intervention, even among the highest risk patients [10, 11]. Similar issues have been shown with trauma scoring systems [12]. Some surgically-based scoring systems predict the need for a massive transfusion protocol with variable prediction accuracy [13]. Tools that target massive transfusion protocol activation do so as a surrogate for predicting large volume blood loss. Unfortunately, massive transfusion protocols in trauma are often initiated by trauma surgeons [14], thus protocol activation may be subject to some variability between (and within) hospitals.

It is unclear whether surrogate markers for global tissue hypoperfusion, such as lactate, can predict outcomes in trauma patients [15, 16]. Observational studies have shown that neither an isolated lactate [15] nor lactate clearance [16] was correlated with outcome. Kaplan and Kellum demonstrated that hyperlactatemia is neither sensitive nor specific for mortality prediction after traumatic injury: 33 % of survivors had lactic acidosis upon admission; conversely, 42 % of non-survivors had normal lactate levels [15]. The authors showed that the strong ion difference was strongly correlated to mortality [15]. However, it would be useful for clinicians to identify occult hemorrhage prior to signs of tissue hypoperfusion.

Dynamic Changes in Physiology are Important Early Markers of Hypovolemia

Currently, no model exists to detect ongoing hypovolemia or bleeding. There is an intuition that dynamic changes, rather than static factors would have important detection power. Indeed, disease states reflect the dynamic interaction of pathological processes and the adaptive responses of the host to minimize the detrimental effects of those processes. Thus, dynamic interactions of vital sign measurements dependent on these interactions should be useful in defining developing pathological states and the host's response to them. For instance, patients presenting with trauma or gastrointestinal hemorrhage could have intermittent episodes of bleeding that cannot be captured by a static vital sign measurement. One study showed 22 % mortality among elderly patients presenting to the hospital with normal vital signs, defined as a systolic blood pressure between 120 and 130 mmHg and a heart rate between 60 and 90 beats per minute [17]. Another retrospective emergency department-based study of trauma patients showed that the initial shock index – calculated as the initial heart rate divided by initial systolic blood pressure – was a poor measure to identify patients with major injury, with an area under the curve (AUC) of the receiver-operator characteristics (ROC) analysis of 0.58 [18]. The initial shock index also performed poorly in a subgroup of patients with normal vital signs (AUC 0.56) [18]. In practice, clinicians use changes in data to gauge suspicion of a process that may not be immediately obvious. Tools used to identify occult hypovolemia or bleeding should reflect this practice.

While dynamic changes in vital signs can be useful for early identification of developing hypovolemia, such as ongoing bleeding, the dynamics of other physiologic parameters have been shown to identify hypovolemia in various disease processes. Tracking changes in central venous oxygen saturation ($ScvO_2$) is a useful surrogate for the changes in mixed venous saturation (SvO_2); the latter is an invasive measure of the balance between oxygen consumption and oxygen delivery [19]. $ScvO_2$ has been shown to have diagnostic implications in many hypovolemic states [19].

Capturing the changes in the interactions of certain physiologic parameters by incorporating blood flow dynamics and the use of functional hemodynamic monitoring will add another useful dimension to the detection of occult bleeding. These modalities can help us distinguish different disease processes before they are clinically apparent. Patients in whom a clinician suspects occult bleeding may have another cause for any subtle changes in status. For instance, a patient who had recent abdominal surgery could have mild tachycardia because of pain, hypovolemia from occult bleeding or fluid deficit, decreased vasomotor tone from sepsis, or a combination of all these processes. Blood flow to tissues, as estimated by cardiac output, is only adequate if the body's consumptive demands are met [20]. Therefore, understanding the changing interactions between cardiac output, $ScvO_2$, vital signs, and other hemodynamic variables should be useful in occult bleeding identification, and should distinguish bleeding from other processes.

Central venous pressure (CVP), as a mean value, is another commonly used hemodynamic parameter. CVP is not a grossly inadequate marker for circulating blood volume [21] or volume responsiveness [22]. This is not surprising since CVP is simply the back-pressure to, and not synonymous with venous return [20]. Venous return normally increases during spontaneous inspiration as a function of decreased intrathoracic pressure. This inspiratory decrease in CVP with decreased intrathoracic pressure in a spontaneously breathing patient can predict volume responsiveness [20]. This is because any associated decrease in CVP must equate to a lack of over-filling of the right ventricle, hence identifying a volume-responsive state. Hemodynamic parameters interpreted within the context of other physiologic processes may markedly improve their utility in identifying pathological cardiovascular states, such as occult hemorrhage.

Cardiac output, arterial pressure, CVP, and other hemodynamic parameters are easier to measure in recent years with the advent of new minimally invasive and non-invasive technologies. Traditionally, many of these variables were measured using a pulmonary artery catheter (PAC), an invasive procedure with questionable value and cost-benefit [23, 24]. There are a number of non-invasive devices that can be used in current practice [18, 25, 26]. Velmahos et al. showed good correlation between cardiac index (CI) measurements using thermodilution and non-invasive thoracic bioimpedance in a cohort of patients with severe blunt trauma [26]. Incidentally, survivors in that study had an increase in CI after resuscitation when compared with non-survivors, indicating the importance of blood flow as a dynamic parameter in trauma patients.

Changes in global blood flow will be accompanied by regional changes in tissue blood flow and tissue oxygen concentration and reciprocal changes in CO_2 concentration. These metrics have shown promise as early detection signals in occult bleeding. Surrogate markers of sublingual or skeletal muscle blood flow such as tissue pH, PCO_2, and oxygen saturation can identify hemorrhage in both animal models [27, 28] and humans [29]. In some cases, changes in some of these metrics can precede overt shock [29]. We would expect tissue PCO_2 to increase and PO_2 to decrease because of decreased tissue blood flow during hemorrhage. Measurement ease and feasibility may hinder immediate clinical translation of some of these metrics, but others may have potential utility in the near future. Velmahos et al. showed that the ratio of transcutaneous oxygen tension-to-inspired oxygen concentration, along with other measures of metabolic consumption/delivery balance were normal in survivors and higher in non-survivors of severe blunt trauma [26].

Derived Physiologic Parameters: Pulse Contour and Variability Analysis

When hemodynamic parameters are collected on a beat-to-beat basis, clinicians are able to quantify additional metrics that could be used to identify occult hemorrhage early. Mechanical ventilation induces cyclical changes in many hemodynamic parameters by changes in intrathoracic pressure. A positive pressure breath will increase afterload and decrease venous return, which in turn decreases preload in the left ventricle. The resulting changes in the arterial waveform – pulse pressure variation (PPV), stroke volume variation (SVV), and systolic pressure variation (SPV) – during the respiratory cycle will be exaggerated in the hypovolemic state. One meta-analysis of over 500 patients showed that SVV was a sensitive measure to detect volume responsiveness [30]. Michard et al. found that a PPV of 13 % or more predicted a CI increase of more than 15 % with a sensitivity of 94 % and specificity of 98 % [31]. Although the patients they studied had tidal volumes of 8–12 ml/kg, their findings were later validated in patients with acute respiratory distress syndrome (ARDS) receiving lower tidal volumes and high positive end-expiratory pressure (PEEP) [32]. Thus, pulse contour analyses (PPV, SVV, and SPV) allow us to calculate derived parameters which may further improve our ability to identify hypovolemic states such as occult bleeding.

Time varying, or dynamic variability analysis could also be useful for early detection of occult bleeding, although these analyses are often more difficult to perform at the bedside without the aid of computational devices. Organ-organ interaction between the brain, cardiovascular, endocrine and respiratory systems, and modulation of any aspect of this organ cross-talk during trauma or shock could be manifested by changes in vital sign variability [33, 34]. Adjustments in autonomic tone is one proposed explanation for decreased heart rate variability (HRV) in critical illness [35], but there could be additional explanations related to other aspects of organ-organ interaction [33] acting at vastly different time scales. HRV is assessed on a beat-to-beat basis and can, therefore, be acquired (using appropriate computer software) from any available monitoring system that continuously assesses R-R interval length or beat-to-beat heart rate measurements.

Empirical evidence linking decreased HRV and poor outcome, cardiovascular mortality in particular, is several decades old [36] and has stimulated research in other disease processes. Many of these conditions have a hypovolemic component, and trigger elaborate host responses with similar changes in organ-organ interaction to those seen in occult hemorrhage [37]. Griffin et al. showed that heart rate characteristics specific to the neonatal population – reduced variability and transient decelerations – could predict culture-positive and culture-negative sepsis up to

5 days prior to the clinical suspicion of sepsis in a neonatal ICU using traditional vital sign measurements [37]. Furthermore, Moorman et al. demonstrated a decrease in neonatal mortality when heart rate characteristics were monitored clinically, particularly among those patients at highest risk for sepsis [38].

Evidence suggests that variability analysis could be applied to occult bleeding detection, although there is a paucity of clinical data. Using a swine model, Batchinsky et al. showed that many HRV indices predictably decreased during a 30 ml/kg controlled bleed, and increased after resuscitation [39]. These authors found statistically significant decreases in HRV indices after 10 ml of blood loss, compared with tachycardia after 20 ml of blood loss. Decreased HRV is associated with mortality among trauma patients, and can predict outcomes hours in advance [40]. One study showed that among a cohort of trauma patients without severe injury, pathological changes in autonomic function occurred prior to tachycardia [41]. However, it is unclear from these studies who among these trauma patients experienced bleeding, and which bleeding events were occult. While variability analysis may be useful, it needs to be confirmed through prospective observational studies in medical, surgical, and trauma patients at risk of occult bleeding.

There are some potential challenges before variability analysis could be used as a practical bedside tool. Measurement of beat-to-beat intervals is not a routine function of bedside monitors, although the algorithms to compute this time series are accessible [42]. HRV and respiratory rate variability (RRV) can be affected by medications and sedation. However, one study showed that HRV and RRV could still be reliably identified in mechanically ventilated patients on sedation [43]. Also, HRV is not a single metric but a summary of dozens of different derived indices assessing autonomic function. One review paper mentions over 70 different indices of HRV, and this list was not exhaustive [44]. Table 1 shows some HRV features that can be extracted. It is not clear whether one (or more) index is the best. Finally, variability analysis can be derived from other parameters besides heart rate, including respiratory rate, blood pressure, temperature and continuous blood glucose. Performing variability analyses on all of these continuous measurements would lead to hundreds of new derived indices. If all of them are included as markers for the detection of occult bleeding, then methods for optimal data utilization need to be developed and implemented. One study showed that multiorgan variability analysis is feasible in the ICU setting, yet the technical investment necessary to achieve this real-time comprehensive analysis is considerable [43].

'Featurized' Physiologic Parameters: Waveform Analysis

The time series in variability analysis is information extracted on an interval basis – e. g., the R-R interval in HRV– but there are potentially many features embedded in physiologic waveforms themselves that could be used to detect occult bleeding. Harmonic analysis deconstructs waveforms into basic waves suitable for signal processing to extract useful information. One can then compare features of a physiologic waveform at different timepoints to detect any changes in physiology that

Table 1 Common heart rate variability (HRV) groupings and selected metrics

Group	Overview	Selected indices
Statistical domain	Describes statistical features of time-series data; assumes data comes from a stochastic process	SDNN, RMSSD, NN50, pNN50, IQRNN, SDSD
Frequency domain	Deconstructs a sequence of R-R intervals into its spectral components to obtain information about the power distribution of the time series	Total power, ULF, VLF, LF, HF, LF/HF
Geometric domain	Constructs a "shape" out of a histogram representation of an R-R interval series (e. g., NN distribution of interval lengths). Histograms created by grouping NNs according to some property of the NNs (see selected indices)	Distribution of NN interval length, differential index, Lorenz plot of NN intervals, TINN, HTI
Information domain	Characterizes the regularity of the R-R time series	SampEn, ApEn, Kolmogorov entropy, Shannon entropy
Non-linear methods	Describes properties that demonstrate fractality, and other characteristics that do not vary in time and space	DFA, FDDA, FDCL, Poincare sections, Lyapunov exponents

NN: the interval between two normal R-waves (i.e., from non-ectopic beats); SDNN: standard deviation of the NN interval; RMSSD: root mean square of the successive differences; NN50: number of interval differences of successive NN intervals > 50 ms; pNN50: proportion derived by diving NN50 by the total NN intervals; IQRNN: interquartile range of NN; SDSD: standard deviation of the first derivative of the time series; ULH: "ultralow" frequency (≤ 0.003 Hz); VLF: very low range (0.003–0.04 Hz); LF: low frequency (0.04–0.15 Hz); HF: high frequency (0.15–0.4 Hz); TINN: triangular interpolation of NN interval histogram; HTI: HRV triangular index; SampEn: sample entropy; ApEn: approximate entropy; DFA: detrended fluctuation analysis; FDDA: fractal dimension by dispersion analysis; FDCL: fractal dimension of the signal

would identify hemorrhage early. Fourier transform is one signal processing approach that has been used on physiologic waveforms [45]. Fourier transform can deconstruct a waveform at a given timepoint and window length into a combination of complex sinusoids, allowing us to then see how features of a hemodynamic waveform (e. g., CVP) change with time. If different time window lengths are processed for a given timepoint – 20 seconds, 40 seconds, 60 seconds, 120 seconds, etc. – one can extract features that are dependent on different harmonic frequencies. For instance, it is necessary to use longer sampling windows for Fourier transform to extract changes in the CVP waveform caused by respiratory rate, compared to sampling windows needed to identify changes in CVP imposed by heart rate, since the respiratory rate is slower. Once waveform data is featurized for patients during time periods deemed important for occult bleeding identification, and harmonic analysis is performed on all available physiologic waveforms at different window lengths, an entire library of useful hemodynamic information could be uncovered.

Putting it all Together: Hemodynamic Monitoring Parsimony and Machine Learning

If the immense breadth of information extracted from dynamic physiology is to play a role in occult hypovolemia detection, it needs an organizational framework. Physiologic variables and derived features, simple and complex, will change as a patient experiences progressive hypovolemia. Data organization is also necessary because a number of devices can be used for data measurement and extraction, each with their own associated risks, sampling frequencies and inaccuracies. Building an organizational framework would help establish hemodynamic monitoring parsimony; it would be possible to know the minimum number of parameters (and devices) needed to detect occult hemorrhage as early as possible. This concept reflects the same process that clinicians go through every day whenever they provide patient care. However, in this case the process would need to be automated since it would be impractical for physicians to account for the utility of hundreds of derived and featurized parameters in real time. Organizing patient data could inform clinicians if more parameters – and thus devices – are necessary. How does one begin to build such a framework? One answer could be found through machine learning.

Data-driven machine learning approaches would be applicable to a broad scope of acute care settings – including emergency department triage and critical illness management – and specifically to diseases characterized by hypovolemia like acute bleeding. Many animal and human studies have used machine learning to identify hemorrhage in a timely fashion [46–48]. There are a number of approaches available (Table 2), but a common methodology is shown in Fig. 1: Clearly, any machine learning approach chosen for early occult bleeding identification requires primary data from a robust patient cohort. Derived and featurized parameters can be extracted from primary data, and the machine learning technique will 'train' from all available information in a derivation cohort. It selects the most useful variables to accurately classify subjects in a training dataset as 'bleeding' or 'not bleeding' at every specified timepoint. The derived model is internally validated in a validation cohort and then tested in a 'new' subject. Some machine learning algorithms classify new subjects by predicting their expected course based on the training dataset; a subject is classified as exhibiting abnormal behavior – in this case, bleeding – based on deviation from that predicted course [49]. Moreover, if a subject is classified as 'bleeding' under controlled experimental conditions, machine learning approaches can also quantify the amount of blood loss with reasonable accuracy [46]. Machine learning approaches can identify a bleeding subject at any point in the process of hemorrhage because it has a library of all available data at every point in the process. When given a new subject exhibiting certain physiologic feature patterns, the model can simply reference its data library to match those patterns with others in its repository. The model may not only be able to identify bleeding, but also how far it is in the process. Another potential benefit of a machine learning approach is that the classification process could be iterative when applied in a clinical context. Figure 1 illustrates an adaptive detection tool – one that incorporates new data into its library to refine its training model for use

Table 2 Common machine learning approaches

Algorithm	Properties
Regression analysis (e. g., logistic regression)	Trains on one or more independent variables in a cohort of subjects to determine the conditional expectation of a dependent variable. Dependent variables can be a classification (e. g., logistic regression) or continuous (e. g., linear regression). May assume a linear relationship between the dependent and independent variables (e. g., logistic and linear regression), or non-linear relationship (e. g., polynomial regression).
Decision tree learning (e. g., CART, C4.5)	Generates classifiers by decision trees. Trees are constructed using a "divide-and-conquer" algorithm. When a set of observations is presented, the algorithm determines the single most informative attribute, and splits the dataset according to this attribute. This splitting is represented by branching in the decision tree. This process is repeated recursively to build the complete decision tree. Overfitting is common; it is prevented by pruning algorithms.
Support vector machine (SVM)	The SVM algorithm is based on linear optimization; subjects are classified in a way that maximizes the hyperplane margin (the minimum distance between the observations and the separation hyperplane). The SVM deals with non-linear problems with a 'kernel trick'. The kernel trick is an efficient way to project data with non-linear mapping, without having to actually compute the mapping.
k-nearest neighbor (kNN)	Takes an unlabeled observation, looks for the k most similar observations in the training set (k and the distance's definition are two user parameters), and returns the most represented class of those labeled observations.
Artificial neural networks (ANN) (e. g., multi-layer perceptron with back-propagation algorithm)	Biologically-inspired models with three basic parts: 'Neurons' (nodes), the weights applied to different input connections, and the transfer function that produces the neuron output. These components form a network based on training data by adjusting input weights and building or destroying connections. Exhibit complex/nonlinear behavior based on the connection network. Used for both supervised and unsupervised learning.
Naive Bayesian classifier	Applies the Bayes theorem while considering all input to be independent. It classifies subjects based on a cut-off score and then assigns a future subject to a class based on its score relative to the cut-off value. Simple to construct, and generally very robust for many types of classification tasks. May assume independent contribution of predictors (naive Bayes)
Ensemble learning algorithms (e. g., AdaBoost, random forest of decision trees)	Learns sets of classifiers and merges their outputs. Each classifier is trained independently on a specifically prepared set of training observations. In boosting, each subsequent training set emphasizes the importance of training samples that have been problematic for the models that are already part of the ensemble. Random Forest is an example of bagging (bootstrap aggregation) approach. A separate decision tree is learned from an independently drawn sample of the training data, and multiple random data samples yield the ensemble of models. Random sampling can either apply to the records of the training set, or to data attributes selected from the original training sample.

Fig. 1 Data organization
through machine learning

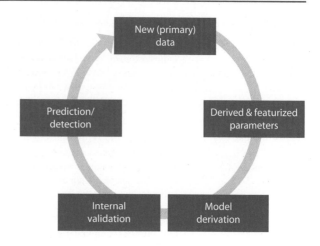

in future patient encounters. Thus, machine learning approaches could mirror good clinical practice.

Challenges may exist when machine learning is implemented. Small training samples could lead to over-fitting, but many machine learning approaches have algorithms in place to handle this limitation. For example, decision-tree learning uses pruning algorithms to prevent overfitting (Table 2). If a tree 'leaf' does not decrease the classifier error rate, then the leaf is removed ('pruned') to minimize information from the training set that is used in test dataset classification. Missing values in a time series is a major issue as well, but different techniques could be used to minimize this problem. A classification and regression tree (CART) algorithm (a type of decision-tree analysis) uses training data to build a classifier tree; if a split ('branch') point must reference a missing datapoint in training or testing data, it uses other branch points as surrogates to aid in the classification process [50]. One can also impute data into empty portions of the dataset. Finally, it may be difficult to convince hospitals and clinicians that machine learning approaches to common clinical problems like occult hypovolemia are a useful adjunct to care. They may be skeptical of a technology that could be viewed as a 'replacement' for human decision-making, or does not add to the ability of an experienced clinical decision-maker. Large-scale observational and intervention studies are necessary – using many of the available dynamic monitoring parameters previously discussed – to affirm feasibility and utility of machine-learning application in occult bleeding detection.

Conclusion

Clinical decisions are made about patients at-risk for hypovolemia using static, sub-optimal measures of patient physiology. If hypotension, hyperlactatemia or other signs of end-organ injury have developed before a diagnosis is made and definitive treatment is implemented, patients may have suffered irreversible damage. Healthcare providers require dynamic physiologic parameters that assess global and regional changes in flow and vascular tone, as well as metabolic metrics, such as tissue PCO_2. These variables should ideally be measured at the highest frequency to extract derived and featurized parameters from raw data, and to assess real-time changes in hemodynamics prior to overt signs of tissue injury. Machine learning approaches can identify patterns in patient hemodynamic features by comparing them to known patterns in an existing data repository. It may also be possible to identify how far patients are in the bleeding process. Future studies in this area should: (1) Check robustness of machine learning classification using different known hypovolemic stressors (in animal models); (2) utilize all currently available dynamic and featurized parameters from high frequency data (in animal and human studies); and (3) investigate how coagulopathy could change detection algorithms. Furthermore, observational and intervention-based studies are needed to confirm that machine-learning approaches could change therapeutic timing and patient outcomes in occult bleeding.

Acknowledgement

This work was supported in part by NIH grants HL07820 and NR013912

References

1. Kauvar DS, Lefering R, Wade CE (2006) Impact of hemorrhage on trauma outcome: An overview of epidemiology, clinical presentations, and therapeutic considerations. J Trauma 60:S3–S11
2. Cooper GS, Chak A, Way LE, Hammar PJ, Harper DL, Rosenthal GE (1999) Early endoscopy in upper gastrointestinal hemorrhage: associations with recurrent bleeding, surgery, and length of hospital stay. Gastrointest Endosc 49:145–152
3. Wysocki JD, Srivastav S, Winstead NS (2012) A nationwide analysis of risk factors for mortality and time to endoscopy in upper gastrointestinal hemorrhage. Aliment Pharmacol Ther 36:30–36
4. American College of Surgeons Trauma Committee (2008) Advanced trauma life support for doctors. 8th edn. American College of Surgeons, Chicago
5. Gomez H, Mesquida J, Hermus L et al (2012) Physiologic responses to severe hemorrhagic shock and genesis of cardiovascular collapse: Can irreversibility be anticipated? J Surg Res 178:358–369
6. Zimmerman JE, Kramer AA, McNair DS, Malila FM (2006) Acute Physiology and Chronic Health Evaluation (APACHE) IV: hospital mortality assessment for today's critically ill patients. Crit Care Med 34:1297–1310
7. Boyd CR, Tolson MA, Copes WS (1987) Evaluating Trauma Care: The TRISS Method. J Trauma 27:370–378
8. Moller MH, Engebjerg MC, Adamsen S, Bendix J, Thomsen RW (2012) The Peptic Ulcer Perforation (PULP) score: a predictor of mortality following peptic ulcer perforation. A cohort study. Acta Anaesthesiol Scand 56:655–662
9. Sinuff T, Adhikari NKJ, Cook DJ et al (2006) Mortality predictions in the intensive care unit: Comparing physicians with scoring systems. Crit Care Med 34:878–885

10. Chen I, Hung M, Chiu T, Chen J, Hsiao C (2007) Risk scoring systems to predict need for clinical intervention for patients with nonvariceal upper gastrointestinal bleed. Am J Emerg Med 25:774–779
11. Wang C, Chen Y, Young Y, Yang C, Chen I (2013) A prospective comparison of 3 scoring systems in upper gastrointestinal bleeding. Am J Emerg Med 31:775–778
12. Brockamp T, Nienaber U, Mutschler M et al (2012) Predicting on-going hemorrhage and transfusion requirement after severe trauma: a validation of six scoring systems and algorithms on the TraumaRegister DGU. Crit Care 16:R129
13. Ranucci M, Castelvecchio S, Frigiola A, Scolleta S, Giomarelli P, Biagioli B (2009) Predicting transfusions in cardiac surgery: the easier, the better: the Transfusion Risk and Clinical Knowledge score. Vox Sanguinis 96:324–322
14. Schuster KM, Davis KA, Lui FY, Maerz LL, Kaplan LJ (2010) The status of massive transfusion protocols in United States trauma centers: massive transfusion or massive confusion? Transfusion 50:1545–1551
15. Kaplan LJ, Kellum JA (2008) Comparison of acid-base models for prediction of hospital mortality after trauma. Shock 29:662–666
16. Jansen TC, van Bommel J, Mulder PG et al (2009) Prognostic value of blood lactate levels: Does the clinical diagnosis at admission matter? J Trauma 66:377–385
17. Hefferman DS, Thakkar RK, Monaghan SF et al (2010) Normal vital signs are unreliable in geriatric trauma victims. J Trauma 69:813–820
18. Paladino L, Subramanian RA, Nabors S, Sinert R (2011) The utility of shock index in differentiating major from minor injury. Eur J Emerg Med 18:94–98
19. Rivers EP, Ander DS, Powell D (2001) Central venous oxygen saturation monitoring in the critically ill patient. Curr Opin Crit Care 7:204–211
20. Pinsky MR, Payen D (2005) Functional hemodynamic monitoring. Crit Care 9:566–572
21. Kumar A, Anel R, Bunnell E et al (2004) Pulmonary artery occlusion pressure and central venous pressure fail to predict ventricular filling volume, cardiac performance, or the response to volume infusion in normal subjects. Crit Care Med 32:691–699
22. Marik PE, Baram M, Vahid B (2008) Does central venous pressure predict volume responsiveness? A systematic review of the literature and the tale of seven mares. Chest 134:172–178
23. Rajaram SS, Desai NK, Karla A, et al (2013) Pulmonary artery catheters for adult patients in intensive care. Cochrane Database Syst Rev CD003408
24. Clermont G, Kong L, Weissfeld LA et al (2011) The effect of pulmonary artery catheter use on costs and long-term outcomes in acute lung injury. PLoS One 6:e22512
25. Hadian M, Kim HK, Severyn DA, Pinsky MR (2010) Cross-comparison of cardiac output trending accuracy of LiDCO, PiCCO, FloTrac, and pulmonary artery catheters. Crit Care 14:R212
26. Velmahos GC, Wo CCJ, Demetriades D, Shoemaker WC (1999) Early continuous noninvasive hemodynamic monitoring after severe blunt trauma. Injury 33:209–214
27. Clavijo-Alvarez JA, Sims CA, Pinsky MR, Puyana JC (2005) Monitoring skeletal muscle and subcutaneous tissue acid-base status and oxygenation during hemorrhagic shock and resuscitation. Shock 24:270–275
28. Pellis T, Weil MH, Tang W, Sun S, Csapozi P, Castillo C (2005) Increases in both buccal and sublingual partial pressure of carbon dioxide reflect decreases of tissue blood flows in a porcine model during hemorrhagic shock. J Trauma 58:817–824
29. Soller BR, Yang Y, Soyemi OO et al (2008) Noninvasively determined muscle oxygen saturation is an early indicator of central hypovolemia in humans. J Appl Physiol 104:475–481
30. Zhang Z, Lu B, Sheng X, Jin N (2011) Accuracy of stroke volume variation in predicting fluid responsiveness: a systematic review and meta-analysis. J Anesth 25:904–916

31. Michard F, Boussat S, Chemla D et al (2000) Relation between respiratory changes in arterial pulse pressure and fluid responsiveness in septic patients with acute circulatory failure. Am J Respir Crit Care Med 162:143–138
32. Huang C, Fu J, Hu H et al (2008) Prediction of fluid responsiveness in acute respiratory distress syndrome patients ventilated with low tidal volume and high positive end-expiratory pressure. Crit Care Med 36:2810–2816
33. Godin PJ, Buchman TG (1996) Uncoupling of biological oscillators: a complementary hypothesis concerning the pathogenesis of multiple organ dysfunction syndrome. Crit Care Med 24:1107–1116
34. Seely AJE, Christou NV (2000) Multiple organ dysfunction syndrome: Exploring the paradigm of complex nonlinear systems. Crit Care Med 28:2193–2200
35. Task Force of the European Society of Cardiology and the North American Society of Pacing and Electrophysiology (1996) Heart rate variability: standards of measurement, physiological interpretation, and clinical use. Circulation 93:1043–1065
36. Kleiger RE, Miller JP, Bigger JT Jr, Moss AJ (1987) Decreased heart rate variability and its association with increased mortality after acute myocardial infarction. Am J Cardiol 59:256–262
37. Griffin MP, O'Shea TM, Bissonette EA, Harrell FE Jr, Lake DE, Moorman JR (2003) Abnormal heart rate characteristics preceding neonatal sepsis and sepsis-like illness. Pediatr Res 53:920–926
38. Moorman JR, Carlo WA, Kattwinkel J et al (2011) Mortality reduction by heart rate variability characteristic monitoring in very low birth weight neonates: A randomized controlled trial. J Pediatr 159:900–906
39. Batchinsky AI, Cooke WH, Kuusela T, Cancio LC (2007) Loss of complexity characteristics the heart rate response to experimental hemorrhagic shock in swine. Crit Care Med 35:519–525
40. Norris PR, Morris JA, Ozdas A, Grogan EL, Williams AE (2005) Heart rate variability predicts trauma patient outcomes as early as 12 hours: Implications for military and civilian triage. J Surg Res 129:122–128
41. Fathizadeh P, Shoemaker WC, Wo CCJ, Colombo J (2004) Autonomic activity in trauma patients based on variability of heart rate and respiratory rate. Crit Care Med 32:1300–1305
42. Kasaoka S, Nakahara T, Kawamura Y, Tsuruta R, Maekawa T (2010) Real-time monitoring of heart rate variability in critically ill patients. J Crit Care 25:313–316
43. Bradley B, Green GC, Batkin I, Seely AJE (2012) Feasibility of continuous multiorgan variability in the intensive care unit. J Crit Care 27:218.e9–218.e20
44. Bravi A, Longtin A, Seely AJE (2011) Review and classification of variability analysis techniques with clinical applications. BioMed Engineer 10:90
45. Scheuer ML, Wilson SB (2004) Data analysis for continuous EEG monitoring in the ICU: seeing the forest and the trees. J Clin Neurophysiol 21:353–378
46. Glass TF, Knapp J, Ambrun P et al (2004) Use of artificial intelligence to identify cardiovascular collapse in a model of hemorrhagic shock. Crit Care Med 32:450–456
47. Chen L, McKenna TM, Reisner AT, Gribok A, Reifman J (2007) Decision tool for the early diagnosis of trauma patient hypovolemia. J Biomed Inform 41:469–478
48. Convertino VA, Grudic G, Mulligan J, Moulton S (2013) Estimation of individual-specific progression to impending cardiovascular instability using arterial waveforms. J Appl Physiol 115:1196–1202
49. Dubrawski A (2011) Detection of events in multiple streams of surveillance data: Multivariate, multi-stream and multi-dimensional approaches. In: Zeng D, Chen H, Castillo-Chavez C, Lober WB, Thurmond M (eds) Infectious disease informatics and biosurveillance. Springer, New York, pp 145–171
50. Wu J, Roy J, Stewart WF (2010) Prediction modeling using EHR data: Challenges, Strategies, and a comparison of machine learning approaches. Med Care 48:S106–S113

Optimizing Intensity and Duration of Oral Antithrombotic Therapy after Primary Percutaneous Coronary Intervention

G. Biondi-Zoccai, E. Romagnoli, and G. Frati

Introduction

The most serious type of acute coronary syndrome (ACS) is acute myocardial infarction with persistent ST-segment elevation (STEMI) or new left bundle branch block (LBBB), which actually qualifies as a true medical emergency. Notwithstanding the historically ominous outlook of patients with STEMI, constant improvement in the management of STEMI, including emergency services, means of reperfusion, medical devices, and pharmacologic therapy have significantly ameliorated the short and long-term prognosis of this condition. Whereas short-term case fatality could be as high as 13 % in the placebo arm of a megatrial in 1986 [1], today it can be as low as 4 % for up to 1 year in those receiving state of the art care [2].

Despite such favorable developments and improvements, several questions remain regarding the most appropriate choice of devices and drugs to achieve reperfusion while minimizing the risk of early or late adverse events. We have previously summarized in this and other venues how evidence-based stent choice can maximize efficacy and safety in this clinical setting [3–5], and focus this present view on how to optimize the intensity and duration of oral antithrombotic therapy in patients undergoing primary percutaneous coronary intervention (PCI).

Scope of the Problem

ACSs, which span from unstable angina to STEMI, are typically caused by atherosclerotic plaque instability (i. e., plaque rupture or plaque erosion) due to

G. Biondi-Zoccai ✉ · G. Frati
Department of Medico-Surgical Sciences and Biotechnologies, Sapienza University of Rome, 04100 Latina, Italy
e-mail: giuseppe.biondizoccai@uniroma1.it

E. Romagnoli
Division of Cardiology, Policlinico Casilino, 00169 Rome, Italy

J.-L. Vincent (Ed.), *Annual Update in Intensive Care and Emergency Medicine 2014*, 569
DOI 10.1007/978-3-319-03746-2_42, © Springer International Publishing Switzerland 2014

superimposed coronary thrombosis. Accordingly, pre-, peri-, and post-procedural medical therapy, including antithrombotic agents, has been a cornerstone in the care of these patients since the landmark megatrials performed in the 1980s [1]. A naïve approach to this issue could be based on simple administration of very potent anticoagulants and antiplatelet agents at maximum dosage, but a delicate balance must be found between minimizing the risk of thrombosis and the risk of bleeding. Indeed, the last few years have been characterized by a shift from a prevalent emphasis on ischemic events only (e. g., major adverse cardiac or cerebrovascular events [MACE or MACCE], typically defined as death, myocardial infarction, stroke, and/or repeat revascularization) to a composite endpoint of net adverse clinical events (NACE), based on major adverse cardiac and cerebrovascular events plus bleeding (typically major ones only) [6].

Oral antithrombotic agents, which can be operatively distinguished into agents that inhibit platelet activation or aggregation (i. e., antiplatelet agents) and those that inhibit the coagulation cascade (i. e., anticoagulants), represent only one of the ingredients of the optimal recipe for successful antithrombotic treatment in patients with STEMI, because parenteral anticoagulants and antiplatelet agents are also routinely used. These agents fall outside the scope of this viewpoint, however, as their choice and monitoring is usually reserved to the clinicians directly responsible for patient triage or invasive treatment. However, it may be useful to briefly recall them:

- Unfractionated heparin (UFH) is a highly sulfated glycosaminoglycan that activates antithrombin III. It has mainly anticoagulant activity and is typically administered intravenously before and/or during PCI;
- Low-molecular weight heparin (LMWH) is a group of antithrombin III activators with prevalent anticoagulant activity, which can also be used before, during, or after coronary revascularization, although the bulk of evidence lies with enoxaparin [7];
- Bivalirudin is a direct thrombin inhibitor with prevalent anticoagulant activity that can be administered during or after intervention [8];
- Glycoprotein IIb/IIIa inhibitors are potent antiplatelet agents which can be administered intravenously before, during or shortly after coronary revascularization;
- Cangrelor is a an antiplatelet agent that blocks the platelet P2Y12 adenosine-diphosphate (ADP) receptor, which can be administered before or during angioplasty;
- Aspirin, which is mainly used as an oral antiplatelet agent in this clinical setting, can be administered perioperatively by means of intravenous bolus [9].

As the present work focuses rather on the optimal intensity and duration of oral antithrombotic therapy in those undergoing primary PCI, it is best to further characterize these important concepts. The intensity of oral antithrombotic therapy has to do with its antiplatelet efficacy, its anticoagulant efficacy, or a combination of these factors. It should also be remembered that several of these agents have pleiomorphic actions, such as aspirin, the anti-neoplastic effect of which has recently been demonstrated. The intensity of a given regimen can generally be appraised according to dose (in mg) per day, with or without adjustment for specific features

(e. g., body weight, gender, history of prior stroke or transient ischemic attack). Otherwise, formal laboratory assays can be employed, such as platelet aggregation tests [10]. It is less straightforward to compare the intensity of two or more different regimens with various combinations of the available agents (e. g., it is unclear whether high-dose aspirin plus standard-dose ticagrelor is more potent than low-dose aspirin plus low-dose rivaroxaban). Indeed, the bulk of research and attention is currently focused on the best dual antiplatelet therapy, e. g., the combination of aspirin and an oral P2Y12 inhibitor (i. e., clopidogrel, prasugrel, or ticagrelor) or triple antiplatelet therapy, e. g., the combination of aspirin, an oral P2Y12 inhibitor, and an oral anticoagulant.

Duration of oral antithrombotic therapy can be distinguished as recommended duration at discharge from the hospital and at subsequent visits versus actual duration. Accordingly, it is important to highlight the concepts of discontinuation or disruption of antiplatelet therapy, which have been shown to be harbingers of adverse events [11, 12]. Planned or recommended withdrawal of antithrombotic therapy under a physician's supervision can be operatively defined as discontinuation, whereas unplanned or unsupervised withdrawal for non-compliance or bleeding can be identified as disruption. Whereas discontinuation has been blamed for increased rates of adverse events in several reports, disruption is typically much more ominous.

Another crucial aspect impacting, especially in the short-term, on the complex set of decisions regarding antithrombotic management in patients undergoing primary PCI is the choice of the most appropriate arteriotomy access site [6]. Indeed, faced with the possibility of using transradial versus transfemoral access, clinicians should be aware that transradial access is associated with much less bleeding (potentially leading also to fewer deaths) [13]. Thus, those undergoing coronary revascularization by the transradial route can also be treated more aggressively with more potent antithrombotic agents.

Finally, the overall impact concerning the multifaceted set of decisions regarding antithrombotic management in patients undergoing primary PCI has modified not only the clinical outcome of these patients, but also the horizon of the cardiac surgeon, because a significant number of patients require surgical revascularization after primary PCI and may be at increased risk of bleeding complications, especially when emergency or urgent cardiac surgery is mandatory. Indeed, non-surgical bleeding is responsible for 50 to 60 % of surgical reopening, and bleeding complications following cardiac surgery are mainly related to the use of antithrombotic drugs, to the onset of fibrinolysis platelet dysfunction, or a combination of these factors as platelets are partially activated by heparin and are diluted, destroyed, and modified during cardiopulmonary bypass (CPB) because of their adhesion to circuit surfaces, aggregation, and activation [14]. Thus, the main concern for the urgent treatment of these patients is the potential for increased risk of bleeding caused by this class of agents [15]. Recent studies have suggested the value of preoperative *in vitro* platelet aggregometry to determine perioperative bleeding risk in cardiac surgery for patients requiring emergency surgery despite recently received antithrombotic therapy, as an assessment of *in vitro* platelet aggregation might permit recognition of patients at higher risk of perioperative hemorrhage with a 70 %

inhibition of platelet aggregation cut-off of predictive value for bleeding and transfusion requirement. Accordingly an update of the Society of Thoracic Surgeons guidelines suggests point-of-care (POC) platelet function testing may be exploited in order to asses bleeding risk for patients receiving antithrombotic drugs before surgery [16, 17]. Nevertheless, the intra- and perioperative management of patients who have recently received antithrombotic drugs (particularly dual antiplatelet therapy) and require urgent surgery still remains a challenge. However, it is safe to assume that at least 5 days should pass since the last dose of clopidogrel, rivaroxaban, or ticagrelor before cardiac surgery is performed, with even longer periods for prasugrel and warfarin [18, 19].

Oral Antithrombotic Agents

Oral antithrombotic agents suitable for patients undergoing primary PCI can be divided into three broad classes: Non-P2Y12-blocking antiplatelet agents (e. g., aspirin), P2Y12-blocking antiplatelet agents (e. g., clopidogrel), and oral anticoagulants (e. g., rivaroxaban). We present the key features of the most important ones (Table 1, Fig. 1).

Table 1 Oral antithrombotic agents suitable for patients undergoing primary percutaneous coronary intervention

Agent	Aspirin	Clopidogrel	Prasugrel	Rivaroxaban	Ticagrelor	Warfarin
Class	Salicylate	Thieno-pyridine	Thieno-pyridine	Oxazolidi-none	Nucleoside analog	Dicoumarol derivative
Onset	<1h	>2h	<1h	>2h	<1–2h	>1 day
Action	Irreversibly inhibits COX	Irreversibly inhibits P2Y12r	Irreversibly inhibits P2Y12r	Reversibly inhibits factor Xa	Reversibly inhibits P2Y12r	Inhibits the synthesis of VKD coagulation factors
Pros	Well-tested safety and efficacy; prevents colon cancer	Well-tested safety and efficacy; wide therapeutic window	Established efficacy; prolonged effect	Established efficacy; decreases risk of stroke/embolism	Established safety and efficacy	Well-tested safety and efficacy profile; intensity adjustable
Cons	Limited potency; variability in response	Limited potency; variability in response	Narrow therapeutic window	Narrow therapeutic window	Less prolonged effect; dyspnea	Narrow therapeutic window; interactions; INR monitoring

COX: cyclooxygenase; INR: international normalized ratio; P2Y12r: P2Y12 receptor; VKD: vitamin K-dependent

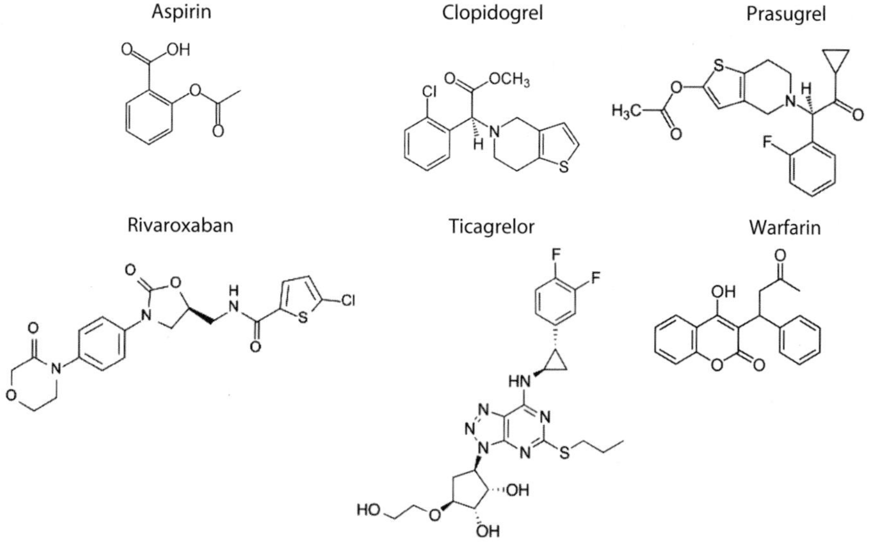

Fig. 1 Chemical structure of aspirin, clopidogrel, prasugrel, rivaroxaban, ticagrelor, and warfarin, the most important oral antithrombotic agents suitable for patients undergoing primary percutaneous coronary intervention

Aspirin

Aspirin (acetylsalicylic acid) is an irreversible cyclooxygenase (COX) inhibitor, which prevents the platelet production of thromboxane and its ensuing platelet activating effects. It is a drug with a long clinical history, proven risk-benefit balance in a variety of settings, and important favorable effects in primary as well as secondary prevention of arterial and venous cardiovascular events [20]. Aspirin also has beneficial anti-neoplastic actions [21]. Intense research has focused on the optimal dose, with European practitioners favoring a low-dose regimen ($\leq 100\,\mathrm{mg}$ daily), which is considered to be associated with the most beneficial risk-benefit balance, despite recent challenges to this view [20]. Aspirin is accordingly considered a mandatory component of any antiplatelet regimen, from antiplatelet monotherapy, to dual antiplatelet therapy (e. g., aspirin plus clopidogrel), and triple antithrombotic therapy (e. g., aspirin, clopidogrel, and warfarin). However, even this custom has been recently questioned, at least in patients requiring long-term oral anticoagulation [22]. Indeed, response to aspirin is highly variable, such that several authors have tried to develop the concept of aspirin resistance [10].

Clopidogrel

Clopidogrel is a thienopyridine with irreversible inhibiting effects on the P2Y12 receptor. It is a pro-drug requiring hepatic conversion into its active metabolite. Despite its remarkable safety profile compared to the first thienopyridine, ticlopidine, clopidogrel elicits variable responses in patients and an unsatisfactory time to achieve peak activity, such that progressively increasing loading doses have been used over time [23]. Although clopidogrel is remarkably safe, it is still theoretically more potent than aspirin alone [24], and their combination is clearly associated with a measurable increase in the risk of bleeding events [25, 26]. Nonetheless, it is clearly more beneficial in reducing the risk of ischemic events when combined with aspirin compared to aspirin alone.

Conversely, some patients respond poorly to clopidogrel or still experience thrombotic events despite complying with clopidogrel-based regimens [27]. This, and the recent patent expiration for this drug, is why novel alternatives to clopidogrel have been recently developed and tested formally in clinical trials [28, 29].

Prasugrel

Prasugrel is a thienopyridine, similar in its main features and mechanisms of action to clopidogrel. However, it is much more potent (at least in the regimens that underwent formal testing) and has a much faster time to peak activity on platelet function. It has been shown to be beneficial in patients with STEMI, given its association with a lower risk of ischemic events, despite an obvious and statistically significant incremental effect on bleeding [29]. Accordingly, it is currently and routinely prescribed in patients with ACS undergoing percutaneous coronary revascularization. Its benefits in those not undergoing revascularization or those in whom revascularization is being postponed are less clear [30, 31].

Rivaroxaban

Rivaroxaban is an oxazolidinone which inhibits coagulation factor Xa and has a favorable risk-benefit profile in patients requiring oral anticoagulation instead of warfarin (e. g., those with atrial fibrillation or venous thromboembolism) [32]. Its use in patients with ACS, on top of dual or single antiplatelet therapy, has been recently tested formally in two trials [33, 34]. Notably, in the ATLAS ACS 2-TIMI 51 study, rivaroxaban proved remarkably beneficial, being associated with significant reductions in the risk of fatal and non-fatal ischemic events, despite an obvious increase in the rate of bleeding [34]. Care should be taken when prescribing novel oral anticoagulants in patients with mechanical cardiac valves, because dabigatran was associated with more adverse events than warfarin in this setting [35].

Ticagrelor

Ticagrelor is a novel non-thienopyridine nucleoside analog that directly and reversibly inhibits the P2Y12 receptor. It has a fast onset and offset of action, does not require hepatic activation, and may be associated with a more favorable risk-benefit balance than prasugrel in patients with ACS [27, 36]. This is in addition to its clear superiority versus clopidogrel, with significant reductions in all cause death, non-fatal ischemic events, and major bleedings related to cardiac surgery despite an obvious increase in the risk of major bleeding (either overall or unrelated to cardiac surgery) [29].

Warfarin

Oral anticoagulants acting as antivitamin K agents (first and foremost warfarin) represent a common tool in the antithrombotic armamentarium, given their inhibitory effect on the synthesis of factors II, VII, IX and X, as well as protein C, S, and Z. Despite their established role in cardiovascular therapy, they have a narrow therapeutic index, require periodic monitoring, and may interact with several foods and drugs. Nonetheless, when thrombotic risk is particularly high, warfarin and similar agents continue to be prescribed, with favorable clinical results. The most common indications in patients with a recent STEMI are left ventricular thrombus, atrial fibrillation, and venous thromboembolism. In this setting, warfarin is typically prescribed on top of aspirin and clopidogrel, in a cocktail regimen often referred to as triple therapy. The WOEST trial has, however, challenged this custom, showing that bleeding risk was significantly higher with triple therapy than with dual therapy (i. e., the combination of clopidogrel and warfarin), whereas thrombotic events were not in favor of the aspirin-including regiment (they actually favored the dual therapy group) [22]. Similar findings have been recently reported by Lamberts and colleagues in a nationwide Danish observational study comparing different oral antithrombotic regimens in patients with an indication for oral anticoagulation. Specifically, these authors reported that the combination of clopidogrel and oral anticoagulants (without aspirin) provided the most favorable risk-benefit balance in patients with atrial fibrillation after myocardial infarction or PCI [37].

Optimizing Intensity

Having clarified which agents are available for oral antithrombotic therapy in patients undergoing primary PCI, and having briefly reported their main pros and cons, we tentatively suggest a pragmatic approach to optimization of oral antithrombotic therapy (Table 2). Clinicians should individualize their approach according to the specific patient's risks of bleeding and thrombosis, which may vary considerably.

Patients at low bleeding and low thrombotic risk can be reasonably prescribed aspirin and clopidogrel for the first 12 months after the acute event, continuing aspirin

Table 2 Key studies on novel oral antithrombotic agents suitable for patients undergoing primary percutaneous coronary intervention

Study	ATLAS ACS 2-TIMI 51 [34]	Biondi-Zoccai et al. [27]	CURRENT-OASIS 7 [43]	PLATO [29]	TRITON-TIMI 38 [28]	WOEST [22]
Year	2012	2011	2010	2009	2007	2013
Design	RCT of rivaroxaban (2.5 mg or 5.0 mg twice daily) vs placebo	NMA of clopidogrel, prasugrel and ticagrelor	RCT of 600 mg loading then 150 mg/day for 7 days followed by 75 mg daily vs. 300 mg loading followed by 75 mg daily clopidogrel and 300–325 mg vs. 75–100 mg daily aspirin	RCT of clopidogrel vs. ticagrelor	RCT of clopidogrel vs. prasugrel	RCT of aspirin, clopidogrel and warfarin vs. clopidogrel and warfarin
Patients	15,526 with ACS	32,893 with ACS	25,086 with ACS	18,624 with ACS	13,608 with ACS	573 undergoing PCI
Findings	Rivaroxaban ↓ MACE, but ↑ major bleeding	Prasugrel and ticagrelor had similar efficacy and safety, but prasugrel ↓ ST, while ↑ major bleeding	There was no difference in MACE between groups	Ticagrelor ↓ MACE, but ↑ non-procedural bleeding	Prasugrel ↓ MACE, but ↑ major bleeding	Clopidogrel without aspirin ↓ bleeding complications, without ↑ thrombotic events

ACS: acute coronary syndrome; MACE: major adverse cardiac event; NMA: network meta-analysis; RCT: randomized clinical trial

lifelong thereafter [26]. Nonetheless, even in this setting, prasugrel and ticagrelor may prove risk-beneficial, if not cost-beneficial [27]. Patients at low bleeding but high thrombotic risk should be routinely prescribed aspirin plus prasugrel or ticagrelor, unless specific contraindications are present. Twelve months after the index event, aspirin alone can be continued indefinitely.

When a concomitant indication to oral anticoagulation is present, the bulk of high-quality evidence suggests that clopidogrel and warfarin may constitute the most favorable regimen, at least up to mid-term [22]. However, rivaroxaban could be considered in the future instead of warfarin, either in combination with aspirin and clopidogrel, or with aspirin or clopidogrel monotherapy [34]. It remains an object of speculation whether it is possible to safely discontinue clopidogrel in exchange for aspirin after the first 6–12 months in those on dual therapy including an antiplatelet agent and an anticoagulant.

Optimizing Duration

The optimal duration of oral antithrombotic therapy in those undergoing primary PCI is a focus of intense research, with, hitherto, few trials formally able to informing decision makers (Table 3). Indirect evidence suggests that a 12-month clopidogrel regimen is more risk-beneficial than a shorter regimen, irrespective of the revascularization technique [25, 26]. Indeed, recent randomized trials and observational studies have questioned the wisdom of prolonged dual antiplatelet regimens (e. g., those lasting 1 year, 18 months, or more), which had been, in the past, emphatically recommended, especially after drug-eluting stent implantation [38–42].

Pragmatically, we suggest prescribing short-term (3 month) dual antiplatelet regimens only to those at very high bleeding risk and not receiving drug-eluting stents, whereas mid-term (6–12 months) regimens can be recommended after drug-eluting stenting or in those without a severe bleeding risk. Some evidence suggests that novel drug-eluting stents are safer than bare-metal stents, even in those with STEMI, thus indirectly implying that short-term dual antiplatelet therapy could also be safe when these devices are used [4, 5]. However, further trials testing this paradigm-shifting hypothesis in a formal fashion are required before changing time-tested management protocols.

The usefulness of long-term (> 12 months) regimens is to date unproven, and they should be considered only in very selected patients with very high thrombotic risk or who have had recurrent events despite complying with the recommended antithrombotic prescription.

Table 3 Key studies on optimal duration of oral antithrombotic therapy suitable for patients undergoing primary percutaneous coronary intervention (PCI)

Study	Cassese et al. [41]	CREDO [25]	EXCELLENT [44]	Park et al. [40]	PRODIGY [39]	RESET [45]
Year	2012	2002	2012	2010	2012	2012
Design	PMA of short – vs. long-term DAPT (16.8 vs. 6.2 months)	RCT of 300 mg loading plus 12-month vs. 75 mg loading plus 1-month clopidogrel	RCT of 6- vs. 12-month DAPT	RCT of 12- vs. 19-month DAPT	RCT of 6- vs. 24-month DAPT	RCT of 3- vs. 12-month DAPT
Patients	8,158 undergoing PCI with DES	2,116 undergoing PCI with BMS	1,443 undergoing PCI with DES	2,701 undergoing PCI with DES	2,013 undergoing PCI with BMS or DES	2,117 undergoing PCI with DES
Findings	Long vs. short DAPT ↑ major bleeding, without ↓ MACE	12-month clopidogrel ↓ MACE, whereas 300 mg did not	No difference in MACE between groups	No difference in MACE between groups	No difference in MACE between groups	No difference in MACE or major bleeding between groups

BMS: bare-metal stent; DAPT: dual antiplatelet therapy including aspirin and a thienopyridine; DES: drug-eluting stent; MACE: major adverse cardiac event; PMA: pairwise meta-analysis; RCT: randomized clinical trial

Conclusions

The management of STEMI has changed dramatically during the last few decades thanks to concomitant improvements in medical therapy and developments in mechanical reperfusion. Whereas individualization of treatment remains the safest and most effective management strategy, we believe that all such patients should be considered for dual antiplatelet therapy with prasugrel or ticagrelor on top of aspirin for the first year, with aspirin continued lifelong thereafter. Aggressive antithrombotic regimens shorter or longer than 12 months, as well as different combinations of these or other antithrombotic agents (e. g., clopidogrel versus rivaroxaban or warfarin) can also be considered, but only in carefully selected cases, based on, respectively, increased bleeding or increased thrombotic risk.

References

1. Gruppo Italiano per lo Studio della Streptochinasi nell'Infarto Miocardico (GISSI) (1986) Effectiveness of intravenous thrombolytic treatment in acute myocardial infarction. Lancet 1:397–402
2. Sabate M, Cequier A, Iñiguez A et al (2012) Everolimus-eluting stent versus bare-metal stent in ST-segment elevation myocardial infarction (EXAMINATION): 1 year results of a randomised controlled trial. Lancet 380:1482–1490
3. Biondi-Zoccai G, Peruzzi M, Frati G (2013) Stent choice in patients undergoing primary per-cutaneous coronary intervention. In: Vincent J-L (ed) Annual Update in Intensive Care and Emergency Medicine 2013. Springer, Berlin, pp 313–330
4. Palmerini T, Biondi-Zoccai G, Della Riva D et al (2012) Stent thrombosis with drug-eluting and bare-metal stents: evidence from a comprehensive network meta-analysis. Lancet 379:1393–1402
5. Palmerini T, Biondi-Zoccai G, Della Riva D et al (2013) Clinical outcomes with drug-eluting and bare-metal stents in patients with ST-segment elevation myocardial infarction: evidence from a comprehensive network meta-analysis. J Am Coll Cardiol 62:496–504
6. Romagnoli E, Biondi-Zoccai G, Sciahbasi A et al (2012) Radial Versus Femoral Random-ized Investigation in ST-Segment Elevation Acute Coronary Syndrome: The RIFLE-STEACS Study. J Am Coll Cardiol 60:2481–2489
7. Silvain J, Beygui F, Barthélémy O et al (2012) Efficacy and safety of enoxaparin versus unfractionated heparin during percutaneous coronary intervention: systematic review and meta-analysis. BMJ 344:e553
8. Bertrand OF, Jolly SS, Rao SV et al (2012) Meta-analysis comparing bivalirudin versus heparin monotherapy on ischemic and bleeding outcomes after percutaneous coronary intervention. Am J Cardiol 110:599–606
9. Bhatt DL, Stone GW, Mahaffey KW et al (2013) Effect of platelet inhibition with cangrelor during PCI on ischemic events. N Engl J Med 368:1303–1313
10. Biondi-Zoccai G, Lotrionte M (2008) Aspirin resistance in cardiovascular disease. BMJ 336:166–167
11. Biondi-Zoccai GG, Lotrionte M, Agostoni P et al (2006) A systematic review and meta-analysis on the hazards of discontinuing or not adhering to aspirin among 50,279 patients at risk for coronary artery disease. Eur Heart J 27:2667–2674
12. Mehran R, Baber U, Steg PG et al (2013) Cessation of dual antiplatelet treatment and cardiac events after percutaneous coronary intervention (PARIS): 2 year results from a prospective observational study. The Lancet 382:1714–1722
13. Biondi-Zoccai G, D'Ascenzo F, Mancone M et al (2013) Can we predict which patients with ST-elevation myocardial infarction benefit most from radial access? Evidence from frequentist and Bayesian meta-regressions of randomized trials. Int J Cardiol 168:4931–4934
14. Woodman RC, Harker LA (1990) Bleeding complication associated with cardiopulmonary bypass. Blood 76:1680–1697
15. Bizzarri F, Scolletta S, Tucci E et al (2001) Perioperative use of tirofiban hydrochloride does not increase surgical bleeding after emergency or urgent coronary artery bypass grafting. J Thorac Cardiovasc Surg 122:1181–1185
16. Held C, Asenblad N, Bassand JP et al (2011) Ticagrelor versus clopidogrel in patients with acute coronary syndromes undergoing coronary artery bypass surgery: results from the PLATO (Platelet Inhibition and Patient Outcomes) trial. J Am Coll Cardiol 57:672–684
17. Ferraris VA, Saha SP, Oestreich JH et al (2012) Update to the Society of Thoracic Surgeons guideline on use of antiplatelet drugs in patients having cardiac and noncardiac operations. Ann Thorac Surg 94:1761–1781
18. Smith PK, Goodnough LT, Levy JH et al (2012) Mortality benefit with prasugrel in the TRITON-TIMI 38 coronary artery bypass grafting cohort: risk-adjusted retrospective data analysis. J Am Coll Cardiol 60:388–396

19. Fitchett D, Eikelboom J, Fremes S et al (2009) Dual antiplatelet therapy in patients requiring urgent coronary artery bypass grafting surgery: a position statement of the Canadian Cardiovascular Society. Can J Cardiol 25:683–689
20. Lotrionte M, Biondi-Zoccai GG (2008) The hazards of discontinuing acetylsalicylic acid therapy in those at risk of coronary artery disease. Curr Opin Cardiol 23:487–493
21. Rothwell PM, Price JF, Fowkes FG et al (2012) Short-term effects of daily aspirin on cancer incidence, mortality, and non-vascular death: analysis of the time course of risks and benefits in 51 randomised controlled trials. Lancet 379:1602–1612
22. Dewilde WJ, Oirbans T, Verheugt FW et al (2013) Use of clopidogrel with or without aspirin in patients taking oral anticoagulant therapy and undergoing percutaneous coronary intervention: an open-label, randomised, controlled trial. Lancet 381:1107–1115
23. Lotrionte M, Biondi-Zoccai GG, Agostoni P et al (2007) Meta-analysis appraising high clopidogrel loading in patients undergoing percutaneous coronary intervention. Am J Cardiol 100:1199–1206
24. CAPRIE Steering Committee (1996) A randomised, blinded, trial of clopidogrel versus aspirin in patients at risk of ischaemic events (CAPRIE). Lancet 348:1329–1339
25. Steinhubl SR, Berger PB, Mann JT 3rd et al (2002) Early and sustained dual oral antiplatelet therapy following percutaneous coronary intervention: a randomized controlled trial. JAMA 288:2411–2420
26. Yusuf S, Zhao F, Mehta SR, Chrolavicius S, Tognoni G, Fox KK (2001) Effects of clopidogrel in addition to aspirin in patients with acute coronary syndromes without ST-segment elevation. N Engl J Med 345:494–502
27. Biondi-Zoccai G, Lotrionte M, Agostoni P et al (2011) Adjusted indirect comparison meta-analysis of prasugrel versus ticagrelor for patients with acute coronary syndromes. Int J Cardiol 150:325–331
28. Wiviott SD, Braunwald E, McCabe CH et al (2007) Prasugrel versus clopidogrel in patients with acute coronary syndromes. N Engl J Med 357:2001–2015
29. Cannon CP, Harrington RA, James S et al (2010) Comparison of ticagrelor with clopidogrel in patients with a planned invasive strategy for acute coronary syndromes (PLATO): a randomised double-blind study. Lancet 375:283–293
30. Montalescot G, Bolognese L, Dudek D et al (2013) Pretreatment with prasugrel in non-st-segment elevation acute coronary syndromes. N Engl J Med 369:999–1010
31. Roe MT, Armstrong PW, Fox KA et al (2012) Prasugrel versus clopidogrel for acute coronary syndromes without revascularization. N Engl J Med 367:1297–1309
32. Biondi-Zoccai G, Malavasi V, D'Ascenzo F et al (2013) Comparative effectiveness of novel oral anticoagulants for atrial fibrillation: evidence from pair-wise and warfarin-controlled network meta-analyses. HSR Proc Intensive Care Cardiovasc Anesth 5:40–54
33. Mega JL, Braunwald E, Mohanavelu S et al (2009) Rivaroxaban versus placebo in patients with acute coronary syndromes (ATLAS ACS-TIMI 46): a randomised, double-blind, phase II trial. Lancet 374:29–38
34. Mega JL, Braunwald E, Wiviott SD et al (2012) Rivaroxaban in patients with a recent acute coronary syndrome. N Engl J Med 366:9–19
35. Eikelboom JW, Connolly SJ, Brueckmann M et al (2013) Dabigatran versus warfarin in patients with mechanical heart valves. N Engl J Med 369:1206–1214
36. Alexopoulos D, Galati A, Xanthopoulou I et al (2012) Ticagrelor versus prasugrel in acute coronary syndrome patients with high on-clopidogrel platelet reactivity following percutaneous coronary intervention: a pharmacodynamic study. J Am Coll Cardiol 60:193–199
37. Lamberts M, Gislason GH, Olesen JB et al (2013) Oral anticoagulation and antiplatelets in atrial fibrillation patients after myocardial infarction and coronary intervention. J Am Coll Cardiol 62:981–989
38. Grines CL, Bonow RO, Casey DE Jr et al (2007) Prevention of premature discontinuation of dual antiplatelet therapy in patients with coronary artery stents: a science advisory from the American Heart Association, American College of Cardiology, Society for Cardiovascular

Angiography and Interventions, American College of Surgeons, and American Dental Association, with representation from the American College of Physicians. Circulation 115:813–881

39. Valgimigli M, Borghesi M, Tebaldi M, Vranckx P, Parrinello G, Ferrari R (2013) Should duration of dual antiplatelet therapy depend on the type and/or potency of implanted stent? A pre-specified analysis from the PROlonging Dual antiplatelet treatment after Grading stent-induced Intimal hyperplasia studY (PRODIGY). Eur Heart J 34:909–919

40. Park SJ, Park DW, Kim YH et al (2010) Duration of dual antiplatelet therapy after implantation of drug-eluting stents. N Engl J Med 362:1374–1382

41. Cassese S, Byrne RA, Tada T, King LA, Kastrati A (2012) Clinical impact of extended dual antiplatelet therapy after percutaneous coronary interventions in the drug-eluting stent era: a meta-analysis of randomized trials. Eur Heart J 33:3078–3087

42. Kedhi E, Stone GW, Kereiakes DJ et al (2012) Stent thrombosis: insights on outcomes, predictors and impact of dual antiplatelet therapy interruption from the SPIRIT II, SPIRIT III, SPIRIT IV and COMPARE trials. EuroIntervention 8:599–606

43. Mehta SR, Bassand JP, Chrolavicius S et al (2010) Dose comparisons of clopidogrel and aspirin in acute coronary syndromes. N Engl J Med 363:930–942

44. Gwon HC, Hahn JY, Park KW et al (2012) Six-month versus 12-month dual antiplatelet therapy after implantation of drug-eluting stents: the Efficacy of Xience/Promus Versus Cypher to Reduce Late Loss After Stenting (EXCELLENT) randomized, multicenter study. Circulation 125:505–513

45. Kim BK, Hong MK, Shin DH et al (2012) A new strategy for discontinuation of dual antiplatelet therapy: the RESET Trial (REal Safety and Efficacy of 3-month dual antiplatelet Therapy following Endeavor zotarolimus-eluting stent implantation). J Am Coll Cardiol 60:1340–1348

The Utility of Thromboelastometry (ROTEM) or Thromboelastography (TEG) in Non-bleeding ICU Patients

K. Balvers, M.C. Muller, and N.P. Juffermans

Introduction

A hypocoagulable state is highly prevalent in critically ill patients. An international normalized ratio (INR) of > 1.5 occurs in 30 % of patients and is associated with increased mortality [1]. Moreover, up to 40 % of critically ill patients develop thrombocytopenia during their intensive care unit (ICU) stay [2–4], associated with increased length of stay, need for transfusion of blood products and increased mortality [5]. Disseminated intravascular coagulation (DIC) develops in 10 to 20 % of ICU patients. A hypercoagulable state is associated with increased thromboembolic events [6], contributes to organ failure and is associated with a high mortality, ranging from 45 to 78 % [7].

Coagulopathy is thought to result from an imbalance between activation of coagulation and impaired inhibition of coagulation and fibrinolysis. Activation is triggered by tissue factor, which is expressed in reaction to cytokines or endothelial damage. Impaired inhibition of coagulation is the consequence of reduced plasma levels of antithrombin (AT), depressed activity of the protein C system and decreased levels of tissue factor pathway inhibitor (TFPI). A decrease in fibrinolysis is due to increased levels of plasminogen activator inhibitor type 1 (PAI-1) [8, 9]. This disturbance between components of the coagulation system leads to a variable clinical picture, ranging from patients with an increased bleeding tendency (hypocoagulable state) to those with DIC with (micro-) vascular thrombosis (hypercoagulable state).

Assessment of coagulation status in patients is complex. Global coagulation tests, including activated partial thromboplastin time (aPTT) and prothrombin time (PT), are used clinically. However, these tests are of limited value and their abil-

K. Balvers · M.C. Muller · N.P. Juffermans ✉
Department of Intensive Care, Academic Medical Center, University of Amsterdam,
Amsterdam, Netherlands
e-mail: n.p.juffermans@amc.uva.nl

J.-L. Vincent (Ed.), *Annual Update in Intensive Care and Emergency Medicine 2014*,
DOI 10.1007/978-3-319-03746-2_43, © Springer International Publishing Switzerland
2014

ity to accurately reflect *in vivo* hypocoagulable states is questioned [10]. Also, aPTT/PT reflects a part of the coagulation system and does not provide information on the full balance between coagulation, anticoagulation and fibrinolysis. Hypercoagulable state can be assessed by increased levels of D-dimers, but specificity is limited [10]. Impaired function of the anticoagulant system can be diagnosed by measuring plasma levels of the naturally occurring anticoagulant factors, AT, protein C and TFPI. However, these are not readily available for clinical use. Apart from the DIC score, there are no diagnostic tests which evaluate a hypercoagulable state. Markers of activity of the fibrinolytic system are also not used at the bedside [10].

TEG/ROTEM Tests

Rotational thromboelastography (TEG/ROTEM) is a point-of-care test, which evaluates whole clot formation and degradation. The thromboelastogram arises through movement of the cup (TEG) or the pin (ROTEM). As fibrin forms between the cup and the pin, this movement is influenced and converted to a specific trace. The trace reflects different phases of the clotting process. Major parameters are R (reaction/clotting) time, the period from the initiation of the test until the beginning of clot formation. K-time is the period from the start of clot formation until the curve reaches an amplitude of 20 mm. Kinetics of fibrin formation and cross-linking are expressed by the α-angle, which is the angle between the baseline and the tangent to the TEG/ROTEM curve. Clot strength is represented by the maximal amplitude of the trace. The degree of fibrinolysis is reflected by the difference between the maximal amplitude and the amplitude measured after 30 and/or 60 minutes. To describe these visco-elastic changes, both systems have their own terminology (Table 1). Both generate similar data. The technique was developed in the 1940s, but, until recently, clinical application has been limited. However, technical developments have led to standardization and improved reproducibility of the method [11]. Also, the availability for bedside evaluation and a changing view regarding the use of blood and hemostatic therapy in massive bleeding, have both contributed to a renewed interest in this technique.

TEG/ROTEM may also facilitate diagnosis of clotting abnormalities in the critically ill. By detecting a hypocoagulable state, TEG/ROTEM may be a useful tool in the assessment of the risk of bleeding perioperatively or prior to an invasive procedure. This could lead to a more tailored transfusion strategy, with an efficient use of blood products.

TEG/ROTEM can also diagnose a hypercoagulable state. With TEG/ROTEM, a hypercoagulable state can be detected by high maximal amplitude, shortened reaction time, increased alfa angle and total clot strength, G (defined as $(5000 \times A)/(100-A)$, Table 2). Assessment of a hypercoagulable state could lead to prognostication of multiple organ failure (MOF) and risk for thromboembolic events. Another potential advantage could be a more tailor-made administration of therapies that interfere with the coagulation system. Difficulties in identifying responders from

Table 1 TEG and ROTEM parameters

	ROTEM	TEG
Time to initial fibrin formation (to 2 mm amplitude)	CT	R
Clot strengthening, rapidity of fibrin build up	CFT α	K α
Clot strength, represents maximum dynamics of fibrin and platelet bonding	MCF	MA
Clot breakdown, fibrinolysis at fixed time (min)	LI30, LI45, LI60	CL30, CL60

MA: maximal amplitude; CFT: clot formation time; MCF: maximum clot firmness; LI: lysis index; CT: clotting time; R: reaction time; CL: clot lysis

Table 2 Normal ranges, hypercoagulable state and hypocoagulable state of ROTEM and TEG

Parameters	Normal ranges for ROTEM	Normal ranges for TEG*	Hypercoagulable state	Hypocoagulable state
Reaction time, R or CT	INTEM 137–246 sec EXTEM 42–74 sec FIBTEM 43–69 sec	4–8 min	Shortened	Prolonged
Clot formation time, K or CFT	INTEM 40–100 sec EXTEM 46–184 sec NA	0–4 min	Shortened	Prolonged
Alpha angle, angle or α	INTEM 71–82° EXTEM 63–81° NA	47–74	Increased	Decreased
Maximum amplitude, MA or MCF	INTEM 52–72 mm EXTEM 49–71 mm FIBTEM 9–25 mm	54–72 mm	Increased	Decreased

A hypercoagulable state is defined as the presence of at least two of the following: Shortened reaction time, increased alpha angle or increased maximum amplitude [46]; * Values for kaolin- or celite-activated TEG

non-responders may in part have contributed to conflicting results from trials evaluating the effect of strategies that interfere with the coagulation system [12–15].

Utility of TEG/ROTEM to Detect Sepsis-induced Coagulopathy

ROTEM clearly demonstrates a hypercoagulable state during endotoxemia [16]. Endotoxin-induced hypercoagulability was demonstrated *in vitro* using TEG. In experiments in which lipopolysaccharide (LPS) was infused in healthy volunteers, a hypercoagulable state measured by TEG had a strong correlation with plasma levels of prothrombin fragments F1 + F2 [17, 18]. In sepsis patients however, TEG/ROTEM measurements have shown conflicting results. Several studies observed no changes in parameters [19–22]; other studies reported a hypercoagulable [23] or hypocoagulable state [24]. A few studies also reported patients showing both a hyper- and hypocoagulable state [25–28]. Taken together, results are heterogeneous. Also, there is a lack of clarity on interpretation of the test results.

To date, no studies have compared conventional coagulation tests such as PT/aPTT to TEG/ROTEM in sepsis patients. However, the utility of TEG to detect DIC has been evaluated. Patients with DIC present with a hypocoagulable state [26]. This may be due to a decrease in coagulation factors used for formation of microthrombi. In support of this concept, sepsis patients who met the International Society on Thrombosis and Hemostasis (ISTH) DIC criteria showed a hypocoagulable state when compared to healthy controls, whereas patients without DIC showed a non-significant trend towards hypercoagulation [25]. Patients with an underlying disease known to be associated with DIC and ISTH DIC scores >5 had significantly prolonged reaction and K times and decreased α-angle and maximal amplitude (signs of a hypocoagulable state) compared to patients with low ISTH DIC scores. The authors developed a score, defined as the total number of parameters (R, K, maximal amplitude, and α) that were deranged in the direction of a hypocoagulable state. With this score, the discriminatory value of thromboelastometry to detect DIC improved [29]. Impaired fibrinolysis in sepsis may contribute to a hypercoagulable state. Inhibition of the fibrinolytic system was found to discriminate sepsis from postoperative controls [19, 28, 30].

In terms of prognostication, a hypercoagulable state was not found to be a predictor of outcome. In contrast, the finding of a hypocoagulable state has repeatedly been shown to be associated with a poor outcome. The TEG maximal amplitude value is an independent predictor for 28-day mortality on admission [27]. Hospital mortality was predicted by a hypocoagulable state due to a deficit in thrombin generation [30]. A hypocoagulable state measured with TEG has been found to be associated with a pro-inflammatory response [19, 24]. The degree of hypocoagulable state is also associated with severity of organ failure in sepsis [19, 22].

Taken together, results are heterogeneous. Timing of measurements may be relevant to these observations, as a hypocoagulable state may be more marked in the acute phase of sepsis and return to normal values towards discharge of ICU, or even to enhanced clot formation.

Use of TEG/ROTEM to Guide Anticoagulant Treatment in Sepsis Patients

In sepsis, activation of coagulation is a crucial step in the pathophysiological cascade of sepsis, with concomitant low levels of circulating natural anticoagulants [8, 9]. From this perspective, various treatment modalities that interfere with the coagulation system have been studied (e. g., recombinant activated protein C [rhAPC], AT and heparin) [12–15]. However, efficacy has been questioned. It can be hypothesized that TEG/ROTEM may help to identify patients likely to respond to therapies that target coagulopathy. To date, there are no studies that have addressed this question. Only a few small patient series evaluated TEG/ROTEM measurement during anticoagulant medication; ROTEM parameters did not change during anticoagulant medication. Moreover, treatment with antithrombin did not induce changes in the ROTEM measurements [23].

Use of TEG/ROTEM in Patients with Induced Hypothermia

Induced hypothermia is a common therapy in survivors of a cardiac arrest [31–33]. However, hypothermia is associated with coagulopathy, prolongation of aPTT and PT [33, 34] and an increased risk of bleeding [35]. A test that reliably detects hypothermia-induced coagulopathy would be helpful in identifying patients who have an increased bleeding risk while being cooled and sedated. Unfortunately, little is known about the value of TEG/ROTEM in these patients.

Spiel et al. observed that ROTEM measurements showed a prolonged clotting time at 1 hour after infusion of 4 °C cold crystalloid solution. All other parameters remained within reference values. An important limitation of this study was that all measurements were performed at 37 °C [33]. TEG parameters were evaluated also in patients after cardiac arrest. The TEG was performed at isothermal conditions and a hypocoagulable state was detected by TEG [36].

Use of TEG/ROTEM in Patients with Brain Injury

After severe traumatic brain injury and neurosurgery, up to 45 % of patients develop a coagulopathy [37–39]. Given the serious consequences of intracranial bleeding, instant assessment of coagulation status is desirable. Two small trials have studied the value of TEG to detect coagulopathy in these patients, and mostly found test results within reference values. However, the functional response of platelets as measured in a platelet mapping™ (TEG-PM) assay, was significantly lower in brain injury patients than in control groups, with a particularly low response in those patients who developed bleeding complications [40]. Furthermore, a hypocoagulable state on admission to the ICU is associated with worse outcome in patients with traumatic brain injury and intracranial bleeding [41].

Utility of TEG to Detect a Hypercoagulable State and Prognosticate Organ Failure in Trauma Patients

Patients who survive the acute phase of trauma are prone to develop a hypercoagulable state with increased risk of thromboembolic events and DIC [1]. Conventional coagulation tests are not able to detect such a hypercoagulable state. There is also debate as to whether the syndrome DIC is applicable to coagulation abnormalities in trauma. With TEG/ROTEM, a hypercoagulable state can be detected by high maximal amplitude and shortened reaction time (Table 1). Several reports have demonstrated a hypercoagulable state in severely injured patients with TEG/ROTEM. In trauma and burn patients admitted to the ICU, TEG was found to be more sensitive in detecting a hypercoagulable state than conventional clotting assays [42, 43]. A high maximal amplitude was found to be an independent contributor to mortality in multiple logistic regression analysis [42]. A hypercoagulable state measured by TEG predicted the development of thromboembolic events in trauma patients [44] although not all studies have confirmed this finding [45]. It should be noted that the finding of a hypercoagulable state is not specific for deep venous thrombosis (DVT).

A study on the use of ROTEM to prognosticate the occurrence of multiple organ failure in a cohort of trauma patients is currently underway.

Considerations

In several non-bleeding critically ill patient populations, evidence supporting the use of TEG/ROTEM to diagnose a hypocoagulable or hypercoagulable state is limited at this stage, mostly because of heterogeneity of the included studies in design, use of control groups and chosen endpoints. Heterogeneity of results can also be caused by differences in disease severity, as changes were more marked during severe illness. Timing of TEG/ROTEM measurements may greatly influence results, as coagulopathy is a dynamic process, e. g., evolving from subtle activation of coagulation to overt DIC in sepsis and from a hypocoagulable to a hypercoagulable state in trauma. Performing sequential measurements will probably provide better insight into the development of coagulation derangements.

Another important issue is that no uniform definitions exist for hypocoagulable or hypercoagulable states. Reference values for non-bleeding patients with disorders of coagulation are not widely assessed and cut-off values are often not defined in studies. To compare patient categories and possibly investigate therapeutic interventions in the coagulation system, validated universal reference values and definitions are essential. A study on TEG reference intervals has been recently completed (NCT01357928).

Conclusions

TEG/ROTEM can detect coagulopathy in the critically ill. Whether these tests are useful as diagnostic tools remains to be investigated when reference values and clear definitions have been established. TEG/ROTEM may be useful for prognostication of outcome. A hypocoagulable status seems to be an independent predictor for organ failure and mortality in sepsis, even after correction for disease severity. In patients with brain injury, a hypocoagulable state on admission to the ICU is also associated with worse outcome. In patients who survive the acute phase of trauma, a hypercoagulable state as detected by TEG/ROTEM is a common finding. These tests could be helpful in identifying those patients at risk of thromboembolic complications, because a hypercoagulable state predicted the development of thromboembolic events in the majority of studies. Further research on this topic is forthcoming.

References

1. Walsh TS, Stanworth SJ, Prescott RJ, Lee RJ, Watson DM, Wyncoll D (2010) Prevalence, management, and outcomes of critically ill patients with prothrombin time prolongation in United Kingdom intensive care units. Crit Care Med 38:1939–1946
2. Crowther MA, Cook DJ, Meade MO et al (2005) Thrombocytopenia in medical-surgical critically ill patients: prevalence, incidence, and risk factors. J Crit Care 20:348–353
3. Strauss R, Wehler M, Mehler K, Kreutzer D, Koebnick C, Hahn EG (2002) Thrombocytopenia in patients in the medical intensive care unit: bleeding prevalence, transfusion requirements, and outcome. Crit Care Med 30:1765–1771
4. Vanderschueren S, De Weerdt A, Malbrain M et al (2000) Thrombocytopenia and prognosis in intensive care. Crit Care Med 28:1871–1876
5. Hui P, Cook DJ, Lim W, Fraser GA, Arnold DM (2011) The frequency and clinical significance of thrombocytopenia complicating critical illness: a systematic review. Chest 139:271–278
6. Shackford SR, Davis JW, Hollingsworth-Fridlund P, Brewer NS, Hoyt DB, Mackersie RC (1990) Venous thromboembolism in patients with major trauma. Am J Surg 159:365–369
7. Singh B, Hanson AC, Alhurani R et al (2013) Trends in the incidence and outcomes of disseminated intravascular coagulation in critically ill patients (2004–2010): a population-based study. Chest 143:1235–1242
8. Dempfle CE (2004) Coagulopathy of sepsis. Thromb Haemost 91:213–224
9. Levi M, Ten CH (1999) Disseminated intravascular coagulation. N Engl J Med 341:586–592
10. Levi M, Meijers JC (2011) DIC: which laboratory tests are most useful. Blood Rev 25:33–37
11. Reikvam H, Steien E, Hauge B et al (2009) Thrombelastography. Transfus Apher Sci 40:119–123
12. Bernard GR, Vincent JL, Laterre PF et al (2001) Efficacy and safety of recombinant human activated protein C for severe sepsis. N Engl J Med 344:699–709
13. Afshari A, Wetterslev J, Brok J, Moller A (2007) Antithrombin III in critically ill patients: systematic review with meta-analysis and trial sequential analysis. BMJ 335:1248–1251
14. Abraham E, Reinhart K, Opal S et al (2003) Efficacy and safety of tifacogin (recombinant tissue factor pathway inhibitor) in severe sepsis: a randomized controlled trial. JAMA 290:238–247
15. Jaimes F, De La Rosa G, Morales C et al (2009) Unfractioned heparin for treatment of sepsis: A randomized clinical trial (The HETRASE Study). Crit Care Med 37:1185–1196
16. Schochl H, Solomon C, Schulz A et al (2011) Thromboelastometry (TEM) findings in disseminated intravascular coagulation in a pig model of endotoxinemia. Mol Med 17:266–272
17. Spiel AO, Mayr FB, Firbas C, Quehenberger P, Jilma B (2006) Validation of rotation thrombelastography in a model of systemic activation of fibrinolysis and coagulation in humans. J Thromb Haemost 4:411–416
18. Zacharowski K, Sucker C, Zacharowski P, Hartmann M (2006) Thrombelastography for the monitoring of lipopolysaccharide induced activation of coagulation. Thromb Haemost 95:557–561
19. Brenner T, Schmidt K, Delang M et al (2012) Viscoelastic and aggregometric point-of-care testing in patients with septic shock – cross-links between inflammation and haemostasis. Acta Anaesthesiol Scand 56:1277–1290
20. Durila M, Kalincik T, Jurcenko S, Pelichovska M, Hadacova I, Cvachovec K (2010) Arteriovenous differences of hematological and coagulation parameters in patients with sepsis. Blood Coagul Fibrinolysis 21:770–774
21. Altmann DR, Korte W, Maeder MT et al (2010) Elevated cardiac troponin I in sepsis and septic shock: no evidence for thrombus associated myocardial necrosis. PLoS One 5:e9017
22. Daudel F, Kessler U, Folly H et al (2009) Thromboelastometry for the assessment of coagulation abnormalities in early and established adult sepsis: a prospective cohort study. Crit Care 13:R42
23. Gonano C, Sitzwohl C, Meitner E, Weinstabl C, Kettner SC (2006) Four-day antithrombin therapy does not seem to attenuate hypercoagulability in patients suffering from sepsis. Crit Care 10:R160

24. Viljoen M, Roux LJ, Pretorius JP, Coetzee IH, Viljoen E (1995) Hemostatic competency and elastase-alpha 1-proteinase inhibitor levels in surgery, trauma, and sepsis. J Trauma 39:381–385

25. Sivula M, Pettila V, Niemi TT, Varpula M, Kuitunen AH (2009) Thromboelastometry in patients with severe sepsis and disseminated intravascular coagulation. Blood Coagul Fibrinolysis 20:419–426

26. Collins PW, Macchiavello LI, Lewis SJ et al (2006) Global tests of haemostasis in critically ill patients with severe sepsis syndrome compared to controls. Br J Haematol 135:220–227

27. Ostrowski SR, Windelov NA, Ibsen M, Haase N, Perner A, Johansson PI (2013) Consecutive thrombelastography clot strength profiles in patients with severe sepsis and their association with 28-day mortality: a prospective study. J Crit Care 28:317 e1–e11

28. Adamzik M, Langemeier T, Frey UH et al (2011) Comparison of thrombelastometry with simplified acute physiology score II and sequential organ failure assessment scores for the prediction of 30-day survival: a cohort study. Shock 35:339–342

29. Sharma P, Saxena R (2010) A novel thromboelastographic score to identify overt disseminated intravascular coagulation resulting in a hypocoagulable state. Am J Clin Pathol 134:97–102

30. Massion PB, Peters P, Ledoux D et al (2012) Persistent hypocoagulability in patients with septic shock predicts greater hospital mortality: impact of impaired thrombin generation. Intensive Care Med 38:1326–1335

31. Hypothermia after Cardiac Arrest Study Group (2002) Mild therapeutic hypothermia to improve the neurologic outcome after cardiac arrest. N Engl J Med 346:549–556

32. Bernard SA, Gray TW, Buist MD et al (2002) Treatment of comatose survivors of out-of-hospital cardiac arrest with induced hypothermia. N Engl J Med 346:557–563

33. Spiel AO, Kliegel A, Janata A et al (2009) Hemostasis in cardiac arrest patients treated with mild hypothermia initiated by cold fluids. Resuscitation 80:762–765

34. Reed RL, Bracey AW Jr., Hudson JD, Miller TA, Fischer RP (1990) Hypothermia and blood coagulation: dissociation between enzyme activity and clotting factor levels. Circ Shock 32:141–152

35. Nielsen N, Sunde K, Hovdenes J et al (2011) Adverse events and their relation to mortality in out-of-hospital cardiac arrest patients treated with therapeutic hypothermia. Crit Care Med 39:57–64

36. Cundrle I Jr, Sramek V, Pavlik M, Suk P, Radouskova I, Zvonicek V (2013) Temperature corrected thromboelastography in hypothermia: is it necessary? Eur J Anaesthesiol 30:85–89

37. Sun Y, Wang J, Wu X et al (2011) Validating the incidence of coagulopathy and disseminated intravascular coagulation in patients with traumatic brain injury – analysis of 242 cases. Br J Neurosurg 25:363–368

38. Lustenberger T, Talving P, Kobayashi L et al (2010) Time course of coagulopathy in isolated severe traumatic brain injury. Injury 41:924–928

39. Stein SC, Smith DH (2004) Coagulopathy in traumatic brain injury. Neurocrit Care 1:479–488

40. Nekludov M, Bellander BM, Blomback M, Wallen HN (2007) Platelet dysfunction in patients with severe traumatic brain injury. J Neurotrauma 24:1699–1706

41. Windelov NA, Welling KL, Ostrowski SR, Johansson PI (2011) The prognostic value of thrombelastography in identifying neurosurgical patients with worse prognosis. Blood Coagul Fibrinolysis 22:416–419

42. Park MS, Salinas J, Wade CE et al (2008) Combining early coagulation and inflammatory status improves prediction of mortality in burned and nonburned trauma patients. J Trauma 64:S188–S194

43. Gonzalez E, Kashuk JL, Moore EE, Silliman CC (2010) Differentiation of enzymatic from platelet hypercoagulability using the novel thrombelastography parameter delta (delta). J Surg Res 163:96–101

44. Schreiber MA, Differding J, Thorborg P, Mayberry JC, Mullins RJ (2005) Hypercoagulability is most prevalent early after injury and in female patients. J Trauma 58:475–480

45. Park MS, Martini WZ, Dubick MA et al (2009) Thromboelastography as a better indicator of hypercoagulable state after injury than prothrombin time or activated partial thromboplastin time. J Trauma 67:266–275
46. Kaufmann CR, Dwyer KM, Crews JD, Dols SJ, Trask AL (1997) Usefulness of thrombelastography in assessment of trauma patient coagulation. J Trauma 42:716–720

Sodium in Critical Illness: An Overview

Y. Sakr, C. Santos, and S. Rother

Introduction: Physiology of Sodium and Water Homeostasis

Water accounts for around 60 % of body weight in humans. Total body water is distributed between the extra- and intra-cellular compartments (Fig. 1). The intra-cellular space is the largest fluid compartment and contains up to two thirds of the total body water, i. e., around 30–40 % of the body weight. The extracellular compartment comprises one third of the total body water, mainly in the interstitium; only 25 % of the extracellular fluid is present in the intravascular space, i. e., 5 % of body weight. The distribution of electrolytes varies widely between the extra- and intra-cellular compartments.

Fig. 1 Fluid compartments and intra- and extracellular sodium concentrations; IVF: intravascular fluid; [Na$^+$]: Sodium concentration

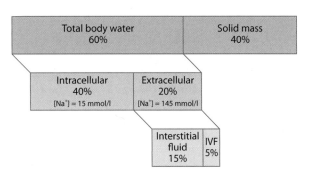

Y. Sakr ✉
Department of Anesthesiology and Intensive Care, Uniklinikum Jena, Jena, Germany
e-mail: Yasser.Sakr@med.uni-jena.de

C. Santos
Department of Intensive Care, Cassiano Antônio de Moraes University Hospital, Maruípe, Vitória-ES, Brazil

S. Rother
Department of Neurology, Helios Hanseklinikum Stralsund, 18435 Stralsund, Germany

J.-L. Vincent (Ed.), *Annual Update in Intensive Care and Emergency Medicine 2014*, DOI 10.1007/978-3-319-03746-2_44, © Springer International Publishing Switzerland 2014

Sodium is an essential electrolyte in the human organism and can be regarded as the most important extracellular cation in this compartment in terms of osmotic effect [1]. Despite fluctuations in sodium and water intake, serum sodium concentration is usually maintained within the physiologic range of 135–145 mmol/l. The concentration of extracellular sodium is 10 times greater than the intracellular sodium concentration. This concentration gradient is an important prerequisite of the transmembranous excitation process and many active transport functions of the cell membrane. To maintain this gradient, sodium is actively transported from the intracellular to the extracellular compartments by Na^+/K^+-ATPase, an ion transporter present in the cell membrane. Sodium and water homeostasis are closely related. Serum sodium concentration and subsequently serum osmolality are controlled through programmed manipulations of water homeostasis.

Sodium and its related anions, mainly bicarbonate and chloride, are responsible for approximately 86 % of the osmotic activity in blood plasma and the extracellular compartment [2]. Serum sodium concentration is crucial, therefore, for maintaining extracellular tonicity, which controls diffusion of water through the cell membrane and thus regulates extracellular volume [3, 4]. Glucose is another osmolyte that contributes to serum tonicity. Because it is not membrane-permeable, glucose remains in the extracellular compartment and is, therefore, able to draw free water from the intracellular to the extracellular compartments. In contrast, other substances, such as ethanol, methanol, and urea, are regarded as ineffective osmolytes because they can freely cross the cell membrane and hence do not produce significant fluid shifts [5]. Homeostatic mechanisms maintain serum osmolality within a narrow physiologic range between 275–290 mosmol/kgH$_2$0 [6]. The osmolality of blood plasma can be estimated using the following equation [7]:

$$\text{osmolality (mosmol/kgH}_2\text{O)} \approx 2 \times \text{sodium (mmol/l)} + \text{glucose (mmol/l)}$$
$$+ \text{ urea (mmol/l)}.$$

Regulatory Mechanisms

Water homeostasis is determined by the balance between fluid intake and fluid excretion, both of which are influenced by controlled and uncontrolled elements. Uncontrolled water intake arises from nutrition containing various amounts of water, whereas controlled water intake is adjusted by thirst sensation. Water excretion occurs in an uncontrolled fashion through the kidney during the excretion of nitrogen compounds and extrarenally in the form of insensible water loss from the skin and the respiratory tract as well as through the gastrointestinal tract. In contrast, renal excretion of free water is strictly controlled under the influence of antidiuretic hormone (ADH) [1, 8]. The controlled mechanisms of water intake and excretion are responsible for maintaining water homeostasis and compensating for the uncontrolled water intake or loss [5]. Detection of changes in serum osmolality and fluctuations in circulating blood volume are crucial in the regulation of water homeostasis.

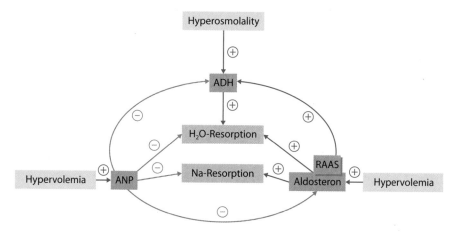

Fig. 2 Overview of the main interactions of the hormones involved in sodium and water balance. ADH: antidiuretic hormone, ANP: atrial natriuretic peptide, H₂O: water, Na: sodium, RAAS: renin-angiotensin-aldosterone system; $\longrightarrow \oplus$ Stimulation; $\longrightarrow \ominus$ Inhibition

Sodium homeostasis is strictly regulated by the kidney and through the interaction of several neuro-hormonal mechanisms (Fig. 2). These interactions involve the renin-angiotensin-aldosterone-system (RAAS), the sympathetic nervous system, atrial natriuretic peptide (ANP) and the B-type natriuretic peptide (BNP) [9] to maintain the balance between sodium intake and excretion, although regulation of sodium excretion is the key aspect of this process [5]. About 95 % of sodium excretion takes place through the kidneys and this function plays an important role in regulating extracellular volume and the related physiologic functions of various organs. This regulation is achieved mainly through the secretion of aldosterone and ANP. Other factors that have been suggested to play a minor role in this process include angiotensin II, ADH, dopamine, sympathetic activity and renal prostaglandins [5].

Disturbances of Sodium Homeostasis

Disturbance of the regulatory mechanisms mentioned above leads to deviations in serum sodium concentrations from the normal physiologic range of 135–145 mmol/l. These disturbances are generally referred to as dysnatremia, which includes both hypo- and hypernatremia, and commonly reflect disturbances in water homeostasis. Dysnatremia is one of the most commonly occurring electrolyte disturbances in hospitalized patients [2], especially in critically ill patients requiring intensive care [10].

Hyponatremia

Hyponatremia is defined as a decrease in serum sodium concentration to less than 135 mmol/l [9, 11].

Epidemiology

Hyponatremia is the most commonly occurring electrolyte disturbance in hospitalized patients, reported in up to 40 % of patients on hospital admission [12]. In critically ill patients, the reported incidence of hyponatremia was up to 30 % [13]. The frequency of hyponatremia is especially high in some subgroups of ICU patients, including neurosurgical patients with subarachnoid hemorrhage [14] and those with liver cirrhosis [15].

Etiology

Hyponatremia is characterized by a reduced proportion of sodium in relation to extracellular water. This condition essentially occurs as a result of relative or absolute excess in total body water in relation to the dissolved solutes in the extracellular compartment [5]. Two forms of hyponatremia can occur: Hypotonic and non-hypotonic.

Hypotonic Hyponatremia

Hypotonic or hypo-osmolar hyponatremia is characterized by an excess of free water in relation to the extracellular sodium content. It can, therefore, also be described as dilutional hyponatremia and represents the most common form of electrolyte disturbance in ICU patients [9]. Hypotonic hyponatremia occurs either because of water retention with subsequent dilution of electrolytes in the extracellular compartment or water depletion disproportionate to the degree of loss of electrolytes. These effects lead to hypo-osmolality and hypotonicity [16]. In the clinical setting, three main forms of hypotonic hyponatremia may occur depending on the intravascular volume: Hypovolemic, euvolemic, and hypervolemic.

*Hypo*volemic hyponatremia occurs because of deficits in both total body water and sodium content with higher sodium deficits in relation to water losses. This type of hyponatremia can have renal and extrarenal causes (Table 1). Measurement of urinary sodium concentration may be useful in identifying the underlying etiology; urinary sodium concentrations > 20 mmol/l favor renal causes and lower concentrations favor extrarenal causes [17]. Excessive use of diuretics, especially thiazide diuretics, is one of the most common causes of hypovolemic hponatremia. Osmotic diuresis is another possible cause of hypovolemic hyponatremia and commonly occurs because of hyperglycemia with glucosuria or after mannitol infusion. In patients with diabetes mellitus, ketonuria may also occur with subsequent renal sodium excretion [17]. Primary adrenal insufficiency associated with Addison's disease is characterized by aldosterone and glucocorticoid deficiency with subsequent hyponatremia from excessive sodium loss. Increased bicarbonate excretion occurs in patients with renal tubular acidosis type 2 because of deficiency of carbonic anhydrase with subsequent sodium loss. Salt-wasting nephropathy may also occur

Table 1 Etiology of hypotonic hyponatremia

1. Hypovolemic hypotonic hyponatremia	
Renal causes	Diuretic administration Primary adrenal insufficiency Cerebral salt wasting syndrome Salt losing nephropathy Osmotic diuresis (e. g., ketonuria)
Extrarenal causes	Vomiting Diarrhea Excessive sweating Third space fluid loss (e. g., burns)
2. Euovolemic hypotonic hyponatremia	
	Hypothyroidism Syndrome of inappropriate ADH secretion (SIADH) Hypophyseal insufficiency Psychiatric diseases (e. g., acute psychosis) Postoperative stress Drugs – ADH-similar (desmopressin, oxytocin) – ADH-releasing or promoting its renal effect: cyclophosphamide, carbamazepine, clofibrate, nicotine, morphine, tricyclic antidepressants, selective serotonin reuptake inhibitors, omeprazole, oral antidiabetics, ecstasy – Inhibit prostaglandin synthesis and hence increase ADH action: non-steroidal anti-inflammatory, acetylsalicylic acid, interferon vincristine – Diuretics: thiazides
3. Hypervolemic hypotonic hyponatremia	
Renal causes	Acute and chronic renal failure
Extrarenal causes	Heart failure Liver cell failure

in chronic renal diseases, such as polycystic kidneys, analgesic-induced nephropathy, or chronic pyelonephritis [17]. A clinically relevant syndrome that produces hypovolemic hyponatremia is the cerebral salt-wasting syndrome that occurs following disturbance of the hypothalamic-renal axis [18]. This rather rare syndrome occurs primarily in neurosurgical ICU patients, especially those with subarachnoid hemorrhage, traumatic brain injury, or after neurosurgical interventions [19]. The pathophysiological mechanism underlying this syndrome is not fully understood. Cerebral injury probably increases ANP and BNP release with subsequent natriuresis and polyuria leading to hypovolemia and hyponatremia [19].

Other extrarenal causes of hypovolemic hyponatremia include excessive water loss from excessive sweating, increased insensible water loss due to fever, or fluid loss into the so-called third space, which may occur in patients with inflammatory conditions, such as pancreatitis, peritonitis, intestinal obstruction, and burn injuries [16].

Clinical manifestations of hypovolemic hyponatremia are mainly related to decreased extracellular volume and include orthostatic hypotension, tachycardia, dryness of skin mucous membranes, loss of weight, and thirst sensation.

*Eu*volemic hyponatremia is characterized by a mild increase in extracellular volume with relatively normal sodium content. Diagnosis of this clinical entity is difficult because of the lack of signs of hypo- or hypervolemia. Several clinical conditions may be associated with euvolemic hyponatremia (Table 1). The syndrome of inappropriate ADH secretion (SIADH) is one of the common causes of this electrolyte disturbance and may lead to severe hyponatremia in ICU patients, with serum sodium concentrations < 120 mmol/l [20]. SIADH is characterized by increased ADH secretion as a result of suppressed osmotic or hypovolemic stimulation [21]. Several diseases may induce SIADH, including diseases of the central nervous system, such as meningitis, encephalitis, intracranial hemorrhage, traumatic brain injury, demyelinating processes, cerebrovascular accidents; lung diseases, such as pneumonia, tuberculosis; and neoplasm, such as small cell bronchial carcinoma, duodenal malignancy, or neuroblastoma [1, 16]. Disturbances at the level of the central nervous system lead to excessive ADH release, whereas peripheral diseases, such as malignant tumors, may lead to ectopic ADH production [17]. Drug-induced SIADH may also occur (e. g., carbamazepine or vincristine). The diagnosis of SIADH should be established after exclusion of other possible causes of increased ADH secretion [11]. The major diagnostic criteria include a decrease in the effective osmolality of the extracellular fluid (< 270 mosmol/kg water), inadequate urinary concentration (urine osmolality > 100 mosmol/kg water despite normal renal function), euvolemia, increased urinary sodium excretion despite normal salt and water intake, and the absence of other euovolemic hyposmolar conditions [21]. Minor diagnostic criteria include an abnormal water challenge test, demonstrating the inability to excrete 90 % of an enteral water load (20 ml/kg) within 4 hours or failure to dilute urine to < 100 mosmol/kg water, a high ADH plasma level despite low plasma osmolality, and no improvement in hyponatremia after volume expansion but improvement after volume restriction [22].

Other disease entities may also be associated with euvolemic hyponatremia (Table 1). Hypothyroidism, hypophyseal insufficiency with secondary adrenal insufficiency and glucocorticoid deficiency can be overlooked causes of euvolemic hyponatremia. Postoperative stress may also play an important role in the development of hyponatremia in surgical ICUs [23]. Several drugs may also stimulate ADH secretion or promote its renal effects [7].

*Hyper*volemic hyponatremia is a condition in which both extracellular volume and sodium content are increased, but the increase in extracellular volume is more pronounced than the increase in sodium content. The underlying etiology is advanced heart failure, liver cell failure, or nephrotic syndrome. The underlying pathophysiology is a disturbance in hypothalamic osmotic regulation. Impairment of renal tubular function, e. g., in patients with acute or chronic renal failure, leads to inadequate water and sodium excretion and predisposes to hypervolemic hyponatremia [11]. The clinical presentation is characterized by edema, ascites, and pleural effusion.

Non-hypotonic Hyponatremia

Pseudohyponatremia is a rare condition characterized by normal serum osmolality and may be observed in patients with hyperlipidemia or paraproteinemias (e. g., multiple myeloma and hypergammaglobulinemia) due to a relative increase in the solid phase of plasma, which leads to artificially low measured serum sodium concentrations [9]. Infusion of solutions with an isotonic character, such as mannitol, which do not produce a transcellular water shift may also lead to hyponatremia with normal serum osmolality [16].

Hyperosmolar or translocational hyponatremia is another rare form of non-hypotonic hyponatremia in which total body water remains unaltered. Serum osmolality increases because of the presence of additional osmotically active particles, such as glucose in advanced hyperglycemia, hypertonic mannitol, or intravenous contrast substances, with subsequent water shift from the intracellular to the extracellular compartments and hyponatremia [11]. Hyperglycemia is the most common cause of translocational hyponatremia [16]. The so-called transuretheral resection syndrome (TUR-syndrome) may also predispose to translocational hyperosmolar hyponatremia because of the osmotically active particles (e. g., mannitol, glycin, sorbitol) in the urethral irrigation solution, which produce water shift.

Clinical manifestations

Mild hyponatremia (130–135 mmol/l) is usually asymptomatic, but further decrease in serum sodium concentration leads to non-specific symptoms in the form of concentration deficits, apathy, loss of appetite, headache, dizziness, nausea, and vomiting. With increased severity of hyponatremia, clinical manifestations of encephalopathy become evident in the form of lethargy, restlessness, disorientation, muscle cramps, and hyporeflexia [16, 24].

Cerebral manifestations dominate the clinical picture of hyponatremia and can be referred to as hyponatremic encephalopathy [25]. Extracellular hypo-osmolality leads to water diffusion into the brain cells with a concomitant increase in intracellular volume. Cellular swelling (brain edema) can occur within a few minutes. However, adaptive mechanisms are present in the brain cells to maintain intracellular volume constant and prevent the development of brain edema. A rapid adaptive response (1–3 seconds) occurs due to the increase in the interstitial pressure, allowing part of the extracellular volume to be transmitted to the cerebrospinal fluid and back to the systemic circulation [11]. Solutes, such as sodium and potassium (salts), are transported actively outside the brain cells within hours with subsequent water shift to the extracellular compartment [26]. Another adaptive process that occurs over days involves active transport of organic osmolytes (phosphocreatine, myoinositol, glutamate, and taurine) outside the brain cells with secondary water diffusion [11, 26]. The net result of these adaptive mechanisms is a reduction in brain volume and reduction in brain edema. Under the effect of hypo-osmolality and with a delay in the previously described adaptive mechanisms, the increase in brain volume may lead to increased intracranial pressure (ICP) because of the limited intracranial space. The increased ICP may produce life-threatening complications due to brain injury [27].

The severity of the clinical presentation is not only related to the severity of the hyponatremia but also to the duration over which hyponatremia develops [2].

Therapeutic approaches

The presence and severity of clinical manifestations as well as the duration of development of hyponatremia are the main factors that influence therapeutic decisions. Causal therapy is also important, especially in patients with adrenal insufficiency or hypothyroidism. Acute hyponatremia, occurring within 48 hours and accompanied by neurologic symptoms, requires immediate therapy to prevent possible complications related to brain edema. In such patients, hyponatremia should be corrected with the aim of increasing serum sodium concentration at a rate of 1–2 mmol/l/h over the first few hours until improvement of clinical symptoms. Daily correction rates should not exceed 8–10 mmol/l over the first 24 hours or 18–25 mmol/l over the first 48 hours [28].

Chronic hyponatremia should be corrected slowly to avoid osmotic demyelinating syndromes [16, 29]. The osmotic stress related to therapy induces osmolyte and water shifts from the intracellular to the extracellular compartments and shrinkage of brain cells with subsequent demyelination of the pontine and extrapontine neurons. This leads to increased neurological manifestations with additional symptoms related to the severity and the site of lesions, including convulsions, pseudobulbar paralysis, dysarthria, tetraplegia, coma, and death [16, 24]. Central pontine (CPM) or extrapontine myelinosis (IPM) are the most common clinical variants and occur 2–3 days after correction of hyponatremia [30]. Common predisposing factors for these syndromes include alcohol intake, female sex, nutritional deficiency, hypokalemia, burn injuries, and thiazide therapy [31].

The amount of sodium to be administered can be calculated according to the following formula:

$$\text{Na}^+ \text{ administered (mEq)} = [\text{Na}^+ \text{ desired}]$$
$$- [\text{Na}^+ \text{ measured} \times \text{total body water (TBW)}]$$

with TBW = 0.6 × weight (kg) for men, and 0.5 × weight (kg) for women [32].

The choice of therapy should take into consideration the underlying pathophysiology and the clinical variant of hyponatremia [33]. The main therapeutic options include hypertonic (3 %) and isotonic (0.9 %) sodium chloride solutions, fluid restriction, ADH receptor antagonists (vaptans, urea, and demeclocycline) [34]. In cases of hypervolemia, loop diuretics (e. g., furosemide) may also be used [33]. Hypertonic solutions can be used to correct acute hyponatremia with serious neurologic manifestations, whereas isotonic solutions are recommended in patients with volume depletion. Fluid restriction can be useful to correct chronic asymptomatic hyponatremia (euvolemic or hypervolemic) in which negative fluid balance is targeted to raise serum sodium concentrations. In patients with reduced compliance to fluid restriction, demeclocycline (ADH antagonist), urea (osmotic diuresis of free water) or a vaptan can be considered as alternative therapeutic options [11]. Vaptans are non-peptide oral ADH receptor antagonists, e. g., tolvaptan, which selectively binds V2-receptors in the distal nephron with subsequent excretion of solute-free water [35]. Tolvaptan is recommended for the therapy of euvolemic (SIADH) and hypervolemic hyponatremia as well as in patients with heart or liver cell failure [36].

Hypernatremia

Hypernatremia is defined as a serum sodium concentration greater than 145 mmol/l [3].

Epidemiology
Hypernatremia occurs less commonly than does hyponatremia. The prevalence of hypernatremia in hospitalized patients has been reported as between 0.2 and 1 % [37, 38]. Hospital-acquired hyponatremia occurs in 0.6–2.1 % of patients [39, 40]. In ICU patients, the incidence of hypernatremia is 2–52 % [41, 42]. Several factors predispose to hypernatremia in ICU patients, including disturbed consciousness, sedation, severe brain injury, increased fluid loss (gastrointestinal, drainage fluids, open wounds, and insensible fluid loss due to fever or mechanical ventilation), the use of osmotic diuretics using mannitol to reduce ICP, or the use of hypertonic and salt-containing fluids. Neurosurgical patients are at especially high risk of developing hypernatremia because many of these factors are present simultaneously in these patients [1, 43].

Etiology
Hypernatremia occurs due to an absolute or relative deficit of total body water relative to its sodium content, mainly because of disturbances in the body's defense mechanisms against hyperosmolarity, i. e., ADH secretion and thirst sensation. The perception of thirst can be impaired or absent as a result of disturbed consciousness, structural hypothalamic lesions in the thirst center, or extreme age [9]. The common underlying pathophysiology is a combination of impaired water intake and excessive fluid loss [37]. Three clinical entities can be differentiated according to the extracellular volume status: hypovolemic, euvolemic, and hypervolemic.

Hypovolemic Hypernatremia
Hypovolemic hypernatremia occurs due to loss of both water and sodium with predominant hypotonic water loss. Renal and extrarenal causes may be responsible for this condition (Table 2). Clinical manifestations of hypovolemia are evident in these patients, and include orthostatic hypotension, tachycardia, decreased skin turgor, dry mucous membranes, and sometimes disturbance of consciousness [17].

Euovolemic Hypernatremia
Euovolemic hypernatremia is the most common form of hypernatremia in clinical practice [1]. It occurs due to pure water loss without concomitant sodium excretion

Table 2 Etiology of hypernatremia

1. Hypovolemic hypernatremia	
Renal losses	Osmotic and loop diuretics
	Post-obstructive diuresis
	Polyuric phase of acute tubular necrosis
	Intrinsic renal diseases
Extrarenal losses	Gastrointestinal losses
	– Diarrhea
	– Vomiting
	– Nasogastric reflux
	– Entro-cutaneous fistulas
	– Oral administration of osmotically active drugs
	Excessive sweating
	Burn injuries
	Open surgical wounds
2. Euovolemic hypernatremia	
Renal losses	Diabetes insipidus (central or nephrogenic)
	Hypodipsia
Extrarenal losses	Insensible water loss
	– Cutaneous
	– Respiratory
3. Hypervolemic hypernatremia	
	Hypertonic fluid administration (NaCl 3 %)
	$NaHCO_3$ infusion or salt-rich emetics
	Excessive sodium intake (e. g., salt tablets)
	Hypertonic dialysis
	Primary hyperaldosteronism (Conn's syndrome)
	Cushing's syndrome

and is particularly common in ICU patients. Several conditions are associated with euovolemic hypernatremia in hospitalized patients (Table 2).

Diabetes insipidus (DI) is an important cause of euovolemic hypernatremia in ICU patients [25]. The clinical picture of this syndrome is characterized by hypo-osmolar polyuria and polydipsia due to impairment of the ability of the kidney to concentrate urine. Two clinical variants can be differentiated: Central and nephrogenic DI. Central DI occurs as a result of ADH deficiency. Structural damage of the hypothalamic core region, injury to the tractus supraptic-hypophysis or destruction of the posterior lobe of the pituitary gland play an important role in the pathogenesis of this syndrome [44]. Congenital forms of central DI can occur due to autosomal dominant gene mutation (ADH-neurophysin) [5]. Acquired central DI may also occur for various reasons, including traumatic brain injury, neoplasia (meningioma, hypophyseal tumors, lymphoma, and cerebral metastases), infectious diseases (meningitis and encephalitis), infiltrative conditions (sarcoidosis, histocytosis, and tuberculosis), vascular injuries (aneurysmal subarachnoid and intracranial hemorrhage and cerebrovascular accidents), and drug-induced (ethanol and phenytoin) [5, 9].

Nephrogenic DI is characterized by a defective renal response to ADH stimulation. Severe forms are rare and occur mostly in congenital renal diseases [5, 9]. More common, mild forms occur in acquired nephrogenic DI [17]. The most common cause of acquired DI is long term lithium treatment and electrolyte disturbances such as hypercalcemia and hypokalemia [45]. Diagnostic criteria for DI are urine osmolality > 800 mosmol/kg H_2O with concomitantly increased serum osmolality > 295 mosmol/kg H_2O or hypernatremia > 145 mmol/l [9]. Administration of ADH or desmopressin (a V_2-receptor agonist that increases urinary osmolality only in central DI) [46] and measurement of ADH serum levels (low in cerebral but normal or high in nephrogenic DI) may help differentiate between central and nephrogenic forms of DI.

Hypervolemic Hypernatremia

Hypervolemic hypernatremia is a rather rare form of hypernatremia, which occurs because of an increase in sodium content following infusion of excessive amounts of hypertonic fluids containing sodium, i. e., iatrogenic, or because of excessive salt intake [1, 24].

Clinical manifestations

Hypernatremia is mainly characterized by neurologic disturbances. Acute hypernatremia leads to water shift from the intracellular to the extracellular fluid compartments because of hyperosmolality with subsequent cellular dehydration, cellular shrinkage, and decreased cell volume. Brain cells are able to react to decreased cell volume with adaptive responses to prevent cellular dehydration and its consequences. These responses occur through intracellular accumulation of osmotically active particles, such as sodium, potassium, and chloride ions [47]. In cases of a persistent increase in plasma osmolality, organic osmolytes, such as polyoles (sorbitol, myoinositol), aminoacids or aminoacid-derivates (alanine, glutamine, glutamate, taurine), and methylamine (glyceryl phosphorylcholine, beataine), accumulate intracellularly [47]. Accumulation of organic compounds takes a few hours to occur, however, because this process involves transcription and synthesis of organic osmolytes [47]. The adaptive mechanisms aim at increasing intracellular osmolality with subsequent restoration of cellular volume.

Similar to hyponatremia, the severity of hypernatremia and the rate of increase in serum sodium levels together determine the severity of the clinical presentation [8, 9]. Initial symptoms are non-specific and include loss of appetite, restlessness, nausea, vomiting, muscle weakness, and lethargy [2, 9]. Severe symptoms occur mostly in acute severe hypernatremia with serum sodium levels > 160 mmol/l and include hyperreflexia, spasticity, disturbed consciousness, and coma. If the brain cells fail to adapt rapidly to the extracellular hyperosmolality, severe complications may occur due to decreased cell volume, which may ultimately lead to rupture of meningeal blood vessels with subsequent intracranial or subarachnoid hemorrhage and brain injury [48]. Osmotic myelinolysis is a serious complication of hypernatremia that has been reported in experimental models and in clinical settings [30, 49].

Persistent hypernatremia and the resulting hyperosmolality may also negatively influence organ function. Cardiac dysfunction may occur because of reduced left ventricular contractility [50]. Impaired glucose metabolism has also been reported in association with severe hypernatremia with increased insulin-resistance and hyperglycemia [51] or impaired hepatic gluconeogenesis and lactate clearance [52]. The immunological function of leukocytes may also be suppressed by hypernatremia [53], and severe hypernatremia may produce rhabdomyolysis and acute renal failure [54].

In patients with hypernatremia of long duration, rapid correction with hypotonic fluids induces rapid intracellular fluid shift and may lead to life-threatening brain edema, coma, and death [55].

Therapeutic approaches

Treatment of hypernatremia should be oriented to the etiology, severity, and the rate of increase in serum sodium concentration [6]. Causal therapy is based on preventing further fluid losses with, for example, use of antipyretic therapy, treatment of infectious diseases, adequate substitution and prevention of gatrointestinal losses, treatment of hyperglycemia and associated electrolyte disturbances (hypokalemia and hypercalcemia), in addition to termination of any therapy that may be responsible for hypernatremia, such as diuretics, lactulose, or salt-rich infusions.

In symptomatic acute hypernatremia (onset < 48 hours), correction can be relatively rapid with a maximal correction rate of 2–3 mmol/l per hour over the first hours of therapy and should not exceed 12 mmol/l per day [56]. These correction rates can be tolerated by the brain cells as the adaptive mechanisms to cellular dehydration require longer periods of time [57]. However, chronic hypernatremia (onset > 48 hours) requires slow correction with a rate not exceeding 0.5 mmol/l per hour and a maximal daily rate of 10 mmol/l [3].

The water deficit can be calculated using the following formula:

$$\text{Water deficit (L)} = \text{TBW} \times [1 - (\text{desired Na}^+/\text{serum Na}^+)]$$

with TBW = 0.6 × weight (kg) for men and 0.5 × weight (kg) for women [32].

Correction of hypernatremia varies according to the underlying pathophysiology (fluid loss or excess sodium intake) and the status of the extracellular volume (hypovolemia, euvolemia, or hypervolemia) but can be basically achieved using hypotonic fluids (electrolyte free solutions e. g., 5 % glucose solutions or 0.45 % sodium chloride solution) [3]. In hypovolemic hypernatremia associated with hemodynamic instability, isotonic 0.9 % sodium chloride solutions may also be used to correct hypovolemia and replace fluid loss. After hemodynamic stabilization, correction of water deficit can be performed using 5 % glucose or 0.45 % sodium chloride solutions [17]. In patients with hyperglycemia, 0.45 % sodium chloride is the treatment of choice to correct hypertonicity rather than 5 % glucose solutions [56]. In patients with euvolemic hypernatremia, water deficits should also be replaced by hypotonic solutions. The treatment of central DI also includes the use of desmopressin (intranasal, oral, or subcutaneous) [58]. Nephrogenic DI is treated by correction of hypokalemia and termination of any drugs that may be responsible for the syndrome [6, 17]. The treatment of hypervolemic hypernatremia should focus on the elimination of excess sodium. Sodium-containing infusions should be discontinued with restriction of salt intake. Loop diuretics can be used to promote renal sodium excretion and achieve euvolemia. In addition, hypotonic solutions should be used concomitantly to maintain fluid homeostasis and correct hyperosmolality, preferably using 5 % glucose solutions [17]. In the specific situation in which hypernatremia occurs in a patient with renal failure due to increased sodium intake, renal replacement therapies, such as hemofiltration, hemodialysis, or peritoneal dialysis can be considered [25].

Dysnatremia and Outcome

Symptomatic hyponatremia associated with neurologic manifestations has been reported to be associated with mortality rates of 50 % [59]. Mortality rates for patients with primary hyponatremia, present on hospital admission, are cited as between 3.4–22.5 % [60, 61], whereas for those who develop hyponatremia during the ICU stay rates of 2.9–15 % have been reported [60, 62]. Critically ill patients admitted to the ICU are especially at risk of worse outcome from hyponatremia. Mortality rates ranging from 23.8–73.1 % [15, 63] and from 10.5–28 % [10, 64] were reported in ICU patients suffering from primary and secondary hyponatremia, respectively.

Hypernatremia has also been reported to be associated with worse outcomes in hospitalized patients, especially those admitted to the ICU [37, 40, 41, 65]. Hospitalized geriatric patients suffering from hypernatremia have mortality rates ranging from 26–79.2 % [61, 66]. Acquired hypernatremia in unselected hospitalized patients is also associated with mortality rates ranging from 41–66 % [37, 67]. Mortality rates between 23–43 % have been reported in patients with hypernatremia on ICU admission [41, 68] and 13.6–48 % in patients with ICU-acquired hypernatremia [64, 65].

The high mortality rates in patients with dysnatremia may be explained, at least in part, by the increased severity of illness, associated comorbidities, and associated neurological complications in these patients. Nonetheless, dysnatremia is independently associated with a higher risk of death in ICU patients, especially surgical ICU patients [69].

In the ICU setting, several factors predispose to changes in serum sodium level, both disease-related and as an effect of therapeutic interventions. This effect may lead to considerable fluctuations in serum sodium concentrations. Some 3.6–6.4 % of ICU patients will have both hypo- and hypernatremia at some time during the ICU stay [10, 64], and mixed dysnatremia may be associated with mortality rates of up to 42 % [70]. Moreover, in postoperative ICU patients there is a dose-effect relationship between fluctuation in serum sodium levels and outcome [64, 69]. Indeed, even fluctuations in serum sodium concentrations within the normal range have been reported to be associated with a higher risk of death in surgical ICU patients [69].

Conclusions

Sodium homeostasis is strictly regulated by the kidney and through the interaction of several neuro-hormonal mechanisms. Dysnatremia is one of the most commonly occurring electrolyte disturbances in hospitalized patients, especially in critically ill patients requiring intensive care, and is associated with poor outcome in these patients. Hyponatremia is characterized by a reduced proportion of sodium in relation to extracellular water. Hypernatremia occurs due to an absolute or relative deficit of total body water relative to its sodium content. Cerebral manifestations dominate the clinical picture of dysnatremia. The severity of the clinical presentation is related to both the severity of the dysnatremia and the duration over which dysnatremia develops. The presence and severity of clinical manifestations and the underlying etiology as well as the duration of development of dysnatremia are the main factors that influence therapeutic decisions.

References

1. Tisdall M, Crocker M, Watkiss J, Smith M (2006) Disturbances of sodium in critically ill adult neurologic patients: a clinical review. J Neurosurg Anesthesiol 18:57–63
2. Reynolds RM, Padfield PL, Seckl JR (2006) Disorders of sodium balance. BMJ 332:702–705
3. Adrogue HJ, Madias NE (2000) Hypernatremia. N Engl J Med 342:1493–1499
4. Weiss-Guillet EM, Takala J, Jakob SM (2003) Diagnosis and management of electrolyte emergencies. Best Pract Res Clin Endocrinol Metab 17:623–651
5. Verbalis JG (2003) Disorders of body water homeostasis. Best Pract Res Clin Endocrinol Metab 17:471–503
6. Kraft MD, Btaiche IF, Sacks GS, Kudsk KA (2005) Treatment of electrolyte disorders in adult patients in the intensive care unit. Am J Health Syst Pharm 62:1663–1682
7. Lichtwarck-Aschoff M, Dietrich B, Breitschaft D (2009) Disorders of water and sodium balance in intensive care patients. Anaesthesist 58:543–560
8. Gennari FJ (1984) Current concepts. Serum osmolality. Uses and limitations. N Engl J Med 310:102–105
9. Bagshaw SM, Townsend DR, McDermid RC (2009) Disorders of sodium and water balance in hospitalized patients. Can J Anaesth 56:151–167
10. Stelfox HT, Ahmed SB, Khandwala F, Zygun D, Shahpori R, Laupland K (2008) The epidemiology of intensive care unit-acquired hyponatraemia and hypernatraemia in medical-surgical intensive care units. Crit Care 12:R162
11. Schrier RW, Bansal S (2008) Diagnosis and management of hyponatremia in acute illness. Curr Opin Crit Care 14:627–634
12. Hoorn EJ, Lindemans J, Zietse R (2006) Development of severe hyponatraemia in hospitalized patients: treatment-related risk factors and inadequate management. Nephrol Dial Transplant 21:70–76
13. DeVita MV, Gardenswartz MH, Konecky A, Zabetakis PM (1990) Incidence and etiology of hyponatremia in an intensive care unit. Clin Nephrol 34:163–166
14. Hasan D, Wijdicks EF, Vermeulen M (1990) Hyponatremia is associated with cerebral ischemia in patients with aneurysmal subarachnoid hemorrhage. Ann Neurol 27:106–108

15. Jenq CC, Tsai MH, Tian YC et al (2010) Serum sodium predicts prognosis in critically ill cirrhotic patients. J Clin Gastroenterol 44:220–226
16. Adrogue HJ, Madias NE (2000) Hyponatremia. N Engl J Med 342:1581–1589
17. Kumar S, Berl T (1998) Sodium. Lancet 352:220–228
18. Cort JH (1954) Cerebral salt wasting. Lancet 266:752–754
19. Betjes MG (2002) Hyponatremia in acute brain disease: the cerebral salt wasting syndrome. Eur J Intern Med 13:9–14
20. Anderson RJ, Chung HM, Kluge R, Schrier RW (1985) Hyponatremia: a prospective analysis of its epidemiology and the pathogenetic role of vasopressin. Ann Intern Med 102:164–168
21. Bartter FC, Schwartz WB (1967) The syndrome of inappropriate secretion of antidiuretic hormone. Am J Med 42:790–806
22. Verbalis JG (1997) The syndrome of inappropriate antidiuretic hormone. In: Schrier RW, Gottschalk CW (eds) Diseases of the Kidney, 6th edn. Little Brown & Co, Boston, p 2400
23. Chung HM, Kluge R, Schrier RW, Anderson RJ (1986) Postoperative hyponatremia. A prospective study. Arch Intern Med 146:333–336
24. Pokaharel M, Block CA (2011) Dysnatremia in the ICU. Curr Opin Crit Care 17:581–593
25. Moritz ML, Ayus JC (2004) Dysnatremias in the critical care setting. Contrib Nephrol 144:132–157
26. Gullans SR, Verbalis JG (1993) Control of brain volume during hyperosmolar and hypoosmolar conditions. Annu Rev Med 44:289–301
27. Arieff AI, Llach F, Massry SG (1976) Neurological manifestations and morbidity of hyponatremia: correlation with brain water and electrolytes. Medicine (Baltimore) 55:121–129
28. Ellison DH, Berl T (2007) Clinical practice. The syndrome of inappropriate antidiuresis. N Engl J Med 356:2064–2072
29. Sterns RH, Riggs JE, Schochet SS Jr (1986) Osmotic demyelination syndrome following correction of hyponatremia. N Engl J Med 314:1535–1542
30. Brown WD (2000) Osmotic demyelination disorders: central pontine and extrapontine myelinolysis. Curr Opin Neurol 13:691–697
31. Lauriat SM, Berl T (1997) The hyponatremic patient: practical focus on therapy. J Am Soc Nephrol 8:1599–1607
32. Nacul FE (2010) Disorders of electrolytes. In: O'Donnell JM, Nacul FE (eds) Surgical Intensive Care Medicine. Springer Science & Business Media, New York, pp 439–451
33. Hoorn EJ, Zietse R (2008) Hyponatremia revisited: translating physiology to practice. Nephron Physiol 108:46–59
34. Verbalis JG, Goldsmith SR, Greenberg A, Schrier RW, Sterns RH (2007) Hyponatremia treatment guidelines 2007: expert panel recommendations. Am J Med 120:S1–S21
35. Schrier RW, Gross P, Gheorghiade M et al (2006) Tolvaptan, a selective oral vasopressin V2-receptor antagonist, for hyponatremia. N Engl J Med 355:2099–2112
36. Verbalis JG (2002) Vasopressin V2 receptor antagonists. J Mol Endocrinol 29:1–9
37. Palevsky PM, Bhagrath R, Greenberg A (1996) Hypernatremia in hospitalized patients. Ann Intern Med 124:197–203
38. Liamis G, Tsimihodimos V, Doumas M, Spyrou A, Bairaktari E, Elisaf M (2008) Clinical and laboratory characteristics of hypernatraemia in an internal medicine clinic. Nephrol Dial Transplant 23:136–143
39. O'Connor KA, Cotter PE, Kingston M, Twomey C, O'Mahony D (2006) The pattern of plasma sodium abnormalities in an acute elderly care ward: a cross-sectional study. Ir J Med Sci 175:28–31
40. Snyder NA, Feigal DW, Arieff AI (1987) Hypernatremia in elderly patients. A heterogeneous, morbid, and iatrogenic entity. Ann Intern Med 107:309–319

41. Lindner G, Funk GC, Schwarz C et al (2007) Hypernatremia in the critically ill is an independent risk factor for mortality. Am J Kidney Dis 50:952–957
42. Maggiore U, Picetti E, Antonucci E et al (2009) The relation between the incidence of hypernatremia and mortality in patients with severe traumatic brain injury. Crit Care 13:R110
43. Aiyagari V, Deibert E, Diringer MN (2006) Hypernatremia in the neurologic intensive care unit: how high is too high? J Crit Care 21:163–172
44. Shucart WA, Jackson I (1976) Management of diabetes insipidus in neurosurgical patients. J Neurosurg 44:65–71
45. Garofeanu CG, Weir M, Rosas-Arellano MP, Henson G, Garg AX, Clark WF (2005) Causes of reversible nephrogenic diabetes insipidus: a systematic review. Am J Kidney Dis 45:626–637
46. Robinson AG (1985) Disorders of antidiuretic hormone secretion. Clin Endocrinol Metab 14:55–88
47. McManus ML, Churchwell KB, Strange K (1995) Regulation of cell volume in health and disease. N Engl J Med 333:1260–1266
48. Arora SK (2013) Hypernatremic disorders in the intensive care unit. J Intensive Care Med 28:37–45
49. Soupart A, Penninckx R, Namias B, Stenuit A, Perier O, Decaux G (1996) Brain myelinolysis following hypernatremia in rats. J Neuropathol Exp Neurol 55:106–113
50. Lenz K, Gossinger H, Laggner A, Druml W, Grimm G, Schneeweiss B (1986) Influence of hypernatremic-hyperosmolar state on hemodynamics of patients with normal and depressed myocardial function. Crit Care Med 14:913–914
51. Bratusch-Marrain PR, DeFronzo RA (1983) Impairment of insulin-mediated glucose metabolism by hyperosmolality in man. Diabetes 32:1028–1034
52. Druml W, Kleinberger G, Lenz K, Laggner A, Schneeweiss B (1986) Fructose-induced hyperlactemia in hyperosmolar syndromes. Klin Wochenschr 64:615–618
53. Kuroda T, Harada T, Tsutsumi H, Kobayashi M (1997) Hypernatremic suppression of neutrophils. Burns 23:338–340
54. Rosa EC, Lopes AC, Liberatori Filho AW, Schor N (1997) Rhabdomyolysis due to hyperosmolarity leading to acute renal failure. Ren Fail 19:295–301
55. Oh MS, Carroll HJ (1992) Disorders of sodium metabolism: hypernatremia and hyponatremia. Crit Care Med 20:94–103
56. Lindner G, Funk GC (2013) Hypernatremia in critically ill patients. J Crit Care 28:216.e11–216.e20
57. Lien YH, Shapiro JI, Chan L (1990) Effects of hypernatremia on organic brain osmoles. J Clin Invest 85:1427–1435
58. Richardson DW, Robinson AG (1985) Desmopressin. Ann Intern Med 103:228–239
59. Arieff AI (1988) Osmotic failure: physiology and strategies for treatment. Hosp Pract 23:173–174
60. Wald R, Jaber BL, Price LL, Upadhyay A, Madias NE (2010) Impact of hospital-associated hyponatremia on selected outcomes. Arch Intern Med 170:294–302
61. Whelan B, Bennett K, O'Riordan D, Silke B (2009) Serum sodium as a risk factor for in-hospital mortality in acute unselected general medical patients. QJM 102:175–182
62. Herrod PJ, Awad S, Redfern A, Morgan L, Lobo DN (2010) Hypo- and hypernatraemia in surgical patients: is there room for improvement? World J Surg 34:495–499
63. Funk GC, Lindner G, Druml W et al (2010) Incidence and prognosis of dysnatremias present on ICU admission. Intensive Care Med 36:304–311
64. Stelfox HT, Ahmed SB, Zygun D, Khandwala F, Laupland K (2010) Characterization of intensive care unit acquired hyponatremia and hypernatremia following cardiac surgery. Can J Anaesth 57:650–658

65. Hoorn EJ, Betjes MG, Weigel J, Zietse R (2008) Hypernatraemia in critically ill patients: too little water and too much salt. Nephrol Dial Transplant 23:1562–1568
66. Bhatnagar D, Weinkove C (1988) Serious hypernatraemia in a hospital population. Postgrad Med J 64:441–443
67. Mandal AK, Saklayen MG, Hillman NM, Markert RJ (1997) Predictive factors for high mortality in hypernatremic patients. Am J Emerg Med 15:130–132
68. Wu CJ, Li CS (2009) The impact of iatrogenic hypernatremia on the prognosis of critical patients. Zhongguo Wei Zhong Bing Ji Jiu Yi Xue 21:474–477
69. Sakr Y, Rother S, Ferreira AM et al (2013) Fluctuations in serum sodium level are associated with an increased risk of death in surgical ICU patients. Crit Care Med 41:133–142
70. Neithercut WD, Spooner RJ (1988) Nosocomial dysnatremia. Clin Chem 34:2239–2240

Continuous Glucose Monitoring Devices for Use in the ICU

R. T. M. van Hooijdonk, J. H. Leopold, and M. J. Schultz

Introduction

Many critically ill patients are treated with insulin for shorter or longer periods during their stay in the intensive care unit (ICU) [1]. Intensive monitoring of the blood glucose level is a prerequisite for efficient and safe insulin titration in these patients [2]. Glucose levels are currently monitored manually in the ICU by intermittent measurements of the blood glucose level in central laboratories or using laboratory-based blood gas analyzers and/or glucose strips at the bedside [3]. Intermittent manual glucose monitoring, however, is impractical and expensive, time and blood consuming [4], and could even cause dangerous insulin titration errors in critically ill patients [5].

Glucose monitoring through so-called continuous glucose monitoring (CGM) could overcome some of the shortcomings and drawbacks of intermittent manual glucose monitoring. Specifically, CGM could allow for smoother insulin adjustments based on trends of the glucose level visualized on a monitor [3]. Several CGM devices for use in the ICU are being developed. These all require thorough accuracy testing in diverse cohorts of critically ill patient before they can be implemented in daily ICU practice.

This chapter provides an overview of the diverse CGM techniques and CGM devices intended for use in the ICU. This chapter also deals with how point and trend accuracy of CGM systems could be studied in critically ill patients and how accuracy results could be reported.

R. T. M. van Hooijdonk ✉ · J. H. Leopold · M. J. Schultz
Department of Intensive Care, Academic Medical Center, University of Amsterdam, Amsterdam, Netherlands
e-mail: r.t.vanhooijdonk@amc.uva.nl

J.-L. Vincent (Ed.), *Annual Update in Intensive Care and Emergency Medicine 2014*, 613
DOI 10.1007/978-3-319-03746-2_45, © Springer International Publishing Switzerland 2014

Search Strategy

We searched MEDLINE (1966–2013) using the following search terms: ('intensive care'[MeSH Terms] OR 'intensive care'[tiab]) OR 'critical care'[MeSH Terms] OR 'critical care'[tiab] OR ('critical illness'[MeSH Terms] OR 'critical illness'[tiab]) AND 'glucose'[tiab] AND ('continuous glucose monitoring'[tiab] OR 'continuous glucose measurement'[tiab] OR 'CGM'[tiab]). Retrieved articles, and cross-referenced studies from those articles, were screened for pertinent information. Articles were selected if they evaluated a CGM device intended for use in ICU patients. Articles reporting on studies in animals were excluded, as were articles reporting on studies of CGM in populations other than ICU patients. Revisions and articles that did not report outcomes of interest were also excluded, and if duplicate articles of the same study were found in abstract form or other articles, we considered the most complete data set.

We then performed an internet search, using similar search terms in Google™. We visited commercial websites identified by this search and looked for pertinent information. We also visited websites of medical congresses for information and abstracts of studies that had not yet been published.

In August 2013, the two searches identified several CGM devices that were already available for use, as well as devices that were in a developmental phase (Table 1). Studies concerning CGM accuracy in critically ill patients were very limited, and the results of most studies were only available on commercial websites or in abstracts presented at medical congresses.

CGM Devices

Common to all CGM devices is that they measure glucose levels continuously, or intermittently but frequently, but in different body fluids (i. e., whole blood, plasma, dialysate, or interstitial fluid) using dissimilar procedures (e. g., automated blood draws, or no blood draws at all) and distinctive measurement techniques (i. e., based on a chemical reaction, or using fluorescence or spectroscopy) (Table 1).

Measurement in plasma is considered the 'gold standard' for intermittent glucose measurements in the ICU setting, but of all the CGM devices only one device is reported to measure glucose levels in automated bedside-prepared plasma (OptiScanner). Other devices measure glucose levels in whole blood (GlySure, GluCath, and GlucoClear), dialysate from blood (Eirus and Diramo) or interstitial body fluids (Sentrino, Symphony, and GlucoDay).

CGM devices are reported to measure the glucose level in venous blood via a sensor inserted through a peripheral venous catheter (GluCath) or a central venous catheter (GlySure). Other CGM devices automatically draw venous blood via a central venous catheter (OptiScanner) or via a peripheral venous catheter (GlucoClear). For measurements of the glucose level in subcutaneous tissue, one single sensor or a set of sensors is used (Symphony, Sentrino). Systems that measure glucose levels in dialysate, prepare dialysate in a catheter designed for this pur-

Table 1 Overview of continuous glucose monitoring (CGM) devices intended for use in intensive care unit (ICU) patients

Device Name	Manufacturer	Glucose is measured in:	Sampling technique	Measurement technique	Frequency of measurements
OptiScanner	OptiScan Biomedical Corporation	plasma created from central venous whole blood	blood drawn via a central venous catheter	mid-infrared	15 minutes
GlySure	GlySure Limited	central venous whole blood	blood sensor-based	fluorescence	not reported
Eirus	Maquet	central venous whole blood	dialysate	glucose oxidase	1 minute
Diramo	Flowsion AS	central venous or peripheral arterial whole blood	dialysate	glucose oxidase	1 second
GluCath	GluMetrics Incorporated	peripheral venous or arterial whole blood	blood sensor-based	fluorescence	10 seconds
GlucoClear	Edwards Lifesciences	peripheral venous whole blood	blood sensor-based	glucose oxidase	5 minutes
Symphony	Echo Therapeutics	interstitial fluid	transdermal biosensor	glucose oxidase through hydrogel	1 minute
Sentrino	Medtronic Incorporated	interstitial fluid	fluid sensor-based	glucose oxidase	not reported
GlucoDay	A. Menarini Diagnostics	interstitial fluid	dialysate	glucose oxidase	3 minutes

pose and inserted into a central vein (Eirus, Diramo) or into the subcutis (Gluco-Day).

CGM devices measure glucose levels by using the glucose oxidase test (Eirus, Diramo, GlucoClear, Symphony, Sentrino and GlucoDay), fluorescence (GlySure and GluCath) or spectroscopy (OptiScanner). The glucose oxidase test is based on an enzymatic reaction, which uses glucose oxidase as a catalyst to bind glucose to water and oxygen to form gluconic acid and hydrogen peroxide. When there is more glucose, more hydrogen peroxide will be released, which can subsequently be measured [6]. The fluorescence technique is based on emission of light by a substance after absorbing light. Fluorescent chemistry is sensitive to glucose. When the glucose level increases, the fluorescent signal increases, which is detected with an optical fiber [7]. The spectroscopy technique is based on the characteristic absorption of vibrational nodes of different molecules, including glucose. Mid-infrared spectroscopy can be used because the glucose spectral peaks are in the mid-infrared region [8].

Potential Drawbacks

Glucose levels in plasma are higher than in whole blood, demanding a conversion factor that depends on the hematocrit level [9]. Furthermore, arterial blood glucose levels are higher compared to peripheral venous glucose levels (difference of ~0.2 mmol/l) and central venous glucose levels (difference of ~0.3 to 0.4 mmol/l) [10]. Glucose levels in dialysate tend to be slightly lower compared to glucose levels in surrounding fluids from which the dialysate is created [11]. Glucose levels in subcutaneous tissues are dependent on the speed by which glucose diffuses from the blood compartment to the interstitial spaces, as well as the rate at which glucose is taken up by cells in the subcutaneous compartment [12]. Users may take these drawbacks into account when using GCM devices in daily practice, but researchers certainly will need to correct for this when determining GCM accuracy.

A potential disadvantage of any biosensor is the buildup of body fluid deposits on sensor surfaces, for which repeated calibrations and eventually sensor replacements are needed [13]. Need for repeated replacements of (parts of the) system is not limited to sensor-based devices, though, because all CGM devices need replacement of other parts of the system, such as cartridges, and/or dialysate-membranes. Furthermore, with the exception of CGM using a transdermal sensor (Symphony), all CGM devices must be considered 'invasive', and as such could cause infections and/or bleeding. Additionally, all CGM devices that measure the blood glucose level in a vein are at risk of presenting erroneous glucose levels when glucose, or other substances that interfere with the measuring technique, are infused through the same catheter or close to that catheter.

Finally, the oxygen level and the pH could affect measurements by both the glucose oxidase test and the fluorescence technique [6, 7]. Drugs can interfere with the glucose oxidation reaction through molecules oxidizing with hydrogen peroxide [6] and mid-infrared spectroscopy by producing spectrums of molecules other than glucose [8]. Users need to be aware of these drawbacks when using GCM devices in their practice.

Point and/or Trend Accuracy

All CGM devices need accuracy testing in cohorts of patients in which they will be used. Two different types of accuracy can be tested: 'point accuracy' and 'trend accuracy'. Point accuracy is the accuracy of intermittent measurements at a static point. Trend accuracy is the accuracy to detect changes in glucose levels.

Several point accuracy metrics have been used to report accuracy, including correlation coefficients, mean absolute difference (MAD) or mean absolute relative difference (MARD), and Bland-Altman plots [14, 15]. A high correlation coefficient (close to 1 or −1) means that paired glucose measurements (measurement by the device versus measurement by a reference test) lie along any straight line – but this line may not lie along the line of equality where differences between paired measurements are zero. Both MAD and MARD summarize all paired glucose measurements in a single number, but unfortunately this process causes loss of important information. Another frequently used metric to demonstrate point accuracy is presenting all collected paired glucose measurements, with bias (the mean overall difference between the paired measurements) and limits of agreement (mean difference ± 1.96 * standard deviation) in Bland-Altman plots [16].

Fig. 1 The Clarke error grid. Paired measurements are plotted; measurements are most accurate in zones A and least accurate in zone E, where measurements are erroneous. See text for more details

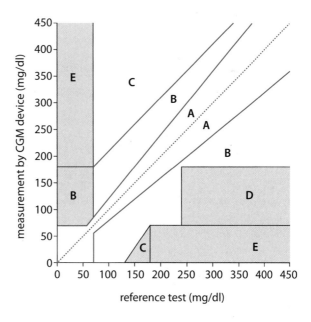

Fig. 2 The continuous glucose error grid with the 'rate error grid' (panel **a**), the 'point error grid' (panel **b**) and the 'error matrix' (panel **c**). The rate error grid is divided into zone Ar-Er, with Ar being the most accurate zone and Er being the least accurate (erroneous) zone; the point error grid has similar zones to the Clark error gird (CEG, Fig. 1), but the limits are dependent on rates of change: When there is no significant glucose change, zones are similar to the original CEG; with declining reference glucose levels upper limits change; with increasing reference glucose levels the lower limits change (see *arrows* in panel **b**); the results of the point error grid and rate error grid are put into an error matrix (panel **c**) with 3 zones; accurate readings (□), benign errors (///) and erroneous readings (=). See text for details

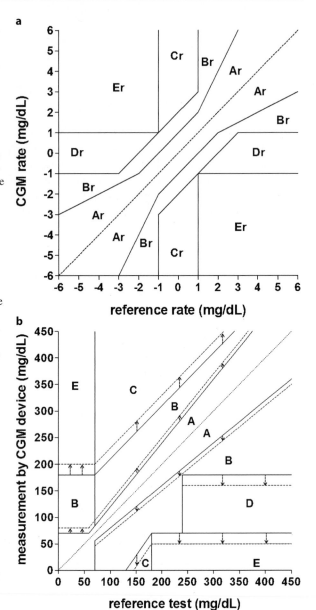

Fig. 2 *Continued*   c

		Point Error Grid zones										
		hypoglycemia glucose ≤ 70 mg/dL			normoglycemia 70 < glucose ≤ 180 mg/dL			hyperglycemia glucose > 180 mg/dL				
		A	D	E	A	B	C	A	B	C	D	E
Rate Error Grid zones	Ar											
	Br											
	upper Cr											
	lower Cr											
	upper Dr											
	lower Dr											
	upper Er											
	lower Er											

Reports on studies testing the accuracy of home glucose meter commonly use so-called Clark error grids (CEG) (Fig. 1). A CEG visualizes information by presenting all collected paired glucose measurements and 'scoring' clinical accuracy [17]. For this, a CEG is divided into five paired 'zones': Zones A (measurement within 20 % of the reference or glucose levels < 70 mg/dl); zones B (measurement more than 20 % different from the reference but still clinically acceptable as it would not cause change in the rate of insulin infusion); zones C (measurement that would lead to unnecessary changes in insulin infusion, i. e., overcorrecting acceptable glucose levels); zones D (potentially dangerous hypo- or hyperglycemic events are missed); and zones E (levels that would lead to a decision opposite to that required, i. e., treatment for hypoglycemia instead of hyperglycemia). General consensus is that 95 % of the values should be in zones A and 5 % in zones B [14].

It must be noted that the CEG was originally designed for testing accuracy of home glucose meters, not ICU meters. At the moment, it is uncertain whether the CEG zones are useful in the ICU setting. As an alternative to the CEG, an insulin titration-error grid has been proposed [18]. In this grid, very much like the original CEG, accuracy zones are based on a specific guideline for insulin titration. As guidelines for insulin titration differ (extensively) between ICUs worldwide, it could be difficult to compare results of accuracy testing of CGM devices using these grids.

R-deviation (RD) and absolute R deviation (ARD) have been proposed as rate accuracy metrics [15]. RD is defined as the difference between rates of change of measurements by the device and the reference test, divided by the time interval [15]. The ARD is the absolute value of RD [15]. Unfortunately, as for MAD and MARD, reporting only RD or ARD causes loss of important information.

More recently, the 'continuous glucose-error grid analysis' (CG-EGA) has been proposed for testing rate accuracy of CGM devices (Fig. 2) [19]. The CG-EGA

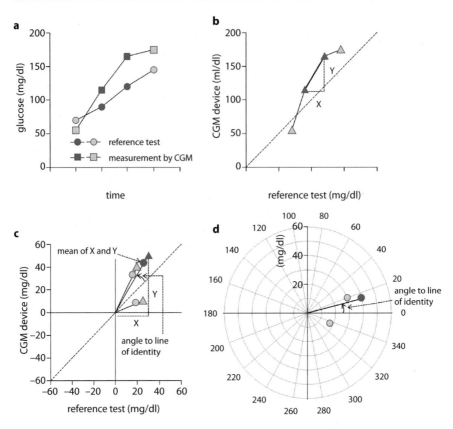

Fig. 3 A polar plot. The 4 panels indicate how a polar plot is constructed. Panel **a** shows four paired glucose measurements. Panel **b** visualizes the same measurements with continuous glucose monitoring (CGM) measurements on the Y-axis and reference test measurements on the X-axis (note that the solid dots and squares in panel **a** represent the same measurements as solid triangles in panel **b**); a line is drawn between the consecutive measurements. In panel **c**, the difference between two consecutive readings (or the rate of change) by the CGM device is plotted on the Y-axis against the difference (or the rate of change) between two readings by the reference test on the x-axis (note how the rates of change make a particular angle with the line of identity, which is the line where the rate of change detected by the CGM device and by the reference test is the same). The radius is calculated as the mean of the rates measured by the CGM device and the reference test (dots in panel **c**). The angle with the line of identity is one coordinate in the polar plot with the radius being the other coordinate. The transformation to the polar plot is made in panel **d**, with the dark blue dot representing the same dark blue dot in panel **c**. Measurements with a large angle, i. e., a large difference between the rate of change measured with CGM and the reference test, are less accurate. Criteria for defining good and poor trend accuracy for the polar plot are uncertain

combines point accuracy with rate accuracy though a rate error grid, a point error grid, and an error matrix. The rate error grid plots the rate of change of the glucose level measured by the CGM device and the reference test. A bit similar to the original CEG, the rate error grid is divided into 5 paired 'zones': Zones

Ar (rate, the accurate zone) and Br (the benign error zone) – in these zones errors do not cause inaccurate adjustments; zones Cr (over- or underestimation of the rate of change); zones Dr (reference test detects a change, which is undetected by the CGM device); and zones Er (reference test detects a change, but an opposite change is detected by the CGM device). The point error grid looks like the original CEG, but also takes glucose changes into account. Indeed, in this adjusted grid, zones are defined depending on the speed of change of glucose levels. When there is no significant glucose change, zones are similar to the original CEG, but when reference glucose levels are decreasing, the upper limits change, and when reference glucose levels are increasing, the lower limits change. Finally, results from the point and error grids are put into an error matrix with three regions, one for hypoglycemic range, one for normoglycemic range and one for hyperglycemic range. The CG-EGA is a complex tool and creation of a CG-EGA requires (very) frequent sampling to come to meaningful conclusions. However, one should keep in mind that the rate of sampling has an important effect on the results [20].

An alternative for the CG-EGA could be the polar plot, originally developed for testing trend accuracy of cardiac output monitors (Fig. 3) [21]. A polar plot shows the agreement between measurements by a device and measurements by a reference test as the angle made with the line of identity (where the difference between the measurements is zero) and the magnitude of change as the radian [21]. This method of accuracy testing has, however, not yet been used for testing accuracy of CGM devices.

Reported Accuracies of CGM Devices

Studies on point accuracy of CGM devices for use in the ICU are very scarce (Table 2). The search in Medline identified only two point accuracy studies in ICU patients (Eirus [11] and GlucoDay [22]). The internet search identified several point accuracy studies presented as abstracts (Glysure [23], GluCath [24], Symphony [25] and Sentrino [26]) or on commercial websites (OptiScanner [27], Diramo [28] and GlucoClear [29]). Most studies were rather small in terms of the number of patients as well as the number of paired measurements. Notably, accuracy was sometimes only tested in 'less severely ill' patient populations, e. g., patients in the ICU after (cardiac) surgery [11, 25, 26, 28, 29].

Two studies tested trend accuracy (GlucoDay [22], Symphony [25]). In the study on GlucoDay, a paired sample was obtained in five medical ICU patients every 15 minutes. The error matrix of the CG-EGA showed that all samples in the hypoglycemic range were in zone A, in the hyperglycemic range 88 % were in zone A and B and in the normoglycemic range 94 % were in zone A and B [22]. In the study of Symphony in post-cardiac surgery patients, paired samples were obtained only every 30–60 minutes. Although not specified for the range of glucose levels, 100 % of the samples were in the A and B zones [25].

Table 2 Overview of studies of continuous glucose monitoring (CGM) devices in intensive care unit (ICU) patients

Device	Patients studied	Number of paired samples	Point accuracy	Trend accuracy
OptiScanner [27]	63 medical or surgical ICU patients	Not reported	CEG analysis: 100 % in zones A+B	–
GlySure [23]	16 medical or surgical ICU patients	296	CEG analysis: 99.6 % in zones A+B	–
Eirus [11]	30 perioperative cardiac surgery patients	607	CEG analysis: 100 % in zones A+B; MARD 5.6 %	–
Diramo [28]	10 postoperative cardiac surgery patients	359	CEG analysis: 100 % in zones A+B; MARD 4.1 %	–
GluCath [24]	5 postoperative cardiac surgery	202	MARD 5.5 %	–
GlucoClear [29]	10 postoperative surgical ICU patients	1393	CEG analysis: 100 % in zones A+B; MARD 5.0 %	–
Symphony [25]	15 perioperative cardiac surgery	>600	MARD 12.3 %	CG-EGA: 99.6 % in zones A+B of the error matrix (not specified for which range)
Sentrino [26]	21 postoperative cardiac surgery patients	864	MARD 12.2	–
GlucoDay [22]	50 medical ICU patients (5 patients were included for trend accuracy)	N = 820 (for 2-point calibration) N = 555 (for 6-point calibration)	CEG analysis: 95 % in zones A+B for 2 point calibration; 97 % in zones A+B for 6 point calibration	CG-EGA: 100 % in zones A of hypoglycemic range, 88.1 % in zones A+B of hyperglycemic range, 93.8 % in zones A+B of normoglycemic range

CEG: Clark error grid; MARD: mean absolute relative difference; CG-EGA: continuous glucose error grid analysis; –: no data

Discussion

The most frequently suggested potential benefit of CGM in ICU patients is a reduction in time spent by nurses measuring glucose levels [30]. Whether CGM truly reduces time spent on glucose monitoring has, however, not yet been demonstrated. CGM devices could indeed reduce the number of manual measurements. However, initiation, repeated manual calibrations and replacement of (parts of) the system could also use up nursing time. Whether time spent with using CGM weighs against the burden of intermittent manual measurement in central laboratories or using laboratory-based blood gas analyzers and/or strips at the bedside could be the subject of future studies.

Intermittent manual glucose monitoring is usually seen as expensive [4]. It is questionable, however, whether use of CGM will reduce costs associated with glucose monitoring. Indeed, CGM devices will come at a price, as do the disposables used with these devices. Costs for glucose monitoring should never be considered in isolation, but together with potential financial benefits and other healthcare costs (e. g., cost prevented by reducing the incidence of dysglycemia). Therefore, health-economy analyses could accompany future studies of CGM in critically ill patients.

It has been suggested that CGM could prevent dangerous insulin titration errors in critically ill patients [5]. One trial of glucose control confirmed that CGM prevented hypoglycemia, but overall glucose control did not improve [31]. One trial of closed-loop CGM-insulin titration did show improved glucose control [32]. Of note, these two trials used a home CGM device and frequent intermittent manual glucose measurements were still necessary.

The number of studies assessing the accuracy of CGM devices is surprisingly small. In addition, the numbers of patients studied in each investigation are low and most studies have been performed only in a highly selected ICU population (e. g., patients after cardiac surgery). It could be questioned whether accuracy is also good in 'more severely ill' patients, such as patients with severe sepsis or septic shock.

Point accuracy of some CGM devices is low. The question is whether such CGM devices are useless in the ICU setting. One advantage of CGM is that there will be many more glucose readings than with manual intermittent glucose monitoring. Thus, the user could detect trends, and trend accuracy may be more important than point accuracy. An analogy that supports use of CGM devices with poor point accuracy is the comparison between camcorders versus still cameras, as previously pointed out by Kovatchev et al. [19], "Still cameras produce highly accurate snapshots at random sparse points in time, and camcorders generally offer lower resolution of each separate image but capture the dynamics of the action. Thus, it would be inappropriate to gauge the accuracy of still cameras and camcorders using the same static measure of the number of pixels in a single image. Similarly, it is inappropriate to gauge the precision of [...] devices using the same measures and to ignore the temporal characteristics of the observed process."

Conclusions

Implementation of CGM devices in daily ICU practice is at hand. Several CGM devices, using different body fluids and diverse sample and measuring techniques, have been or are being developed. These devices all need accuracy testing. The number of studies assessing the accuracy of CGM devices is still limited, and most studies have included only low numbers of highly selected ICU patients.

References

1. Schultz MJ, Spronk PE, van Braam Houckgeest F (2009) Glucontrol, no control, or out of control? Intensive Care Med 36:173–174
2. Schultz MJ, Harmsen RE, Spronk P (2010) Clinical review: Strict or loose glycemic control in critically ill patients-implementing best available evidence from randomized controlled trials. Crit Care 14:223
3. Finfer S, Wernerman J, Preiser JC et al (2012) Clinical review: Consensus recommendations on measurement of blood glucose and reporting glycemic control in critically ill adults. Crit Care 17:229
4. Aragon D (2006) Evaluation of nursing work effort and perceptions about blood glucose testing in tight glycemic control. Am J Crit Care 15:370–377
5. Karon BS, Boyd JC, Klee GG (2010) Glucose meter performance criteria for tight glycemic control estimated by simulation modeling. Clin Chem 56:1091–1097
6. Dungan K, Chapman J, Braithwaite SS, Buse J (2007) Glucose measurement: confounding issues in setting targets for inpatient management. Diabetes Care 30:403–409
7. Klonoff DC (2012) Overview of fluorescence glucose sensing: a technology with a bright future. J Diabetes Sci Technol 6:1242–1250
8. Magarian P, Sterling B (2009) Plasma-generating glucose monitor accuracy demonstrated in an animal model. J Diabetes Sci Technol 3:1411–1418
9. D'Orazio P, Burnett RW, Fogh-Andersen N et al (2006) Approved IFCC recommendation on reporting results for blood glucose: International Federation of Clinical Chemistry and Laboratory Medicine Scientific Division, Working Group on Selective Electrodes and Point-of-Care Testing (IFCC-SD-WG-SEPOCT). Clin Chem Lab Med 44:1486–1490
10. Finfer S, Wernerman J, Preiser JC et al (2013) Clinical review: Consensus recommendations on measurement of blood glucose and reporting glycemic control in critically ill adults. Crit Care 17:229
11. Schierenbeck F, Owall A, Franco-Cereceda A, Liska J (2013) Evaluation of a continuous blood glucose monitoring system using a central venous catheter with an integrated microdialysis function. Diabetes Technol Ther 15:26–31
12. Cengiz E, Tamborlane WV (2009) A tale of two compartments: interstitial versus blood glucose monitoring. Diabetes Technol Ther 11:S11–S16
13. Rice MJ, Coursin DB (2012) Continuous measurement of glucose: facts and challenges. Anesthesiology 116:199–204
14. Krouwer JS, Cembrowski GS (2010) A review of standards and statistics used to describe blood glucose monitor performance. J Diabetes Sci Technol 4:75–83
15. Clarke WL, Kovatchev B (2007) Continuous glucose sensors: Continuing questions about clinical accuracy. J Diabetes Sci Technol 1:669–675
16. Bland JM, Altman DG (1986) Statistical methods for assessing agreement between two methods of clinical measurement. Lancet 1:307–310
17. Clarke WL, Cox D, Gonder-Frederick LA, Carter W, Pohl SL (1987) Evaluating clinical accuracy of systems for self-monitoring of blood glucose. Diabetes Care 10:622–628

18. Ellmerer M, Haluzik M, Blaha J et al (2006) Clinical evaluation of alternative-site glucose measurements in patients after major cardiac surgery. Diabetes Care 29:1275–1281
19. Kovatchev BP, Gonder-Frederick LA, Cox DJ, Clarke WL (2004) Evaluating the accuracy of continuous glucose-monitoring sensors: continuous glucose-error grid analysis illustrated by TheraSense Freestyle Navigator data. Diabetes Care 27:1922–1928
20. Wentholt IM, Hoekstra JB, Devries JH (2006) A critical appraisal of the continuous glucose-error grid analysis. Diabetes Care 29:1805–1811
21. Critchley LA, Lee A, Ho AM (2010) A critical review of the ability of continuous cardiac output monitors to measure trends in cardiac output. Anesth Analg 111:1180–1192
22. De Block C, Manuel YKB, Van Gaal L, Rogiers P (2006) Intensive insulin therapy in the intensive care unit: assessment by continuous glucose monitoring. Diabetes Care 29:1750–1756
23. Mulavisala K, Gopal P, Crane B, Mackenzie A (2012) Preliminary ICU experience of a novel intravascular blood glucose sensor. Crit Care 16:P175 (abst)
24. Bird S, Macken L, Flower O et al (2013) Continuous arterial and venous glucose monitoring by quenched chemical fluorescence in ICU patients after cardiac surgery. Crit Care 17:P461 (abst)
25. Nasraway SA, Ehsan A, Melanson AM et al (2012) Accuracy of a novel non-invasive trans-dermal continuous glucose monitor in critically ill patients. Crit Care Med 40:S305 (abst)
26. Kosiborod M, Gottlieb R, Sekella J et al (2013) Performance of the Medtronic Sentrino(R) continuous glucose management system in the cardiac ICU. Crit Care 17:P462 (abst)
27. Optiscan (2013) OptiScan Biomedical presents study results demonstrating optis-canner's excellent glucose monitoring accuracy in critically ill ICU patients. Available at: http://www.optiscancorp.com/OptiScan%20MANAGE%20Study%20Data%20Press%20Release%20-%20FINAL.pdf. Accessed Nov 2013
28. Flowsion. http://www.flowsionmedical.com/ Accessed Nov 2013
29. Foubert L (2012) Clinical experience with the GluCoclear continuous glucose monitoring system. Available at: http://www.esicm.org/flash-conferences-sponsorised/lisbon-2012 Accessed Nov 2013
30. Miller M, Skladany MJ, Ludwig CR, Guthermann JS (2007) Convergence of continuous glucose monitoring and in-hospital tight glycemic control: closing the gap between caregivers and industry. J Diabetes Sci Technol 1:903–906
31. Holzinger U, Warszawska J, Kitzberger R et al (2010) Real-time continuous glucose monitoring in critically ill patients: a prospective randomized trial. Diabetes Care 33:467–472
32. Leelarathna L, English S, Thabit H et al (2013) Feasibility of fully automated closed-loop glucose control utilizing continuous subcutaneous glucose measurements in critical illness: a randomised controlled trial. Crit Care 17:R159

Nutritional Therapy in the Hospitalized Patient: Is it better to Feed Less?

S. A. McClave

Introduction

These are turbulent times in clinical nutrition. Recent studies have generated the clinical impression that it is better to feed less when a patient is admitted to the intensive care unit (ICU) [1–3]. Some investigators have pressed further to suggest that no "forced mandatory feeding" should be provided during the first week of hospitalization [4]. The implication from these comments is that nutrition is less important than previously thought, that providing sustenance to critically ill patients has a lower priority than before. A number of dangerous misconceptions are present in this line of thinking, which may lead to suboptimal care of those patients in the hospital who are most in need of such therapy.

Trophic feeding, defined as 10–15 ml/hr of an enteral formula, is a concept that was introduced over four decades ago. To put it in perspective, trophic feeding provides just over one tablespoon of formula per hour. Whether or not trophic feeding is appropriate for patients in the critical care setting is influenced by two principles. First, the benefit of nutrition therapy in the hospitalized patient is due entirely to early enteral nutrition (EN) [5]. The role of parenteral nutrition (PN) is unclear, as it is difficult to identify a benefit of PN outside the setting of intestinal failure or short bowel syndrome [6, 7]. Second, the need to aggressively feed a patient in the ICU is determined by nutritional risk, which is derived from components of both poor nutritional status and disease severity [8, 9]. Patients at high nutritional risk may need provision of nutrition therapy as close to goal as possible. Those with mild to moderate risk may be more appropriate candidates for trophic feeding or, in fact, may not need any specialized nutrition therapy over the first week of hospitalization.

S. A. McClave ✉

Division of Gastroenterology, Hepatology and Nutrition, University of Louisville School of Medicine, Louisville, Kentucky 40202, USA

e-mail: samcclave@louisville.edu

J.-L. Vincent (Ed.), *Annual Update in Intensive Care and Emergency Medicine 2014*,   627
DOI 10.1007/978-3-319-03746-2_46, © Springer International Publishing Switzerland
2014

Impact of Surviving Sepsis Campaign Recommendations

In 2009, the American Society of Parenteral and Enteral Nutrition (ASPEN) and the Society of Critical Care Medicine (SCCM) published Guidelines for the Provision and Assessment of Nutritional Support Therapy in the Adult Critically Ill Patient [10]. These guidelines, similar to the Canadian Clinical Practice Guidelines [11] and the European Society for Clinical Nutrition and Metabolism (ESPEN) guidelines [12], emphasized the importance of providing EN in the hospitalized patient, starting early after admission to the ICU and aggressively pushing to goal as soon as tolerated. Although no guidelines are perfect and a number of criticisms were made with regard to these guidelines, the concepts were not seriously challenged until the publication of the Surviving Sepsis Campaign Guidelines for the Management of Severe Sepsis and Septic Shock: 2012 in February 2013 [3]. In the third edition of this guideline series, the Surviving Sepsis Campaign committee provided nutritional recommendations for the first time. In those guidelines, they suggested starting oral diet or EN within 48 hours of the diagnosis of sepsis. They recommended avoiding "mandatory full feeds", and instead, giving 500 kcal/d over the first week [3]. Finally, they recommended using 5 % intravenous dextrose with EN, providing no exclusive PN or supplemental PN added to the enteral tube feeding over the first week. These recommendations surprised the nutrition community. The recommendation of trophic feeding over the first week of hospitalization in septic ICU patients seemed to contradict the recommendations provided in the ASPEN/SCCM, Canadian, and ESPEN clinical practice guidelines [10–12]. The Surviving Sepsis Campaign committee appeared to have a unique perspective in reviewing the nutrition literature, that focusing solely on recent large randomized controlled trials (RCTs) was most important, even if they contradicted the results of previous observational studies, small RCTs, and meta-analyses. Understanding this perspective helps explain how the committee focused on the ARDSNet trophic feeding study [1] and the Casaer EPaNIC study [13].

Differentiating the Role of Enteral from Parenteral Nutrition in the ICU

The EPaNIC study, published in 2011, evaluated the difference between the early and late initiation of supplemental PN for patients already receiving enteral tube feeding [13]. Results of the study indicated that those patients randomized to early supplemental PN started on day 3 had significantly worse outcome with increased infection, hospital length of stay, duration of renal replacement therapy (RRT) and mechanical ventilation, healthcare costs, and a lower likelihood of being discharged alive than those patients randomized to receive late supplemental PN on day 8. Subsequently, this study was criticized for the use of tight glucose control, infusion of a large intravenous glucose load in the two days prior to starting PN in the early group, and the impression that study patients were only moderately critically ill and would not require PN at most other institutions. In November 2012, Casaer et al. published a post-hoc reanalysis of the EPaNIC study addressing these early complaints [4]. Ranking the patients by increasing range of Acute Physiology and Chronic Health Evaluation (APACHE) II score, the reanalysis showed that the deleterious effects of early supplemental PN were worse with increasing severity of disease. Those patients at higher ranges of APACHE II score were less likely to be discharged alive if they received PN on day 3 than if it was withheld until day 8. The likelihood of acquiring a new nosocomial infection again was worse with increasing disease severity if PN was provided on day 3 compared to day 8 [4].

The reanalysis also showed that the deleterious effects of early supplemental PN could not be attributed to an infusion of intravenous glucose [4]. The likelihood of being discharged alive was no different if intravenous glucose was provided early or late in the first week of hospitalization. Surprisingly, increased receipt of protein on day 3 reduced the likelihood of patients being discharged alive compared to its receipt on day 5 or day 7. The difference in the effect between provision of these two macronutrients would suggest that it was not the practice of intravenous glucose loading, but the early nutrition therapy that accounted for the mortality effect seen in this study. The reanalysis showed that when all patients were combined, those patients who received nutrition therapy closer to target goal on day 3 were less likely to be discharged alive. Although a similar pattern was seen again on day 5, the differences did not reach statistical significance. These findings led the investigators to conclude that "forced mandatory feeding" in ICU patients resulted in worse, not better outcome [4].

Schetz, Casaer and Van den Berghe proposed a physiologic mechanism to explain these findings, that early nutrition therapy suppressed autophagy [2]. Clinicians have been aware of the concept of autophagy for over four decades, but its complexity is poorly understood [14]. Autophagy is an important protective mechanism of the cell in situations of increasing oxidative stress and inflammation. With increasing dysfunction of the endoplasmic reticulum, unfolded proteins accumulate which can lead to insulin resistance, loss of structural integrity, apoptosis, and eventually necrosis of the cell. Autophagy helps clear unfolded proteins through a process of vesicle formation that ultimately degrades the protein to individual amino acids, promoting new protein synthesis and maintenance of cell structure [2, 14]. The impression that feeding suppresses autophagy is suggested by the fact that autophagy is highest in periods of fasting, where the ability to degrade dysfunctional protein and stimulate protein synthesis would help maintain lean body mass and cell structure [2]. This line of thinking quickly leads to apparent contradictions. Is lean body mass better preserved by supporting autophagy and starving the patient, or by providing exogenous nutrients to stimulate protein synthesis? Glutamine is a known stimulant of autophagy, which would contradict the notion that feeding would lead to suppression [14]. The concept that preserving autophagy in order for the cell to better manage oxidative stress and inflammation is offset by the evidence that provision of early EN reduces inflammation and hastens recovery from the systemic inflammatory response syndrome (SIRS) [5].

A closer evaluation of the EPaNIC trial shows that on every day of the study, the early and late PN groups received an equal number of enteral calories from tube feeding [13]. Any difference in outcome therefore has to be attributed to the difference in parenteral calories delivered to each group. This point was emphasized by the subset of patients in whom EN was surgically contraindicated because the bowel was in discontinuity. Even in this group of patients, early receipt of supplemental PN was associated with increased infection and less likelihood of being discharged alive than late receipt of PN [13]. The reanalysis separates the early from the late PN group in the evaluation of percent of target goal calories delivered and its effect on outcome [4]. The correlation between feeding closer to goal and the lower likelihood of being discharged alive is seen only in the early PN group on days 3 and 5; those differences were not present on day 7 in this group. In the late PN group (for whom only enteral calories were provided on day 3, day 5 and day 7), no such adverse effect from providing calories closer to target goal was seen on likelihood of being discharged alive [4].

Two additional studies provided evidence that questioned whether any clinical benefit resulted from use of PN in the ICU setting. In the Swiss Supplemental Parenteral Nutrition (SPN) trial, patients determined to be at high risk in a medical ICU with a functional gut and expected to stay in the ICU for > 5 days were placed on enteral tube feeding [6]. At day 3, if EN was providing < 60 % of measured energy expenditure, patients were randomized to receive either supplemental PN added to the EN in the experimental group, or to receive continued EN alone in controls. When abstracts from this study were first presented at the European Society of Intensive Care Medicine (ESICM) Congress in October 2011, 275 patients had been entered, with results showing that supplemental PN given to study patients reduced new infection, duration of mechanical ventilation, and hospital length of stay compared to controls who received EN alone. However, with the final publication of the study (at which point 300 patients had been entered in the study), two of these end-points were lost [6]; only a difference in nosocomial infection was significantly different between the two groups. Surprisingly, occurrence of major infections, such as bacteremia, pneumonia, and abdominal abscesses, was no different between groups. The experimental supplemental PN group sustained fewer "other" infections (nose, skin, ear, etc.) compared to controls only after day 9 [6]. In a second study by Gordon Doig and colleagues, critically ill patients with a short-term contraindication to EN (expected not to get tube feeding for at least three days) were randomized in a multicenter trial to receive PN or standard therapy (no additional specialized nutrition therapy) [7]. Nearly 1400 patients were entered into the study, with results showing that the provision of early PN succeeded only in reducing the duration of mechanical ventilation by 1.2 days compared to receipt of standard therapy. No other outcome parameter was different between the two groups [7].

Interpretation of these three large studies (EPaNIC, SPN, and the Doig PN study) [6, 7, 13] has varied among different groups within the global nutrition community. Interpretation by North Americans and some Europeans was that these studies indicate that enteral and parenteral calories are not equal, that there is a difference in their risk:benefit ratio, and that although PN can be provided safely, its benefit in the hospitalized patient (particularly in the ICU) is not clear; therefore,

PN should be used on a case-by-case basis. Doig and some others of the European community continue to believe that PN, if given properly, can benefit the patient and should be used readily if EN is insufficient [7]. Casaer et al., through their interpretation of these study results, maintain that mandatory forced feeding causes worse outcome in the hospitalized patient and that no nutrition therapy should be provided until after the first week of hospitalization [4].

Impact of the ARDSNet Trophic Feeding Study

The second largest study that seemed to provide the basis for the recommendations of the Surviving Sepsis Campaign committee was the initial trophic vs. full enteral feeding in patients with acute lung injury (ALI) study by the ARDSNet group [1]. Patients with acute respiratory distress syndrome (ARDS) or ALI in a medical ICU setting were randomized to receive trophic feeding at 10–20 ml/h for 6 days and then advanced to goal versus full feeding at 100 % of goal calories from time of admission. Throughout the study, those patients randomized to trophic feeding received approximately 25 % of goal calories, whereas those randomized to full feeding ended up receiving 80 % of goal calories. Surprisingly, there was no difference in outcome between the two groups with regard to mortality, ventilator-free days, organ failure, or nosocomial infection [1]. Although these results surprised the nutrition community, a number of reasons may explain why trophic feeding performed as well with respect to outcome as full feeding in this particular patient population. Patients in this setting were moderately critically ill, with an average age of 52 years, a higher than normal average body mass index (BMI) at 30, and a short stay in the ICU of < 5–6 days. Of the 8000 patients who were screened (to get the 1000 patients included in the study), 7000 patients were excluded because of increased disease severity. If patients had underlying liver disease, lung disease, low BMI, or severe shock, they were excluded from the study [1]. It is possible that 25 % of goal calories may have been sufficient to achieve the outcome benefits of EN, as suggested in another study by Rubinson et al. in which receipt of > 25 % of goal calories succeeded in preventing nosocomial bloodstream infection [15]. Dose may be less important than timing of initiation of feeding and the degree to which interruptions in delivery of EN are minimized. In this trial, EN was initiated within six hours of randomization [1]. In the single center trial at Vanderbilt [16] that preceded the multicenter ARDSNet study [1], it was shown that nurses forgot that the trophic feedings were still being infused in the experimental group, resulting in less cessation of EN than the infusion of full feeding in controls. Nurses were less likely to turn off the EN for nursing care, bedside procedures, or diagnostic tests. Because of trophic feeding, study patients in the ARDSNet trial received 1.5 liters less fluid per day than controls randomized to full feeding [1]. Research from the ARSDNet group in the past has shown that conservative fluid management yields better outcome than aggressive volume resuscitation. With the reported average BMI range, these patients may represent a group less likely to see an impact on outcome from nutrition therapy than patients at a much lower or much higher range of BMI. A study by Alberda et al. showed that patients with a BMI range below 20 or above 35 were more likely to see a reduction in mortality with increased delivery of nutrition therapy [17]; however, those patients with a BMI of 25–35 showed no change in mortality with greater receipt of calories.

Are the findings of this study unique to this specific population of patients? Would the same strategy of trophic feeding be just as effective in patients with severe pancreatitis or major burns? In a dangerous extrapolation of these results, some clinicians tend to think that if trophic feeding of as little as 10–20 ml/hr achieves the same endpoint as full feeding, maybe no nutrition therapy is really needed. Other clinicians believe that trophic feeding is better than full feeding. These study results show that they are simply equivalent. Any nutritional prescription that is made in the ICU setting must also take into account the fact that often only 50–80 % of prescribed calories are actually delivered to the patient [18].

Does the Literature Support the Notion that Feeding Less is Better?

There are five distinct bodies of literature in the public record that contradict the notion that feeding less is better in the first week of hospitalization in an ICU setting. First, those studies evaluating early versus delayed EN have shown that feeding initiated within 36 hours of admission to the ICU reduced infection by 55 %, hospital length of stay by 1.2 days, and mortality by 64 % compared to late EN started after that point in time [19, 20]. These findings have been demonstrated in a variety of patient populations, ranging from patients in a general ICU to those with burns, trauma, and head injury. Second, those studies comparing early EN to standard therapy (where no specialized nutrition therapy is provided) have shown value of early feeding. In 14 studies involving elective surgery and surgical critical care and two studies in severe acute pancreatitis (where patients were being operated on for complications of pancreatitis), aggressive use of the oral route or tube feeding initiated the day after surgery significantly reduced infection by 28 %, hospital length of stay by 0.84 days, and mortality by 4 % compared to standard therapy [21, 22]. In the pancreatitis studies, mortality was reduced from 25.6 to 6.2 %, but this difference just missed statistical significance (p = 0.06) [23]. The third body of literature involves the concept of caloric deficit, or the notion that with patients expending calories in the ICU every day, any delay in initiating nutrition therapy generates a large caloric deficit. Early studies three decades ago focused on the association between a caloric deficit of 10,000 calories and increased adverse outcome. But more recent studies from Europe have suggested that a caloric deficit of as little as 4000 calories is associated with increased incidence of ARDS, renal failure, sepsis, need for surgery, and total complications [24, 25]. This body of literature provides the weakest argument, because the sicker the patient, the more difficult it is to provide EN therapy. This finding is supported, however, by the fourth body of literature which involves the impact of nurse-driven feeding protocols [26, 27]. In these studies (which range in design from randomized trials to before/after implementation of protocols), invariably more patients receive a greater volume of EN within the first week of admission to the ICU. Although not every study shows an impact on outcome, those that do show reduced infection, total complications, length of stay, and even mortality compared to those patients for whom no protocol is in place [26, 27]. The fifth body of literature is represented by three decades of studies providing mechanistic support for a benefit of EN in reducing oxidative stress, attenuating SIRS, hastening recovery, and improving clinical outcome [5]. These mechanisms range from maintaining gut integrity, modulating both innate and acquired immunity, and suppressing the gut/lung access of inflammation (where cytokines from the gastrointestinal tract are delivered directly through lymphatics to the pulmonary system), to supporting the role of commensal bacteria [5].

Clinicians have interpreted the findings of the ARDSNet trophic feeding study in two ways. One interpretation, which most reflects that of the nutrition community, is that brief trophic feeding is appropriate in this particular population of patients with a moderate degree of critical illness. The other interpretation is represented by clinicians who now believe that the concept of 'feeding less is better' is not limited to patients with ARDS or ALI (as suggested by the ARDSNet data) or sepsis (as recommended by the Surviving Sepsis Campaign committee) [1, 3]. These clinicians have extrapolated these data and recommendations to imply that trophic feeding is the appropriate strategy for all ICU patients.

Who Benefits from Nutrition Therapy?

The concept of 'malnutrition' has always been nebulous, poorly-defined, and difficult to quantify. An International Consensus Committee redefined malnutrition in 2010 into three states: Starvation-related, chronic disease-related, and acute disease or injury-related malnutrition [28]. The unique contribution of this revised definition was acknowledging the effect of inflammation on nutritional status. However, the true nature of malnutrition still could not be clarified to any degree. In contrast, Kondrup et al., in the development of the Nutritional Risk Score (NRS)-2002, described the concept of "nutritional risk", which is much more readily defined and easily quantified [9]. In this report, nutritional risk is determined by both nutritional state and disease severity. In the NRS-2002, points are accumulated for evidence of poor nutritional status based on weight loss $>5\%$ over 1–3 months, BMI <20, or reduced food intake prior to admission. Patients are then evaluated for disease severity, accumulating points depending upon whether they have a mild (e. g., chronic obstructive pulmonary disease [COPD], cirrhosis, hip fracture), moderate (e. g., stroke or pneumonia), or severe (e. g., head injury, bone marrow transplant, or critical illness with APACHE II scores > 10) disease process. Age >70 years adds an additional point (Table 1) [9]. Patients who generate a score of ≥ 3 points should be considered for specialized nutrition therapy. Those patients with a score of ≥ 5 are identified as being at high nutritional risk. Heyland et al. developed a similar assessment tool to identify level of nutritional risk, measuring disease severity

Table 1 Nutrition assessment scoring system using the Nutrition Risk Score (NRS)-2002 [9] to determine nutrition risk

Impaired Nutritional Status		Severity of Disease	
Absent **Score 0**	Normal nutritional status	**Absent** **Score 0**	Normal nutritional requirements
Mild **Score 1**	Wt loss > 5 % in 3 months OR food intake below 50–75 % of normal requirement in preceding week	**Mild** **Score 1**	Hip fracture Chronic patients in particular with acute complications: cirrhosis, COPD Chronic hemodialysis, diabetes, oncology
Moderate **Score 2**	Wt loss > 5 % in 2 months OR BMI 18.5–20.5 + impaired general condition OR food intake 25–50 % of normal requirement in preceding week	**Moderate** **Score 2**	Major abdominal surgery Stroke Severe pneumonia, hematologic malignancy
Severe **Score 3**	Wt loss > 5 % in 1 month (15 % in 3 mos) OR BMI < 18.5 + impaired general condition OR food intake < 25 % of normal requirement in preceding week	**Severe** **Score 3**	Head injury Bone marrow transplantation Intensive care patients (APACHE II $\geq$ 10)

Note: If age $\geq$ 70 years, add 1 point
Total score = (Points for nutritional status) + (Points for disease severity) + (Points for age)
COPD: chronic obstructive pulmonary disease; Wt: weight; BMI: body mass index; APACHE: Acute Physiology and Chronic Health Evaluation.

and nutritional status to determine an overall NUTRIC score [8]. Six parameters are used to determine the NUTRIC score: Age, APACHE II score, sequential organ failure assessment (SOFA) score, number of comorbidities, days from hospital admission to ICU admission (the sole marker of poor nutritional status), and interleukin-6 levels (Table 2) [8, 29]. Higher NUTRIC scores are associated with increased nutritional risk and greater mortality [8].

In a prospective study, Jie et al. used the NRS-2002 to evaluate nutritional risk in patients undergoing a major elective operation [30]. "Sufficient" nutrition therapy was defined as receiving > 10 kcal/kg/d for at least 7 full days preoperatively. Out of 1,085 patients, 120 were identified to be at high nutritional risk with an NRS-2002 score of $\geq$ 5. The increased severity of disease in these patients was indicated by the fact that they had a 20 % incidence of pneumonia, 20 % incidence of abdominal infection, and 10 % incidence of an anastomotic leak. At the end of the study, those patients at high nutritional risk who received sufficient preoperative nutrition showed a reduction in overall complications from 50.6 % to 25.6 %, and a reduction in nosocomial infection from 33.8 % to 15.3 %, compared to those high risk patients who received "insufficient" nutrition therapy. Surprisingly, in those patients with

Table 2 Nutrition assessment scoring system using the NUTRIC Score to determine nutrition risk [8]

Factors	NUTRIC Points			
	0	1	2	3
Age (yrs)	<50	500–74	≥75	–
APACHE II Score	<15	15–19	20–27	28
Baseline SOFA Score	<6	6–9	≥10	–
# Comorbidities	0–1	≥2	–	–
Days in hospital to ICU admit	0	≥1	–	–
Interleukin-6 (μ/ml)	0–399	≥400	–	–

Total Score = (Total of six separate factors)
APACHE: Acute Physiology and Chronic Health Evaluation
SOFA: Sequential Organ Failure Assessment

NRS-2002 scores of < 5, there was no difference in outcome whether they received sufficient or insufficient feeding [30]. Using the NUTRIC Score, Heyland et al. showed that patients at low nutritional risk with NUTRIC scores of 0–5, showed no change in mortality over a range of delivery from 0–100 % of goal calories [8]. However, for those patients at high nutritional risk with NUTRIC scores of 6–10, increasing delivery of nutrition therapy over a range up to 100 % of goal target calories was associated with a steady significant reduction in mortality [8]. These studies show that patients at high nutritional risk are those who need aggressive delivery of early EN to achieve desired outcome benefits. For these patients, having an institutional structure in place to deliver the nutrition therapy, such as volume-based feeding, "Top-Down" or "Pep-Up" clinical pathways, nurse-driven protocols, or bundling nutritional elements into a set of action statements, are all strategies by which to provide aggressive early nutrition therapy to those patients at highest risk [31, 32].

When is it Appropriate to Intentionally or Permissively Underfeed Patients?

There are three scenarios where the literature supports appropriate underfeeding of patients in a critical care setting. In the first scenario, patients with ARDS or ALI on mechanical ventilation may receive trophic feeding over the first six days of therapy [1]. Trophic feeding at 20 ml/h should provide 25 % of goal calories, and this patient population should experience the same clinical endpoints as would be expected with full feeding. However, the clinician must be careful to identify that there are no extremes of age, BMI, or disease severity, because disparate outcomes may result.

In a second scenario, obese critically ill patients with BMI > 30 are appropriate candidates to receive high protein hypocaloric feeding [33]. In these patients, aggressive delivery of protein at a dose of 2.0–2.5 gm/kg ideal body weight/d is assured, while providing approximately 60–70 % of caloric requirements as measured by indirect calorimetry. When indirect calorimetry is not available, use of simplistic weight-based equations (11–14 kcal/kg actual body weight/d for those patients with BMI of 30–40, or 22–25 kcal/kg ideal body weight/d for those with BMI > 40) provides an adequate estimate of the value representing 60–70 % of energy expenditure [34]. This strategy has been shown in physiologic studies to maintain lean body mass while depleting the fat mass.

In the third scenario, any critically ill patient placed on PN should be given hypocaloric feeding over the first week of ICU admission [35]. Prescribing 80 % of caloric requirements with full protein provision in these patients avoids the dangers of overfeeding from PN and may improve insulin sensitivity. In a meta-analysis of five studies in a surgical ICU setting, hypocaloric (20 kcal/kg/d) compared to eucaloric (25 kcal/kg/d) PN successfully reduced infectious complications by 40 %, and hospital length of stay by 2.49 days [35].

What Direction Are We Going?

In late September 2013, at the annual meeting of the Surgical Infection Society in the United States, Dr. Eric Charles from the University of Virginia presented the results of a prospective randomized controlled trial of 84 patients in a surgical ICU setting, randomized to receive either hypocaloric feeding at 12.5–15 kcal/kg/d or eucaloric feeding at 25–30 kcal/kg/d (with normal provision of protein at 1.5 g/kg/d in both groups) [36]. Although the formal results of the study were not yet available, the abstract presented appeared to show no difference between groups with regard to ICU or hospital length of stay, infectious complications, or mortality. The President of the Surgical Infection Society, Dr. William Cheadle, was quoted to say "The risks of providing nutrition therapy were lessened if the amount of calories needed were less than the traditional amounts. This study shows that feeding less in the ICU may be better" [36]. Certainly there is a risk that this study could suffer from a type II error, in which a true difference between the two groups could not be shown with this small number of patients. Nonetheless, a consistent impression is being delivered to clinicians – that feeding less may be the optimal strategy.

Conclusions

The benefit of early nutrition in the hospitalized ICU patient is due primarily to EN. The risk:benefit ratio of PN is narrower and its benefit to patients over the first week of hospitalization outside the setting of intestinal failure or short bowel syndrome is not clear. As a result, PN should be used in high risk patients on a case-by-case basis. In clinical practice, malnutrition is poorly understood and difficult to define. In contrast, nutritional risk can be readily identified and easily measured. High nutritional risk is determined by both disease severity and poor nutritional status. Aggressive strategies increase delivery of EN and improve the chances for optimal patient outcome. Such strategies reduce the need for PN in hospitalized patients. Clinicians need to remain flexible in their understanding and interpretation of these studies as this is an evolving field and our understanding is bound to change in the future as new literature becomes available.

References

1. Rice TW, Wheeler AP, Thompson BT et al (2012) Initial trophic vs full enteral feeding in patients with acute lung injury: The EDEN randomized trial. JAMA 307:795–803
2. Schetz M, Casaer MP, Van den Berghe G (2013) Does artificial nutrition improve outcome of critical illness? Crit Care 17:302–309
3. Dellinger RP, Levy MM, Rhodes A et al (2013) Surviving sepsis campaign: International guidelines for management of severe sepsis and septic shock: 2012. Crit Care Med 41:580–637
4. Casaer MP, Wilmer A, Hermans Wouters GP, Mesotten D, Van den Berghe G (2013) Role of disease and macronutrient dose in the randomized controlled EPaNIC trial, a post-hoc analysis. Am J Respir Crit Care Med 187:247–255
5. McClave SA, Heyland DK (2009) The physiologic response and associated clinical benefits from provision of early enteral nutrition. Nutr Clin Pract 24:305–315
6. Heidegger CP, Berger MM, Graf S et al (2013) Optimisation of energy provision with supplemental parenteral nutrition in critically ill patients: A randomised controlled clinical trial. Lancet 381:385–393
7. Doig GS, Simpson F, Sweetman EA et al (2013) Early parenteral nutrition in critically ill patients with short term contraindications to early enteral nutrition: A randomized controlled trial. JAMA 309:2130–2138
8. Heyland DK, Dhaliwal R, Jiang X, Day AG (2011) Identifying critically ill patients who benefit the most from nutrition therapy: The development and initial validation of a novel risk assessment tool. Crit Care 15:R268–R279
9. Kondrup J, Rasmussen HH, Hamberg O, Stanga Z, Ad Hoc ESPEN Working Group (2003) Nutritional risk screening (NRS 2002): A new method based on an analysis of controlled clinical trials. Clin Nutr 22:321–336
10. McClave SA, Martindale RG, Vanek VW et al (2009) Guidelines for the provision and assessment of nutrition support therapy in the adult critically ill patient: Society of Critical Care Medicine (SCCM) and American Society for Parenteral and Enteral Nutrition (A.S.P.E.N.). JPEN J Parenter Enteral Nutr 33:277–316
11. Heyland DK, Dhaliwal R, Drover JW, Gramlich L, Dodek P (2003) Canadian critical care clinical practice guidelines committee: Canadian clinical practice guidelines for nutrition support in mechanically ventilated, critically ill adult patients. JPEN J Parenter Enteral Nutr 27:355–373
12. Kreyman KG, Bereger MM, Deutz NEP et al (2006) ESPEN guidelines on enteral nutrition: Intensive care. Clin Nutr 25:210–223
13. Casaer MP, Mesotten D, Hermans G et al (2011) Early versus late parenteral nutrition in critically ill adults. N Engl J Med 365:506–517
14. Heyland DK, Wischmeyer P (2013) Does artificial nutrition improve outcome of critical illness? An alternative viewpoint! Crit Care 17:324–326
15. Rubinson L, Diette GB, Song X, Brower RG, Krishnan JA (2004) Low calorie intake is associated with nosocomial bloodstream infections in patients in the medical intensive care unit. Crit Care Med 32:350–357
16. Rice TW, Mogan S, Hays MA, Bernard GR, Jensen GL, Wheeler AP (2011) A randomized trial of initial trophic versus full-energy enteral nutrition in mechanically ventilated patients with acute respiratory failure. Crit Care Med 39:967–974

17. Alberda CA, Gramlich L, Jones NE et al (2009) The relationship between nutritional intake and clinical outcomes in critically ill patients: Results of an international multicenter observational study. Intensive Care Med 35:1728–1737

18. McClave SA, Sexton LK, Spain DA et al (1999) Enteral tube feeding in the intensive care unit: Factors impeding adequate delivery. Crit Care Med 27:1252–1256

19. Marik PE, Zaloga GP (2001) Early enteral nutrition in acutely ill patients: A systematic review. Crit Care Med 29:2264–2270

20. Doig GS, Heighes PT, Simpson F, Sweetman EA, Davies AR (2009) Early enteral nutrition, provided within 24 h of injury or intensive care unit admission, significantly reduces mortality in critically ill patients: a meta-analysis of randomised controlled trials. Intensive Care Med 35:2018–2027

21. Lewis SJ, Egger M, Sylvester PA, Thomas S (2001) Early enteral feeding versus "nil by mouth" after gastrointestinal surgery: Systematic review and meta-analysis of controlled trials. BMJ 323:773–776

22. Lewis SJ, Andersen HK, Thomas S (2009) Early enteral nutrition within 24 h of intestinal surgery versus later commencement of feeding: A systematic review and meta-analysis. J Gastrointest Surg 13:569–575

23. McClave SA, Chang WK, Dhaliwal R, Heyland DK (2006) Nutrition support in acute pancreatitis: A systematic review of the literature. JPEN J Parenter Enteral Nutr 30:143–156

24. Dvir D, Cohen J, Singer P (2006) Computerized energy balance and complications in critically ill patients: An observational study. Clin Nutr 25:37–44

25. Villet S, Chiolero RL, Bollmann MD et al (2005) Negative impact of hypocaloric feeding and energy balance on clinical outcome in ICU patients. Clin Nutr 24:502–509

26. Taylor SJ, Fettes SB, Jewkes C, Nelson RJ (1999) Prospective, randomized, controlled trial to determine the effect of early enhanced enteral nutrition on clinical outcome in mechanically ventilated patients suffering head injury. Crit Care Med 27:2525–2531

27. Martin CM, Doig GS, Heyland DK et al (2004) Multicentre, cluster-randomized clinical trial of algorithms for critical-care enteral and parenteral therapy (ACCEPT). CMAJ 170:197–204

28. Jensen GL, Mirtallo J, Compher C et al (2010) Adult starvation and disease-related malnutrition: A proposal for etiology-based diagnosis in the clinical practice setting from the international consensus guideline committee. JPEN J Parenter Enteral Nutr 34:156–159

29. Faisy C, Lerolle N, Dachraoui F et al (2009) Impact of energy deficit calculated by a predictive method on outcome in medical patients requiring prolonged acute mechanical ventilation. Br J Nutr 101:1079–1087

30. Jie B, Jiang ZM, Nolan MT, Zhu SN, Yu K, Kondrup J (2012) Impact of preoperative nutritional support on clinical outcome in abdominal surgical patients at nutritional risk. Nutrition 28:1022–1027

31. McClave SA, Saad M, Jotautas A, Franklin G, Heyland D, Anderson M (2011) Volume-based feeding in the critically ill patient. JPEN J Parenter Enteral Nutr 35:134–135

32. Heyland DK, Cahill NE, Dhaliwal R et al (2011) Enhanced protein-energy provision via the enteral route in critically ill patients: A single center feasibility trial of the PEP uP protocol. Crit Care 14:R78

33. Choban P, Dickerson R, Malone A, Worthington P, Compher C (2013) A.S.P.E.N. Clinical guidelines: Nutrition support of hospitalized adult patients with obesity. JPEN J Parenter Enteral Nutr 37:714–734

34. McClave SA, Kushner R, Van Way C et al (2011) Nutritional therapy of the severely obese critically ill patient: Summation of conclusions and recommendations. JPEN J Parenter Enteral Nutr 35:88S–96S

35. Jiang H, Sun MW, Hefright B, Chen W, Lu CD, Zeng J (2011) Efficacy of hypocaloric parenteral nutrition for surgical patients: A systematic review and meta-analysis. Clin Nutr 30:730–737

36. Frangou C (2013) Limited calorie diet may have same benefits as eucaloric in ICU. Gen Surg News 40:1–3

Glutamine Supplementation to Critically Ill Patients?

J. Wernerman

Introduction

A recent study (Reducing Deaths due to Oxidative Stress, REDOXS) reported harm in critically ill patients who received glutamine supplementation [1]. This is in contrast to a number of earlier studies reporting beneficial effects or failing to demonstrate any effect [2, 3]. Naturally, this finding raises a number of questions, which are not answered by combining all existing studies into a large meta-analysis. This overview will discuss existing clinical data, including dosing and selection of patients. In addition, suggested mechanisms will be discussed from a clinical perspective. Finally, possibilities for future research will be outlined.

Rationale for Supplementation

The background to the suggestion that critically ill patients should receive glutamine supplementation is that plasma glutamine concentration at intensive care unit (ICU) admission is an independent predictor of an unfavorable outcome [4, 5]. Empirically, a plasma concentration of 420 µmol/l has repeatedly been reported as a cut-off for a low plasma glutamine concentration associated with a higher risk of mortality in adults [4, 5]. In principle, the same effect applies in critically ill pediatric patients, but here the low mortality rates have not made it possible to demonstrate a mortality disadvantage, although a morbidity disadvantage has been reported [6]. Approximately one third of ICU admissions are consistently found to have a low plasma glutamine concentration, and this is independent from conventional risk-scoring [1, 4–6]. In a study from Stockholm, the mortality associated

J. Wernerman ✉
Department of Anesthesia and Intensive Care Medicine, Karolinska University Hospital
Huddinge, Stockholm, Sweden
e-mail: jan.wernerman@karolinska.se

J.-L. Vincent (Ed.), *Annual Update in Intensive Care and Emergency Medicine 2014*,   639
DOI 10.1007/978-3-319-03746-2_47, © Springer International Publishing Switzerland
and BioMed Central Ltd. 2014

with a low ICU admission glutamine concentration was to a large extent due to the post-ICU mortality within 6 months from ICU admission [5].

In addition to the predictive value of a low plasma glutamine concentration at ICU admission for an unfavorable outcome, there seem to be a similar prediction also for high plasma glutamine concentrations at admission [5]. This group of patients, however, is much smaller, and the evidence for this prediction is mostly in form of case series. It has been reported that acute liver failure is quite often associated with high or very high plasma glutamine concentrations [7]. Chronic liver insufficiency and acute-on-chronic liver failure are not accompanied by high plasma glutamine concentrations. In single cases, it has been observed that terminal patients with multiple organ failure (not necessarily including advanced liver failure) have very high plasma glutamine concentrations. One can speculate that this observation may relate to impaired cellular integrity in general.

In parallel to the association between a low plasma glutamine and an unfavorable outcome, there is an extensive literature about the essential role of glutamine in a number of experimental systems, including whole animals. Cell division demands an increase in nucleotide production, and glutamine is a main precursor for this type of synthesis. Cell culture media usually contain a much higher free glutamine concentration than does human plasma, and lowering of glutamine concentration in cell culture media is associated with a lower rate of cell division. Many cultured cells prefer glutamine over glucose as their main energy source, and imposing stressful events to the cell culture is reported to enhance the preference for glutamine over glucose as energy substrate. In tissues and whole animals, it is the rapidly replicating cells that seem to be particularly dependent on glutamine availability. Enterocytes in the gastrointestinal tract and immune-competent cells are reported to be particularly sensitive to glutamine depletion. Histological changes and bacterial translocation in the gut occur when there is glutamine shortage, and provision of glutamine can reverse this effect. Similarly, for immune-competent cells, markers of immune function deteriorate during glutamine shortage, to return back to normal upon restoration of glutamine availability.

Targets for Supplementation

With this background, the suggestion that glutamine shortage should be compensated for by supplementation is not far-fetched and consequently a number of clinical studies have been performed, mainly in critically ill patients. Behind the suggestion to supplement there are two different philosophies: To substitute a deficiency or to administer a pharmacological agent (pharmaconutrition). It is recommended that these two philosophies be separated because the target for treatment is different in the two cases. To supplement to normal levels would mean adding supplementation in order to reach normal plasma concentrations, or normal availability in tissues if more invasive monitoring is possible. To administer a pharmaconutrition agent on the other hand, would mean that a dose-response relation is presumed and that the desired response effect can be defined. This effect may be in terms of plasma glutamine concentrations, but may also be in terms of other measureable effects related to glutamine intake.

When determining the target for dosing of exogenous glutamine supplementation, small studies of intravenous supplementation restoring hypoglutaminemia back to normoglutaminemia are usually cited [8, 9]. These data have also been applied to enteral administration of supplementation, although enteral doses only marginally affect plasma concentration [10–12]. If the pharmaconutrition philosophy is applied, higher doses are usually given, although the rationale for doses beyond what may be needed to restore a low plasma concentration is purely hypothetical. Finally, the effect of treatment on glutamine availability is only very rarely defined in the available clinical studies. At best, articles report the success of administering the intended dose, but sometimes not even that is communicated in the article.

Available data make it highly unlikely that all critically ill patients are depleted in glutamine, as only approximately one third of patients admitted to the ICU have a plasma glutamine concentration $< 420\,\mu mol/l$. Furthermore, a higher risk of an unfavorable outcome indicated by a high APACHE II score or a high sequential organ failure assessment (SOFA) score is not statistically associated with glutamine depletion. In contrast, glutamine depletion at admission is not associated with risk scoring [4, 5]. However, the risk for a given patient may be increased if a low admission glutamine concentration is present (Fig. 1). As pointed out by Rodas et al. this additional risk may be most pronounced for the group of patients with a moderate mortality risk [5]. If patient recruitment in a study focuses on patients with high mortality risk or low mortality risk, the additional risk associated with concomitant glutamine depletion will be less pronounced.

If exogenous glutamine supplementation aims to compensate for an additional risk imposed on patients with glutamine depletion, the target group should be critically ill patients with a moderate mortality risk, with low admission plasma glutamine concentration, who are in need of nutrition support for, for example, not less than 5 days. The more a study population deviates from this target group in which a beneficial effect can be hypothesized, the less likely it will be that the study will show an effect of exogenous glutamine supplementation attributable to glutamine supplementation.

If, on the other hand, the hypothesis is that a pharmacological provision of glutamine may be beneficial, the target group should be patients with a high mortality risk with a pathology likely to respond to effects associated with providing a surplus of glutamine. To just combine all available studies of glutamine supplementation in critically ill patients in a meta-analysis will not contribute to answering the question whether exogenous glutamine supplementation may be beneficial or may cause harm. It should be recognized that different studies are based on very different assumptions of the involved mechanisms.

Additional information on glutamine status in the individual patient, in addition to the plasma concentration, can be obtained from studies about glutamine turnover. Available techniques use isotopically-labeled glutamine to estimate the endogenous rate of appearance of glutamine. A limited number of studies have

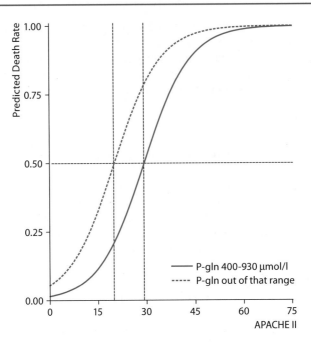

Fig. 1 Simulation of the additional mortality prediction from an out of range plasma glutamine concentration at ICU admittance. The solid line is the APACHE II predicted mortality rate if plasma glutamine concentration is in the range 400–930 µmol/l; the dotted line represents the predicted mortality rate when admittance plasma glutamine concentration is outside that range. The simulation suggests a 50 % mortality risk at APACHE 20 for admittance plasma glutamine concentrations out of range in contrast to a 50 % mortality risk at APACHE 30 for the range 400–930 µmol/h. Reproduced from [5] with permission

been published employing this type of technique. Available data show that the endogenous production of glutamine is in the region of 50–80 g/day in adults [13–16]. Furthermore, in healthy individuals the endogenous rate of appearance is higher in the fed state as compared to the postabsorptive state [13, 14], reflecting that intake of amino acids other than glutamine stimulates glutamine synthesis *de novo* mainly in skeletal muscle. The possible relationship between plasma glutamine concentration, endogenous rate of appearance for glutamine, and outcome in critical illness has so far not been defined. In healthy individuals, as well as in critically ill patients, it has been demonstrated that exogenous glutamine supplementation does not decrease the endogenous rate of appearance, which suggest that there is not a negative feed-back mechanism to decrease *de novo* glutamine synthesis when concentration is high [15, 17]. The absence of such a negative feed-back may be related to the fact that glutamine is an inter-organ transporter of nitrogen from the periphery to the liver. The alternative, free ammonia, is potentially neurotoxic, which glutamine is not. Therefore, it is most likely metabolically sound to synthesize glutamine for this transportation and, in the liver, a surplus of nitrogen will be converted into urea to be eliminated in the urine. These pathways may be compromised in critically ill patients with failure of these organs. Studies of glutamine turnover and elimination in critically ill patients with compromised liver and/or kidney function are, however, not available. To better define the possible role of exogenous glutamine supplementation, more information from studies of glutamine kinetics and turnover are, therefore, needed.

Which Patients are Suitable for Glutamine Supplementation?

The initial studies of glutamine supplementation were small and involved patients who were receiving parenteral nutrition [18, 19]. Results were encouraging in terms of outcome benefits, and although the generalizability of these studies was limited, meta-analyses including these studies indicated mortality benefits and guidelines recommended intravenous supplementation of glutamine when parenteral nutrition was given to critically ill patients [20, 21]. When glutamine was given enterally, the results were much less conclusive, and meta-analyses of these results were not able to demonstrate beneficial effects; consequently guidelines did not recommend enteral glutamine supplementation [20, 22]. Part of this documentation refers to trials that used so-called immune-nutrition, meaning that a number of agents with potential effect on immune function were combined in the supplementation. It goes without saying that the results from such trials do not allow discrimination of the possible contributions for the individual ingredients in the mixtures given. Nevertheless, when given to critically ill patients receiving enteral nutrition, generally beneficial effects have not been demonstrated when glutamine has been the sole supplement or part of a supplemented mixture [2, 3].

It is unfortunate when reviewing the literature that selection of patients, target for dosing, and effect of treatment are often not very well motivated. Critically ill patients included in studies of exogenous glutamine supplementation are usually patients admitted to the ICU, sometimes confined to only those receiving mechanical ventilation. Often a dichotomization is made related to the route of nutrition administration. There is some empiric evidence for such a discrimination [23, 24], but the possible underlying mechanisms are obscure. Risk-scoring of patients at admission or sequentially during the ICU stay does not usually include any estimate of gut function. It is again empiric evidence that successful enteral feeding, indicative of a functional intestinal tract, is associated with a more favorable outcome, also in patients with comparable risk-scoring (only reflecting other organ systems) [25]. Hence, when evaluating the literature it is important to consider that the scales in the risk-scoring instruments are not linear and that the scores for selected subgroups of patients may not directly correspond to the prediction for unselected patient populations for whom the scoring systems were validated.

In this context, there is also reason to comment upon the length of treatment period. In general there is a marked difference between the mean and the median lengths of stay in the ICU. This difference reflects that the vast majority of patients are short-stayers, less than 4–5 days, while a minority of patients stay for a long time in the ICU. Nevertheless, this small group of long-stayers consumes the majority of ICU days in a given unit. The variability in length of ICU stay within the patient population constitutes a problem when inclusion and exclusion criteria are to be defined. Is it feasible that exogenous supplementation to a critically ill patient for 2 days will make a difference?; 3 days?; 5 days?; 7 days? On the other hand, it is often very difficult to foresee the length of stay for the individual patient at ICU admission. It may, therefore, be reasonable to have a predefined subgroup analysis of those patients who are given treatment for a period of time that is found sufficient for an effect to be demonstrated.

Comments on Recent Studies with Glutamine Supplementation

With this background, it is quite clear that studies including patients with a high mortality risk, who are poorly fed and supplied with pharmacological doses of glutamine are not very likely to produce results on how glutamine supplementation may be beneficial for critically ill patients. Indeed, this strategy turned out to be harmful, possibly attributable to the pharmacological doses of glutamine used [1]. Because glutamine supplementation given to the right patients in the right doses may be helpful, this result imposes the risk of 'killing' the glutamine supplementation concept. To just look upon the critically ill patient as a 'black box', and to pour in pharmacological doses of glutamine without proper nutritional support and without knowledge of whether or not glutamine deficiency is present is obviously not a very good idea [26].

A neutral or non-conclusive effect, which was the result of the Scottish glutamine study, would have been the logical result also in the REDOXS study; therefore, a number of important differences between these studies should be highlighted. The Scottish SIGNET study included well-fed patients with a pragmatic protocol [27]. The study has been criticized for the relatively low dose of glutamine given, for not communicating how much of the intended dose the patients were actually given, and for the limited time period of treatment. The REDOXS study, on the other hand, was not neutral in terms of outcome, rather it demonstrated harm [1]. It is the first study to demonstrate harm related to provision of exogenous glutamine in critically ill patients. Earlier a report of possible harm was published in a case series of hematological patients with insufficient comparability between patients who received extra glutamine and those who did not [28].

A closer look at the comparability of patients in the REDOXS study, also reveals a difference between the patient groups that may offer an alternative explanation for the result of harm. The inclusion criterion was patients with ≥ 2 organ failures according to SOFA scoring, and the group given glutamine had a similar mean SOFA to the group not given glutamine; so far so good. However, if the two groups are compared in patients with > 2 organ failures, suddenly there is a statistically significant difference between them (Fig. 2). To disregard this finding, the risk prediction by SOFA scoring must be assumed to be linear, but there is actually no evidence for such a linearity. On the contrary, there is evidence that mortality rate

Fig. 2 Calculations of the likelihood of occurrence of three or more organ failures and of 30-day mortality rate in the REDOXS study related to whether randomized to glutamine (GLN) supplementation or not [1]

Gln group	n = 611		
No Gln group	n = 607		

3 or more organ failures	424	187	Chi²
	459	148	p = 0.015
28-day mortality	413	198	chi²
	442	165	p = 0.046

increases logarithmically with the number of organ failures [29]. Actually the level of statistical significance attributable to the skewed distribution of patients with > 2 organ failures is larger than the level of significance for the harm of pharmacological doses of glutamine. This is not a scientific comparison, but the investigators of the REDOXS study could perform a multiple stepwise regression analysis to address this possible bias in patient selection.

If the increased mortality in the glutamine group of the REDOXS study can be associated with a difference between the two groups other than the glutamine supply, we are suddenly in quite a different position. The expected non-conclusive result of the study, according to the chosen study population, would then no longer disqualify studies with protocols aimed at evaluating supplementation of an actual glutamine deficiency. If on the other hand, no other difference than the supply of 50 g glutamine daily can be found between the two groups in REDOXS, the mechanism behind the increased mortality must be looked for. Could short-term use of a bodily substance lead to intoxication? At this time-point, we do not know whether the patients that died in the REDOXS study did so with high glutamine concentrations. In the small subgroup of patients in REDOXS in which plasma glutamine concentrations were recorded, no information over outcome was communicated. The endogenous production of glutamine is some 50–80 g/24 h; will an exogenous provision of similar magnitude cause toxicity? This effect has been reported in patients with liver encephalopathy, but in that situation the effect is not specific for glutamine but is reported for amino acids or proteins in general when given at high doses [30].

Suggestions for Future Research

It is obvious that more studies are needed, but it may not currently be possible to randomize patients to be given extra glutamine. At least, it cannot be considered ethical to give glutamine supplementation without monitoring plasma concentrations. However, quite large doses can be given enterally with only marginal effect on plasma concentration. Still toxic? Obviously more observational studies are needed and in addition the toxicity of glutamine must be characterized. Is the toxicity related to plasma concentration?

In general, provision of glutamine by the enteral route only marginally influences plasma concentration, whereas intravenous provision immediately leads to an increased plasma concentration [8]. Moreover, with a high rate of intravenous glutamine infusion, a steady state will be reached [8, 9]. The suggested relationship between a high plasma glutamine concentration at admission and an unfavorable outcome is based on a very limited number of observations, and needs to be further explored by observational studies. The connection between a high plasma glutamine level and acute fulminant hepatic insufficiency is well known [7], but whether a relation between glutamine level and outcome in this specific group exists is not known [30]. In chronic liver disease and in acute-on-chronic liver failure, high plasma glutamine concentrations are not observed. The manufacturer of glutamine containing dipeptides for intravenous use does not recommend supplementation to patients with liver and/or kidney insufficiency. This recommendation is mainly based on the very limited documentation for this patient group, rather than actual data about glutamine toxicity in liver failure or kidney failure. The relationship between kidney failure and mortality in REDOXS is more difficult to interpret [1]. As kidney failure is most often the third organ failure, increased mortality is seen with kidney failure in critical illness. Again we come back to the possibility of a skewed distribution between the randomized groups in that particular study.

Can clinical use of glutamine supplementation be recommended today after REDOXS? Clearly not to critically ill patients with two (or three) organ failures in the acute phase, but what about other situations? It is speculated that the route of glutamine administration, enteral or parenteral, should make a difference. The handling of glutamine is clearly different with different routes of administration as reflected by the effect on plasma concentration [8, 12], but is possible toxicity related to route of administration? It can also be speculated that it is the pharmacological dose of glutamine that is harmful. Are moderate doses safe? These doses were used in the Scottish SIGNET study as well as in the Scandinavian glutamine study [27, 31]. Is glutamine combined with parenteral nutrition safe, while combination with enteral nutrition is harmful? This has recently been argued in meta-analyses in which published studies are divided according to how patients were fed [2], but is there a mechanistic rational for such a suggestion?

Conclusions

The result of the REDOXS study raises concern about whether or not large doses of glutamine can cause harm in critically ill patients. A number of peculiarities in the protocol of the study and in the patient selection should be clarified. This clarification can be done by the REDOXS investigators and by observational studies of critically ill patients. In addition, more research is needed to characterize the relation between endogenous production of glutamine and exogenous supplementation of glutamine in critically ill patients. Finally, glutamine substitution to normalize plasma glutamine concentrations in critically ill patients should be evaluated in well-conducted randomized controlled trials. Meanwhile, it is recommended that use of glutamine supplementation be restricted to situations in which a safety protocol is used or within clinical studies.

References

1. Heyland D, Muscedere J, Wischmeyer PE et al (2013) A randomized trial of glutamine and antioxidants in critically ill patients. N Engl J Med 368:1489–1497
2. Bollhalder L, Pfeil AM, Tomonaga Y, Schwenkglenks M (2013) A systematic literature review and meta-analysis of randomized clinical trials of parenteral glutamine supplementation. Clin Nutr 32:213–223
3. Novak F, Heyland DK, Avenell A, Drover JW, Su X (2002) Glutamine supplementation in serious illness: a systematic review of the evidence. Crit Care Med 30:2022–2029
4. Oudemans-van Straaten HM, Bosman RJ, Treskes M, van der Spoel HJ, Zandstra DF (2001) Plasma glutamine depletion and patient outcome in acute ICU admissions. Intensive Care Med 27:84–90
5. Rodas PC, Rooyackers O, Hebert C, Norberg A, Wernerman J (2012) Glutamine and glutathione at ICU admission in relation to outcome. Clin Sci (Lond) 122:591–597
6. Ekmark L, Rooyackers O, Wernerman J, Flaring U (2009) Plasma glutamine correlates with multiple organ failure in critically ill children. Clin Nutr Suppl 4:174 (abst)
7. Clemmesen JO, Kondrup J, Ott P (2000) Splanchnic and leg exchange of amino acids and ammonia in acute liver failure. Gastroenterology 118:1131–1139
8. Berg A, Rooyackers O, Norberg A, Wernerman J (2005) Elimination kinetics of L-alanyl-L-glutamine in ICU patients. Amino Acids 29:221–228
9. Tjader I, Rooyackers O, Forsberg AM, Vesali RF, Garlick PJ, Wernerman J (2004) Effects on skeletal muscle of intravenous glutamine supplementation to ICU patients. Intensive Care Med 30:266–275
10. Houdijk AP, Rijnsburger ER, Jansen J et al (1998) Randomised trial of glutamine-enriched enteral nutrition on infectious morbidity in patients with multiple trauma. Lancet 352:772–776
11. Dechelotte P, Darmaun D, Rongier M, Hecketsweiler B, Rigal O, Desjeux JF (1991) Absorption and metabolic effects of enterally administered glutamine in humans. Am J Physiol 260:G677–G682
12. Melis GC, Boelens PG, van der Sijp JR et al (2005) The feeding route (enteral or parenteral) affects the plasma response of the dipeptide Ala-Gln and the amino acids glutamine, citrulline and arginine, with the administration of Ala-Gln in preoperative patients. Br J Nutr 94:19–26
13. Darmaun D, Matthews DE, Bier DM (1986) Glutamine and glutamate kinetics in humans. Am J Physiol 251:E117–E126
14. Matthews DE, Marano MA, Campbell RG (1993) Splanchnic bed utilization of glutamine and glutamic acid in humans. Am J Physiol 264:E848–E854
15. Rooyackers O, Prohn M, Van Riel N, Wernerman J (2005) Bolus injection on 13 C-glutamine to study glutamine metabolism in humans. Clin Nutr 24:575–576
16. van Acker BA, Hulsewe KW, Wagenmakers AJ, Soeters PB, von Meyenfeldt MF (2000) Glutamine appearance rate in plasma is not increased after gastrointestinal surgery in humans. J Nutr 130:1566–1571
17. van Acker BA, Hulsewe KW, Wagenmakers AJ, von Meyenfeldt MF, Soeters PB (2000) Response of glutamine metabolism to glutamine-supplemented parenteral nutrition. Am J Clin Nutr 72:790–795

18. Goeters C, Wenn A, Mertes N et al (2002) Parenteral L-alanyl-L-glutamine improves 6-month outcome in critically ill patients. Crit Care Med 30:2032–2037
19. Griffiths RD, Jones C, Palmer TE (1997) Six-month outcome of critically ill patients given glutamine-supplemented parenteral nutrition. Nutrition 13:295–302
20. McClave SA, Martindale RG, Vanek VW et al (2009) Guidelines for the provision and assessment of nutrition support therapy in the adult critically ill patient: Society of Critical Care Medicine (SCCM) and American Society for Parenteral and Enteral Nutrition (A.S.P.E.N.). JPEN J Parenter Enteral Nutr 33:277–316
21. Singer P, Berger MM, Van den Berghe G et al (2009) ESPEN Guidelines on Parenteral Nutrition: intensive care. Clin Nutr 28:387–400
22. Kreymann KG, Berger MM, Deutz NE et al (2006) ESPEN Guidelines on Enteral Nutrition: Intensive care. Clin Nutr 25:210–223
23. Doig GS, Heighes PT, Simpson F, Sweetman EA, Davies AR (2009) Early enteral nutrition, provided within 24 h of injury or intensive care unit admission, significantly reduces mortality in critically ill patients: a meta-analysis of randomised controlled trials. Intensive Care Med 35:2018–2027
24. Heyland DK, MacDonald S, Keefe L, Drover JW (1998) Total parenteral nutrition in the critically ill patient: a meta-analysis. JAMA 280:2013–2019
25. Doig GS, Heighes PT, Simpson F, Sweetman EA (2011) Early enteral nutrition reduces mortality in trauma patients requiring intensive care: a meta-analysis of randomised controlled trials. Injury 42:50–56
26. Preiser JC, Wernerman J (2013) REDOXS: Important answers, many more questions raised! JPEN J Parenter Enteral Nutr 37:566–567
27. Andrews PJ, Avenell A, Noble DW et al (2011) Randomised trial of glutamine, selenium, or both, to supplement parenteral nutrition for critically ill patients. BMJ 342:d1542
28. Pytlik R, Benes P, Patorkova M et al (2002) Standardized parenteral alanyl-glutamine dipeptide supplementation is not beneficial in autologous transplant patients: a randomized, double-blind, placebo controlled study. Bone Marrow Transplant 30:953–961
29. Moreno R, Vincent JL, Matos R et al (1999) The use of maximum SOFA score to quantify organ dysfunction/failure in intensive care. Results of a prospective, multicentre study. Working Group on Sepsis related Problems of the ESICM. Intensive Care Med 25:686–696
30. Amodio P, Bemeur C, Butterworth R et al (2013) The nutritional management of hepatic encephalopathy in patients with cirrhosis: International Society for Hepatic Encephalopathy and Nitrogen Metabolism Consensus. Hepatology 58:325–336
31. Wernerman J, Kirketeig T, Andersson B et al (2011) Scandinavian glutamine trial: a pragmatic multi-centre randomised clinical trial of intensive care unit patients. Acta Anaesthesiol Scand 55:812–818

Part XVI
Sedation

Early Goal-directed Sedation in Mechanically Ventilated Patients

Y. Shehabi, R. Bellomo, and S. Kadiman

Introduction

The use of sedative drugs in intensive care is ubiquitous. Every year, more than 3 million patients worldwide, 50,000 patients in Australia and New Zealand [1, 2] and nearly 800,000 in the United States receive mechanical ventilation and sedation with an in-hospital mortality (2005) of 34.5 %. The estimated US national cost per annum reached nearly $US27 billion in 2005 [3]. In Ontario, in 1992, the number of mechanically ventilated patients was 221/100,000 population with the estimated number of ventilated patients across Canada likely to exceed 75,000 per annum [4]. The number of ventilated patients per 100,000 population is likely to be similar in Europe. Projections suggests that this number is expected to rise by 31 % over the next decade [5]. Almost all ventilated patients receive sedative agents in one form or another [6]. Sedation is given to promote tolerance of endotracheal intubation and associated life-sustaining interventions, including mechanical ventilation, and to relieve anxiety and reduce distress [6]. Thus, sedation is considered vital to patient comfort and safety.

Despite significant advances in the management of critically ill patients, the crude 30-day adjusted mortality in ventilated patients in Ontario increased from 27 % in 1992 to 32 % in 2000 [4]. This presents a significant concern, considering

Y. Shehabi
Clinical School University of New South Wales, Intensive Care Research, The Prince of Wales Hospital, 2031 Randwick, Australia
e-mail: y.shehabi@unsw.edu.au

R. Bellomo
Department of Intensive Care, Austin Hospital and Monash University, Studley Road, 3084 Heidelberg, Australia

S. Kadiman
Department of Anesthesiology, National Heart Institute (Institut Jantung Negara), 50400 Kuala Lumpur, Malaysia

J.-L. Vincent (Ed.), *Annual Update in Intensive Care and Emergency Medicine 2014*, DOI 10.1007/978-3-319-03746-2_48, © Springer International Publishing Switzerland 2014

the widespread application of mechanical ventilation and sedative therapy. Sedative drugs and the strategy of delivering sedation may be an important factor in determining survival after an episode of mechanical ventilation. The impact of etomidate infusion on trauma-related mortality is a stark reminder of the possible link between sedation and mortality [7]. It is extraordinary that many of the commonly used sedative and analgesic agents used in intensive care units (ICUs) today have not undergone long-term safety evaluation. Despite its ubiquitous use and contribution to comfort and safety, sedation carries significant risk [8].

Sedative and analgesic drug-related increase in the risk of death is multifactorial; it can be mediated via several direct and indirect effects. In the context of critical illness with impaired liver and kidney function, sedative drugs and their active metabolites can accumulate, leading to prolonged deep sedation (unintended drug-induced coma), respiratory depression, immune suppression, and hypotension [9, 10]. Prolonged sedation contributes to immobility, weakness and prolongation of mechanical ventilation with attendant need for tracheostomy and extended ICU stay [11]. Subsequent cessation of sedative medications, after prolonged exposure, can lead to drug withdrawal syndromes [12]. These shortcomings expose ICU patients to other major complications, such as agitation requiring physical restraints [12], nosocomial infection [13], pressure sores, critical illness neuropathy and myopathy [11], vascular thrombosis and, in some patients, sepsis, multiple organ failure and death. The incidence and severity of these problems is rising in association with the increasing complexity of surgery and admission of older patients with multiple comorbidities to intensive care [14]. Furthermore, older patients with high severity of illness undergoing complex interventions are at high risk of associated delirium [15, 16]. Delirium and its duration are independently associated with increased mortality [17].

Over the last decade, however, clinical practice has moved towards the use of lighter levels of sedation whenever clinically safe, better management of pain, and recognition that delirium occurs commonly in patients with critical illness [18]. This change in practice is supported by the 2013 Society of Critical Care Medicine (SCCM) Clinical Practice Guidelines on Pain, Agitation and Delirium [19].

Different strategies have been recommended to achieve light sedation including protocolized sedation, sedative interruption, opioid-based sedation and benzodiazepine minimization. Early goal-directed sedation is a strategy that aims to achieve optimal sedation shortly after initiation of mechanical ventilation, using a systematic algorithm which combines the three dimensions of sedative interventions, assessment, titration and the optimal choice of sedative agents. In this chapter, we present the rationale, the key elements, the algorithm, the early experience and future of early goal-directed sedation as a process-of-care for sedation of mechanically ventilated ICU patients.

Early Goal-directed Sedation: Rationale

Early Deep Sedation is Common

The Sedation Practice in Intensive Care Evaluation (SPICE) program included three prospective, multicenter, multinational, longitudinal observational cohort studies in 25 ICUs in Australia and New Zealand (ANZ, n = 251), 11 ICUs in Malaysia (n = 259) and 7 ICUs in Singapore (n = 198), with a total of more than 8000 ICU days of follow-up. All patients were followed up to 180 days for survival [20, 21]. The patients in the ANZ cohort were highly representative of general mixed ICU patients with a mean age of 62 years, a mean APACHE II score of 20.8, a median duration of mechanical ventilation of 5.1 days, a hospital mortality of 21 %, and 180 day mortality of 26 %. These studies found that traditional sedatives (midazolam and propofol) are still almost universally used with one third of patients receiving dexmedetomidine. It also found two important and potentially modifiable elements of sedation therapy: A high prevalence (76 %) of deep sedation especially in the first 48 hours and a high incidence of delirium (50.7 % of all assessable patients), which increased substantially with longer ICU stay [20]. At first assessment, 191/251 patients were deeply sedated and more than 50 % of patients continued to score deep sedation at least once till day 4. Adjusted multivariable analysis showed that early deep sedation was strongly and independently associated with longer time to extubation, hospital death and 180-day mortality but not associated with increased delirium or time to first delirium episode [20].

Sedation Trials Ignored Early Deep Sedation

Over the last decade, sedation minimization strategies have become the focus of strong research interest. Most randomized trials, by virtue of design and need for consent, did not take into account early deep sedation. Amongst many other limitations, this has been a significant drawback of most sedation trials. Therefore, the potential benefits of any strategy that targets light sedation are significantly diminished by late randomization, which allows non-systematic non-protocolized interventions and undetermined duration of deep sedation following initiation of mechanical ventilation.

One way to minimize sedation depth may be the use of planned sedation interruptions. Daily sedation interruption became a key strategy after Kress and colleagues reported significant reductions in ventilation time and ICU stay in a single center 128-patient randomized trial [22]. Patients, however, were recruited into this trial after 48 hours of mechanical ventilation.

While daily sedation interruption has many potential advantages it is not clear whether it offers any advantages compared with a sedation strategy that targets light sedation. A multicenter randomized trial compared protocolized sedation with protocolized sedation plus daily sedation interruption in 423 critically ill, mechanically ventilated medical and surgical patients [23]. There was no difference in the duration of mechanical ventilation, ICU and hospital lengths of stay between the groups.

Despite the limitations of a before-and-after study design, this approach may overcome the problem of late randomization. A before-and-after study of protocolized analgesia and sedation resulted in reduced sedative-induced coma rates, from 18.1 % to 7.1 %, with reduced total doses of sedative and opioids and reduced ventilation and ICU time [24]. This study also showed an absolute risk reduction in hospital mortality of 6.5 %.

The above observations suggest that a strategy that reduces early deep sedation would have the potential to improve relevant and clinically important clinical outcomes, such as mortality.

Key Elements of Early Goal-directed Sedation

Taking into consideration the limitations of previous ICU sedation studies and the failure to account for early deep sedation, it is imperative that any future sedation strategy should have the following principal elements: First, it should be delivered early, within less than 6 hours of initiation of sedation and mechanical ventilation; second, it should rely on an integrated process of targeting light sedation through frequent assessment of sedation levels; and, finally, it should incorporate the use of sedative agents known to promote wakefulness and arousal and/or agents with favorable pharmacokinetic profile, such as short onset and offset time. The 2013 SCCM guidelines [19] recommend early and adequate analgesia, routine use of targeted light sedation and suggested that sedation strategies using non-benzodiazepine sedatives (such as propofol or dexmedetomidine) may be preferred over benzodiazepines. This has strengthened the choice of dexmedetomidine and/or propofol as the sedative agents to be used in early goal-directed sedation. The alpha$_2$ agonist, dexmedetomidine, has emerged over the last 15 years as a viable alternative to traditional sedatives for mechanically ventilated patients with growing evidence that dexmedetomidine facilitates arousable sedation, shortens ventilation time, and attenuates the occurrence of delirium [25, 26].

Based on the above considerations, we recognize that key elements of any plausible strategy directed at improving patient-centered outcomes through reduction of early deep sedation must include:

1. Early effective analgesia titrated to effect according to standardized pain assessment; this assessment is part of a systematic patient evaluation for analgesic need.
2. Early delivery of sedative agents including dexmedetomidine as a primary sedative as needed, shortly after initiating mechanical ventilation;
3. Tight targeting of light sedation early, from the time of initiation, with regular and frequent assessment of patient wakefulness/sedative state and titration of sedative infusions;

4. Avoidance of benzodiazepines and minimization of other sedatives, opioids and antipsychotics;
5. Reduced overall sedation depth with targeted light sedation.

The Early Goal-directed Sedation Algorithm

Early goal-directed sedation is designed to be delivered by bedside clinicians; it is simple, pragmatic and emulates real life sedation management in concordance with the SCCM 2013 guidelines [19]. While the description of the algorithm follows a step-by-step flow for clarity, the algorithm is designed to be delivered as a package and many interventions administered simultaneously (Fig. 1).

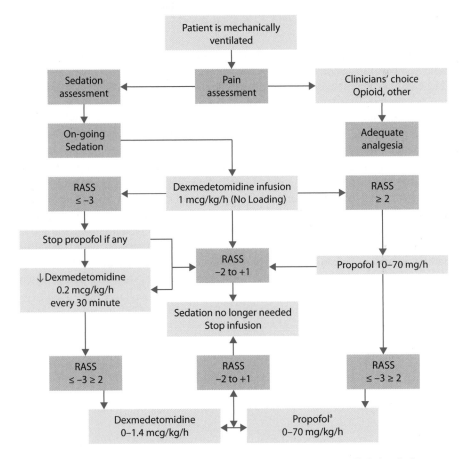

Fig. 1 Early goal-directed sedation algorithm. RASS: Richmond Agitation Sedation Scale; [a] recommend weaning/titrating propofol to the lowest dose before reducing dexmedetomidine

Once a patient is ventilated, pain assessment should be performed; a Numeric Reporting Scale 0–10 is an accepted and validated assessment tool for patients who are able to report pain. The Critical Care Pain Observation Tool (CPOT) [27] is a validated and effective assessment tool in patients who are unable to report pain.

The provision of adequate analgesia using opiates by infusion or incremental boluses is the commonest and most effective pain management in most patients. Agents such as low dose ketamine (4–8 mg/hour) and/or paracetamol can also be used. Care should be taken not to use opiates or ketamine for the purpose of providing sedation but rather to alleviate pain only.

As pain is assessed and treated, sedation level is assessed using any of the validated sedation scales. In our algorithm, we use the Richmond Agitation Sedation scale (RASS) [28]. The target sedation level is light sedation defined as an RASS range between -2 and $+1$.

Pain and sedation assessment is a continuous process that should be done at least every hour and on need basis. This will guide the use and titration of analgesic and sedative agents.

During early goal-directed sedation, we recommend the use of dexmedetomidine as a first line sedative agent starting at 1 mcg/kg/hour without a loading dose. The onset of the sedative effect for dexmedetomidine is about 45–60 minutes. During this period, if sedation is required, then propofol can be given by infusion at 10–70 mg/hour or small boluses of 10–30 mg/hour. The use of propofol should be scaled back to the lowest dose at all times to achieve the target RASS of -2 to $+1$. In more than 75 % of patients, dexmedetomidine as a sole agent would be adequate. If the RASS score is -3 to -5 (moderate to deep sedation), propofol should be stopped first, followed by a gradual reduction in dexmedetomidine infusion by 0.2 mcg/kg/hour every 30 minutes. The process of titration is also a continuous process guided by RASS assessments.

We recommend caution in applying early goal-directed sedation using the above algorithm in patients with head injury, renal failure and in patients with acute liver failure. Dexmedetomidine has not been adequately assessed in these patients.

A summary of patient selection and appropriateness for the early goal-directed sedation algorithm is provided in Table 1.

Table 1 Early goal-directed sedation: Patient selection

Patients who are suitable for the early goal-directed sedation algorithm
Mechanically ventilated patients who are expected to be ventilated and need ongoing sedation for longer than 24 hours
Patients in whom the early goal-directed sedation algorithm is not appropriate
1. Patients where deep sedation is indicated, such as:
a. Traumatic brain injury,
b. Extracorporeal support,
c. High frequency oscillation,
d. Continuous neuromuscular blockade.
2. Patients with a contraindication to dexmedetomidine:
a. Acute fulminant liver failure,
b. High grade atrioventricular block,
c. Heart rate <50/min not induced by adrenergic blockade
d. Heart rate <50/min in the absence of a functioning pacemaker.
e. Systolic blood pressure <85 mmHg despite adequate resuscitation and vasopressor therapy
3. Patients who need palliative therapy

Managing Emergent Agitation during Early Goal-directed Sedation

A common problem associated with critical illness is breakthrough agitation. In early goal-directed sedation, we recommend the following algorithm to manage agitation and/or delirium:

1. Increase the dose of dexmedetomidine to an acceptable maximum dose of up to 1.4 mcg/kg/hour.
2. If dexmedetomidine is at the maximum dose, the use of small boluses or infusion of propofol, in particular to control acute emergent agitation, is recommended at a dose of 10–70 mg/hour by infusion or blouses of 10–50 mg/hour.
3. For persistent agitation, we recommend the use of quetiapine at a starting dose of 12.5 mg twice daily and up to 50 mg twice daily [29].
4. If agitation persists, we suggest the addition of haloperidol 2.5–5 mg blouses every 4–6 hours.
5. For refractory agitation, we recommend further investigation such as an electro-encephalogram (EEG) and/or a computed tomography (CT) scan to rule out organic lesions. We suggest adding a benzodiazepine, such as midazolam, boluses only, 1–3 mg as needed.

Once agitation has resolved, we recommend the withdrawal of all agents in reverse sequence with dexmedetomidine weaned last.

Is Early Goal-directed Sedation Feasible?

The premise of early goal-directed sedation is the provision of adequate analgesia and optimal sedation soon after the initiation of mechanical ventilation. The feasibility of early goal-directed sedation is thus tested through the assessment of key objectives. First, how soon can early goal-directed sedation be effectively delivered? Second, how effective is early goal-directed sedation in providing optimal and preventing early deep sedation? Third, is early goal-directed sedation only effective with a dexmedetomidine based algorithm? Fourth, is early goal-directed sedation achievable outside high intensity bedside nursing such as Australian-based intensive care practice? And finally, is early goal-directed sedation feasible in the context of randomized clinical trials?

We tested the feasibility of delivering a process-of-care sedative intervention that had the above design features in a pilot randomized trial comparing early goal-directed sedation with standard sedation in Australian ICUs [30]. Randomization occurred within a median [interquartile range] of 1.1 [0.46–1.9] hours after intubation or ICU admission for out of ICU intubation. A significantly higher proportion of patients were lightly sedated on days 1, 2 and 3 in the early goal-directed sedation than in the standard care group (12/19 [63.2 %], 19/21 [90.5 %] and 18/20 [90 %], respectively, compared with 2/14 [14.3 %], 8/15 [53.3 %] and 9/15 [60 %], p = 0.005, 0.011, 0.036, respectively). More RASS assessments were between -2 and $+1$ in the first 48 hours in the early goal-directed sedation group than in the standard sedation group (203/307 [66 %] vs. 74/197 [38 %], p = 0.01). Early goal-directed sedation patients received midazolam on 6/173 (3.5 %) study days while standard sedation patients received dexmedetomidine on 4/114 (3.5 %) patient-days. Propofol was given to 16/21 (76 %) of the early goal-directed sedation patients compared to 16/16 (100 %) of the standard sedation patients (p = 0.04). Early goal-directed sedation patients required significantly less physical restraints than did standard sedation patients (1 [5 %] vs 5 [31 %], p = 0.03). There were no differences in vasopressor use and self-extubation [30]. These data support the feasibility of the early goal-directed sedation concept in representative ICUs in Australia.

We also conducted a similar pilot in 10 ICUs in Malaysia (n = 60) and concluded in May 2013. This pilot was designed to test the feasibility of achieving early goal-directed sedation using conventional sedatives and in addition test the feasibility of early goal-directed sedation in ICUs outside an Australian-based ICU practice. The study showed that even with targeted protocol, early goal-directed sedation could not be delivered with conventional sedatives. Midazolam and/or propofol achieved light sedation in the first 48 hours in 68 % of participants vs. 96 % being lightly sedated with a dexmedetomidine-based algorithm. Furthermore, this pilot proved that early goal-directed sedation is a concept that can be delivered in tertiary, regional and rural ICUs.

The results of the Australian and the Malaysian early goal-directed sedation pilot studies provide concrete evidence on the applicability of early goal-directed sedation in the context of randomized multicenter trials.

Early Goal-directed Sedation: A Global Trial

Despite the comprehensive review undertaken, the 2013 SCCM Guidelines called for definitive studies to inform the practice of sedation in critical illness. The paucity of data on long-term and patient centered outcomes is a stark reminder for the need of adequately powered well-designed clinical trials into sedation practice. There are many limitations of previous sedation trials [31] that limited the external validity and general applicability of the evidence produced in different care settings.

Over the last 3 years, we have led a structured sedation research program to address the limitations of previous trials and test an innovative strategy of early goal-directed sedation in a large scale randomized controlled trial. The necessity and value of testing early goal-directed sedation is strong and the strengths of the proposed strategy are clear. First, early goal-directed sedation is aligned with current actual practice as identified by our recent observational longitudinal cohort study and in line with international guidelines. Second, early goal-directed sedation mimics clinical reality and delivers an intervention that combines potentially safer drugs and beneficial light sedation targets. Third, early goal-directed sedation mandates frequent monitoring of patient responsiveness ('wakefulness'), sedation depth, and delirium. Fourth, all interventions are delivered soon after initiation of mechanical ventilation maximizing their potential benefits. Fifth, our planned primary outcomes will be patient-centered and long-term. Finally, as therapy is delivered by bedside nurses, early goal-directed sedation will be applicable to currently practiced ICU models of care.

Our group is leading a large collaborative of researchers worldwide, including more than 50 ICUs in Australia, New Zealand, Canada, Asia, the Middle East and Europe. The Sedation Practice in Intensive Care Evaluation (SPICE Program) is now funded and will deliver many answers to inform worldwide sedation practice in the critically ill. The SPICE program is the largest sedation research program to be launched so far.

Conclusions

Current sedation practice, supported by the 2013 SCCM Guidelines on Pain, Agitation and Delirium, promotes the provision of light sedation whenever clinically safe. Sedation trials in large did not account for the first 48 hours of mechanical ventilation, which represent at least 33 % of total ventilation time in most patients [20]. Deep sedation commonly occurs early after initiation of mechanical ventilation and is a strong independent predictor of time to extubation and long-term mortality. A strategy to reduce early deep sedation through a process of care named early goal-directed sedation has been developed and tested in two pilot randomized trials in 16 ICUs in two different care settings. These pilot trials have confirmed the feasibility, efficacy and safety of the proposed strategy. These results pave the way for a large scale global-reach randomized control trial assessing the clinical effectiveness of early goal-directed sedation on long-term and patient-centered outcomes.

References

1. Australian and New Zealand Intensive Care Society (2011) The Australian and New Zealand Intensive Care Society Clinical Outcome and Resource Evaluation 2010 Annual Report. Australian and New Zealand Intensive Care Society, Melbourne
2. Craven J, Hicks P (2010) Intensive Care Resources and Activity in Australia and New Zealand Annual Report 2009/2010. Anzics Centre for Outcome and Resource Evaluation, Carlton
3. Wunsch H, Linde-Zwirble WT, Angus DC, Hartman ME, Milbrandt EB, Kahn JM (2010) The epidemiology of mechanical ventilation use in the United States. Crit Care Med 38:1947–1953
4. Needham DM, Bronskill SE, Sibbald WJ, Pronovost PJ, Laupacis A (2004) Mechanical ventilation in Ontario, 1992–2000: Incidence, survival, and hospital bed utilization of noncardiac surgery adult patients. Crit Care Med 32:1504–1509
5. Needham DM, Bronskill SE, Calinawan JR, Sibbald WJ, Pronovost PJ, Laupacis (2005) Projected incidence of mechanical ventilation in Ontario to 2026: Preparing for the aging baby boomers. Crit Care Med 33:574–579
6. Wunsch H, Kahn JM, Kramer AA, Rubenfeld GD (2009) Use of intravenous infusion sedation among mechanically ventilated patients in the United States. Crit Care Med 37:3031–3039
7. Ledingham IMA, Watt I (1983) Influence of sedation on mortality in critically ill multiple trauma patients. Lancet 1:1270
8. Devlin JW, Mallow-Corbett S, Riker RR (2010) Adverse drug events associated with the use of analgesics, sedatives, and antipsychotics in the intensive care unit. Crit Care Med 38:S231
9. Devlin JW (2008) The pharmacology of over sedation in mechanically ventilated adults. Curr Opin Crit Care 14:403–407
10. Devlin JW, Roberts RJ (2011) Pharmacology of commonly used analgesics and sedatives in the ICU: benzodiazepines, propofol, and opioids. Anesthesiol Clin 29:567–585
11. Foster J (2005) Complications of sedation and critical illness. Crit Care Nurs Clin North Am 17:287–296
12. Woods JC, Mion LC, Connor JT et al (2004) Severe agitation among ventilated medical intensive care unit patients: frequency, characteristics and outcomes. Intensive Care Med 30:1066–1072
13. Nseir S, Makris D, Mathieu D, Durocher A, Marquette CH (2010) Intensive care unit-acquired infection as a side effect of sedation. Crit Care 14:R30
14. Marik PE (2006) Management of the critically ill geriatric patient. Crit Care Med 34:176–182
15. Ouimet S, Kavanagh BP, Gottfried SB, Skrobik Y (2007) Incidence, risk factors and consequences of ICU delirium. Intensive Care Med 33:66–73
16. Gunther ML, Morandi A, Ely EW (2008) Pathophysiology of delirium in the intensive care unit. Crit Care Clin 24:45–65
17. Shehabi Y, Riker RR, Bokesch PM, Wisemandle W, Shintani A, Ely EW (2010) Delirium duration and mortality in lightly sedated, mechanically ventilated intensive care patients. Crit Care Med 38:8
18. Patel SB, Kress JP (2012) Sedation and analgesia in the mechanically ventilated patient. Am J Respir Crit Care Med 185:486–497

19. Barr J, Fraser GL, Puntillo K et al (2013) Clinical practice guidelines for the management of pain, agitation, and delirium in adult patients in the intensive care unit. Crit Care Med 41:263–306

20. Shehabi Y, Bellomo R, Reade MC et al (2012) Early intensive care sedation predicts long-term mortality in ventilated critically ill patients. Am J Respir Crit Care Med 186:724–731

21. Shehabi Y, Chan L, Kadiman S et al (2013) Sedation depth and long-term mortality in mechanically ventilated critically ill adults: a prospective longitudinal multicentre cohort study. Intensive Care Med 39:910–918

22. Kress JP, Pohlman AS, O'Connor MF, Hall JB (2000) Daily interruption of sedative infusions in critically ill patients undergoing mechanical ventilation. N Engl J Med 342:1471–1477

23. Mehta S, Burry L, Cook D et al (2012) Daily sedation interruption in mechanically ventilated critically ill patients cared for with a sedation protocol a randomized controlled trial. JAMA 308:1985–1992

24. Skrobik Y, Ahern S, Leblanc M, Marquis F, Awissi DK, Kavanagh BP (2010) Protocolized intensive care unit management of analgesia, sedation, and delirium improves analgesia and subsyndromal delirium rates. Anesth Analg 111:451–463

25. Jakob SM, Ruokonen E, Grounds RM et al (2012) Dexmedetomidine vs midazolam or propofol for sedation during prolonged mechanical ventilation: two randomized controlled trials. JAMA 307:1151–1160

26. Riker RR, Shehabi Y, Bokesch PM et al (2009) Dexmedetomidine vs midazolam for sedation of critically ill patients: a randomized trial. JAMA 301:489–499

27. Gélinas C, Fillion L, Puntillo KA, Viens C, Fortier M (2006) Validation of the critical-care pain observation tool in adult patients. Am J Crit Care 15:420–427

28. Sessler CN, Gosnell MS, Grap MJ et al (2002) The Richmond agitation–sedation scale validity and reliability in adult intensive care unit patients. Am J Respir Crit Care Med 166:1338–1344

29. Devlin JW, Roberts RJ, Fong JJ et al (2010) Efficacy and safety of quetiapine in critically ill patients with delirium: A prospective, multicenter, randomized, double-blind, placebo-controlled pilot study. Crit Care Med 38:419

30. Shehabi Y, Bellomo R, Reade MC et al (2013) Early goal directed sedation vs standard care sedation in mechanically ventilated critically ill patients, randomized controlled trial. Crit Care Med 41:1983–1991

31. Shehabi Y, Bellomo R, Mehta S, Riker R, Takala J (2013) Intensive care sedation: The past, present and the future. Crit Care 17:322

Assessment of Patient Comfort During Palliative Sedation: Is it always Reliable?

R. Deschepper, J. Bilsen, and S. Laureys

Introduction

"When death knocks at the door of our ward, we do not easily open the door", an intensivist once said. In the intensive care unit (ICU) and emergency department, care is strongly focused on cure and resuscitation. Notwithstanding the technological progress made in intensive and emergency medicine, a substantial number of the patients admitted to the ICU cannot be saved. In these cases, it is important to make a timely shift from curative efforts to palliative care, so that futile and burdensome interventions can be avoided. When death becomes imminent, a major concern of the family members and caregivers is to assure maximal comfort during the dying process. A central aspect of good end-of-life care is to keep the patient, as much as possible, free of pain and other kinds of distress. However, many critically ill patients often suffer from symptoms such as pain and delirium. More than 50 % of critically ill patients in the ICU experience moderate to severe pain and pain in critically ill patients often remains untreated [1].

On some occasions, patients are unable to communicate or give signs of discomfort and in these circumstances ensuring comfort is very challenging. This is the case, for example, with patients who are in a coma and patients in a vegetative/unresponsive state. Communication is also limited with patients who have been diagnosed as minimally conscious, locked-in syndrome or late-stage dementia and with newborns. Patients may also be unable to communicate because of treatments, such as intubation and administration of neuromuscular blocking agents. In all these patients, assessment of comfort is challenging. Although it might sound obvious, it is important not to overlook the fact that the inability to communicate,

R. Deschepper · J. Bilsen
Department of Public Health, Vrije Universiteit Brussel, 1090 Brussel, Belgium

S. Laureys ✉
Coma Science group, Cyclotron Research Centre and Neurology Department, University and University Hospital of Liège, Sart Tilman B35, 4000 Liège, Belgium
e-mail: steven.laureys@ulg.ac.be

J.-L. Vincent (Ed.), *Annual Update in Intensive Care and Emergency Medicine 2014*,   663
DOI 10.1007/978-3-319-03746-2_49, © Springer International Publishing Switzerland 2014

verbally or non-verbally, does not negate the possibility that an individual is experiencing pain or other kinds of distress and is in need of appropriate treatment to ensure optimal comfort.

Box 1:

Core Elements in Guidelines on Palliative Sedation

- **Indications for palliative sedation**
  - Refractory symptoms leading to unbearable suffering such as intolerable pain, dyspnea and delirium [11, 12, 23, 35]
- **Types of palliative sedation**
  - Degree: mild, intermediate and deep [15]
  - Continuity: from intermittent to continuous [15]
- **Ethical principles**
  - Palliative sedation is normal medical practice and must be clearly distinguished from the termination of life [35]
  - Proportionality: the degree of sedation must not be deeper than necessary to relief suffering [11, 12, 23, 35]
  - Palliative sedation will not (usually) hasten death (and that is certainly not the intention) [12, 15]
- **Administration of drugs**
  - Titration to the minimum level of consciousness reduction necessary to render symptoms tolerable [16, 23, 24]
  - Lack of consensus
    - "No good evidence exists to strongly recommend one medication over any other of those commonly used in continuous palliative sedation therapy" [16]
    - "Midazolam is the drug of first choice" [24]
- **Monitoring of palliative sedated patients**
  - Aspects requiring monitoring: [16]
    - Relief of suffering
    - Level of consciousness (depth of sedation)
    - Adverse effects of sedation
  - Guidelines' evaluations of the usefulness of monitoring scales
    - "There are no scales available to assess the patient's comfort during continue sedation" [24]
    - "Monitoring (observational) scales exist but the usefulness of these scales has not been proven" [16]
    - "Presently no particular scale can be recommended" [16, 24]
  - "Scales involving administration of painful stimuli are not acceptable" [16]
  - Frequency of monitoring: every 20 minutes until adequate sedation has been reached

Patient comfort can often be achieved by 'conventional' pharmacological drugs such as opioids or other symptom-controlling drugs. However, in cases of severe pain caused by withdrawal of life-sustaining treatment, for example, or where refractory symptoms lead to unbearable suffering such as intolerable pain, dyspnea and delirium, a more drastic option may be chosen, known as palliative sedation (Box 1). In these cases, comfort is sought by reducing the patient's level of consciousness [2, 3]. Palliative sedation is ethically controversial because it is viewed by some as a kind of 'slow euthanasia' and because patients are not always involved in the decision-making. Another point of controversy is whether or not palliative sedation has a life-shorting effect and therefore should be considered to be an end-of-life decision [4].

Some studies have pointed out that palliative sedation is an effective method that does not shorten survival time, but the topic creates controversy [2, 5]. However, the practice of palliative sedation has increased substantially and seems to have established its place in end-of-life care. The incidence of palliative sedation is not easily measured, partly because there are several definitions and alternative terms in use, such as 'terminal sedation' and 'continuous sedation until death', to describe this practice [6]. However, available studies indicate that the practice of palliative sedation is increasing in hospitals, nursing homes and the home care setting. The overall reported incidences vary between 7 % and 17 % of all deaths [7]. It is assumed that patients who are sedated according to the current standards of care and the guidelines for palliative sedation are unaware of their clinical situation and, therefore, do not experience symptoms of discomfort, such as dyspnea, delirium, and other distressing conditions that are common during the terminal phase. However, a critical evaluation based on more recent evidence raises the question of whether the current assessments of suffering and awareness are accurate enough. Our concerns are based on three types of problem. First, the assessment of comfort in dying patients is challenging; second, patients are sometimes mistakenly considered to be unaware, and, third, the titration of drugs is difficult.

Problems with Assessment of Comfort in Dying Patients

Pain is always subjective. Therefore, the gold standard for detecting distress is patient self-reporting. However, in the case of palliative sedation, patients are usually unable to communicate whether or not they are still in distress or still (partially) aware of what is happening around them. In these cases, caregivers have to rely on observable signs, such as facial expression. In newborns, for instance, tongue protrusion and licking the lips can be considered a positive affective expression, whereas brow wrinkling and opening the eyes wide are usually considered as facial expressions of negative affect [8]. To achieve a more reliable assessment, several instruments, such as the Visual Analog Scale for pain, are based on these observable signs. Some scales have been developed for non-communicative patients as well, including the Critical Care Pain Observational Tool (CCPOT) [9], the Behavioral Pain Scale (BPS) [10], and the Richmond Agitation-Sedation Scale (RASS) [11] but several problems have been reported. A well-documented problem is that these scales cannot detect pain and awareness in all patients, for example because they depend on inferences made from patients' motor responses [12, 13].

Another problem is that these scales have only been partially validated for dying patients, and in most cases not at all [14]. In the guidelines on palliative sedation it is acknowledged that the efficacy and safety of palliative sedation is not sufficiently understood and that the usefulness of these observational scales has not been proven [15, 16]. These findings cause even more concern considering the evidence that family members of patients often have different perceptions of the patient's comfort and his/her quality of dying during palliative sedation than do caregivers. While family members tend to overestimate pain, caregivers often underestimate it [17]. Furthermore, assessment discrepancies between nurses and physicians often occur [18, 19]. Moreover, non-clinical factors, such as characteristics of both the patient and the caregiver, play a role. For example, paramedical professionals, religious correspondents and older caregivers more often believe that patients in vegetative or minimally conscious states may be experiencing pain [19]. In a study of patients coming to the emergency department with pain-related complaints, older men were less likely than younger men to receive an analgesic or an opioid regardless of pain severity. Older adults were generally less likely to receive pain treatment. However, older women with severe pain were more likely to receive treatment than younger women with severe pain. These results suggest an interaction between age, gender, and pain severity on pain treatment [20].

Physiological parameters such as respiratory frequency, heart rate, blood pressure, pupillary diameter and skin conductance, are also often used as indicators for discomfort but these are not always reliable either [21]. Furthermore, once a decision has been made to provide only palliative care, measuring these parameters is usually considered to be a futile and therefore unnecessary intervention, which is likely to be considered more of an obstacle to a quiet dying process than helpful for the patient.

When patients are considered completely unconscious, they are often considered unable to experience any kind of pain or emotion [22]. However, this topic is still controversial and poses clinical and ethical challenges [8]. In cases of painful interventions and especially after decisions to withdraw life-sustaining support, such as mechanical ventilation or artificial hydration and nutrition, these patients are, therefore, sometimes left without administration of opioids or other analgesic. Mistakenly considering a patient as unaware is a pitfall that may deprive a patient of optimal comfort medication. Therefore, the premise of unawareness is a crucial aspect in critically ill or dying patients.

Problems with Assessment of Awareness

Given the importance of the status of unawareness in comfort care, a reliable assessment of awareness is pivotal. However, in recent years, doubts have arisen as to whether patients labeled 'unconscious' really are completely insensate and unaware. Studies in different types of patient and setting, which critically reviewed awareness, have consistently reported that persons were, in contrast to what was assumed by the caregivers, not always (completely) unaware. For example, several studies showed that patients diagnosed as being in a vegetative state (now also called 'unresponsive wakefulness syndrome') did show (minimal) clinical signs of conscious awareness in about 40 % of cases [23]. In some cases, the purportedly unconscious patient could even reliably generate appropriate electroencephalographic (EEG) responses to two distinct commands [24] and occasionally was even able to establish basic communication with 'yes' or 'no' answers using functional magnetic resonance imaging (fMRI) [25]. These observations proved that some minority of clinically diagnosed unresponsive patients displayed some residual cognitive function and conscious awareness that even skilled caregivers were not able to recognize [26].

Furthermore, patients with locked-in syndrome may be mistakenly considered unconscious. In a survey of 44 patients with locked-in syndrome, the time elapsed between brain insult and the diagnosis of locked-in syndrome was on average 2.5 months (78 days). Several patients had not been diagnosed correctly for more than 4 years. It has been stated that this delay in the diagnosis of locked-in syndrome mainly reflected initial misdiagnosis [27].

In rare cases, patients also have reported awareness during general anesthesia. Light anesthesia has been suggested as a risk factor for this frightening phenomenon [28].

As is the case with perception of pain, a patient's awareness is perceived differently by caregivers and family members. In a study on patients in a persistent vegetative state, 90 % of these patients were considered by family members to have some awareness of the family member's presence and of pain [29]. The study on patients with locked-in syndrome also showed that the first person to realize the patient was conscious and could communicate with eye movements was most often a family member (55 % of cases) and not the treating physician (23 % of cases) [27].

The above examples show how difficult it is to recognize unambiguous signs of conscious perception of the environment and the self. This also applies to the assessment of awareness and communication in non-verbally expressive end-stage palliative sedation patients, who traditionally do not benefit from detailed neurological examinations.

In contrast to palliative care settings, in which advanced monitoring equipment is avoided, in the ICU bispectral (BIS) monitors are usually available. The BIS monitor is a reliable instrument for assessment of the level of sedation. Low BIS index values are known to correlate negatively with higher sedative concentrations. It has to be remembered that assessment of anesthetic depth is not the same as assessment of comfort [30]. Some studies suggest that use of BIS monitoring may be useful, especially in patients who have been administered blocking agents [9]. As mentioned above, behavioral observation is unreliable in these patients because even patients in severe pain may show no observable signs of distress. In a study in non-verbal ICU patients who were mechanically ventilated and sedated, the BIS index seemed to be an indicator for pain during procedures known to be painful. However, further research is needed before this technique can be used for the detection of pain in non-communicative patients [9].

Based on these findings, we have to realize that 'traditional' clinical tools and procedures to assess comfort and awareness in dying non-communicative patients have important methodological limitations. It should be noted that the problems with assessments are not to be ascribed to lack of competence on the part of the caregivers but are of a much more fundamental nature: The absence of reliable tools. The developers of guidelines for palliative sedation are aware of these limitations and rightly point out that there is a lack of evidence (Box 1). Some guidelines mention that "there are no scales available to assess the patient's comfort" [31] and the authors of a recent guideline conclude that "presently no particular scale can be recommended" [16]. Sometimes guidelines refer to sedation scales but point out that these scales are "not intended to measure the effect of sedation but to make clear when the sedation is too deep" [31]. The current guidelines for palliative sedation are therefore limited to suggesting "a daily visit by the physician" and "continue attention to possible expressions of discomfort (e. g., facial expressions, movements etc.)" [31, 32]. Not surprisingly, people who have more intensive contact with the patient, such as nurses and family members, should also play an important role in signaling discomfort in sedated patients [31].

Problems with the Titration of Drugs

Since the aim of palliative sedation is to give optimal comfort but not to hasten death, the principle of proportionality is a pivotal aspect of this treatment. Hence, the guidelines state that sedation should be "no deeper than necessary to avoid suffering" [15, 16, 31, 32]. To meet this principle of proportionality, caregivers should carefully titrate the doses of the drugs so that they are high enough to provide comfort but should not hasten death. Studies have shown that palliative sedation does not usually affect survival time [5]. However, the fact that palliative sedation is considered by some to be 'slow euthanasia' may lead physicians to be 'extra careful' with the use of high doses of sedative medication [4]. Several studies have reported underuse of medicines because of a lack of knowledge, unwarranted beliefs, to avoid the perception of giving 'excessive' doses and even because of fear among caregivers of being accused of 'killing' the patient [33, 34]. In a Dutch study among nurses, sedation was considered insufficiently effective by 42 % of the respondents [35].

Recent Advances Changing Our View of Palliative Sedation

In recent years important progress has been made that has forced us to review our opinions about comfort during palliative sedation. We will report here on some major breakthroughs in the assessment of pain, the assessment of consciousness and the mechanisms of sedation.

An important insight with regard to pain perception and brain activity is that several areas in the brain (thalamus, S1, and the secondary somatosensory or insular, frontoparietal, and anterior cingulate cortices) are activated by pain. This neurological signature of pain is also known as the pain matrix [36]. In a study with patients in a minimally conscious state, patients in a persistent vegetative state and healthy volunteers, Boly and colleagues investigated brain activation induced by noxious stimulation [37]. A remarkable finding was that in minimally conscious state patients, no area of the pain matrix was less activated than in the healthy control group. Since cerebral correlates of pain processing are found in a similar network in controls and patients with minimally conscious state, it is plausible that patients in a minimally conscious state experience pain. An important benefit of this method is that it provides objective evidence of potential pain perception and does not require communication with the patient. This method is also promising because cerebral activity is not only a good indicator for physical pain but can also be considered as an objective indicator for other kinds of suffering, such as emotional suffering caused by feelings of rejection [36]. This may be important because in palliative care all the dimensions of suffering, i. e., physical, social, emotional and spiritual suffering, must be evaluated.

A second breakthrough to be mentioned occurred in the field of awareness. Despite its widespread use, little is known about how anesthesia produces loss of consciousness. Over the past five years, significant progress has been made in understanding what happens in the brain as consciousness departs and returns [38]. Studies based on neuroimaging and electroencephalography have found evidence to support the integrated information theory. This theory states that consciousness depends on the brain's capacity to sustain complex patterns of internal communication [39, 40]. Hence, if we are able to measure communication between different brain areas, this may be an indication of the degree of consciousness. A possible method of establishing communication between brain areas is based on the use of transcranial magnetic stimulation (TMS) and high density EEG. Based on this idea, a recent study introduced a theory-driven index of the level of consciousness, called the perturbational complexity index. This index was tested on a large data set of TMS-evoked potentials recorded with high density EEG in healthy patients and patients with consciousness disorders. The index that resulted from this study can potentially be used for objective determination of the level of consciousness at the bedside [41].

In a study by Boly et al. with healthy volunteers, high density EEG recordings were made during gradual induction of and emerging from unconsciousness with propofol. The study revealed structured EEG patterns that mark the transition between consciousness and unconsciousness induced by propofol. These findings provide precise, neurophysiologically principled markers that can be used to monitor the state of a patient's unconsciousness under propofol general anesthesia [42].

Given the important ethical and clinical aspects related to the depth of sedation, adequate sedation is considered a crucial aspect of palliative sedation and all the guidelines highlight its importance (Box 1). Since the guidelines all seems to rely on behavioral observation, they are based on an important premise, i. e., that the unresponsiveness of the patient is proof of unawareness, and hence of the absence of distress. However, it appears that this premise should be questioned. In an important publication, Sanders et al. concluded that unresponsiveness was not the same as unconsciousness [13]. Unresponsiveness sometimes provides unreliable information about the probability of consciousness. To achieve optimal titration during palliative sedation, i. e., to ensure that the patient is comfortable and to avoid unnecessarily high levels of sedation, we need to make a distinction between three separate concepts: Consciousness, connectedness and responsiveness.

Consciousness can be connected or disconnected. In the latter case, a person can be conscious without experiencing the external world. An example of this is dreaming during natural sleep, but dreaming also seems to occur in more than a quarter of patients anesthetized with propofol or desflurane [43]. Another finding reported by Sanders et al. is based on the isolated forearm technique (IFT). In the IFT, anesthesia is followed by the inflation of a cuff on the arm before neuromuscular blockade is induced. The cuff prevents paralysis of the hand and hence allows a simple kind of communication through predefined hand movements, for instance, squeezing the hand if the answer to a question is "yes". A literature review of IFT studies found that positive responses were observed in a median of 37 % of patients, which is evidence of connected consciousness [13]. Strikingly, also, EEG monitors based on the depth of anesthesia, such as the BIS monitor, could not reliably distinguish between responders and non-responders to the IFT [44, 45].

The above findings have practical implications for anesthesia and palliative sedation, e. g., for monitoring the depth of sedation and the titration of drugs used for palliative sedation. One implication is that consciousness should not always be a clinical problem in which the subjective experience of pain and other kinds of distress is disconnected. If we do not make the distinction between the three concepts – responsiveness, consciousness and connectedness – we risk either administering doses of sedatives that may be too low, entailing the risk of an uncomfortable death, or too high, entailing the risk that this act is perceived as life-shortening or even euthanasia. An example of a case in which insufficient sedation may occur is in patients who are unresponsive but may nevertheless retain some kind of consciousness and hence are able to feel pain and distress. An example in which patients do not necessarily need higher levels of sedation, notwithstanding the fact that they do have some kind of consciousness, may occur when their consciousness is disconnected, which implies that they do not experience their suffering. In theory, this may happen when (palliative) sedated patients are dreaming. Such an event can be detected with an EEG showing the typical pattern of rapid eye movement (REM) sleep, which is similar to the EEG pattern when people are awake. However, we do not have sufficient understanding of how and when consciousness becomes connected to the environment, especially in dying, palliative sedated patients who are very difficult to include in studies on this topic. Moreover, patients on palliative sedation eventually die and will by definition not be able to remember their experience.

Another problem is that palliative sedated patients have not been involved in any of the above studies. This is understandable, because it is ethically delicate to include such patients in these studies. However, given the possible impact, efforts should be made to design studies that do not impose too much extra burden on these patients so that they can be included. Even studies with a limited number of selected patients would be very useful.

How Can the Assessment of Suffering in Palliative Sedated Patients be Improved?

Until now, studies of the efficacy of palliative sedation to relieve pain and discomfort have been based on observational scales or subjective assessments by caregivers [35]. Although some efforts have been made to validate the observation scales, as far as we know all these attempts are based on the same paradigm, i. e., that all kinds of distress in all patients can be measured by observation of the patient and that this is the only available method.

As illustrated in the above studies, new insight and technologies, such as fMRI and EEG, have proven to be promising technologies for detecting awareness and pain that cannot be observed or detected by 'traditional' methods [25]. Although these technologies also have their limitations and should not be regarded as a perfect surrogate for self-reporting, they provide valuable objective and quantifiable indicators of awareness and pain in non-communicative patients. Strikingly, they have not yet been used to check whether the current assessments of palliative sedated patients are reliable. It is remarkable that, given the increasing incidence of palliative sedation, there is so little concern about the risks that patients may experience an uncomfortable dying phase in which they are unable to signal their suffering. An assessment tool that would allow clinicians to determine the appropriate doses of medications more accurately would also encourage more vigorous symptom management in the dying.

Paradoxically, the inability to report distress might also be aggravated or even blocked by the use of drugs that may abolish potential further communication and even facial expressions [12]. Hence, some patients might have subjective phenomenological awareness or suffering with very limited, fluctuating or absent behavioral motor signs of distress [13]. The fact that neuroimaging or electrophysiology recordings have not been used so far to validate the assessment tools for distress in non-communicative patients, even when doubts about these tools have arisen, may be related to the reluctance in palliative and end-of-life care to bother patients with high-tech equipment as, in most cases, patients have already experienced a long treatment period.

Conclusions

A problem in monitoring the depth of palliative sedation and the titration of sedatives is that caregivers still have to make use of very rudimentary assessment tools,
which do not take into account the above described new insights. Uncommunicative
dying patients are a vulnerable population and, therefore, we should do everything possible to assure them a comfortable death, free of pain and distress. We,
therefore, urgently need a triangulation of methods in which existing observational
scales, subjective assessments of caregivers and family, and neuroimaging and/or
electrophysiological techniques are combined (Fig. 1). The latter are non-invasive
procedures which should not burden the patient and his/her family too much. Because of its complexity and intensity, this integrated mixed method is intended for
research and not (yet) for everyday clinical assessments. It can be used for the
validation of existing clinical tools for the assessment of distress in palliative sedated patients. Each of the three methods has its potentials and limitations but, in
combination, they can be used to achieve the best possible assessments.

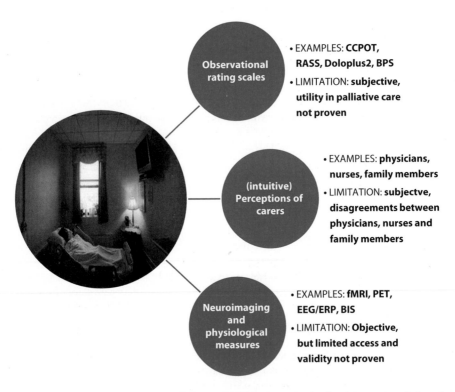

Fig. 1 Triangulation of assessment of distress in the non-communicative dying patient (adapted
from [2] with permission). CCPOT: Critical Care Pain Observational Tool; RASS: Richmond
Agitation-Sedation Scale; BPS: Behavioral Pain Scale; fMRI: functional magnetic resonance
imaging; PET: positron emission tomography; ERP: event related potential; EEG: electroencephalography; BIS: bispectral index

Acknowledgements

Supported by a grant from the Research Council of the Vrije Universiteit Brussel (Project HOA 27). SL is Research Director at the Belgian National Fund for Scientific Research (FRS). The authors also want to thank Said Hachimi-Idrissi, Jan Poelaert and Wim Distelmans for their valuable input.

References

1. Gelinas C (2007) Management of pain in cardiac surgery ICU patients: have we improved over time? Intensive Crit Care Nurs 23:298–303
2. Deschepper R, Laureys S, Hachimi-Idrissi S, Poelaert J, Distelmans W, Bilsen J (2013) Palliative sedation: Why we should be more concerned about the risks that patients experience an uncomfortable death. Pain 154:1505–1508
3. Kirk TW, Mahon MM (2010) National Hospice and Palliative Care Organization (NHPCO) position statement and commentary on the use of palliative sedation in imminently dying terminally ill patients. J Pain Symptom Manage 39:914–923
4. Claessens P, Menten J, Schotsmans P, Broeckaert B (2012) Level of consciousness in dying patients. The role of palliative sedation: a longitudinal prospective study. Am J Hosp Palliat Care 29:195–200
5. Maltoni M, Scarpi E, Rosati M et al (2012) Palliative sedation in end-of-life care and survival: a systematic review. J Clin Oncol 30:3429
6. Rys S, Mortier F, Deliens L, Deschepper R, Battin MP, Bilsen J (2013) Continuous sedation until death: moral justifications of physicians and nurses – a content analysis of opinion pieces. Med Health Care Philos 16:533–542
7. Anquinet L, Rietjens JA, Seale C, Seymour J, Deliens L, van der Heide A (2012) The practice of continuous deep sedation until death in Flanders (Belgium), the Netherlands, and the U.K.: a comparative study. J Pain Symptom Manage 44:33–43
8. Demertzi A, Racine E, Bruno MA et al (2013) Pain perception in disorders of consciousness: neuroscience, clinical care, and ethics in dialogue. Neuroethics 6:37–50
9. Gelinas C, Tousignant-Laflamme Y, Tanguay A, Bourgault P (2011) Exploring the validity of the bispectral index, the Critical-Care Pain Observation Tool and vital signs for the detection of pain in sedated and mechanically ventilated critically ill adults: a pilot study. Intensive Crit Care Nurs 27:46–52
10. Ahlers SJ, van der Veen AM, van Dijk M, Tibboel D, Knibbe CA (2010) The use of the Behavioral Pain Scale to assess pain in conscious sedated patients. Anesth Analg 110:127–133
11. Arevalo JJ, Brinkkemper T, van der Heide A et al (2012) Palliative sedation: reliability and validity of sedation scales. J Pain Symptom Manage 44:704–714
12. Brown JE, Chatterjee N, Younger J, Mackey S (2011) Towards a physiology-based measure of pain: patterns of human brain activity distinguish painful from non-painful thermal stimulation. PLoS One 6:e24124
13. Sanders RD, Tononi G, Laureys S, Sleigh JW (2012) Unresponsiveness not equal unconsciousness. Anesthesiology 116:946–959
14. Brinkkemper T, van Norel AM, Szadek KM, Loer SA, Zuurmond WW, Perez RS (2013) The use of observational scales to monitor symptom control and depth of sedation in patients requiring palliative sedation: a systematic review. Palliat Med 27:54–67
15. de Graeff A, Dean M (2007) Palliative sedation therapy in the last weeks of life: a literature review and recommendations for standards. J Palliat Med 10:67–85
16. Dean MM, Cellarius V, Henry B, Oneschuk D (2012) Framework for continuous palliative sedation therapy in Canada. J Palliat Med 15:870–879

17. Kappesser J, Williams AC (2010) Pain estimation: asking the right questions. Pain 148:184–187
18. Breau LM, McGrath PJ, Stevens B et al (2006) Judgments of pain in the neonatal intensive care setting: a survey of direct care staffs' perceptions of pain in infants at risk for neurological impairment. Clin J Pain 22:122–129
19. Demertzi A, Schnakers C, Ledoux D et al (2009) Different beliefs about pain perception in the vegetative and minimally conscious states: a European survey of medical and paramedical professionals. Prog Brain Res 177:329–338
20. Platts-Mills TF, Hunold KM, Weaver MA et al (2013) Pain treatment for older adults during prehospital emergency care: variations by patient gender and pain severity. J Pain 14:966–974
21. Halliburton JR (1998) Awareness during general anesthesia: new technology for an old problem. CRNA 9:39–43
22. Laureys S (2005) Science and society: death, unconsciousness and the brain. Nature Rev Neurosci 6:899–909
23. Schnakers C, Vanhaudenhuyse A, Giacino J et al (2009) Diagnostic accuracy of the vegetative and minimally conscious state: clinical consensus versus standardized neurobehavioral assessment. BMC Neurol 9:35
24. Cruse D, Chennu S, Chatelle C et al (2011) Bedside detection of awareness in the vegetative state: a cohort study. Lancet 378:2088–2094
25. Monti MM, Vanhaudenhuyse A, Coleman et al (2010) Willful modulation of brain activity in disorders of consciousness. N Engl J Med 362:579–589
26. Laureys S, Schiff ND (2012) Coma and consciousness: paradigms (re)framed by neuroimaging. Neuroimage 61:478–491
27. Laureys S, Pellas F, Van Eeckhout P et al (2005) The locked-in syndrome: what is it like to be conscious but paralyzed and voiceless? Prog Brain Res 150:495–511
28. Ghoneim MM, Block RI, Haffarnan M, Mathews MJ (2009) Awareness during anesthesia: risk factors, causes and sequelae: a review of reported cases in the literature. Anesth Analg 108:527–535
29. Tresch DD, Sims FH, Duthie EH Jr, Goldstein MD (1991) Patients in a persistent vegetative state attitudes and reactions of family members. J Am Geriatr Soc 39:17–21
30. Sackey PV (2008) Frontal EEG for intensive care unit sedation: treating numbers or patients? Crit Care 12:186
31. Royal Dutch Medical Association (KNMG) (2009) Guideline for palliative sedation. Available at: http://www.palliativedrugs.com/download/090916_KNMG_Guideline_for_Palliative_sedation_2009__2_%5B1%5D.pdf. Accessed Nov 2013
32. Cherny NI, Radbruch L (2009) European Association for Palliative Care (EAPC) recommended framework for the use of sedation in palliative care. Palliat Med 23:581–593
33. Jackson DL, Proudfoot CW, Cann KF, Walsh TS (2009) The incidence of sub-optimal sedation in the ICU: a systematic review. Crit Care 13:R204
34. Oldenmenger WH, Sillevis Smitt PA, van Dooren S, Stoter G, van der Rijt CC (2009) A systematic review on barriers hindering adequate cancer pain management and interventions to reduce them: a critical appraisal. Eur J Cancer 45:1370–1380
35. Brinkkemper T, Klinkenberg M, Deliens L et al (2011) Palliative sedation at home in the Netherlands: a nationwide survey among nurses. J Adv Nurs 67:1719–1728
36. Wager TD, Atlas LY, Lindquist MA, Roy M, Woo CW, Kross E (2013) An fMRI-based neurologic signature of physical pain. N Engl J Med 368:1388–1397
37. Boly M, Faymonville ME, Schnakers C et al (2008) Perception of pain in the minimally conscious state with PET activation: an observational study. Lancet Neurol 7:1013–1020
38. Bodart O, Laureys S, Gosseries O (2013) Coma and disorders of consciousness: scientific advances and practical considerations for clinicians. Semin Neurol 33:83–90
39. Rosanova M, Gosseries O, Casarotto S et al (2012) Recovery of cortical effective connectivity and recovery of consciousness in vegetative patients. Brain 135:1308–1320

40. Demertzi A, Soddu A, Laureys S (2013) Consciousness supporting networks. Curr Opin Neurobiol 23:239–244
41. Casali AG, Gosseries O, Rosanova M et al (2013) A theoretically based index of consciousness independent of sensory processing and behavior. Sci Transl Med 14:198ra105
42. Boly M, Moran R, Murphy M et al (2012) Connectivity changes underlying spectral EEG changes during propofol-induced loss of consciousness. J Neurosci 16:7082–7090
43. Leslie K, Sleigh J, Paech M, Voss M, Lim C, Sleigh C (2009) Dreaming and electrographic changes during anesthesia maintained with propofol or desflurane. Anesthesiology 111:547–555
44. Schneider G, Wagner K, Reeker W et al (2002) Bispectral Index (BIS) may not predict awareness reaction to intubation in surgical patients. J Neurosurg Anesthesiol 14:7–11
45. Russell IF (2006) The Narcotrend 'depth of anaesthesia' monitor cannot reliably detect consciousness during general anaesthesia: an investigation using the isolated forearm technique. Br J Anaesth 96:346–352

Part XVII
ICU Organization and Quality Issues

Patient Identification, A Review of the Use of Biometrics in the ICU

M. Jonas, S. Solangasenathirajan, and D. Hett

Introduction

The ability to identify any patient and match them to the correct care pathway and healthcare professional should represent an absolute right for any individual; however, the potential for misidentification is an ever-present risk, especially in the incapacitated or unconscious patient. The technological 'know how' to identify individuals is electronically advanced in the security sector, but as yet undeveloped in healthcare, despite the growth and widespread adoption of electronic health care systems. It is a certain prediction that with the accelerating development of health informatics in hospitals, biometric identification will have to become embedded within our clinical information systems. The progression of both patient and staff 'tagging' and identification, is inevitable.

In 1999, the Institute of Medicine estimated that between 44,000 and 98,000 deaths per year were attributable to avoidable inaccurate patient identification [1]. A decade later, patient misidentification is still a major problem, which could be minimized by replacing the 'human' contribution of identification with a technological approach [2]. Biometric technologies have evolved rapidly, largely in conjunction with security informatics, as a way of combating identity theft and access control. There has been only limited penetration into the heath technology arena and one reason for this is the relative ignorance of biometric systems by healthcare professionals [3].

Biometric Systems

A biometric identification system is a technology that can identify an individual based on a particular biological characteristic that is unique to them [4]. There

M. Jonas ✉ · S. Solangasenathirajan · D. Hett
Dept of Intensive Care, University Hospital Southampton, Southampton, UK
e-mail: maxjonas@me.com

J.-L. Vincent (Ed.), *Annual Update in Intensive Care and Emergency Medicine 2014*,   679
DOI 10.1007/978-3-319-03746-2_50, © Springer International Publishing Switzerland
2014

are an array of different methods of biometric identification currently in use, all of which have advantages and disadvantages. These include facial imaging, facial thermograms, fingerprinting, hand geometry, retinal scanning and, more recently, vein pattern scanning [5–7].

Finger vein authentication in the medical arena is an emerging healthcare biometric technology, which uses a technique of imaging the digital venous patterns of a finger using infrared light [7–9]. This form of identification is robust and accurate, because vein patterns are unique for each finger as well as each person. This makes misidentification extremely unlikely, operating with the same precision as the iris scanner and relying on just a finger probe [9]. This observation has already led to the adoption of 'Finger Vein Scanners' as a means of providing top-level security both in banks and more recently in European security services [10].

The Importance of Correct Identification

Numerous examples of misidentification that jeopardize a patient's safety are recorded annually, meaning that one patient ends up being given a treatment intended for another [11].

Many patients on the intensive care unit (ICU) and emergency pathways are incapacitated/unconscious and unable to confirm their identity in the same way as elective hospitalized patients would when consenting to, or undergoing a procedure. Additionally, these patients can be particularly brittle and unstable and may require therapeutic interventions, which are linked to a chain of other investigations, that are only applicable to that patient. The correct (and immediate) identification of patients is, therefore, crucial [12]. The administration of a drug to the wrong patient, or the wrong blood transfusion, would be life-threatening to any patient, but especially to critically ill and unstable ICU patients. In 2000, UK data suggested that approximately 10 % of NHS admissions in the UK had an adverse event with a significant proportion being identity related. This represents nearly 850,000 patients being involved in some form of patient safety incident [13]. With this denominator, the NHS in the UK has heightened the enhancement of patient safety with a drive to stop misidentification of patients.

The UK Department of Health now considers the wrong identification of a patient as a 'never event', i. e., an occurrence that just should not happen to a patient; 'never events' are centrally reportable occurrences that carry a financial and managerial penalty for the hospital [6]. The pressure is now building to provide a fool proof system of identification that will link not only treatment to identity but also 'tag' healthcare workers to a patient's care record, providing an audit trail for future scrutiny and governance.

Current Identification Systems

The most commonly used identification system is the 'patient wristband', which may include up to five points of the patient's identification: forename, surname, date of birth, first line of their address and their hospital or health system number [11]. Although widely used, there are numerous potential dangers for patient identification using wristbands. The removal of wristbands after they have been applied to the patient is the biggest issue, either by the patient themselves or by one of the medical professionals following a procedure. Additionally they are unsuitable for psychiatric patients or those with learning difficulties in whom other manual methods have been considered, with limited success, such as barcoding and radio frequency [14].

Biometric Identification

Biometric identification is defined as the process of identifying a person based on a distinguishing characteristic, which can either be physiological or behavioral [7]. Behavioral identification analyses and considers the way people carry out particular tasks such as walking, typing and writing [15]. For example, current systems study an individual's gait, keystroke and signature to identify them [16]. Such systems are reliable because human behavior in general cannot be easily recreated and so forgery is deemed to be very difficult. Physiological identification encompasses biological characteristics that are developed during fetal development and in the first years of life. Examples of such characteristics include vein pattern, facial imaging, iris and retinal scanning, fingerprints and hand geometry [15].

How a Biometric Identification System Works

There are two stages in the process of biometric identification: the enrolment phase and the recognition phase. The enrolment phase is the period when the biometric characteristic of the individual is initially scanned by the device acquiring a digital representation. This digital representation is then processed and compacted into the form of a template that then can be stored [5]. During the recognition phase, the biometric reader captures the characteristic again and converts them into another digital representation. This is then compared against all the templates stored on the database to establish the identity of the individual [5].

The Ideal Biometric Identification System

An ideal system will have particular characteristics to function optimally and efficiently. These characteristics include universality, uniqueness, permanence and collectability. The system must be one where all the members of the population will have the particular characteristic that the biometric is trying to identify and so is *universal*. This characteristic must also be different for every person and is therefore *unique* to every individual [16, 17]. The characteristic must also not vary despite the conditions and timing of the collection of data, so has some *permanence* and finally the measurements can be *collected quantitatively* [16, 18].

Current Biometric Systems

Behavioral Biometrics

Keystroke
It is believed that every individual types in their own characteristic way on a keyboard [16]. This system looks at the typing rhythm for an individual and is able to verify the user at the log in stage. There are limitations, because a person may have variations in their own typical typing patterns, which depend on other factors, mood, pressure etc.

Signature
There are two methods in the approach to using signatures as a form of identification: Dynamic and static [5]. The dynamic approach monitors the movement of the pen during the process of writing the signature rather than matching the image of the signature, which is the static approach. This dynamic approach is thought to be characteristic to the individual and has been used in many situations, including government, legal and commercial documents and transactions [16]. The formation of a signature involves a learning process and the speed, velocity and pressure of a signature remain relatively consistent once it has been formed. These techniques are, however, not always permanent and can possibly change over time due to emotional or physical influences. Fraud is a potential problem as signature forgery is relatively easy and can fool the system [16, 19].

Gait
Gait is observing the way an individual walks. It is not as specific as other methods in terms of uniqueness; however, for low security applications it is a simple verification method. It can however, over time, become inconsistent due to variations in body weight, injuries to the joints or brain or possibly due to inebriety. The system uses video-sequence footage to capture the individual's gait, particularly assessing the different movements of the joints [16].

Voice
Voice recognition systems involve physiological and behavioral biometrics to some degree. An individual's voice has many influencing factors, such as the shape and size of the appendages involved, including the vocal tracts, lips, mouth and nasal cavities as well as the actual synthesis of sound. Voice is invariant from individual to individual; however, for the person themselves there can be variance in the voice

due to age, medical conditions and emotional state. Background noise can also be a contributing unfavorable factor in voice recognition as it can interfere with detection of the voice [16].

Physiological Biometrics

Facial recognition
Facial recognition is one of the most common and widely used biometric technologies. The methods of capturing the image are by using video or thermal imaging. Facial imaging analyses the unique shapes, patterns and positioning of all the facial features, whereas facial thermograms look at the underlying vascular pattern in the human face [5, 19]. Facial thermograms are expensive because of the high costs of infrared cameras. For facial imaging there are also some restrictions, because in most cases a fixed and plain background is required. Additionally, if two drastically differing views are captured, the image may not be recognized, as the system will not be able to match it with the stored template. Both methods are non-intrusive and require no contact, which makes them appealing to the user [16].

Fingerprinting
Fingerprinting captures a pattern of the ridges and furrows on the surface of the fingertip. These features are determined during the fetal period of life and remain unchanged throughout adulthood. Fingerprints are different for every finger of an individual and they have been found to be different even in identical twins. However, fingerprints can be altered by mechanical disruption to the surface of the finger, for example, in manual workers in whom they may be subject to cuts and trauma, which can affect the fingerprint pattern [5, 16].

Hand geometry
This system captures a three-dimensional image of the hand by taking a variety of measurements including the shape, length and widths of the fingers. It has been found that this form of identification is relatively cheap and easy to use. In addition, environmental factors, such as dry weather or skin conditions, are not known to affect correct verification using the system. However, the geometry of the hand is not known to be unique for every individual and some limitations, such as restrictions in dexterity, e. g., arthritis, may also affect the fidelity of this system [5, 19].

Iris and retinal scanning
The iris is formed during fetal development and is generally fully developed in the first two years of life [4, 19]. Each iris is distinctive and is different in identical twins, much like fingerprints. It is also very difficult to tamper with the structural integrity of the iris and the system is able to detect designer or colored contact lenses, making fraud very difficult.

Table 1 Evaluation of biometric techniques [14]

Biometric Technique	EER	FAR	FRR	Subjects	Remarks
Face	N/A	1 %	10 %	37,437	Variable conditions, indoors and outdoors
Voice	6 %	2 %	10 %	30	Text dependent and multilingual
Keystrokes	1.8 %	7 %	0.1 %	15	6-month period
Fingerprint	2 %	2 %	2 %	25,000	Rotation and skin distortion
Hand geometry	1 %	2 %	2 %	129	With rings and poor placement
Iris	0.01 %	0.94 %	0.99 %	1224	Indoor environment

Retinal scanning involves the individual looking into an eyepiece and focusing on a specific spot of the visual field; the retinal vasculature is then imaged. Retinal vasculature is unique for every individual and for each eye as well.

There are some major disadvantages to these systems as they require a steady gaze into the eye piece, as well as conscious effort on the part of the user to keep their eye open, which can be difficult to achieve. This is one of the reasons that these scanners are disappearing from airports, as user error is so prevalent [5, 16].

Table 1 lists the various biometric technologies available in practice [14], showing a relatively low false acceptance rate (FAR) and false rejection rate (FRR) for iris scanning compared to other technologies, such as face recognition and voice. This observation indicates the higher fidelity of such a technology making it more applicable for identification purposes. Iris scanning has been compared to finger vein pattern imaging, which does not appear on the table, and both have similar FRR and FARs.

Current Applications of Biometric Identification

Biometric identification is already implemented in a wide range of applications, including forensics, within the government as well as commercial establishments. Commercially, biometrics are used for access control, in e-commerce, security of electronic data, internet banking, ATM and credit cards. These knowledge-based systems effectively use some form of personal identification number (PIN) or password in conjunction with biometrics. Government applications include national identity (ID) cards, driver's licenses, social security and passport control, in which token-based systems are involved, with the use of ID badges and badges alongside the biometric technology. Forensic applications include criminal identification, corpse identification, parental determination and prison security. It is these systems that have adopted biometric systems solely.

Finger Vein Scanner

The ideal biometric identification system has previously been defined as a technique in which the characteristic being measured is universal, distinctive and permanent as well as quantifiably collectable.

Vein patterns are different for each finger as well as for every individual and once they are developed during childhood, remain permanent throughout adulthood thus making them ideal [9, 20]. Vein pattern identification uses near infrared light with the wavelength between 700 nm and 1000 nm. These wavelengths are used because they can pass through human tissue but are absorbed by hemoglobin in blood vessels causing veins alone to appear as dark line shadows, which can be captured as an image [9, 21]. Arteries do not appear on the captured image as they are deeper in the finger and finger tissue scatters the light before it reaches these blood vessels.

There are two methods of capturing the vein image: Light reflection and light transmission. In light reflection, the light sensor and image sensor are on the same side of the finger; when light is transmitted it is reflected off the surface of the finger and is captured by the image sensor. In light transmission, the finger is placed in between the image sensor and the light source and the near infrared light is passed through the finger. The latter technique is most often used due to its high accuracy [9]. Once the image is captured using the camera, the vein pattern is extracted from the image stored as a template, which is later used to enable authentication of the vein patterns [21]. This process can be seen in Fig. 1.

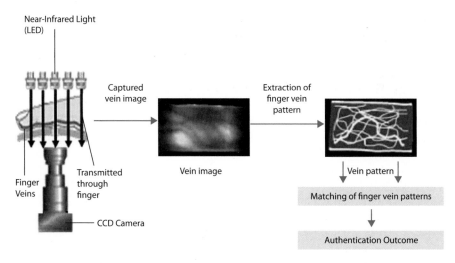

Fig. 1 Authentication process for finger vein scanning

Research and Use of the Vein Scanner

There is limited previous research on medical use of the vein reader; however, in recent years there has been an increasing number of studies as the technology has developed in other arenas [22]. There is concordance among the various studies that the vein reader is highly effective and accurate. Various parameters have been considered in the evaluation of the vein reader, including false acceptance and rejection rates [14]. Once these values have been calculated, it is possible to describe receiver operating characteristics that are used to evaluate the effect of false acceptance or match rates (FMR) and false rejection or non-match rates (FNR) have on each other [23].

The use of vascular biometrics has been evaluated in a number of studies. A near-infrared finger vein scanner was used in 678 volunteers who were scanned and then re-scanned. The results showed that all 678 volunteers were correctly re-identified [24], which carries a concordance with results obtained on the critical care unit at University Hospital Southampton in 150 patients (2012). Yanagawa et al. [20] studied the diversity of the human finger and its potential in personal identification. They scanned right and left index and middle fingers from over 500 volunteers using the vein reader. The fingers were then rescanned to evaluate the false rejection and acceptance rates of the system and the results compared to iris pattern imaging. The authors concluded that the false rejection and acceptance rates reflected a high reliability of the finger vein system. In addition, compared to iris pattern imaging, the standard deviations calculated in both studies were virtually equal and so the vein pattern reader could confidently be used as a personal identification system as well.

Pilot studies are on-going in the UK and US in healthcare and a healthcare system in Carolina, USA, which includes 19 hospitals and 150 clinics, has adopted biometrics using the finger vein reader for identifying patients [10] having enrolled some 180,000 patients in three different counties into the program. The system was found useful in situations where the patient was unable to communicate with the staff in helping to identify the patient and access their health records quickly. In the emergency department, where rapid treatment is essential, the timely identification of a patient was also found to be valuable.

Advantages of the Vein Reader

Most research has shown the vein reader to be reliable and easy to use [8]. Vein patterns are different for each finger and for each person. This was found to be the case even among identical twins and remains constant through the adult years. As the finger veins are hidden underneath the skin's surface, forgery is extremely difficult. In addition, surface conditions, for example, affecting the skin on the hand, have no effect on the vein pattern. The system is able to produce stable and clearly defined images, which would aid rapid and efficient recognition [9]. The finger vein scanner is considered to be hygienic as it is contactless and requires little user training to implement [25]. It also carries fewer stigmas than fingerprinting for example. Additionally venous patterns in the finger are not easily copied, damaged or altered, meaning correct re-identification achievable in virtually every case.

Disadvantages of the Vein Reader

The main disadvantage is the cost involved in the system, not only with the use of the infrared readers but also the implementation of the system. However, these factors are becoming less marked as the costs of this technology fall. Another disadvantage is that the quality of the vein image is reduced in bright lighting conditions and with patient movement, so shielding and immobility are important. Our research suggests that the venous pattern is constant even with hypotension and in the presence of vasotropes.

Conclusions

Biometric identification is an emerging health technology that is being found to be highly useful, secure and effective. Its use could be highly valuable in healthcare where misidentification of patients is a continuous problem Technologies, such as the finger vein reader, have been found to be safe and accurate. The ease of use and simple implementation of such a system potentially make it an ideal tool for the healthcare setting. The limited research and the continuing emergence of new developments highlight the importance of further research into the effectiveness and accuracy of these systems.

References

1. Koshy R (2005) Navigating the information technology highway: computer solutions to reduce errors and enhance patient safety. Transfusion 45:189S–205S
2. Bennardello F, Fidone C, Cabibbo S et al (2009) Use of identification system based on biometric data for patients requiring transfusions guarantees transfusion safety and traceability. Blood Transfus 7:193–203
3. Carlisle P (2011) Natural next step for access biometrics. Hospital Access Management 6:70–72
4. De Luis-Garcia, Alberola-Lopez (2003) Biometric identification systems. Signal Processing 83:2539–2557
5. Jain A, Hong L, Pankanti S (2000) Biometric identification. Commun ACM 2:91–98
6. National health Service (2011) Core list of never events. Available at: http://www.nrls.npsa.nhs.uk/resources/collections/never-events/core-list/ Accessed Nov 2013
7. FastVein™. Available at: http://cssbiometrics.com/fastvein-identity_management.html Accessed Nov 2013
8. Hejtmankova D, Vorak R (2009) A new method of finger vein detection. International Journal of BioScience and BioTechnology 1:11–16
9. Hashimoto J (2006) Finger vein authentication technology and its future. VSLI Circuits, Digest of Technical Papers 5–8

10. Martin Z (2007) A new application for biometrics. Health Data Manag 15:46–48
11. Ranger C, Bothwell S (2004) Making sure the right patient gets the right care. Quality Safety Health Care 13:329
12. Leonard D, Pons A, Asfour S (2009) Realisation of a universal patient identifier for electronic medical records through biometric technology. IEEE Trans Inf Technol Biomed 13:494–500
13. Van der Plog I (2005) Biometric identification technologies: ethical implications of the information of the body. Biometric Technology and Ethics 1:1–19
14. Bhattacharyya D (2009) Biometric authentication: A review. International Journal of Service, Science and Technology 3:13–26
15. Kosmala J, Saeed (2012) Human identification by vascular patterns. In: Saeed K, Nagashima T (eds) Biometrics and Kansei Engineering. Springer, Tokyo, pp 67–87
16. Jain A, Ross A, Prabhakar S (2004) An introduction to biometric recognition. Transactions of Information Technology in Biomedicine 141:4–20
17. El-Bakry H, Mastorakis N (2009) Personal identification through biometric technology. Proceedings of the 9th WSEAS International Conference on Applied Informatics and Technology, p 325–340
18. Phillips PJ, Martin A (2000) An introduction to evaluating biometrics systems. Computer 33:6–63
19. Winter W, Huber L (2000) Part 6: Biometric identification: Limits and possibilities. BioPharm International, Santa Monica
20. Yanagawa T, Aoki S, Ohyama T (2007) Human finger vein images are diverse and its patterns are useful for personal identification. MHF Preprint Series 23–24:1–8
21. Mulyono D, Shi Jinn H (2008) A study of finger vein biometric for personal identification. Proceedings of International Symposium on Biometrics and Security Technologies, p 1–8
22. Pankanti S, Bolle R, Jain A (2000) Biometrics: The future of identification. Computer 33:46–49
23. Deepika CL, Kandaswamy A, Vimal C (2005) Protection of patient identity and privacy using vascular biometrics. International Journal of Security 4:64–84
24. Kono M, Ueki H, Umemura S (2002) Near-infrared finger vein patterns for personal identification. Applied Optic 41:7429–7436
25. Roberts C (2006) Biometric technologies – palm and hand. Centre for Critical Infrastructure Protection 4:1–17
26. Husng B (2010) Finger-vein authentication base on wide line detector and pattern normalisation. 20th International Conference on Pattern Recognition (ICPR), p 1269–1272

Structured Approach to Early Recognition and Treatment of Acute Critical Illness

O. Kilickaya, B. Bonneton, and O. Gajic

Introduction: Global Burden of Critical Illness

Well-known global health priorities (malaria, pneumonia, sepsis, diarrhea, human immunodeficiency virus [HIV], tuberculosis, trauma), although very different threats to an individual's health, share a common consequence: Development of acute, life-threatening illness. In the developed world, such illness is routinely treated in an intensive care unit (ICU) by highly specialized physicians, nurses and support staff. This model of intensive care is spreading rapidly to low and middle income countries and as it spreads, challenges and limitations to this model arise [1].

With an estimated $1000–20,000 per quality-adjusted life year (QALY) gained, critical care support for potentially reversible acute medical or surgical illness should be one of the most cost-effective health care interventions [2, 3]. Unfortunately, incomplete knowledge of the best practices by front-line clinicians and delayed, error-prone care delivery processes are ubiquitous threats to patient safety and commonly offset the potential benefits of critical care support. This is particularly important early in the course of critical illness, when errors and

O. Kilickaya
Department of Internal Medicine, Division of Pulmonary and Critical Care Medicine, Mayo Clinic, Rochester, Minnesota USA
Department of Anesthesiology and Reanimation, Gulhane Military Medical Faculty, Ankara, Turkey

B. Bonneton
Department of Internal Medicine, Division of Pulmonary and Critical Care Medicine, Mayo Clinic, Rochester, Minnesota USA
Department of Emergency Medicine, Rene Arbeltier Hospital, Coulommiers, France

O. Gajic ✉
Department of Internal Medicine, Division of Pulmonary and Critical Care Medicine, Mayo Clinic, Rochester, Minnesota USA
e-mail: gajic.ognjen@mayo.edu

J.-L. Vincent (Ed.), *Annual Update in Intensive Care and Emergency Medicine 2014*, 689
DOI 10.1007/978-3-319-03746-2_51, © Springer International Publishing Switzerland 2014

delays in appropriate care often lead to costly complications and poor outcomes, even in advanced hospital settings. In resource-poor settings, inadequate human resources and training present additional barriers to safe and effective use of life-saving procedures. Simple interventions, such as early recognition and treatment of cardio-respiratory failure, low tidal volume mechanical ventilation, early appropriate antimicrobial treatment, physical therapy, deep vein thrombosis and stress ulcer prophylaxis, require little specialized equipment but are crucial to successful outcome of critically ill patients [4]. Accordingly, these interventions have to be systematically implemented without omission or delay. This seemingly simple and straightforward task has proven to be an enormous challenge and nothing but a distant dream in hospitals worldwide.

Why are Errors and Complications so Prevalent in Acute Care Settings?

Although medical technologies and knowledge are continuously improving, there is overwhelming evidence of persistent error [5] and poor real-world compliance with evidence-based practices in acute care hospitals [6–8]. Critically ill patients are particularly prone to medical errors because of inherent complexity involving multiple organ systems and the immediacy of the decision-making required. Errors of omission are as common as those of commission with cumulative failures in a multi-step process encumbering exponentially on a patient's outcome, inevitably leading to development of costly complications (Table 1).

Within the interdisciplinary nature of intensive care, clinicians permanently face multitasking and interruptions. Data overload, meaningless complexity, interruptions, administrative burden, ineffective regulatory requirements, and fragmented provider-based (rather than patient-based) care are some of the most important barriers to error prevention in hospital environments. Care delivery is further impaired by poor communication, inadequate structure, staffing issues and wrong incentives. These errors persist not because physicians and nurses are ignorant, but because the current systems of care make it very difficult to implement the right decisions [9].

Table 1 The chance for omission or error increases exponentially with the number of steps in a complex multi-step process emphasizing the need for very high reliability in each step. Adapted from [49] with permission

Probability of Success for Each Step in the Process				
Number of Steps	0.95	0.990	0.999	0.999999
1	0.95	0.990	0.999	0.9999
25	0.28	0.78	0.98	0.998
50	0.08	0.61	0.95	0.995
100	0.006	0.37	0.90	0.990

The "Checklist Manifesto": Role of Checklists in Enhancing Patient Safety and Prevention of Medical Error [10]

Studies of human error have identified the key role of cognitive ergonomics and human factors engineering in designing improved care delivery processes and devices [8, 9]. Embracing a safety culture, limiting the number of steps ('less is more'), enhancing and prompting clear prioritized information, patient- and family-centered care delivery (integration of values, beliefs and advanced directives), improved communication and coordination (hand-offs, physician extenders) are all needed for safe and efficient critical care delivery. Considering the exponential spreading of medical knowledge, it appears obvious that clinician memory cannot store and retrieve all of it, particularly during acute care support [9]. Medical textbooks and current guidelines provided by major scientific societies display exhaustive information for best practice, but may be complex to use as an efficient decision support at the point-of-care [11].

Multiple tools have recently been developed, tested and validated to enhance both efficiency and fidelity of acute care delivery. These include: Multidisciplinary rounds, daily goals of care sheets, smart alarms, dashboards and decision supports. Analogous to the complex industry environment (e. g., aviation, nuclear power plants), simplified checklists and care 'bundles' have been recently introduced on a large scale in various medical settings (Table 2) [12, 13].

Worldwide implementation of a relatively simple World Health Organization (WHO) surgical safety checklist led to improved outcomes across three continents [14]. Protocolized procedure bundles have similarly lead to the dramatic reduction in vascular device complications across multiple institutions [12]. The introduction of "goals of care sheet" [15] and checklist prompting during daily rounds [16] have both led to substantial improvements in efficiency and reliability of daily plan of care, and were associated with decreased complications.

In order to be helpful at the point-of-care, checklists and algorithms need to focus on brief prioritized information [17, 18]. Checklist effectiveness also relies on an appropriate display [19] and depends on the integration of the tool into bedside practice. This is often achieved using verbal prompting by the team leader or another designated clinician [20, 21]. Standardized processes spur teams to interact and communicate to find the best strategy in ensuring compliance with each care component [22].

'Golden Hours': The Importance of Error-free Care Early in the Course of Acute Critical Illness

The burden of medical error, omission and waste are especially exacerbated during the early course of critical illness when timely and efficient intervention are of paramount importance for patient outcome. The consequences of inadequate care delivery at the onset of acute critical illness are elegantly summarized in the words

Table 2 Representative examples of the use of checklists in various acute care environments

Settings	Checklist	Author, year [5]	Aim
Operating room	Anesthesia crisis management manual	Runciman, 2005 [36]	24 specific anesthesia crisis management sub-algorithms
	Sepsis during anesthesia management checklist	Myburgh, 2005 [50]	Provide a structured approach for the management of sepsis occurring in association with anesthesia
	Cesarean delivery anesthesia	Hart, 2005 [51]	Improving anesthesia preparation for caesarean delivery
	The WHO surgical safety checklist	Haynes, 2009 [52]	Address key safety steps during perioperative care to reduce rates of death and complications
	SURPASS checklist	De Vries, 2009 [53]	SURgical Patient Safety System: Address surgical errors and adverse events during daily clinical practice, from admission to discharge
	Obstetric safe surgery checklist	Rao, 2010 [54]	WHO surgical safety checklist adapted to obstetric specificities
	Operating room crisis checklists	Ziewacz, 2011 [55]	Improving care during 12 of the most common operating room crises
	Surgical safety	Bliss, 2012 [56]	Implementation of comprehensive surgical checklist
Intensive care unit	Diagnosis of brain death	Young, 1991 [57]	Proper assessment and documentation to the declaration of brain death
	Intensive care delirium screening checklist	Bergeron, 2001 [58]	Quickly identify delirious patient, with earlier diagnosis, earlier intervention and better care
	Improving communication in the ICU	Pronovost, 2003 [15]	Daily goals implementation improve understanding of goals of care and overall patient outcomes
	Room opening checklist	Quinio, 2003 [59]	Improve adequacy of room's equipment endowment
	Weaning from mechanical ventilation in intensive care patients	Walsh, 2004 [60]	Checklist of metabolic, cardiorespiratory and neurological criteria that suggested that patients should start the weaning process (successful weaning from ventilator prediction)
	Catheter-related bloodstream infection (CR-BSI) multifaceted interventions	Berenholtz, 2004 [61]	Eliminate CR-BSIs with staff education, procedure cart, catheter removal daily prompting, evidence-based guidelines checklist
	Improving care for the ventilated patient	Berenholtz, 2004 [62]	Daily rounding checklist to improve mechanically ventilated patient outcome
	Withdrawal of life support (WOLS) standardized process	Hall, 2004 [63]	Improve conduct of end-of-life care
	Catheter-related bloodstream infections	Pronovost, 2006 [12]	Evidence-based intervention to reduce the incidence of infection

Table 2 *Continuation*

Settings	Checklist	Author, year [5]	Aim
Intensive care unit	Daily quality rounding checklist	DuBose, 2008 [21]	Increase compliance to prophylactic measures relative to main ICU complications
	Improving compliance to protocols and objectives in ICU	Byrnes, 2009 [20]	Mandatory verbal review of checklist to improve consideration and implementation of ICU best practices
	Checklist for lung injury prevention (CLIP)	Lee, 2012 [64]	Improving early recognition and utilization of good practices for patients at high-risk for ALI/ARDS
Emergency department	Trauma patient pre-transfer checklist	Harahill, 1990 [65]	Checklist to promptly prepare patient for transfer
	Sepsis treatment checklist	Djogovic, 2012 [66]	Optimize sepsis care in emergency departments
Other acute care settings	Checklists and reminders	Wolff, 2004 [67]	Checklists and reminders in clinical care pathways for inpatients admitted for acute myocardial infarction or stroke (key best practices)
	WHO patient care checklist: new influenza A (H1N1)	WHO, 2009 [68]	Highlights areas of care for the management of new influenza A (H1N1)

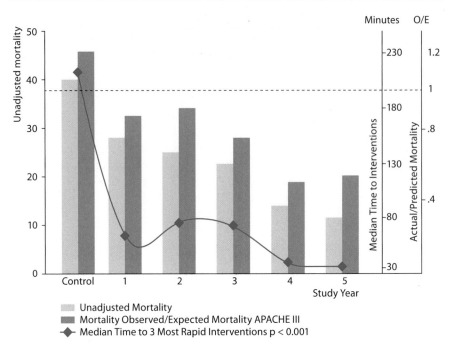

Fig. 1 Golden hours: Importance of minor delays in applying rapid interventions to acutely ill patients in shock. From [28] with permission

of one of the fathers of critical care support, the late Peter Safar: "The most sophisticated intensive care becomes unnecessarily expensive terminal care ..." [23].

This intuitive concept, renowned as the 'Golden Hour', has informed trauma care since the second half of the 20th century [24, 25], but has yet to be widely adopted in most other critical care conditions. The non-linear trajectory and time-sensitive nature of acute critical illness is characteristic of the complex systems [26]. During the vulnerable period immediately prior to 'phase transition', seemingly minor errors, omissions or delays can profoundly alter the patient trajectory. Simple interventions (fluid bolus, oxygen, transfusion, thrombolytic reperfusion), while beneficial during early hours of critical illness may lose effectiveness or even become harmful later in the course of critical illness (after the 'phase transition') [27]. The importance of timely recognition and appropriate treatment of acute critical illness is nicely illustrated in Fig. 1, showing the importance of minute delays in the rapid application of basic critical care support to patients in shock [28]. More recently, a multicenter quality improvement intervention targeting patients with severe sepsis in the emergency department showed that rapid implementation of early bundle elements (i. e., appropriate empiric antimicrobials, fluid bolus, lactate) was associated with aborted progression of organ failures making the patients "ineligible" for subsequent bundle elements (inotropes, steroids, transfusions, low tidal volume ventilation for ARDS) [29].

Regardless of how advanced hospital settings are, expected advantages of critical care support will be impaired if front-line clinicians fail to apply best practices in a timely manner. Therefore, avoiding diagnostic errors and therapeutic delays during these first minutes and hours of the care process ('golden hours') is necessary to prevent costly complications, preventable death and disability [16, 30].

Despite the notion of the importance of 'golden hours, Table 2 shows that the most acute care checklists are concerned with day-to-day care and procedure management. The critical, early period that often occurs outside of the ICU (in the emergency department, hospital ward or recovery room) is largely ignored and checklist use anecdotal. This gap is particularly deep in non-surgical settings where checklists and algorithms generally do not address early recognition and treatment of acute illness, apart from cardiopulmonary resuscitation (CPR) [31], which is often too late!

Structured Approach to Early Recognition and Treatment of Acute Critical Illness

The traditional linear approach, from history and examination to diagnosis and treatment, too often leads to delays in appropriate care and an alternative, iterative approach of addressing life-threatening physiologic disturbances and reviewing the response concurrently with the identification and treatment of underlying condition has been recommended (Fig. 2) [32, 33].

Accurate diagnosis is often elusive during the early stages of critical illness in which vastly different underlying conditions may trigger similar and/or interrelated physiologic disturbances leading to a limited number of acute presentations

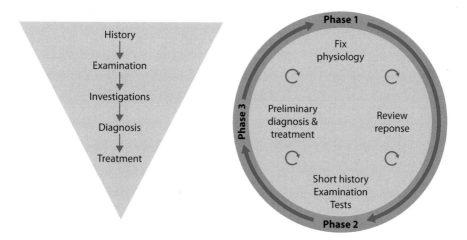

Fig. 2 Contrasting linear vs. iterative approach to initial management of acutely ill patients, adapted from the ESICM PACT module on Clinical Examination [32]

(Box 1) [34]. The timely and appropriate management of these key presentations followed by syndromic diagnoses (shock, respiratory failure, increased intracranial pressure, acute coronary syndrome, etc.), often without full understanding of the underlying condition, constitutes the basics of the acute care of critically ill patients. Keeping in mind the challenges clinicians are facing during early stages of acute critical illness, and the fact that experienced specialist help is often delayed, it is not difficult to imagine the advantages of a systematic and disciplined method that can consistently combine and articulate key diagnostic and therapeutic interventions [35]. Of note, even experienced clinicians are prone to making basic errors during emergency situations exposing patients to harm and clinicians to litigation [36].

Box 1:
Common Presentations of Life-threatening Conditions
- Shortness of breath
- Hypotension
- Chest pain
- Arrhythmia
- Altered mental state
- Abdominal pain
- Sepsis
- Gastrointestinal bleeding
- Trauma
- Intoxication/overdose
- Postoperative

One of the first examples to the systematic and standardized approach to life-threatening illness is the development of the mnemonic 'ABC' by the late Dr. Safar and colleagues in the early 1960s in order to standardize the immediate care of patients with cardiac arrest [37]. In the 1970s, Dr. Styner extended the context of the initial ABC approach for the evaluation of critically injured trauma patients and formed the basis of the Advanced Trauma Life Support courses [38]. The ABCDE approach has been implemented into trauma settings successfully for many years. Box 2 provides an example of the ABCDE checklist suitable for various acute care environments.

Box 2:
Example of an ABCDE checklist

A	Airway compromise Stridor Wheezing
B	Poor air entry Crackles Work of breathing
C	[1]EKG monitor Weak pulse Mottling
D	[2]AVPU Seizure Focal deficit
E	Abdominal distension Bleeding [3]Skin

[1] Sinus, bradycardia, supraventricular tachycardia, ventricular tachycardia, ventricular fibrillation, ST changes
[2] Alert, verbal responsive, pain responsive, unresponsive
[3] Edema, rash, jaundice, wound

The advantage of the structured approach to life-threatening emergencies has been elegantly demonstrated in a recent study [18]. In this study, the use of checklists by operating room teams markedly decreased critical omissions (23 % vs. 6 %, p < 0.001) in a high fidelity simulation of 106 surgical crises scenarios. Unfortunately, apart from CPR, which is too late, a similar checklist approach is largely missing during golden hours outside operating room and trauma settings [36].

Figure 3 outlines the key elements of a structured approach to acute life-threatening illness or injury: Primary survey to address immediate life-threats (need for CPR, ABCDE bundle) followed by secondary survey to assess each organ system, identify relevant syndromes and, in parallel, initiate emergent therapies.

Emerging Technologies: Information Displays, Cloud Computing and Mobile Devices

The advances in information technology, medical informatics and human factors engineering, have provided a tremendous opportunity for the development of novel and user-friendly checklists and decision support tools that can be widely applied in a complex and busy acute care settings [9]. To be successful, these applications need to reduce information overload and the potential for error, facilitate adherence to practice guidelines and enable clear communication and collaborative decision

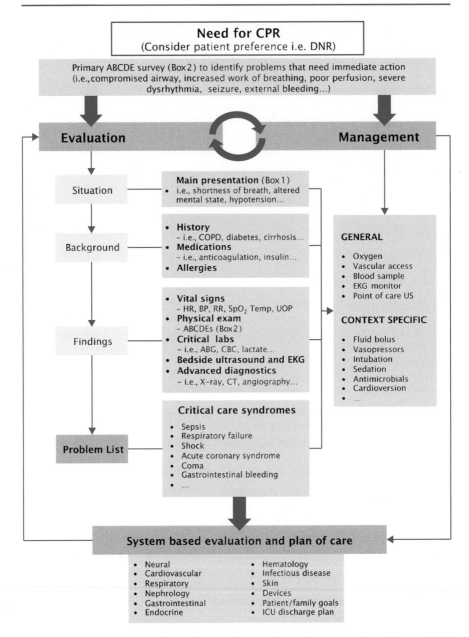

Fig. 3 Outline of the structured approach to early recognition and treatment of acute illness. ABG: arterial blood gases; CBC: complete blood count; COPD: chronic obstructive pulmonary disease; CPR: cardiopulmonary resuscitation; CT: computed tomography; DNR: do-not-resuscitate; ECG: electrocardiography; HR: heart rate; ICU: intensive care unit; RR: respiratory rate; SpO_2: peripheral oxygen saturation; Temp: body temperature; UOP: urine output; US: ultrasound

making between all members of health care team, patients and families. To facilitate high quality, high value health care behaviors, information display and functionality need to be designed using cognitive ergonomic principles and integrated into the clinician workflow in a manner that facilitates, rather than disrupts, care delivery.

Two years of provider surveys and field observation in medical and surgical ICUs of the Mayo Clinic have provided a robust framework for the prioritization of high value data for the management of critically ill patients [39]. The investigators identified no more than 50 data points that are commonly used by ICU experts. These 50 data points are prioritized on the novel user interface depending on the task at hand [40]. Knowledge translation is facilitated by smart alerts and real time access to evidence-based checklists. Collaborative workspace provides a shared view of the plan of care with patient specific tasks, status checks and reminders enabling the clear communication of the goals of care and their status to all members of the multidisciplinary team including the patient and family. Availability of key patient, process and outcome data in an electronic format provides easy access to scheduled and on demand reports of quality metrics and outcomes.

Using real-time data feeds and standardized patient care tasks in a simulated acute care environment, this novel interface was shown to have a significant advantage over the conventional electronic medical record in reducing provider cognitive load and errors [41]. Direct comparisons between electronic and paper checklists have not been done. Despite the potential pitfalls (need for additional training, reliable hardware, software and network) electronic checklists and decision supports offer some compelling advantages including, but not limited to, global access using mobile computing devices, standardized updates based on new knowledge and wide user feedback, versatile display capabilities (hyperlinks, videos and animations) which facilitate the processing of vast patient information and medical knowledge. In addition electronic tools obviate the need for paper products and its transport, thereby reducing associated cost and pollution.

Rapidly increasing access to mobile phones and cellular networks even in remote and resource-poor settings have recently enabled previously unimaginable, successful quality improvement interventions in rural Africa [42]. Cloud computing technology is also evolving swiftly, providing easy shared access to information with an almost unlimited/scalable storage capability increasing the ability for widespread knowledge translation. Using the approach outlined above and inspired by a surgical crisis checklist [17, 18], a multidisciplinary, international team of acute care clinicians is testing the effectiveness of electronic decision support (CERTAIN – Checklist for Early Recognition and Treatment of Acute Illness) in critical care environments across Eastern Europe, Asia, Africa and Central America [43, 44].

Implementing Checklists at the Bedside of Acutely Ill Patients

Regardless of the format (paper vs. electronic), checklist implementation often encounters cultural barriers, particularly among physicians. Perceptions on limitation of autonomous judgment, checklist dependency and questioning someone's seniority, knowledge and skill pose significant challenges to the implementation process [45]. Clinicians are often worried about over-standardized care processes ignoring the critical illness complexity ('cookbook medicine'). But despite these challenges, the checklist approach provides a framework to ensure the best care and a guardrail to avoid errors and omissions during diagnostic and therapeutic courses. Rather than replacing the bedside clinician, these tools are designed to help structure his/her reasoning (focus, precision, reminder, lucidity) and action in spite of facing fatigue and stressful conditions [46].

Assessing the information needs at the point of care is a key prerequisite for designing improved care delivery processes and devices that can fit in clinician workflow. PDSA (Plan-Do-Study-Act) cycles of field observation, surveys, interviews, workflow observations are necessary in order to meet the needs of frontline clinicians. Beta testing and validation of such tools in a simulated environment is essential before implementing them into clinical practice. Similar to any quality improvement projects, the checklist should be reviewed, refined and updated regularly. Senior leadership support is essential to overcome political barriers to the patient-centered (as opposed to the provider-centered) checklist processes. "The model for improvement" [47] is a powerful framework used by many health care organizations to accelerate the improvement of health care processes and outcomes [13, 48].

Conclusions

To fully realize the anticipated patient benefit while treating acute critical illness, clinicians ought to embrace systematic reasoning and a reliable approach to promote early recognition and ensure timely and appropriate treatment. In the current system, much of the effort in critical care is reactionary rather than proactive in implementing best practices aimed at preventing complications. A structured, reliable and error-free approach to the management of acutely ill or injured patients during the early, most vulnerable period is facilitated by point-of-care checklists and algorithms containing brief prioritized information. This approach is rapidly spreading in trauma and operating room settings and other acute care environments should follow soon.

References

1. Adhikari NK, Fowler RA, Bhagwanjee S, Rubenfeld GD (2010) Critical care and the global burden of critical illness in adults. Lancet 376:1339–1346
2. Barie PS, Ho VP (2012) The value of critical care. Surg Clin North Am 92:1445–1462
3. Linko R, Suojaranta-Ylinen R, Karlsson S, Ruokonen E, Varpula T, Pettila V (2010) One-year mortality, quality of life and predicted life-time cost-utility in critically ill patients with acute respiratory failure. Crit Care 14:R60
4. Kumar A, Roberts D, Wood KE et al (2006) Duration of hypotension before initiation of effective antimicrobial therapy is the critical determinant of survival in human septic shock. Crit Care Med 34:1589–1596

5. Kohn LT, Corrigan JM, Donaldson MS (2000) To Err is Human : Building a Safer Health System. National Academy Press, Washington
6. Pronovost PJ, Berenholtz SM, Ngo K et al (2003) Developing and pilot testing quality indicators in the intensive care unit. J Crit Care 18:145–155
7. Ilan R, Fowler RA, Geerts R, Pinto R, Sibbald WJ, Martin CM (2007) Knowledge translation in critical care: factors associated with prescription of commonly recommended best practices for critically ill patients. Crit Care Med 35:1696–1702
8. Moreno RP, Rhodes A, Donchin Y (2009) Patient safety in intensive care medicine: the Declaration of Vienna. Intensive Care Med 35:1667–1672
9. Pickering BW, Litell JM, Herasevich V, Gajic O (2012) Clinical review: the hospital of the future – building intelligent environments to facilitate safe and effective acute care delivery. Crit Care 16:220
10. Gawande A (2010) The Checklist Manifesto : How To Get Things Right, 1st edn. Metropolitan Books, New York
11. Wyer PC, Rowe BH (2007) Evidence-based reviews and databases: are they worth the effort? Developing evidence summaries for emergency medicine. Acad Emerg Med 14:960–964
12. Pronovost P, Needham D, Berenholtz S et al (2006) An intervention to decrease catheter-related bloodstream infections in the ICU. N Engl J Med 355:2725–2732
13. Gawande AA, Arriaga AF (2013) A simulation-based trial of surgical-crisis checklists. N Engl J Med 368:1460
14. Treadwell JR, Lucas S, Tsou AY (2014) Surgical checklists: a systematic review of impacts and implementation. BMJ Qual Saf (in press)
15. Pronovost P, Berenholtz S, Dorman T, Lipsett PA, Simmonds T, Haraden C (2003) Improving communication in the ICU using daily goals. J Crit Care 18:71–75
16. Weiss CH, Moazed F, McEvoy CA et al (2011) Prompting physicians to address a daily checklist and process of care and clinical outcomes: a single-site study. Am J Respir Crit Care Med 184:680–686
17. Gawande A (2007) The checklist: if something so simple can transform intensive care, what else can it do? New Yorker 10:86–101
18. Arriaga AF, Bader AM, Wong JM et al (2013) Simulation-based trial of surgical-crisis checklists. N Engl J Med 368:246–253
19. Lee MJ, Gershengorn HB, Dinkels M et al (2012) Checklist For Lung Injury Prevention (CLIP): A pilot study on implementation across multiple hospitals and multiple clinical areas. American Thoracic Society, San Francisco, A6567 (abst)
20. Byrnes MC, Schuerer DJ, Schallom ME et al (2009) Implementation of a mandatory checklist of protocols and objectives improves compliance with a wide range of evidence-based intensive care unit practices. Crit Care Med 37:2775–2781
21. DuBose JJ, Inaba K, Shiflett A et al (2008) Measurable outcomes of quality improvement in the trauma intensive care unit: the impact of a daily quality rounding checklist. J Trauma 64:22–29
22. Resar R, Pronovost P, Haraden C, Simmonds T, Rainey T, Nolan T (2005) Using a bundle approach to improve ventilator care processes and reduce ventilator-associated pneumonia. Jt Comm J Qual Patient Saf 31:243–248
23. Safar P (1974) Critical care medicine – quo vadis? Crit Care Med 2:1–5
24. Cowley RA (1975) A total emergency medical system for the State of Maryland. Md State Med J 24:37–45
25. Cowley RA (1977) Trauma center. A new concept for the delivery of critical care. J Med Soc N J 74:979–987
26. Dong Y, Chbat NW, Gupta A, Hadzikadic M, Gajic O (2012) Systems modeling and simulation applications for critical care medicine. Ann Intensive Care 2:18
27. Rivers E, Nguyen B, Havstad S et al (2001) Early goal-directed therapy in the treatment of severe sepsis and septic shock. N Engl J Med 345:1368–1377

28. Sebat F, Musthafa AA, Johnson D et al (2007) Effect of a rapid response system for patients in shock on time to treatment and mortality during 5 years. Crit Care Med 35:2568–2575
29. Miller RR 3rd, Dong LNNC et al (2013) Multicenter implementation of a severe sepsis and septic shock treatment bundle. Am J Respir Crit Care Med 188:77–82
30. Pronovost PJ, Berenholtz SM, Needham DM (2008) Translating evidence into practice: a model for large scale knowledge translation. BMJ 337:a1714
31. Nolan JP, Soar J, Zideman DA et al (2010) European Resuscitation Council Guidelines for Resuscitation 2010 Section 1. Executive summary. Resuscitation 81:1219–1276
32. McAuley D, Hillman KM, Bion J (2005) Clinical examination. Ramsay G, Hinds C (eds) European Society of Intensive Care Medicine (ESICM) Patient-centered Acute Care Training (PACT) Module
33. Kortbeek JB, Turki ASA, Ali J et al (2008) Advanced trauma life support, 8th edition, the evidence for change. J Trauma 64:1638–1650
34. Mackenzie R, Sutcliffe RC (2002) Immediate assessment and management of acute medical emergencies. J R Army Med Corps 148:276–287
35. Balas MC, Vasilevskis EE, Burke WJ et al (2012) Critical care nurses' role in implementing the "ABCDE bundle" into practice. Crit Care Nurse 32:35–38
36. Runciman WB, Kluger MT, Morris RW, Paix AD, Watterson LM, Webb RK (2005) Crisis management during anaesthesia: the development of an anaesthetic crisis management manual. Qual Saf Health Care 14:e1
37. Safar P, Brown TC, Holtey WJ, Wilder RJ (1961) Ventilation and circulation with closed-chest cardiac massage in man. JAMA 176:574–576
38. Styner JK (2006) The birth of advanced trauma life support. J Trauma Nurs 13:41–44
39. Pickering BW, Gajic O, Ahmed A, Herasevich V, Keegan MT (2013) Data utilization for medical decision making at the time of patient admission to ICU. Crit Care Med 41:1502–1510
40. Pickering BW, Herasevich V, Ahmed A, Gajic O (2010) Novel representation of clinical information in the ICU: Developing user interfaces which reduce information overload. Appl Clin Inform 1:116–131
41. Ahmed A, Chandra S, Herasevich V, Gajic O, Pickering BW (2011) The effect of two different electronic health record user interfaces on intensive care provider task load, errors of cognition, and performance. Crit Care Med 39:1626–1634
42. Zurovac D, Sudoi RK, Akhwale WS et al (2011) The effect of mobile phone text-message reminders on Kenyan health workers' adherence to malaria treatment guidelines: a cluster randomised trial. Lancet 378:795–803
43. Checklist for early recognition and treatment of acute illness (CERTAIN) official website (2013) Available at http://www.icertain.org. Accessed November 2013
44. The iCertain Project (2013) European Society of Critical Care Medicine (ESICM), Minutes of the Global Intensive Care working group meeting, Brussels. Available at http://www.esicm.org/upload/5191ebaf1b026-protokollmeetingbrusselsmarch2013.pdf. Accessed November 2013
45. Hales BM, Pronovost PJ (2006) The checklist – a tool for error management and performance improvement. J Crit Care 21:231–235
46. Sexton JB, Thomas EJ, Helmreich RL (2000) Error, stress, and teamwork in medicine and aviation: cross sectional surveys. BMJ 320:745–749
47. Langley GL, Nolan KM, Nolan TW, Norman CL, Provost LP (2009) The improvement guide : a practical approach to enhancing organizational performance, 2nd edn. Jossey-Bass Publishers, San Francisco, California
48. Winters BD, Gurses AP, Lehmann H, Sexton JB, Rampersad CJ, Pronovost PJ (2009) Clinical review: checklists – translating evidence into practice. Crit Care 13:210
49. Botwinick L, Bisognano M, Haraden C (2006) Leadership Guide to Patient Safety. Institute for Healthcare Improvement (IHI) Innovation Series white paper. IHI, Cambridge, Massachusetts

50. Myburgh JA, Chapman MJ, Szekely SM, Osborne GA (2005) Crisis management during anaesthesia: sepsis. Qual Saf Health Car 14:e22
51. Hart EM, Owen H (2005) Errors and omissions in anesthesia: a pilot study using a pilot's checklist. Anesth Analg 246–250
52. Haynes AB, Weiser TG, Berry WR et al (2009) A surgical safety checklist to reduce morbidity and mortality in a global population. N Engl J Med 360:491–499
53. de Vries EN, Hollmann MW, Smorenburg SM, Gouma DJ, Boermeester MA (2009) Development and validation of the SURgical PAtient Safety System (SURPASS) checklist. Qual Saf Health Care 18:121–126
54. Rao K, Lucas DN, Robinson PN (2010) Surgical safety checklists in obstetrics. Int J Obstet Anesth 19:235–236
55. Ziewacz JE, Arriaga AF, Bader AM et al (2011) Crisis checklists for the operating room: development and pilot testing. J Am Coll Surg 213:212–217
56. Bliss LA, Ross-Richardson CB, Sanzari LJ et al (2012) Thirty-day outcomes support implementation of a surgical safety checklist. J Am Coll Surg 215:766–776
57. Young GB, Frewen T, Barr HW et al (1991) Checklist for diagnosis of brain death. Can J Neurol Sci 18:104
58. Bergeron N, Dubois MJ, Dumont M, Dial S, Skrobik Y (2001) Intensive Care Delirium Screening Checklist: evaluation of a new screening tool. Intensive Care Med 27:859–864
59. Quinio P, Baczynski S, Dy L, Ferrec G, Catineau J, de Tinténiac A (2003) Evaluation of a medical equipment checklist before intensive care room opening. Ann Fr Anesth Reanim 22:284–290
60. Walsh TS, Dodds S, McArdle F (2004) Evaluation of simple criteria to predict successful weaning from mechanical ventilation in intensive care patients. Br J Anaesth 92:793–799
61. Berenholtz SM, Pronovost PJ, Lipsett PA et al (2004) Eliminating catheter-related bloodstream infections in the intensive care unit. Crit Care Med 32:2014–2020
62. Berenholtz SM, Milanovich S, Faircloth A et al (2004) Improving care for the ventilated patient. Jt Comm J Qual Saf 30:195–204
63. Hall RI, Rocker GM, Murray D (2004) Simple changes can improve conduct of end-of-life care in the intensive care unit. Can J Anaesth 51:631–636
64. Lee MJ, Gershengorn HB, Dinkels M et al (2012) Checklist for lung injury prevention (CLIP): A pilot study on implementation across multiple hospitals and multiple clinical areas. Am J Respir Crit Care Med 185:A6567 (abst)
65. Harrahill M, Bartkus E (1990) Preparing the trauma patient for transfer. J Emerg Nurs 16:25–28
66. Djogovic D, Green R, Keyes R et al (2012) Canadian Association of Emergency Physicians sepsis treatment checklist: optimizing sepsis care in Canadian emergency departments. CJEM 14:36–39
67. Wolff AM, Taylor SA, McCabe JF (2004) Using checklists and reminders in clinical pathways to improve hospital inpatient care. Med J Aust 181:428–431
68. World Health Organization (2009) Patient care checklist. Available at: http://www.who.int/csr/resources/publications/swineflu/ah1n1_checklist.pdf Accessed Nov 2013

Improving Multidisciplinary Care in the ICU

D. M. Kelly and J. M. Kahn

Introduction

Recent efforts to improve outcomes in critical illness have focused on the organization and management of the intensive care unit (ICU) [1]. There is substantial evidence that key elements of ICU organization, including intensivist physician staffing [2], nurse staffing [3], a high volume of critically ill patients [4] and the presence of multidisciplinary care providers, such as clinical pharmacists [5], are associated with improved quality of care in the ICU. Consequently, many recent quality improvement initiatives focus on improving ICU organization by expanding the number of different provider types in the ICU, rather than on the specific care process known to be associated with outcome [6].

Complementing these efforts is the increasing recognition that a well organized ICU is defined not only by the presence of certain provider types, but also by how well those providers work together, so-called "multidisciplinary care" [7]. Modern critical care is extraordinarily complex, and the clinical practices known to save lives are inherently multidisciplinary, with effective implementation requiring a tightly knit team of providers with varying domains of expertise. Thus, it is likely that the next frontier of organization-based quality improvement will involve efforts to better understand, and improve, multidisciplinary care. In this chapter, we will define multidisciplinary care in the context of the modern ICU, review the current evidence and perceived benefits of multidisciplinary care provision, and discuss future challenges to the use of multidisciplinary collaboration as a lever for ICU quality improvement.

D. M. Kelly · J. M. Kahn ✉
University of Pittsburgh School of Medicine, Pittsburgh, PA 15261, USA
e-mail: kahnjm@upmc.edu

J.-L. Vincent (Ed.), *Annual Update in Intensive Care and Emergency Medicine 2014*, 705
DOI 10.1007/978-3-319-03746-2_52, © Springer International Publishing Switzerland
2014

What is 'Multidisciplinary Care'?

A multidisciplinary care model acknowledges the complexities of critical care delivery by incorporating and integrating nurses, physicians, respiratory therapists, pharmacists and other care providers as integral members of the critical care team. Team members work alongside one another and each provider is able to bring their individual expertise and knowledge to the group [8]. In this context, the multidisciplinary care team can be termed the functional unit of the ICU [9]. A well functioning unit is one in which there is both effective communication, i. e., the ability to successfully convey ideas and feelings across team members, and effective collaboration, i. e., the ability for multiple providers to work in partnership to achieve a common goal [10].

A particular distinction is worth noting: Multidisciplinary and interdisciplinary are not synonymous terms. Multidisciplinary is defined as "combining or involving several academic disciplines or professional specializations in an approach to a topic or problem" whereas interdisciplinary is defined as "of or relating to more than one branch of knowledge" [11]. Importantly, interdisciplinary care need not be multidisciplinary – it is possible for multiple provider types to work together in the ICU, but without the effective communication and collaboration that is the hallmark of multidisciplinary care. In these instances, communication is superficial – information is exchanged, but not ideas and feeling; and collaboration is hierarchical – additional providers are not bringing additional expertise. For the purposes of this chapter, we focus specifically on multidisciplinary ICU care, as we aim to discuss how ICUs may improve the ability of disciplines to work together to effectively care for the critically ill.

Potential Benefits of Multidisciplinary Care

There are many potential benefits to improving multidisciplinary care in the ICU. First, all ICUs are not created equal, and although there are many similarities among ICUs, resources vary substantially across hospitals, healthcare systems and countries [12]. Optimizing the ability of the multidisciplinary team to collaborate and function effectively may be most helpful in ICUs that do not have an intensivist on staff, fewer critical care nurses or limited access to respiratory therapy and pharmacy. In this way, multidisciplinary care can potentially overcome staffing deficiencies, making the whole greater than the sum of its parts.

Second, multidisciplinary care harnesses the knowledge, skills and expertise of all providers and disciplines. This is particularly important for extremely sick patients requiring complex care practices proven to save lives. For example, patients in shock in the midst of active resuscitation are likely to receive optimal goal-directed therapy when team members can effectively communicate and collaborate [13]. Patients with severe acute respiratory distress syndrome (ARDS) requiring lung protective ventilation or prone positioning may also benefit from effective multidisciplinary care [14]. These therapies are complex and multi-factorial, involving optimal respiratory care, sedation, pain management and nursing. If all these elements are not working together, the therapies will not be effectively implemented, and outcomes are likely to suffer.

Multidisciplinary care may also allow change in the quality of communication itself, making it more patient-centered. In a qualitative study, researchers compared verbal communication in two ICUs, one in which rounding was single disciplinary (i. e., physicians only) and one using an inter-disciplinary daily rounding approach [15]. These authors followed five patients over a 5-day time period using audio recordings of rounds and provider-to-provider patient handoffs. They found that nurses tended to focus more on data and interventions whereas physicians discussed diagnoses and expectations of clinical care and outcomes, demonstrating the complementary role of multiple disciplines. In regards to ICU nurse-to-nurse handoffs, integration of interventions and clinical goals occurred more in the interdisciplinary ICU than in the single disciplinary ICU, suggesting that interdisciplinary ICUs may allow for a more integrated approach to clinical care.

Finally, multidisciplinary care may facilitate innovation. New ideas and novel treatments are often borne out of conflict, which can only arise when peer collaborators disagree, not in a hierarchical system where the team leader's opinions are the last word [16]. Moreover, effective problem solving occurs when providers bring varying perspectives to the table with the freedom to express dissent [17]. As the old adage goes, "two heads are better than one". Thus, it is likely that the novel treatments of tomorrow will emerge from truly multidisciplinary ICUs rather than traditional hierarchical ICUs.

Review of the Evidence

Early qualitative studies demonstrated that effective, superior ICUs were those that had an emphasis on collaborative approaches to care and good working relationships between nursing and medicine [18]. Since this early work, several studies support the observation that multidisciplinary care is associated with improved outcomes in the ICU, including greater hospital survival, shorter ICU length of stay, and lower costs (Table 1). In this section we will review some of the more important studies and discuss their practical implications for ICU providers.

Most broadly, in a multicenter study in 112 Pennsylvania hospitals, our group found a significantly lower 30-day mortality when medical ICU patients were cared for by a multidisciplinary team that rounded daily (adjusted odds ratio [OR] 0.84, 95 % confidence interval [CI, 0.76, 0.93]) [19]. We also found that patients experienced the lowest odds of death when cared for in an ICU with mandatory or optional intensivist consult and multidisciplinary rounds (adjusted OR 0.78 [0.68, 0.89]) compared to hospitals with low intensivist staffing but without multidisciplinary rounds. These findings suggest that the mortality benefit conferred by having an intensivist present, is explained in part by the presence of multidisciplinary rounds. This is one of the first multicenter studies to indicate that use of a multidisciplinary team during rounds confers a survival benefit.

Table 1 Selected studies of multidisciplinary care models in the intensive care unit

Reference	Study design	Findings
Smrynios [20]	Pre/post, single center, MICU, SICU and CCU	Significant reductions in MV duration, LOS and number of tracheostomies with use of a ventilator management team
Young [21]	Pre/post, MICU/SICU, single center	No difference in mortality but significant reductions in LOS and costs with use of a multidisciplinary care team for ventilator dependent patients
Burns [22]	Pre/post, single center, CCU, MICU, neuro ICU, SICU, CTICU	Significant reductions in MV duration, LOS, costs and mortality after implementation of an 'Outcomes Management' multidisciplinary team
Kaye [26]	Pre/post, four ICUs, single center	Significant reductions in ventilator associated pneumonia with use of a 'Critical Care Bug Team' to manage ventilator dependent patients
Kollef [23]	RCT, MICU and SICU	Protocol-directed ventilator weaning was associated with greater success in weaning than physician-directed weaning protocols
Stone [25]	Pre/post, single center SICU	Found that VAP bundle adherence was improved after implementation of a multidisciplinary ventilator management team

MICU: medical intensive care unit; SICU: surgical intensive care unit; CCU: coronary care unit; RCT: randomized controlled trial; MV: mechanical ventilation; LOS: length of stay; VAP: ventilator associated pneumonia

On a more granular level, multiple studies have examined how multidisciplinary collaboration has improved care or multidisciplinary driven protocols have facilitated weaning from mechanical ventilation. For example, a university hospital implemented a multidisciplinary 'Ventilator Management Team', the primary goal of which was to implement and monitor adherence to a standardized weaning protocol [20]. A dedicated multidisciplinary care team, including two nurses and a pulmonary and critical care specialist, were responsible for monitoring all patients and following up on ventilator management. Two years after implementation, the institution identified significant reductions in the duration of mechanical ventilation compared to the baseline year (23.9 days vs. 17.5 days, $p = 0.004$), significant decreases in hospital and ICU length of stays, as well as a large reduction in the number of patients requiring tracheostomies (61 % to 41 %, $p < 0.0005$).

Similarly, a medical-surgical ICU in a single institution implemented a new multidisciplinary care team that was responsible for coordinating care of ventilator-dependent patients [21]. They evaluated the impact of this care team, which was responsible for using daily multidisciplinary rounds, monthly team meetings as well as ensuring adherence to protocols and guidelines. Although they found no difference in mortality, they demonstrated significant reductions in length of stay (ICU 19.8 days to 14.7 days, $p = 0.001$; hospital 34.6 days to 25.9 days, $p = 0.001$) and lower costs in patients managed by the multidisciplinary care team.

Comparable results were noted when a multidisciplinary 'Outcomes Management' team was created to implement an evidence-based clinical pathway and protocol for ventilator weaning and management in five ICUs in one academic medical center [22]. Data were collected for 20 months. Researchers found that after implementation of the Outcomes Management approach, there were significant reductions in duration of mechanical ventilation, ICU length of stay, hospital length of stay, costs and mortality. The authors concluded that use of a multidisciplinary outcomes management team to design and implement a managed approach to care of the mechanically ventilated improved clinical and financial outcomes in five adult ICUs in an academic medical center.

In addition to these observational studies, some clinical trial evidence suggests that multidisciplinary collaboration is more effective than single disciplinary care in the ICU, particularly for mechanically ventilated patients. In one study, patients were randomly assigned to receive protocol-driven (by a nurse and respiratory therapist) or physician-directed weaning from mechanical ventilation in medical and surgical ICUs in two academic hospitals [23]. Using proportion hazards regression modeling for over 300 patients, the authors found a significantly greater rate of successful weaning in the protocol-driven patients compared to the physician-directed weaning group (hazard ratio 1.31; 95 % CI 1.15 to 1.50) even though mortality was similar in both groups. Other studies have found similar results [24].

Work focusing on using a multidisciplinary team approach to reduce nosocomial infection rates further supports the benefits of multidisciplinary care provision in the ICU. One surgical ICU identified persisting ventilator-associated pneumonia (VAP) rates after implementing a VAP bundle and hypothesized that variation in bundle implementation was to blame [25]. To improve implementation of the VAP bundle, a team of intensivists, nurses, and respiratory therapists reviewed daily patient goals related to ventilator management and the VAP bundle on patient rounds during a 10-month time period for 174 intubated trauma patients. Compared to the 10 months prior to implementation, the team noted significant reductions in VAP rates.

A study describing the impact of a 'Critical Care Bug team' followed a similar design to the previous study; however, these investigators used an even more diverse group of providers: clinical nurse specialists, respiratory therapists, pharmacists, an infection control professional as well as a research specialist [26]. The authors showed significant reductions in VAP in four ICUs in one tertiary care hospital. Although these studies were single site, pre-post study designs, the results are suggestive of the potential for how a multidisciplinary team approach to care of the mechanically ventilated can improve care quality and reduce cost.

Workforce Issues

Despite the evidence in support of multidisciplinary care, health care provider shortages may limit the ability to scale a multidisciplinary model to all ICUs. In many countries, intensivist physicians, nurses and clinical pharmacists are in short supply [27], and it is neither feasible nor practical to put these providers in every ICU. Thus, it is necessary to recognize that effective multidisciplinary care is likely not achievable in the short term for every critically ill patient. That said, multidisciplinary care can, in part, be viewed as a solution to this problem. Studies show that at least a portion of the benefits of intensivist physician staffing are attributable to the presence of a multidisciplinary rounding team [19]. Alternate care models, such as use of nurse practitioner and physician assistants (NP/PAs) in ICUs, may also aid in improving multidisciplinary care in the absence of trained intensivists or highly skilled ICU nurses [28]. Use of NP/PAs in the US is increasingly commonplace since Accreditation Council for Graduate Medical Education regulations limit the amount of hours that residents and fellows can work.

Challenges and Future Directions

Many challenges remain regarding multidisciplinary care and collaboration in the intensive care unit (Table 2). First, the exact mechanism as to how a multidisciplinary approach improves ICU quality has not been fully elucidated. We can speculate that the benefits of multidisciplinary care involve more effective communication and collaboration, but the evidence in this area remains largely anecdotal. Thus, we have few strategies to achieve the benefits of multidisciplinary care in instances when multidisciplinary care teams are not feasible due to staffing shortages. Additionally, we have few data about how to improve the quality of multidisciplinary care. Some teams work well together, and some do not, and we do not necessarily know how to convert an ineffective team into an effective one [29].

For example, a Greek study showed that although ICU clinicians highly valued multidisciplinary care, actualization of collaborative care was difficult to implement mainly due to lack of teamwork skills by the providers [30]. In another example, researchers in Australia found no differences in length of stay, mortality, duration of mechanical ventilation, readmissions or staff satisfaction with care after adding a weekly multidisciplinary team meeting to a general ICU [31]. These data reaffirm the notion that care by multiple disciplines does not equate to multidisciplinary care.

Table 2 What we know and what we need to learn about multidisciplinary care

What we know	What we still need to learn
The addition of interdisciplinary providers to the ICU is associated with improved outcomes	The mechanism by which multidisciplinary care improves outcomes
When interdisciplinary providers work together as multidisciplinary care teams, outcomes are also improved	Strategies to improve multidisciplinary care
Multidisciplinary interventions are especially helpful in management of mechanical ventilated patients	Ways to achieve the benefits of multidisciplinary care in the absence of a full multidisciplinary care team
Collaborative approaches to care can improve outcomes, using existing ICU staff	The role of interprofessional education to facilitate multidisciplinary collaboration?

ICU: intensive care unit

To overcome these challenges, we need high-quality, mixed-methods research designed to elucidate the potential benefits of multidisciplinary care, to understand the barriers and facilitators to multidisciplinary care, and to test novel interventions to improve the quality of multidisciplinary care. One example may be formal inter-professional education, focusing on team science with the goal of building strong teams through effective team building and communication skills [29]. Doing so early on in the healthcare provider educational curriculum would set the stage for future multidisciplinary care, in the hopes of eventually leading to effective communication and collaboration in the ICU and across all healthcare settings.

Another approach might be to facilitate shared understanding of the goals of the multidisciplinary care team, also through education. Lack of a shared understanding of the goals of the multidisciplinary care team in providing effective ICU care can be a major barrier to effective care provision. For example, in five focus groups composed of ICU physicians, nurses and respiratory therapists, researchers explored barriers and motivators for implementing daily interruption of sedation for mechanically ventilated adults [32]. Researchers identified little shared understanding of why daily interruption of sedation would be necessary by the multidisciplinary care team. This lack of shared goals and understanding led to wide variation in daily interruption of sedation for mechanically ventilated patients as well as different approaches to performing sedation interruptions.

Conclusions

The evidence base in support of multidisciplinary care is diverse and evolving. Most studies are single center, pre/post studies evaluating outcomes associated after a multidisciplinary intervention. Few studies examined the mechanism of action of a multidisciplinary team and even fewer focused on how to enhance multidisciplinary collaboration in the ICU. More work is needed to expand our understanding of multidisciplinary collaboration in the ICU. In particular, studies are needed to define the mechanism of action and provide levers for improving multidisciplinary communication and collaboration in a way that affects patient-centered outcomes. These studies will pave the way towards generalizable interventions that work across hospitals and health care settings.

In the meantime, it is clear that multidisciplinary care is an important part of effective and efficient critical care. Extensive research demonstrates that a multidisciplinary team is important for outcomes, particularly for patients requiring mechanical ventilation. Although the mechanism of action is not well understood, and we lack information on how to improve the quality of multidisciplinary care, ICU providers can still take the time to reflect on their own communication and collaboration skills, as this area may be one of the few frontiers left for improving outcomes in the ICU by targeting the organization and management of care.

References

1. Carmel S, Rowan K (2001) Variation in intensive care unit outcomes: a search for the evidence on organizational factors. Curr Opin Crit Care 7:284–296
2. Pronovost PJ, Angus DC, Dorman T, Robinson KA, Dremsizov TT, Young TL (2002) Physician staffing patterns and clinical outcomes in critically ill patients: a systematic review. JAMA 288:2151–2162
3. Tarnow-Mordi WO, Hau C, Warden A, Shearer AJ (2000) Hospital mortality in relation to staff workload: a 4-year study in an adult intensive-care unit. Lancet 356:185–189
4. Kahn JM, Goss CH, Heagerty PJ, Kramer AA, O'Brien CR, Rubenfeld GD (2006) Hospital volume and the outcomes of mechanical ventilation. N Engl J Med 355:41–50
5. Leape LL, Cullen DJ, Clapp MD et al (1999) Pharmacist participation on physician rounds and adverse drug events in the intensive care unit. JAMA 282:267–270
6. Milstein A, Galvin RS, Delbanco SF, Salber P, Buck CR (2000) Improving the safety of health care: the leapfrog initiative. Eff Clin Pract 3:313–316
7. Kahn JM, Rubenfeld GD (2005) Translating evidence into practice in the intensive care unit: the need for a systems-based approach. J Crit Care 20:204–206
8. Slatin C, Galizzi M, Melillo KD, Mawn B (2004) Conducting interdisciplinary research to promote healthy and safe employment in health care: promises and pitfalls. Public Health Rep 119:60–72
9. Manthous CA, Hollingshead AB (2011) Team science and critical care. Am J Respir Crit Care Med 184:17–25
10. Apker J, Propp KM, Zabava Ford WS, Hofmeister N (2006) Collaboration, credibility, compassion, and coordination: professional nurse communication skill sets in health care team interactions. J Prof Nurs 22:180–189
11. Oxford Dictionaries (2010) Oxford Dictionary of English. Oxford University Press, Oxford
12. Wunsch H, Angus DC, Harrison DA et al (2008) Variation in critical care services across North America and Western Europe. Crit Care Med 36:2787–e8
13. Rivers E, Nguyen B, Havstad S et al (2001) Early goal-directed therapy in the treatment of severe sepsis and septic shock. N Engl J Med 345:1368–1377
14. Villar J, Kacmarek RM (2013) What is new in refractory hypoxemia? Intensive Care Med 39:1207–1210
15. Miller A, Scheinkestel C, Limpus A, Joseph M, Karnik A, Venkatesh B (2009) Uni- and interdisciplinary effects on round and handover content in intensive care units. Hum Factors 51:339–353
16. Hülsheger UR, Anderson N, Salgado JF (2009) Team-level predictors of innovation at work: a comprehensive meta-analysis spanning three decades of research. J Appl Psychol 94:1128–1145
17. De Dreu CK, West MA (2001) Minority dissent and team innovation: the importance of participation in decision making. J Appl Psychol 86:1191–1201
18. Zimmerman JE, Shortell SM, Rousseau DM et al (1993) Improving intensive care: observations based on organizational case studies in nine intensive care units: a prospective, multicenter study. Crit Care Med 21:1443–1451
19. Kim MM, Barnato AE, Angus DC, Fleisher LA, Fleisher LF, Kahn JM (2010) The effect of multidisciplinary care teams on intensive care unit mortality. Arch Intern Med 170:369–376
20. Smyrnios NA, Connolly A, Wilson MM et al (2002) Effects of a multifaceted, multidisciplinary, hospital-wide quality improvement program on weaning from mechanical ventilation. Crit Care Med 30:1224–1230
21. Young MP, Gooder VJ, Oltermann MH, Bohman CB, French TK, James BC (1998) The impact of a multidisciplinary approach on caring for ventilator-dependent patients. Int J Qual Health Care 10:15–26

22. Burns SM, Earven S, Fisher C et al (2003) Implementation of an institutional program to improve clinical and financial outcomes of mechanically ventilated patients: one-year outcomes and lessons learned. Crit Care Med 31:2752–2763

23. Kollef MH, Shapiro SD, Silver P et al (1997) A randomized, controlled trial of protocol-directed versus physician-directed weaning from mechanical ventilation. Crit Care Med 25:567–574

24. Ely EW, Baker AM, Dunagan DP (1996) Effect on the duration of mechanical ventilation of identifying patients capable of breathing spontaneously. N Engl J Med 335:1864–1869

25. Stone ME, Snetman D, O'Neill A et al (2011) Daily multidisciplinary rounds to implement the ventilator bundle decreases ventilator-associated pneumonia in trauma patients: but does it affect outcome? Surg Infect (Larchmt) 12:373–378

26. Kaye J, Ashline V, Erickson D et al (2000) Critical care bug team: a multidisciplinary team approach to reducing ventilator-associated pneumonia. Am J Infect Control 28:197–201

27. Ewart GW, Marcus L, Gaba MM, Bradner RH, Medina JL, Chandler EB (2004) The critical care medicine crisis: a call for federal action: a white paper from the critical care professional societies. Chest 125:1518–1521

28. Gershengorn HB, Wunsch H, Wahab R et al (2011) Impact of nonphysician staffing on outcomes in a medical ICU. Chest 139:1347–1353

29. Manthous C, Nembhard IM, Hollingshead AB (2011) Building effective critical care teams. Crit Care 15:307

30. Kydona CK, Malamis G, Giasnetsova T, Tsiora V, Gritsi-Gerogianni N (2010) The level of teamwork as an index of quality in ICU performance. Hippokratia 14:94–97

31. Cheung W, Milliss D, Thanakrishnan G, Anderson R, Tan JT (2009) Effect of implementation of a weekly multidisciplinary team meeting in a general intensive care unit. Crit Care Resusc 11:28–33

32. Miller MA, Bosk EA, Iwashyna TJ, Krein SL (2012) Implementation challenges in the intensive care unit: the why, who, and how of daily interruption of sedation. J Crit Care 27: 218.e1–7

The Role of Autopsy in Critically Ill Patients

G. Berlot, R. Bussani, and D. Cappelli

Introduction

A number of potentially treatable severe conditions different from those determining the hospital admission and/or acquired in the intensive care unit (ICU) can go unnoticed throughout the whole hospital stay and are discovered only at autopsy. Some investigators demonstrated with post-mortem studies that among patients admitted both to regular wards and to the ICU that the rate of major pathological conditions gone undetected during their stay ranged from 12.6 % to 41 % and that their clinical relevance can vary from nil to having been the main cause of death (Table 1) [1–5]. At the same time, the rate of non-legal autopsies of patients who die in the hospital has constantly declined throughout the last decades for a number of reasons, including the need for cost containment, the fear of litigation and the assumption that the unrelenting advances of imaging techniques enable physicians to observe details of almost all conditions many with an accuracy unthinkable only

Table 1 Discrepancies between clinical diagnosis and autopsy findings in ICU patients

First author (year) [ref]	N. autopsies	% Total discrepancies	% Class I discrepancies	% Class II discrepancies
Berlot (1999) [7]	159	41	8	33
Nadrous (2003) [30]	455	21	4	17
Silvfast (2003) [38]	346	6	5	1
Combes (2004) [3]	167	36.5	10	16.5
Pastores (2007) [15]	86	26	54	32
Tejerina (2012) [6]	833	18.5	7.5	11.4

G. Berlot ✉ · D. Cappelli
Dept. of Anesthesia and Intensive Care, University of Trieste, Trieste, Italy
e-mail: berlot@inwind.it

R. Bussani
Dept. of Pathology, University of Trieste, Trieste, Italy

J.-L. Vincent (Ed.), *Annual Update in Intensive Care and Emergency Medicine 2014*, 715
DOI 10.1007/978-3-319-03746-2_53, © Springer International Publishing Switzerland
2014

a few years ago; nevertheless, the rate of pathologic conditions missed during the admission and discovered only at the post-mortem examination seems to be affected only marginally by this progress [3].

The Autopsy as a Diagnostic Tool in Critically Ill Patients

All the above statements apply fully to critically ill patients, in whom a rate of missed *in vivo* diagnoses ranging from 7 to 32 % has been demonstrated in different studies [6]. At a first glance, these findings are somewhat surprising, because patients admitted to the ICU are likely subjected to more clinical investigations than those admitted to regular wards; one possible explanation for these discrepancies consists in the role played by a number of circumstances unique to ICU patients that can contribute to complicate the achievement of a correct diagnosis, including the paucity of information on concomitant diseases different from that/those determining the ICU admission; the sometimes relatively short length of stay in the ICU, which can impede a complete diagnostic workup [7]; the effects of sedation, which prevent patients reporting the occurrence of new disturbances; and the rapidly deteriorating clinical conditions diverting the attention of the physicians more to the symptoms than to their determining factors; moreover, and perhaps more importantly, similar nonspecific symptoms and alterations (e. g., dyspnea, arterial hypotension, metabolic acidosis, fever or anemia of unknown origin, etc.) can be ascribed to different causes requiring specific clinical approaches and treatments. Thus, it appears that autopsy is valuable especially in critically ill patients, as it allows the physician (a) to assess the correctness and completeness of the diagnoses through the identification of pathologic conditions gone undetected during the admission, and (b) to understand if the unexpected autopsy findings could have caused the death, or at least influenced its occurrence [8]. This latter point is particularly relevant as the identification of clinical errors and/or their stem causes could modify the diagnostic workup of forthcoming patients.

With the aim of categorizing the relevance in terms of outcome of the discrepancies between clinical and autopsy diagnoses, the classification proposed by Goldman et al. [9] has been widely adopted, also for ICU patients (Table 1). Major errors include missed relevant underlying conditions with potential negative impact on the outcome and that would have changed the management (Class I) or relevant missed diagnosis without negative effects on the outcome and that would have not changed treatment (Class II). Minor discrepancies include missed minor diagnoses related to the terminal disease but not influencing the outcome (Class III) and, finally, other missed minor diagnosis without any influence on the outcome (Class IV).

However, although this classification can be extremely useful in patients admitted outside the ICU, in critically ill patients the role played by a missed diagnosis must sometimes be interpreted cautiously, because other conditions, including the presence of severe sepsis and septic shock, the occurrence of a multiple organ

Table 2 Discrepancies between clinical and autopsy diagnoses. The rate is calculated on the overall number of discrepancies

Condition	First author (year) [ref]	Class I discrepancy (%)	Class II discrepancy (%)
Pulmonary embolism	Nadrous (2003) [30]	4.5	12
	Silvfast (2003) [38]	0	0
	Pastores (2007) [15]	0	16
	Kakkar (2008) [17]	16	0
	Berlot (2011) [16]	14	0
	Tejerina (2012) [6]	16	0
Acute myocardial infarction	Nadrous (2003) [30]	4.5	0
	Silvfast (2003) [38]	50	n.a.
	Pastores (2007) [15]	8	0
	Tejerina (2012) [6]	5.1	n.a.
Infective and non-infective endocarditis	Nadrous (2003) [30]	0	0
	Silvfast (2003) [38]	0.2	n.a.
	Pastores (2007) [15]	8	8
	Tejerina (2012) [6]	5	n.a.

n.a.: the authors grouped Class I and II discrepancies together.

dysfunction syndrome, etc., can strongly influence the outcome, thus limiting its usefulness.

With these limitations in mind, we will review the studies that have evaluated the discrepancies between clinical and autopsy diagnoses for different conditions, namely pulmonary embolism (PE), acute myocardial infarction (AMI) and infective and non-infective endocarditis, because the recognition of these conditions has been shown to be particularly elusive in critically ill patients admitted to the ICU for different reasons, thus representing a common source of Class I and II errors (Table 2).

Pulmonary Embolism

Critically ill patients are particularly susceptible to the occurrence of venous thromboembolism for several reasons, including prolonged immobilization, use of indwelling central venous catheters and the prothrombotic status associated with sepsis, trauma and postoperative state [10]. Taken together, these factors constitute the classical Virchow's triad, which sets the stage for the occurrence of a deep venous thrombosis (DVT), frequently located in the calf or in the pelvic veins. A number of prophylactic interventions are currently used, basically consisting of the administration of anticoagulative drugs, the use of compressive stockings and, as a last resort in subjects in whom these measures cannot be adopted, the positioning of a filter [11] located in the superior or inferior vena cava. Independent of the type of prophylaxis adopted, the occurrence of either a DVT and/or a PE in critically ill patients is not uncommon: Cook et al. [12] reported an overall incidence of DVT approximating 10 % in a group of medical and surgical critically ill patients and Patel et al. [13] demonstrated an overall incidence of PE of 2 % in a multicenter survey involving more than 12,000 critically ill patients enrolled in 12 different ICUs. Other investigators [14, 15] demonstrated that undiagnosed PE represents a major cause of death in critically ill patients; interestingly, according to Tejerina et al. [6], the rate of missed diagnosis of PE did not vary substantially in the 25-year period of their study. As far as the clinical impact of the missed diagnosis of PE is concerned, Pastores et al. [15] demonstrated that PE represented 16 % of the Class II discrepancies in a group of critically ill cancer patients. In another study, Berlot et al. [16] observed that PE occurred in 84 (14 %) of 600 adult medical and surgical critically ill patients who died in the ICU and was discovered only at autopsy in most of them. This figure is close to that reported by Kakkar and Vasishta [17] who demonstrated a PE in 16 % of a large population of medical adult patients who underwent a post-mortem examination; in both studies, PE was considered as a major cause of death in 80–90 % of patients, thus representing a true Class I error. Other investigators [3] demonstrated that a missed diagnosis of PE accounted for 4.5 % and 12 % of Class I and II errors, respectively. Notably, all patients in the study by Berlot et al. [16] had received full prophylaxis with subcutaneous low molecular weight heparin (LMWH) administered according to the manufacturer's indications. The failure of LMWH to prevent DVT and PE in critically ill patients has been attributed to: (a) the particular prothrombotic status of critically ill patients, especially in the presence of sepsis, possibly leading to the administration of a dose lower than that actually needed; and/or (b) to a number of different factors, including obesity, acute kidney injury (AKI) and the administration of norepinephrine, which reduce the adsorption of LMWH when the preparation is administered via the subcutaneous route [18–20].

Acute Myocardial Infarction

In clinical practice, the use of a 12-lead electrocardiogram (EKG) in combination with repeated measurements of blood troponin (Tn) levels constitute the standard approach for the diagnosis of AMI in patients with suggestive symptoms [21]. However, although this diagnosis can be relatively easy in the majority of cases, in critically ill patients admitted to the ICU for non-cardiac reasons it may not be so straightforward. Several factors account for this observation, including: (a) the attribution of AMI-related hemodynamic derangements to causes other than myocardial ischemia, such as hypovolemia, or the increase in the intrathoracic pressure determined by mechanical ventilation possibly associated with high values of positive end-expiratory pressure (PEEP) ultimately leading to reduced venous return [22]; (b) the conventional 12-lead EKG can be misleading as it can be influenced by non-ischemic conditions, such as certain therapies and the presence of acid-base and electrolyte disorders [10]; (c) the blood levels of cardiac enzymes can be elevated in the absence of cardiac ischemia in a substantial proportion of critically ill patients without coronary artery disease (CAD) [23–26]; increased blood levels of cardiac Tn can be present also in non-ischemic conditions, including myocarditis and pericarditis, heart failure, pulmonary embolism, sepsis, acute stroke, subarachnoid hemorrhage and AKI [27]. Indeed, several studies have shown that 15 % to 70 % of general ICU patients and 31 % to 80 % of septic patients have elevated serum levels of Tn, although the prevalence of AMI is much lower, and ranges, according to different investigators, from 15 % to 36 % [26]. Moreover, some studies [28] demonstrated that histological examination revealed contraction band necrosis in only half of the patients with elevated pre-mortem Tn levels, suggesting that its release does not necessarily indicate myocardial cell necrosis; elevated serum Tn levels in septic patients have been observed despite increased coronary blood flow, decreased extraction of oxygen across the coronary circulation and maintenance of normal high-energy phosphate levels [29]. In a recent study involving 600 patients who died in the ICU for non-traumatic causes and underwent autopsy, Berlot et al. [27] observed that an AMI was present in 75 cases (12.5 %), and in 20 of them, the diagnosis of AMI was obtained only at the post-mortem examination; overall, significant CAD was present in roughly one third of the whole group. At gross examination of the heart it can be difficult to distinguish between an AMI related to CAD or related to the effect of terminal global myocardial underperfusion possibly associated with CAD; in these cases, only microscopic examination can separate patients who died with an AMI from those whose death was caused by this condition. As far as the relevance of a missed diagnosis on outcome is concerned, the missed diagnosis of AMI accounts for 8–16 % of Class I errors in different groups of critically ill patients [6, 15, 30].

Endocarditis

The estimated incidence of infective endocarditis varies from 30 to 100 episodes per million patient-years with a mortality exceeding 30 % [31]; the main risk factors for its occurrence include underlying congenital or degenerative valvular abnormalities, the presence of prosthetic valves, bloodstream infections and intravenous drug use [32, 33]. Different causes account for non-infective endocarditis, including neoplasms, multifactorial pro-coagulative states, long-term hypoxia, chronic low flow states and cachexia [34, 35]. The very same factors are responsible for the occurrence of both forms of endocarditis in the hospital and in critically ill patients admitted to the ICU; these latter patients are particularly prone to bloodstream infection-related endocarditis compared to those admitted to regular wards mainly due to the widespread use of invasive devices, such as indwelling central venous catheters, pulmonary artery catheters (PAC) and intra-arterial lines. The ever-increasing age of critically ill patients with the related burden of disease, the pro-coagulative state associated with sepsis and sepsis-related conditions and the risk factors listed earlier set the stage for non-infective endocarditis [36]. Both infective and non-infective endocarditis can be particularly difficult to recognize in the ICU setting, because: (a) the related cardiovascular symptoms can be attributed to other conditions causing ICU admission or complicating the clinical course, including heart failure, septic shock, etc.; and (b) cerebral embolism-related neurologic signs or symptoms can go undetected because of use of sedatives and neuromuscular blocking agents. Even in specialized units, rates of missed diagnoses of infective and non-infective endocarditis are rather high: According to Saad et al. [37] the clinical diagnosis of infective endocarditis was not made in 27 % of patients admitted to a cardiological hospital. Less is known about the incidence of failed diagnosis of both forms of endocarditis among ICU patients: Infective/non-infective endocarditis was discovered at autopsy in 5–8 % of ICU patients and represented a major source of Class I and II errors [3, 7, 15]. Recently, we discovered infective/non-infective endocarditis in 2.7 % of patients admitted to our ICU who underwent autopsy: interestingly, similar to patients dying with PE, most of these patients had severe sepsis or septic shock.

Conclusions

Worldwide, the rate of autopsies performed in patients dying in the hospital is declining for a number of reasons, including the need for cost containment, the fear of litigation and continuous improvements in imaging techniques. Thus, one could argue that at the present time the autopsy does not play any role in the confirmation of either the diagnostic accuracy or the therapeutic appropriateness, at least in patients who die after a reasonable interval of time during which all the necessary investigations have been carried out. However, different authors have demonstrated that despite all the technological improvements, a number of potentially treatable disorders, including severe infections [3, 7, 15] are detected only at the post-mortem examination, thus making questionable the above quoted assumption. This observation applies particularly to ICU patients, in whom a host of circumstances can make the diagnosis of potentially treatable disorders, including infective and non-infective endocarditis, PE and AMI, particularly challenging.

References

1. Perkins GD, McAuley DF, Davies S, Gao F (2003) Discrepancies between clinical and post-mortem diagnosis in critically ill patients: an observational study. Crit Care 7:R129–R132
2. Tai DYH, El-Bilbeisi H, Tewari S, Masha EJ, Wiedemann HP, Arroliga AC (2001) A study of consecutive autopsies in a medical ICU. A comparison of clinical cause of death and autopsy diagnosis. Chest 119:530–536
3. Combes A, Mokhtari M, Couvelard A et al (2004) Clinical and autopsy diagnosis in the intensive care unit-a prospective study. Arch Intern Med 164:389–392
4. Shojania KG, Burton EC, McDonald KM, Goldman L (2003) Changes in the rate of autopsy detected diagnostic errors over time- a systematic review. JAMA 298:2849–2856
5. Shojania KG, Burton EC (2008) The vanishing nonforensic autopsy. N Engl J Med 358:873–875
6. Tejerina E, Esteban A, Fernandez-Segovian P et al (2012) Clinical diagnoses and autopsy findings: discrepancies in critically ill patients. Crit Care Med 40:842–846

7. Berlot G, Dezzoni R, Viviani M, Silvestri L, Bussani R, Gullo A (1999) Does the length of stay in the intensive care unit influence the diagnostic accuracy? A clinical-pathological study. Eur J Emerg Med 6:227–231
8. Herridge MS (2003) Autopsy in critical illness: it is obsolete. Crit Care 7:407–408
9. Goldman L, Sayson R, Robbins S, Cohn LH, Bettman M, Weisberg M (1983) The vakue of the autopsy in three medical eras. N Engl J Med 308:1000–1005
10. Cook DJ, Crowther MA, Meade MO, Douketis J (2005) Prevalence, incidence and risk factors for venous thromboembolism in medical-surgical intensive care unit patients. J Crit Care 20:309–313
11. Geerts WH, Bergqvist D, Pineo GF et al (2008) Prevention of venous thromboembolism-ACCP EBM-based practice guidelines (8th edition). Chest 133:381S–453S
12. Cook D, Crowther M, Meade M et al (2005) Deep venous thrombosis in medical-surgical critically ill patients: prevalence, incidence and risk factors. Crit Care 33:1565–1571
13. Patel R, Cook DJ, Meade MO et al (2005) Burden of illness in venous thromboembolism in critical care: multicenter observational study. J Crit Care 20:341–347
14. Shorr AF, Jackson WL (2005) Deep vein thrombosis in the intensive care unit: underappreciated, understudied, and undertreated. J Crit Care 20:301–303
15. Pastores SM, Dulu A, Voigt L, Raoof N, Alicea M, Halpern NA (2007) Premortem clinical diagnoses and post-mortem autopsy findings: discrepancies in critically ill cancer patients. Crit Care 11:R48
16. Berlot G, Calderan C, Vergolini A et al (2011) Pulmonary embolism in critically ill patients receiving antithrombotic prophylaxis. A clinical-pathological study. J Crit Care 26:28–33
17. Kakkar N, Vasishta RK (2008) Pulmonary embolism in medical patients: an autopsy-based study. Clin Appl Thrombosis/hemostasis 14:159–167
18. Hirsh J, Warkentin TE, Shaugnessy SG et al (2001) Heparin and low-molecular weight heparin-mechanism of action, pharmacokinetics, dosing, monitoring efficacy and safety. Chest 119:64S–94S
19. Priglinger U, Delle Karth G, Geppert A et al (2003) Prophylactic anticoagulation with enoxaparin: is the subcutaneous route appropriate in the critically ill ? Crit Care Med 31:1405–1409
20. Dörffler-Melly J, de Jonge E, de Pont AC et al (2002) Bioavailability of subcutaneous low-molecular-weigh heparin to patients on vasopressors. Lancet 359:849–850
21. Lim W, Qushmaq I, Cook DJ et al (2005) Elevated troponin and myocardial infarction in the intensive care unit: a prospective study. Crit Care 8:R636–R644
22. Chockalingam A, Mehra A, Dorairajan S, Dellsperger KC (2010) Acute left ventricular dysfunction in the critically ill. Chest 138:198–207
23. Noble JS, Reid AM, Jordan LVM et al (1999) Troponin I and myocardial injury in the ICU. Br J Anaesth 82:41–46
24. Charlson ME, MacKenzie CR, Gold JP et al (1989) The preoperative and intraoperative hemodynamic predictors of postoperative myocardial infarction or ischemia in patients undergoing noncardiac surgery. Ann Surg 210:637–648
25. Spies C, Haude V, Fitzner R et al (1998) Serum cardiac troponin T as a prognostic marker of myocardial injury in early sepsis. Chest 113:1055–1063
26. Arlati S, Brenna S, Prencipe L et al (2000) Myocardial necrosis in ICU patients with acute non cardiac disease : a prospective study. Intensive Care Med 26:31–37
27. Berlot G, Vergolini A, Calderan C, Bussani R, Torelli L, Lucangelo U (2010) Acute myocardial infarction in critically ill patients: a clinical-pathological study. Monaldi Archives Chest Dis 74:164–171
28. Ver Elst KM, Spapen HD, Nguyen DN et al (2000) Cardiac troponins I and T are biological markers of left ventricular dysfunction in septic shock. Clin Chem 46:650–657
29. Merx MW, Weber C (2007) Sepsis and heart. Circulation 116:793–802
30. Nadrous HF, Afesa B, Pfeifer EA, Peters SG (2003) The role of autopsy in critically ill patients. Mayo Clin Proc 78:947–950

31. Hoen B, Duval X (2013) Infective endocarditis. N Engl J Med 368:1425–1433
32. Thury F, Grisoli D, Collart F, Habib G, Raoult D (2012) Management of infective endocarditis: challenges and perspectives. Lancet 379:965–975
33. Moreillon P, Que YO (2004) Infective endocarditis. Lancet 363:139–149
34. Truskinowsky AM, Hutchins GM (2001) Association between nonbacterial thrombotic endocarditis and hypoxigenic pulmonary diseases. Virchows Arch 438:357–361
35. Lee V, Gilbert JD, Byard RW (2012) Marantic endocarditis – not a so benign entity. J Forensic Leg Med 19:312–315
36. Angus DC, van der Poll T (2013) Critical care medicine: severe sepsis and septic shock. N Engl J Med 369:840–851
37. Saad R, Yamada AT, da Pereira RFH, Gutierrez PS, Mansur AJ (2007) Comparison between clinical and autopsy diagnoses in a cardiology hospital. Heart 93:1414–1419
38. Silvfast T, Takkunen O, Kohlo E, Andersson LC, Rosemberg P (2003) Characteristics of discrepancies between clinical and autopsy diagnose in the intensive care unit: a 5-year review. Intensive Care Med 29:321–324

Moral Distress in the ICU

C. R. Bruce, S. Weinzimmer, and J. L. Zimmerman

Introduction

> "[Healthcare professionals] who see themselves as involved in morally significant relationships with sick, vulnerable humans, but have little or no power to respond when what is happening appears to be 'wrong' ... is a serious problem ... One of the most serious aspects of the problem is the tendency of those in power in the clinical setting ... to refuse to treat it as a serious problem [1, 2]."

Moral distress is the inability of a moral agent, a healthcare professional, to act according to his or her core values, professional roles, and perceived obligations due to internal or external constraints [3–5]. When an internal or external constraint prevents a clinician from acting in the way he or she feels is most appropriate, moral integrity and moral conscience are profoundly compromised [6, 7]. William Bartholome advocated developing a comprehensive research agenda on moral distress. As illustrated above, he recognized the importance of studying moral distress and in identifying successful strategies for intervention. He and several other researchers focused their energies on the critical care setting because "the intensive care units (ICUs) are places where the sickest of patients receive the most technologically sophisticated care ... at the brink of death" [8, 9]. There are many opportunities for critical care clinicians to suffer grief from losing patients, but they can also experience moral distress from the complex decisions and disagreements associated with patient care.

C. R. Bruce
Center for Medical Ethics & Health Policy, Baylor College of Medicine, Houston, TX USA
Houston Methodist Biomedical Ethics Program, Houston Methodist Hospital, Houston, TX USA

S. Weinzimmer
Rice University, Houston, TX USA

J. L. Zimmerman ✉
Houston Methodist Biomedical Ethics Program, Houston Methodist Hospital, Houston, TX USA
Weill Cornell Medical College, New York, NY USA
e-mail: janicez@houstonmethodist.com

J.-L. Vincent (Ed.), *Annual Update in Intensive Care and Emergency Medicine 2014*,
DOI 10.1007/978-3-319-03746-2_54, © Springer International Publishing Switzerland
2014

We review the moral distress literature with an emphasis on empirical studies conducted in ICUs. Although moral distress has been studied for nearly thirty years, only recently have efforts shifted from studying nurses' moral distress towards evaluating experiences of other healthcare professionals [7]. We will discuss moral distress research conducted with other critical care clinicians to the extent such studies are available.

Definitional Features

Because of a lack of central agreement on key aspects of moral distress, what was once a narrow definition of a unique phenomenon has broadened to become a complex cluster concept. As part of the cluster concept, related experiences and environments – such as compassion fatigue, moral sensitivity, burnout, ethical climate, and ethical stress – are often treated as synonymous with moral distress. Some authors have focused on the psychological burdens of moral distress and integrated this element into its definition [4, 5, 7], calling moral distress a "psychological disequilibrium," or a "pain affecting the mind, body, or relationships" [10, 11], while others focus on constraints in defining moral distress.

While a lack of conceptual clarity should be expected for newly-discovered phenomena, this lack of consistency and consensus on the definition of moral distress frustrates the ability to systematically study or teach it [12]. To this point, McCarthy and Deady theorized that "uninitiated" persons may well ask: "Is moral distress a situation? A set of beliefs or attitudes? A range of emotions? A group of symptoms?" [7]. Empirical studies based on small qualitative studies and outdated quantitative instruments further confound these issues. The ability to extrapolate generalizable information is undermined by study limitations and variation in terminology.

Despite these limitations in defining and building a comprehensive knowledge base of moral distress, there is agreement on what moral distress is not. Moral distress is different from traditional ethical dilemmas. In the classic ethical dilemma, the healthcare professional recognizes two distinct, mutually-opposing courses of action but cannot identify which of those two courses of action is most ethically supportable. In instances where there is moral distress, the healthcare professional's moral integrity and authenticity is undermined when he or she feels constrained from taking the ethically appropriate courses of action [13].

Moral distress is also different from other forms of emotional distress [12, 14]. When healthcare professionals encounter morally distressing situations, they will likely suffer concomitant psychological or emotional distress, such as anxiety, sleeplessness, irritability, frustration, and detachment. But just because healthcare professionals feel psychological distress, it does not necessarily mean they are experiencing moral distress. In order for there to be moral distress, two elements must be present: (1) The healthcare professional recognizes the ethically preferable course of action to take; and (2) there must be some sort of constraint that prevents the individual from taking that course of action.

Instruments to Measure Moral Distress

The definition of a concept depends significantly on the way it is measured [12]. Corley and colleagues developed the first instrument to measure moral distress. The Moral Distress Scale (MDS) is a 32-item questionnaire in a 7-point Likert format that measures dual dimensions of frequency and intensity of the distress. This instrument was further refined to elucidate sources of distress [7, 15]. Questions are oriented towards the critical care setting, including: Discharging patients before they were ready, working in understaffed conditions, and carrying out treatments perceived to be unnecessary [7, 15, 16]. When applying their instrument, the researchers found that 69 % of nurses experienced moral distress [15, 16]. The MDS is arguably the first instrument and the most widely-used measure for moral distress [12]. It offers the benefit of being validated, reliable, and consistently used with great success in different domains of medicine.

While the revised MDS offers many benefits, several items do not reflect current practices. It is a lengthy, nursing-centric instrument that takes significant time to complete [12]. A major disadvantage of the MDS is that it does not measure real-time distress as it is being experienced by the healthcare professional. Wocial and Weaver recently created a diagnostic instrument that can be used during an ethics consultation to measure real-time moral distress. Their explicit goal in developing the "moral distress thermometer" was to create a quick and easy-to-use visual analog that overcomes the limitations associated with the MDS [17]. Although this development is an important one, we theorize that the instrument might prove to be overly-simplistic in that it overlooks the nuances and complexity of moral distress.

There are several other initiatives being undertaken to broaden the applicability of the MDS to a variety of settings and disciplines. Because consistency in defining moral distress is lacking, it is likely that multiple measures exist that are actually measuring different concepts [12, 18]. In order to foster respect for moral distress and related phenomena, one must be able to correctly diagnose, understand, and mitigate moral distress. This is inextricably linked to deliberative self-examination [2]. To that end, some researchers have highlighted the importance of developing, teaching, and practicing reflective skills in order to mitigate healthcare professionals' moral distress. Bartholome said that healthcare professionals must be able to "describe [the moral distress] ... to discuss the basis for it ... to justify their appeal to it ... to be able to articulate the moral basis of this experience [1, 2]." In order to be able to do this, the clinician must be able to recognize the source (i. e., root cause) of the moral distress.

Root Causes of Moral Distress

A comprehensive knowledge base of root causes likely holds the key to targeting interventions to mitigate moral distress [12, 18]. It is now commonly accepted that moral distress exists across multiple professional healthcare disciplines and is not exclusive to nurses, as was previously thought [19–24]. However, the litera-

Table 1 Summary of current findings concerning root causes of moral distress

	Patient/surrogate vs. clinician dynamics	Clinician vs. clinician dynamics	Unit or system dynamics
Nurses	• Most frequent cause: Aggressive treatments for terminally ill patients • Greater frequency of morally distressing situations compared to other disciplines • Least intense moral distress compared to other disciplines	• Nurses dissatisfied with physician-nurse collaboration and communication • Believed physicians were not collaborating well with nurses • Many nurses believe that ICU physicians withhold diagnostic or prognostic information from patients	• Most successful interventions focus on empowering critical care nurses to maximize their moral agency • To empower nurses: Mandate nurse involvement in family meetings, hold multidisciplinary case reviews, help facilitate code status conversations with patients/surrogates
Physicians	• Most frequent cause: Aggressive treatments for terminally ill patients • Most intense: When providing aggressive life-sustaining interventions believed to be clinically and ethically inappropriate	• Physicians very satisfied with nurse communication • Believed physicians were collaborating well with nurses • Few ICU physicians believe they withhold information	• Call physicians' attention to nurses' perception of poor communication and collaboration

ture varies in relation to sources of moral distress and the way it is experienced by different disciplines.

Some authors focus on external constraints as sources of moral distress, leading to feelings of frustration and powerlessness [3]. Conversely, other authors focus on internal and external constraints as factors leading to self-blame and anxiety [3, 6, 7, 23, 25]. Owing in large part to the recent work by Ann Hamric and colleagues, our understanding of root causes has become considerably better developed. Root causes can be distinguished based on three different sources: The individual, the clinical context, or the unit/hospital culture. The interrelationship between these root causes is not fully understood. For instance, the interconnections between individuals, unit culture, system factors, and clinical or patient characteristics have not been directly evaluated [12]. Table 1 lists further information on root causes of moral distress.

We recognize that the moral distress experienced by a healthcare professional is shaped, not only by characteristics unique to that individual, but also the context in which that person operates on a day-to-day basis. To underscore the importance of relational factors, we describe root causes below in terms of interpersonal dynamics and conflicts.

Patient/Surrogates Versus Healthcare Professional Dynamics

In the beginning of the bioethics movement, ethical conflicts generally occurred between healthcare professionals who insisted on maintenance of aggressive, life-sustaining measures and patients' or surrogates' requests to withdraw it. Conversely, current ethical conflicts generally occur when healthcare professionals believe withdrawing life-sustaining interventions is most appropriate and surrogates request maintenance of it.

Both nurses and physicians clearly feel distress at maintaining aggressive treatments for terminally ill patients [8]. Providing aggressive and non-beneficial treatment has consistently been found to be the most frequent morally distressing situation for healthcare professionals [26]. However, it is presently unclear whether and to what extent moral distress might be experienced differently between disciplines. Houston and colleagues recently surveyed 2700 healthcare professionals representing multiple healthcare disciplines to assess and compare differences in the intensity, frequency, and severity of moral distress [24]. Their findings support previous research suggesting that end-of-life clinical situations produce the highest intensity of moral distress for physicians and nurses, particularly when they believe continued medical treatment is medically inappropriate. Nurses reported greater frequency of morally distressing situations compared to other disciplines, most likely because they are constantly at patients' besides and cannot get relief from the situation [8, 21–24].

A noteworthy contribution of this study is that the investigators were able to elucidate some important distinctions among the disciplines. Chaplains, physicians, and social workers surpassed nurses in relation to the intensity of moral distress. Physicians and residents experienced the greatest moral distress when they provided aggressive life-sustaining interventions they believed were clinically and ethically inappropriate. In contrast, chaplains and social workers experienced the highest moral distress in issues related to complex discharge planning, lack of social support, lengths of stay, and other social justice issues. A reasonable explanation for this difference is that social workers and chaplains are tasked with social support issues, whereas physicians and nurses are responsible for clinical decisions about the level of treatment support. An additional noteworthy feature of this study is that chaplains reported significantly higher moral distress compared to other disciplines when they felt that life-sustaining interventions were prematurely terminated. The authors speculate that chaplaincy training in valuing life and believing in an after-life devoid of human suffering might account for this finding.

The interplay between intensity and frequency should be examined. It is presently unknown whether higher intensity but less frequent moral distress experiences impact a healthcare professional differently than lower intensity but more frequent exposure to morally distressing situations. It is also unclear whether and how moral distress manifests differently between disciplines [24]. For example, it is theorized that repeated exposure to morally distressing situations will lead to physical and emotional detachment from patients and situations, eventually eroding one's sense of moral and professional integrity. This "moral residue" theory, discussed more fully below, is usually discussed in the context of nursing and has not been discussed with other healthcare disciplines.

Healthcare Professional Versus Healthcare Professional Dynamics

Professional interaction refers to the amount of social and professional contacts between two or more people within the job setting [27]. Several studies have found that nurses are dissatisfied with physician-nurse collaboration and communication when they perceive that their contribution to decision making is not valued or permitted by physicians [27, 28]. Professional autonomy is the freedom to make decisions within the roles and duties of one's profession and to act in accordance with that responsibility [29]. Papathanassoglou and colleagues found that lower levels of autonomy were associated with increased frequency and intensity of moral distress, increased intention to leave the nursing profession, and lower perceived nurse-physician collaboration [30]. Conversely, increased autonomy corresponded with higher levels of nurse-physician collaboration and less frequent morally distressing encounters [30].

Moreover, Corley hypothesized that increased moral distress would be associated with lower nurse satisfaction and decreased quality of care. A marker for effective collaboration may include satisfaction from the professional interaction or clinical outcomes. This theory was borne out in a few noteworthy studies. Baggs et al. reported that effective, collaborative relationships between nurses and physicians were associated with significantly better clinical outcomes [31]. Hamric and Blackhall found that ICU nurses with high moral distress scores related to caring for dying patients perceived a more negative environment in their ICU, lower satisfaction with the quality of care, and less collaboration with physicians [8]. Most critical care nurses in this study reported frustration with physician communication (75 % negative), whereas physicians were very satisfied with nurse communication (97 % positive). Physicians believed they were collaborating well, whereas their nursing colleagues disagreed about their collaboration abilities. A significant finding from Hamric and Blackhall's study was that half of the nurses in one of the study sites reported that ICU physicians occasionally or regularly withheld diagnostic or prognostic information from their patients, whereas only 10 % of ICU physicians believed they withheld information on a regular basis. None of these physicians reported that a nurse had expressed concerns to them about physicians' communication with patients or surrogates. These findings are consistent with other studies [21, 22, 32, 33].

Unit or System Dynamics

Collaboration and effective communication are considered integral and necessary for a healthy work environment. A healthy work environment, in turn, is often characterized by team cohesion and role clarity. Ethical climate has been defined as the organizational practices and conditions that promote discussion and resolution of ethical decisions [34]. For an effective work environment, ethical values should be reflected in an organization's strategies, structures, and processes in the way it treats the staff, sets institutional goals, and manages conflicts [34, 35]. Until recently, there had been little study of the ethical dimensions of hospital environments and their bearing on moral distress [36, 37]. It is now known that organizations must have a forum for managing and resolving bioethical tensions. If there is no mechanism like an ethics consultation service or, alternatively, the service has a reputation for being ineffective, moral distress will be experienced more frequently and perhaps more intensely [8, 38].

It is presently unclear how best to improve ICU ethical climates. Hamric and Blackhall suggest that ethical climates can be improved through explicit discussions of moral distress and giving attention to improved collaboration. Yet, as they acknowledge, general exhortations to 'collaboration' will not enhance nurse-physicians interactions if physicians believe they are collaborating well [8]. The most successful interventions often focus on empowering critical care nurses to maximize their sense of autonomy and moral agency. Specifically, these interventions often include a heavy nursing-facilitated communication component. For example, mandating nurses' involvement in family meetings, holding multidisciplinary case reviews, or empowering nurses to facilitate code status conversations with patients or surrogates are all effective ways to empower nurses [32, 39, 40].

Impact of Moral Distress

It is unclear how many healthcare professionals leave their profession because of moral distress. Corley reported that 15 % of nurses said they had left their position because of moral distress, whereas a later study suggested that as many as 26 % reported leaving their profession because of moral distress [16, 25]. These discrepant findings may be attributable to our lack of full appreciation of other contributing factors that influence one's decision to leave a profession.

Some authors are skeptical of the assertion that moral distress directly causes healthcare professionals to leave their profession. These authors argue that moral distress, job dissatisfaction, and physical and emotional burnout are related, but a causal connection between moral distress and leaving the profession has yet to be definitively proven [41, 42]. And while moral distress and a negative ethical climate affect nurses' perception of collaboration, this has not been conclusively linked to nursing turnover. These authors acknowledge, however, that there is a strong correlation between burnout and leaving the profession, and there is a high probability of uncovering a link between moral distress and burnout. If moral distress indeed causes job dissatisfaction and burnout (which is likely), then a connection between moral distress and leaving the profession will likely be found. The degree of causal connection or attenuation between these factors is uncertain.

Two types of moral distress have been described. 'Initial distress' occurs when healthcare professionals cannot pursue what they perceive to be the correct course of action; this distress is associated with feelings of anger, sadness, frustration, and anxiety [5, 43]. 'Reactive distress', is a physical and psychological manifestation of repeated exposure to moral distress and a failure to respond to the initial experience of distress [3, 6, 10, 14]. This distress results in powerlessness, self-criticism, compartmentalization, and detachment. Other physiological responses include crying, lack of sleep, dreaming/having nightmares associated with cases, and a loss of appetite [43].

Epstein and Hamric extend this logic to a concept they call the "crescendo effect [14]." They argue that repeated exposure to morally distressing cases will result in a cumulative building of moral distress (moral residue) if left untreated. This cumulative effect results in a new baseline of moral distress which they call the "crescendo." A crescendo should manifest itself in a healthcare professional's stronger emotional reactions to subsequent interactions, especially when the healthcare professional encounters a situation that reminds them of a situation previously experienced. The crescendo effect causes the healthcare professional to become desensitized. Detachment from troubling cases is exemplified by conscientious objections or other actions indicating a withdrawal from the case [14]. The desensitization could compromise one's moral integrity.

While the crescendo effect may be applicable for some healthcare professionals, we question its generalizability. The crescendo effect has not been directly tested, owing to the lack of an instrument that can directly capture moral residue and crescendos. Further, if the crescendo theory is correct, one would expect to find that older, more experienced nurses should have stronger emotional reactions because of their repeated exposure to untreated moral distress. Our own (unpublished) work suggests the inverse of this: It may be the younger, less experienced nurses who are more susceptible to moral distress and have stronger emotional responses to it. This observation suggests that the crescendo effect is a complex phenomenon that deserves further study.

Interventions

There are few intervention studies on moral distress [12, 44, 45]. Intervention studies typically employ educational interventions to mitigate moral distress, and findings reflect mixed results. The focus on educational interventions is premised on studies suggesting that ethics education can address moral distress. In one study, nurses who experienced ethical conflict and had little (or no) ethics education reported a greater intention to leave their position [46]. In another study, moral distress was found to be a dominant feature in situations where nurses wanted to call for an ethics consultation but felt that they could not or should not [47]. Rogers and colleagues created an education intervention facilitated by the ethics consultation team to address moral distress in the neonatal ICU [45]. These studies suggest that ethics consultation and ethics education are two key interventions that have been advanced to address moral distress.

Other potential strategies have been proposed but have not been systematically studied [12]. Some of these strategies include journaling, developing treatment guidelines to facilitate resolution of complex cases, and teaching or promoting mediation techniques. Clinical ethicists are well-trained in conflict resolution and mediation. Therefore, clinical ethics consultations are thought to be an important vehicle for surfacing feelings and providing case resolution [2]. Ethics rounds have been promoted as another strategy to address moral distress. During these rounds, a clinical ethicist can provide direction to healthcare professionals to help them resolve challenging, morally distressing cases [48]. The effectiveness of these interventions merits further study.

Interventions that promote moral agency or autonomy are likely to be most effective. Towards this goal, some have suggested that debriefing sessions with diverse healthcare professionals present a good forum for talking about and addressing moral distress. The logistics for the debriefing session are a point of discussion and further study. Some have suggested that the debriefing session should be facilitated by an ethicist, who is thought to be in the "unique position of being able to seek out ethical discussion and educate staff to articulate their own ethical problems" [49]. Although it is true that ethicists are trained to elucidate and articulate ethical problems, the assumption that they are best positioned to facilitate a debriefing session may be misguided. For example, what if the ethicist were involved in the case and provided recommendations that are a source of some healthcare professionals' distress? What would be the markers of a 'successful' or 'unsuccessful' debriefing session?

In short, little is known about optimal ways to mitigate moral distress. It can be said with some confidence that interventions should be targeted at the system level (e. g., setting up an ethics consultation service, developing educational initiatives, holding debriefing sessions) as well as the individual level (e. g., journaling, self-care, exercise). A two-pronged approach might be the best way to counter the wide-ranging effects of moral distress.

Conclusions

Moral distress is a complex phenomenon that rightfully deserves more attention in the ICU. Despite the increase in publications related to moral distress, our understanding of moral distress and the empirical study of it remains in formative stages [12, 14]. Further empirical and conceptual clarity on the experiences of moral distress is needed. Using consistent, precise terminology and developing up-to-date, real-time, comprehensive instruments to detect moral distress are needed. The frequency of moral distress and experiences of healthcare professionals beyond nurses have not been adequately studied [13].

Potential differences between critical care contexts deserve some attention. For example, it is conceivable that cardiovascular ICU staff might experience greater frequency or higher intensity of moral distress compared to medical ICU staff. Although entirely speculative, we think healthcare professionals may recognize that

ethically questionable decisions by transplant medicine professionals have consequences that extend far beyond the clinicians involved if the integrity of transplant
medicine is brought into question and donation rates fall [50]. Recognition of these
consequences might engender profound degrees of moral distress.

Perhaps most importantly, the lack of intervention studies is concerning. Studies
have found that nurses feel that physicians do not fully provide prognostic or diagnostic information to patients or surrogates, yet physicians' responses suggest that
nurses do not express these concerns to them. Interventions will only be successful insofar as they do two things: (1) promote moral agency that is necessary for
healthcare professionals to express moral concerns, such as empowering nurses to
talk with physicians about communication concerns; and (2) protect moral integrity
that is vital to being a competent and compassionate healthcare professional. We
believe that moral distress can never be fully eradicated, nor should it be. Moral
distress may reflect an awareness and appreciation of the moral aspects in medicine
but, if left unattended and untreated, it can be destructive.

References

1. Bartholome W (2000) Moral distress. Medical College of Wisconsin Bioethics Discussion.
   Nurs Outlooks Sep-Oct:199–201. doi: online discussion, 10 December 1998, quoted in A.B.
   Hamric, "Moral Distress in Every Day Bioethics"
2. Hamric AB (2000) Moral distress in everyday ethics. Nurs Outlook 48:199–201
3. Jameton A (1984) Nursing practice: the ethical issues. Prentice-Hall, Englewood Cliffs
4. Ulrich CM, Hamric AB, Grady C (2010) Moral distress: a growing problem in the health
   professions? Hastings Cent Rep 40:20–22
5. Jameton A (1993) Dilemmas of moral distress: moral responsibility and nursing practice.
   AWHONNS Clin Issues Perinat Womens Health Nurs 4:542–551
6. Webster, Baylis (2000) Moral residue. In: Rubin SB, Zoloth L (eds) Margin of Error: The
   Ethics of Mistakes in the Practice of Medicine. University Pub. Group, Hagerstown, Md., pp
   217–230
7. McCarthy J, Deady R (2008) Moral distress reconsidered. Nurs Ethics 15:254–262
8. Hamric AB, Blackhall LJ (2007) Nurse-physician perspectives on the care of dying patients in
   intensive care units: collaboration, moral distress, and ethical climate. Crit Care Med 35:422–
   429
9. Angus DC, Barnato AE, Linde-Zwirble WT et al (2004) Use of intensive care at the end of life
   in the United States: an epidemiologic study. Crit Care Med 32:638–643
10. Wilkinson JM (1987) Moral distress in nursing practice: experience and effect. Nurs Forum
    (Auckl) 23:16–29
11. Nathaniel AK (2006) Moral reckoning in nursing. West J Nurs Res 28:419–438
12. Hamric AB (2012) Empirical research on moral distress: issues, challenges, and opportunities.
    HEC Forum Interdiscip J Hosp Ethical Leg Issues 24:39–49
13. Rushton CH (2006) Defining and addressing moral distress: tools for critical care nursing
    leaders. AACN Adv Crit Care 17:161–168
14. Epstein EG, Hamric AB (2009) Moral distress, moral residue, and the crescendo effect. J Clin
    Ethics 20:330–342
15. Corley MC, Elswick RK, Gorman M, Clor T (2001) Development and evaluation of a moral
    distress scale. J Adv Nurs 33:250–256
16. Corley MC (1995) Moral distress of critical care nurses. Am J Crit Care 4:280–285

17. Wocial LD, Weaver MT (2013) Development and psychometric testing of a new tool for detecting moral distress: the Moral Distress Thermometer. J Adv Nurs 69:167–174
18. Hamric AB, Borchers CT, Epstein EG (2012) Development and testing of an instrument to measure moral distress in healthcare professionals. AJOB Prim Res 3:1–9
19. Ulrich C, O'Donnell P, Taylor C, Farrar A, Danis M, Grady C (2007) Ethical climate, ethics stress, and the job satisfaction of nurses and social workers in the United States. Soc Sci Med 65:1708–1719
20. Sporrong SK, Höglund AT, Arnetz B (2006) Measuring moral distress in pharmacy and clinical practice. Nurs Ethics 13:416–427
21. Thomas EJ, Sexton JB, Helmreich RL (2003) Discrepant attitudes about teamwork among critical care nurses and physicians. Crit Care Med 31:956–959
22. Shannon SE, Mitchell PH, Cain KC (2002) Patients, nurses, and physicians have differing views of quality of critical care. J Nurs Scholarsh 34:173–179
23. Kälvemark S, Höglund AT, Hansson MG, Westerholm P, Arnetz B (2004) with conflicts-ethical dilemmas and moral distress in the health care system. Soc Sci Med 58:1075–1084
24. Houston S, Casanova MA, Leveille M et al (2013) The intensity and frequency of moral distress among different healthcare disciplines. J Clin Ethics 24:98–112
25. Corley MC (2002) Nurse moral distress: a proposed theory and research agenda. Nurs Ethics 9:636–650
26. Elpern EH, Covert B, Kleinpell R (2005) Moral distress of staff nurses in a medical intensive care unit. Am J Crit Care 14:523–530
27. Karanikola MNK, Papathanassoglou EDE, Kalafati M, Stathopoulou H (2012) Exploration of the association between professional interactions and emotional distress of intensive care unit nursing personnel. Dimens Crit Care Nurs DCCN 31:37–45
28. Manias E, Street A (2001) Nurse-doctor interactions during critical care ward rounds. J Clin Nurs 10:442–450
29. Varjus SL, Suominen T, Leino-Kilpi H (2003) Autonomy among intensive care nurses in Finland. Intensive Crit Care Nurs 19:31–40
30. Papathanassoglou EDE, Karanikola MNK, Kalafati M, Giannakopoulou M, Lemonidou C, Albarran JW (2012) Professional autonomy, collaboration with physicians, and moral distress among European intensive care nurses. Am J Crit Care 21:e41–e52
31. Baggs JG, Schmitt MH, Mushlin AI et al (1999) Association between nurse-physician collaboration and patient outcomes in three intensive care units. Crit Care Med 27:1991–1998
32. Lilly CM, Sonna LA, Haley KJ, Massaro AF (2003) Intensive communication: four-year follow-up from a clinical practice study. Crit Care Med 31:S394–S399
33. Ferrand E, Lemaire F, Regnier B et al (2003) Discrepancies between perceptions by physicians and nursing staff of intensive care unit end-of-life decisions. Am J Respir Crit Care Med 167:1310–1315
34. Olson LL (1998) Hospital nurses' perceptions of the ethical climate of their work setting. Image J Nurs Sch 30:345–349
35. McDaniel C (1997) Development and psychometric properties of the Ethics Environment Questionnaire. Med Care 35:901–914
36. Olson L (1995) Ethical climate in health care organizations. Int Nurs Rev 42:85–90
37. Rushton CH (1995) Creating an ethical practice environment: a focus on advocacy. Crit Care Nurs Clin North Am 7:387–397
38. Corley MC, Minick P, Elswick RK, Jacobs M (2005) Nurse moral distress and ethical work environment. Nurs Ethics 12:381–390
39. Campbell ML, Guzman JA (2003) Impact of a proactive approach to improve end-of-life care in a medical ICU. Chest 123:266–271
40. Sulmasy DP, He MK, McAuley R, Ury WA (2008) Beliefs and attitudes of nurses and physicians about do not resuscitate orders and who should speak to patients and families about them. Crit Care Med 36:1817–1822

41. Fogel KM (2007) The Relationship of Moral Distress, Ethical Climate, and Intent to Turnover Among Critical Care Nurses. Dissertation, Loyola University
42. Schluter J, Winch S, Holzhauser K, Henderson A (2008) Nurses' moral sensitivity and hospital ethical climate: a literature review. Nurs Ethics 15:304–321
43. Kelly B (1998) Preserving moral integrity: a follow-up study with new graduate nurses. J Adv Nurs 28:1134–1145
44. Beumer CM (2008) Innovative solutions: the effect of a workshop on reducing the experience of moral distress in an intensive care unit setting. Dimens Crit Care Nurs DCCN 27:263–267
45. Rogers S, Babgi A, Gomez C (2008) Educational interventions in end-of-life care: part I: an educational intervention responding to the moral distress of NICU nurses provided by an ethics consultation team. Adv Neonatal Care 8:56–65
46. Hart SE (2005) Hospital ethical climates and registered nurses' turnover intentions. J Nurs Sch 37:173–177
47. Gordon EJ, Hamric AB (2006) The courage to stand up: the cultural politics of nurses' access to ethics consultation. J Clin Ethics 17:231–254
48. Wlody GS (2007) Nursing management and organizational ethics in the intensive care unit. Crit Care Med 35:S29–S35
49. Austin W, Lemermeyer G, Goldberg L et al (2005) Moral distress in healthcare practice: The situation of nurses. HEC Forum 17:33–48
50. Veatch RM (2000) Transplantation ethics. Georgetown University Press, Washington

Specific Diagnoses of Organizational Dysfunction to Guide Mechanism-based Quality Improvement Interventions

T. J. Iwashyna and A. C. Kajdacsy-Balla Amaral

Introduction

Modern health care has endemic quality problems. Our current approach to solving these problems resembles nothing so much as pre-Virchow medicine. Interactions of ill-defined humors are invoked to explain why some organizations prosper, and others fail. 'Culture', 'incentives', 'communication', and 'hierarchy' seem as tangible as phlegm, yellow and black bile once did – clearly capturing something that seems true about our organizations, yet remaining ephemeral. Broad interventions are applied across situations, with little systematic basis on which to match a targeted solution to a specific etiology of a problem. Progress is frustratingly halting, even as evidence of persistent, morbid and expensive quality problems grow.

Here we suggest that quality improvement needs to enter the era of clinico-pathophysiological correlation. We propose that specific organizational lesions should be carefully described and the mechanism by which each lesion generates organizational symptoms elucidated, ideally with an understanding of the environmental contingencies under which lesions become manifest, rather than being compensated around. This approach demands the formulation of explicit differential diagnoses for various organizational dysfunctions and the development of diagnostic tests. The ultimate goal of organizational diagnosis is to guide effective therapy: quality improvement intended as either a lesion-directed cure (i. e., solving the problem) or symptom-directed palliation (i. e., harm mitigation).

T. J. Iwashyna ✉
Pulmonary and Critical Care Medicine, University of Michigan, Ann Arbor, MI USA
e-mail: tiwashyn@umich.edu

A. C. Kajdacsy-Balla Amaral
Sunnybrook Health Sciences Centre, Toronto, Canada

J.-L. Vincent (Ed.), *Annual Update in Intensive Care and Emergency Medicine 2014*,
DOI 10.1007/978-3-319-03746-2_55, © Springer International Publishing Switzerland
2014

Limitations of the Current Approach

Consider two important studies, which, although important advances, have also demonstrated the limits of the current approach to quality improvement and the need for clinico-pathophysiological correlation.

First, our existing quality improvement interventions are broad and untargeted, seemingly hoping to cover everything at once. Consider the Keystone ICU intervention to reduce central line infections [1]. This intervention set up a statewide collaborative, engaged the major attentions of one of the most magnetic leaders in American medicine, required monthly meetings to change the culture of an ICU, each of which required the participation of top hospital executives, and fundamentally changed line insertion practices, introducing significant new equipment into the ICU. This complex intervention was again applied indiscriminately to every ICU in the state, and resulted in dramatic decreases in the median rates of line infection, and was temporally associated with differences in in-hospital (but not 30-day) mortality [2]. This concept seems akin to treating every patient who presents with dyspnea with a package of Lasix, antibiotics, anticoagulation, steroids and nebulizers – many patients will respond to the therapy, but it is hardly efficient or elegant. From an organizational point-of-view, it is possible that many of the institutions involved in this project could improve their rates of infection with a simpler package. In fact, this laborious, indiscriminately applied strategy may lead to unwanted side-effects in the organization, such as inability to implement other practices or poor value for the effort applied [3].

Second, we lack a systematic approach to identifying quality problems, let alone diagnosing their origin. Scales and colleagues conducted a multicenter cluster-randomized trial of interventions to improve compliance with patient-safety practices perceived to be inadequate at 10 hospitals [4]. A complex multi-step intervention including education, reminders and audit and feedback was performed. Statistically significant and clinically meaningful overall improvements in the practices were noted. The authors identified six quality problems by interviewing ICU directors about their perceived problems. Yet when they collected detailed performance during the trial, the authors found that 3 of the 6 practices they targeted had almost perfect pre-intervention performance, and there was in fact no lesion there to correct. By analogy to a clinical trial, 50 % of their cases did not have any disease, yet all of those units underwent a wide-ranging interventional treatment.

A third study further illustrates these challenges. The Institute for Healthcare Improvement (IHI) "100,000 Lives" campaign was one of the signature successes of recent quality improvement. Like the Keystone ICU program, with the help of a charismatic leader, IHI mobilized an unprecedented US-wide attention to patient safety. Both organizations are to be strongly commended for promoting a bias towards action in the face of previous widespread neglect of quality problems. Yet the IHI offered six "planks" as solutions that were adopted by nearly 3000 hospitals (of approximately 6500 total U.S. hospitals). Although it is possible that all these hospitals happened to all suffer from the same problems, it seems plausible that in some cases hospitals may have been distracted from other more pressing problems.

The evaluation of the 100,000 Lives campaign, which helped create the 'fact' that it saved 122,300 lives, was reported in a press release rather than the peer-reviewed medical literature [5], and has been vigorously critiqued even inside the patient safety movement [6]. This may be an example of excellent mass mobilization, but it has clear negatives against efforts to create incremental but thereby cumulative progress.

The Organizational Clinico-pathological Correlation: Symptoms and Lesions

A clinico-pathophysiological correlation-based approach presents an alternative, albeit one in the nascent stage of development. It would require us to work in two directions at once. First, we need many case reports documenting specific organizational pathologies and the diverse symptoms they manifest. This is intrinsically different from the current publication bias towards quality reports of increased compliance or improved outcomes, often without specifying the particular mechanism by which an intervention would improve quality. Akin to clinico-pathological correlations discussed at conferences – that use both difficult diagnosis that were made before death, and cases that died in spite of clinicians' best efforts to diagnose and treat them – organizational clinico-pathological conferences will require data from cases of success, but also from institutions that had delays in diagnosing a problem or were unable to improve performance.

Our goal moving forward is to discover the links from fundamental organizational pathology to visible organizational symptoms, hopefully documenting the environmental contingencies that lead a lesion to manifest itself as symptoms. We define an organizational lesion as the specific problem in terms of specific personnel or technological systems or their interaction that leads to organizational symptoms. We define organizational symptoms as the adverse outcomes for patients and other consumers of services, which may include increased morbidity and mortality, poor costumer satisfaction, or decreased value (less improvement in health per unit cost).

The second arm of this approach is to develop rigorous differential diagnoses of organizational symptoms and systematic approaches to their evaluation. For example, we might consider Stelfox and colleagues' recent finding that rates of do-not-resuscitate (DNR) orders vary with intensive care unit (ICU) occupancy (a symptom of organizational dysfunction) [7]. A differential diagnosis of possible lesions leading to this situation might include: Routine avoidance of end-of-life conversations; fragmentation of care between inpatient and outpatient settings; inappropriate throughput focus that leads to inadequately informed DNR decisions; and others. Each of these organizational diagnoses requires different interventions. What we lack from Stelfox's work is a systematic approach to working through this differential.

A Possible Objection

The fundamental contention of the clinico-pathophysiological correlation is that despite the wide diversity of human experience, there are fundamental regularities in the ways human bodies fail and the symptoms that those failing bodies manifest. When considering the extension to quality improvement, a thoughtful colleague of ours argued: "there is no empiric evidence that quality improvement has lesions which are isolatable from the entire context of patient care that may be identified, modified and corrected without thereby realigning the whole."

To our mind, this resonates with the longstanding holistic complaint that each patient is unique in their suffering and illness, and that to abstract from the patient to a disease is at best dehumanizing, at worse a fundamental misdirection. And while that 'holisticness' has a certain degree of truth, it is also true that methicillin-resistant *Staphylococcus aureus* (MRSA) infections usually respond to vancomycin, but Gram-negative infections do not – and that culture-directed antibiotic therapy can often be effective without a holistic approach to the patient.

Further, there is substantial empirical evidence that there are well-defined and reproducible patterns of organizational failures. Outside medicine, entire fields of organizational studies, institutional sociology, industrial organization, behavioral economics and social psychology have spent years documenting those regularities [8] – just not usually in situations as complex as the average hospital, because hospitals are hard to study. Such regularities are often found to have environmental contingencies, but that does not obviate the fact that there are reproducible underlying problems. (The need to extrapolate from simpler models, but with caution, is familiar to the modern physician.) But we suggest that our current focus on complex quality improvement interventions indicates that the time is ripe to test the alternate hypothesis that hospitals can sometimes have simple diagnoses. Further, this hypothesis holds that there is an art to making such simple unifying diagnoses, and that art needs to refined and tested. When possible, the identification of such simpler diagnoses will allow one to identify narrow, targeted and thereby efficient quality improvement therapies.

A Path to Progress

To move forward, we suggest approaching the categorization of lesions based on the core functions of a given ward or unit, the basic building block of inpatient healthcare. One classification scheme is outlined in Table 1. We offer this as a place to begin; if this line of research and practice is productive, a growing knowledge base will necessitate future revisions. We suspect that organizational lesions may be acute or chronic. Some lesions may cause problems (e. g., presenting symptoms) in all cases, whereas other lesions may be compensated for until presented with particularly stressful situations and environmental demands, or until multiple lesions have accumulated in the organization, reducing its functional reserve.

Table 1 A proposed function-based taxonomy for organizing proposed organizational pathologies. Note that there is not expected to be a 1:1 relationship among specific lesions and specific organizational symptoms, and the focus of this table is on the classes of lesions in column 2. Indeed, the need for a clinico-pathophysiological correlation approach is precisely because a given lesion (column 3) can generate diverse symptoms (column 4) and, as illustrated in Box 2, a given symptom could have a differential diagnosis of alternative possible causes

Functional system	Examples of classes of lesions	Examples of specific lesions	Examples of symptoms generated	Potential interventions to given lesions
Triage	"Not my problem" narrow focus	ICU fellows with a bias towards blocking admissions	Early ICU transfers after ward admissions	Mandatory re-checking on ward "borderline" patients [12]
	Flexibility failure	Rigid criteria for ICU admissions	Inefficient usage of ICU beds with high rate of early discharges to the floor	Reasonable scope for professional judgment in criteria [13]
	Flexibility failure	Rigid criteria for ICU admissions	Patients with severe sepsis and consequent troponin leaks admitted to cardiac intensive care rather than medical intensive care	Reasonable scope for professional judgment in criteria
Monitoring	Lack of closed loop communication	MDs do not explicitly write "contact precautions" orders when MDR pathogens are cultured	Outbreaks of nosocomial MDR-pathogens when contact precautions are delayed	System for confirming alert with nursing when MDR pathogens are cultured
	Coordination	MDs do not have focused handoff reports on transfer out of unit	Excessive mortality or ICU bounce backs for patients discharged at night	Structured interactive handoff conversation [14]
Recognition/ detection	Failure to act ("laissez-faire" lesion)	Poor coordination between outpatient and inpatient attendings	DNR orders on the wards vary with ICU occupancy	Interprofessional team to discuss level of care for target patients at hospital admission [7]
	Systematic coordination failure	Lack of rapid activation protocol for Cath Lab	Prolonged door-to-needle times for STEMI	Development of protocol
Knowledge	Lack of knowledge	MDs failing to prescribe vancomycin for patients with potential healthcare associated pneumonia	High rates of death among patients with nosocomial severe sepsis	Education and auditing, with better screening of hires

Continuation see next page

Table 1 *Continued*

Functional system	Examples of classes of lesions	Examples of specific lesions	Examples of symptoms generated	Potential interventions to given lesions
Response to aberrancy	Communication failure	Lack of interprofessional respect	Late consultation for surgical emergencies or patients dying of potential acute abdomen	House office cross training
	Coordination Failure	Poor systems design that make it easier for users to rewrite things than to readily transfer stable orders	High rates of discontinuation/substitution of active (e. g., antibiotics, heart failure meds) treatment on transfer between units	CPOE, Med Rec, pre-printed order sets, cross-training [15]
	Implementation failure	Pharmacy does not stock antibiotics on the floor	Poor survival rates for immunosuppressed patients developing septic shock	Pre-positioned common antibiotics used for early septic shock [16]
	Flexibility failure	Organizational constipator	Inability to incorporate new evidence into practice.	Change policies for hiring people in middle manager positions [9]
	Efficiency/throughput	Poor hospital discharge practices leading to high floor bed occupancy rates and inability to transfer patients out of ICU to floor	Increased cardiac arrests outside ICU on days of high occupancy	Medical emergency teams
Discharge	Discharge coordination	Poor communication from hospitalists to primary care providers	High rates of unintentional discontinuation of chronic medications	Computerized medicine reconciliation [15]

ICU: intensive care unit; MRD: multidrug resistant; STEMI: ST-segment elevation myocardial infarction; CPOE: computerized physician order entry; Med Rec: medication reconciliation

A clinico-pathophysiological correlation-based approach to improving quality already has important precedents. For example, Krein and colleagues have described the lesion they term the "organizational constipator" [9]. This lesion causes symptoms only when stressed by the need to implement new or innovative approaches to care; in a stable clinical environment it can be well tolerated. They demonstrate that advances in the patient safety agenda with regard to catheter-associated urinary tract infections provide the stressful environment in which an organizational constipator leads to acute organizational dysfunction – manifesting as the symptom of disproportionately slow improvements in catheter-associated urinary tract infection rates. They suggest several pragmatic strategies to management based on their intensive case series of 14 hospitals [9]. Much of this group's work can be understood as an effort to build a complete differential diagnosis for that symptom of disproportionately slow improvements in catheter-associated urinary tract infection rates, and to develop a scientific approach to making the diagnosis and developing lesion-targeted therapies.

The case-based approach to improving quality and safety undergirded the "Quality Grand Rounds" series, which used detailed explorations of single cases as teaching tools [10]. Root-cause analyses (RCA) carefully dig into the underlying pathologies of an organization, but are often kept tightly within the organization [11]. RCAs are also constrained by isolated adverse events, thus focusing on patient safety, while quality improvement problems also arise during the implementation of a new process of care. Business schools have used selective case studies as a teaching tool for years. A clinico-pathophysiological correlation-based approach expands on these previous presentations in three important ways. First, it foregrounds the development of differential diagnoses, making visible and open to argument not only the problems encountered, but the diagnostic and therapeutic reasoning used to explain and remediate those problems. Second, this approach is rooted in the public presentation of these data, reported so that explicit claims about generalizability are made and can then be verified or refuted in future work – to allow the incremental increase in our knowledge. Third, it explicitly encourages the reporting of diverse organizational problems to dramatically increase our communal experience base, soon allowing systematic aggregation.

An approach to reporting the investigation of a quality problem in this spirit is summarized in Box 1. A relatively straightforward case is illustrated in Box 2 to make the application clear. General characteristics of the organization are presented, and the specific problem characterized. The nature of the investigation into alternative etiologies is described; as so often in clinical medicine, this involves a combination of objective data and a careful history informed by a differential diagnosis. An intervention was applied that targeted a specific mechanism for the diagnosis, in this case showing marked improvement. Not all pathologies will be so easy to remedy, but our contention is that these sorts of details matter.

Box 1:

Minimal Components of an Organizational Case Report
- System characteristics
- Symptom manifest
- Evidence that the symptom was not simply expected variation in stable performance
- Differential diagnosis explored
- Proposed underlying pathology
- Processes engaged in to rule-out alternative items on the differential
- Intervention attempted to remedy pathology
- Was intervention intended to be curative or palliative?
- Results of intervention on proposed mechanism
- Results of intervention on manifest symptom
- Comments on generalizability

Box 2:

Example of Minimal Components of an Organizational Case Report (derived from [16])

System characteristics: Pediatric intensive care unit (ICU) in a medium-sized (200) bed, private teaching hospital.

Symptom manifest: Physician director of the pediatric ICU thought that they had excess morbidity, stemming from prolonged time to antibiotics for febrile neutropenia in their unit. There were no data to support this belief, but it had face validity among the staff members.

Evidence that symptom was not simply expected variation in stable performance: An audit of the time to antibiotics over the prior year demonstrated that no patients had received antibiotics within less than 1 hour of admission to the ICU.

Differential diagnoses explored:
1. Lack of knowledge about the importance of timely antibiotics for neutropenic fever
2. Barriers to accessing the required resources
   A. Excessive bureaucracy for authorizing antibiotics by insurance companies
   B. Unit far from central pharmacy where antibiotics were kept
   C. Delays in admitting patients into the e-system to allow for prescribing antibiotics
3. Missed diagnosis (lack of completeness of information to identify specific condition of neutropenic fever)

Proposed underlying pathology: Barriers to accessing the required resources, most likely distance from pharmacy and delays in admitting patients into e-system

Processes engaged in to rule-out alternative items on the differential: Brainstorming with team. No formal data collection. Team had been previously educated on the importance of timely antibiotics.

Intervention attempted to remedy pathology: Availability of first dose of broad-spectrum antibiotics in code-blue cart (which deals both with the distance to pharmacy and the delays in admitting patients into the system as the antibiotic can be given in spite of the patient not being in the system). Authorization from hospital medical director to administer broad spectrum antibiotics before formal authorization by insurance companies.

Was intervention intended to be curative or palliative? Curative

Results of intervention on mechanism: Decreased time to antibiotics for patients with febrile neutropenia, including more than 50 % receiving antibiotics in the first hour

Results of intervention on patient-centered manifest symptom: Not assessed in this trial

Comments on generalizability: While the intervention was tailored to this unit, it is likely the other units that work within similar constraints of availability, technology and bureaucracy may choose to provide some degrees of freedom in the system for processes of care that are dependent on a timely response. The extreme generalization of this would be the resuscitation of a patient with cardiac arrest at the emergency department, where care would be provided independent of the identification of a paying provider or even identification of the name of the patient.

Conclusions

Our goal in this process is to bring the full armamentarium of clinical reasoning and clinical epidemiology to bear on advancing the science of patient care. The quality and safety movement have persuasively argued that we must not hide our errors, but rather that disclosure can bring a powerful impetus to change. Having learned that lesson, we now need a systematic approach to reporting not merely the narratives of the problems, but their systematic investigation. A great strength of medicine has been our nurturing of diagnostic acumen and using careful and precise diagnostic approaches to inform specific selection of therapies. This interplay between the specificity of each story and the generalizable kernel of truth inside it has brought us enormous advances; we suggest that this same rigorous intellectual approach can be used to further improve the quality of our systems of care.

Acknowledgement

This work was supported by K08 HL091249 from the NIH and IIR 11-109 from the VA Health Services Research & Development Service.

References

1. Pronovost PJ, Needham DM, Berenholtz SM et al (2006) An Intervention to Decrease Catheter-Related Bloodstream Infections in the ICU. N Engl J Med 355:2725–2732
2. Lipitz-Snyderman A, Steinwachs D, Needham DM, Colantuoni E, Morlock LL, Pronovost PJ (2011) Impact of a statewide intensive care unit quality improvement initiative on hospital mortality and length of stay: retrospective comparative analysis. BMJ 342:d219
3. Dixon-Woods M, Leslie M, Tarrant C, Bion J (2013) Explaining Matching Michigan: an ethnographic study of a patient safety program. Implement Sci 8:70
4. Scales DC, Dainty K, Hales B et al (2011) A multifaceted intervention for quality improvement in a network of intensive care units: a cluster randomized trial. JAMA 305:363–372
5. Institute for Healthcare Improvement (2006). IHI Announces That Hospitals Participating in 100,000 Lives Campaign Have Saved an Estimated 122,300 Lives 2006. Available from:http://www.ihi.org/about/news/Documents/IHIPressRelease_Hospitalsin100000LivesCampaignHaveSaved122300Lives_Jun06.pdf. Accessed Nov 2013
6. Wachter RM, Pronovost PJ (2006) The 100,000 Lives Campaign: A scientific and policy review. Jt Comm J Qual Patient Saf 32:621–627
7. Stelfox HT, Hemmelgarn BR, Bagshaw SM et al (2012) Intensive care unit bed availability and outcomes for hospitalized patients with sudden clinical deterioration. Arch Intern Med 172:467–474
8. Scott WR, Davis GF (2006) Organizations and Organizing: Rational, Natural and Open Systems Perspectives. Pearson, London
9. Krein SL, Damschroder LJ, Kowalski CP, Forman J, Hofer TP, Saint S (2010) The influence of organizational context on quality improvement and patient safety efforts in infection prevention: a multi-center qualitative study. Soc Sci Med 71:1692–1701
10. Wachter RM, Shojania KG, Saint S, Markowitz AJ, Smith M (2002) Learning from our mistakes: quality grand rounds, a new case-based series on medical errors and patient safety. Ann Intern Med 136:850–852
11. Wu AW, Lipshutz AK, Pronovost PJ (2008) Effectiveness and efficiency of root cause analysis in medicine. JAMA 299:685–687
12. Delgado MK, Liu V, Pines JM, Kipnis P, Gardner MN, Escobar GJ (2013) Risk factors for unplanned transfer to intensive care within 24 hours of admission from the emergency department in an integrated healthcare system. J Hosp Med 8:13–19
13. Das AM, Sood N, Hodgin K, Chang L, Carson SS (2008) Development of a triage protocol for patients presenting with gastrointestinal hemorrhage: a prospective cohort study. Crit Care 12:R57
14. Petersen LA, Orav EJ, Teich JM, O'Neil AC, Brennan TA (1998) Using a computerized sign-out program to improve continuity of inpatient care and prevent adverse events. Jt Comm J Qual Improv 24:77–87
15. Bell CM, Brener SS, Gunraj N et al (2011) Association of ICU or hospital admission with unintentional discontinuation of medications for chronic diseases. JAMA 306:840–847
16. Amado VM, Vilela GP, Queiroz A Jr, Amaral AC (2011) Effect of a quality improvement intervention to decrease delays in antibiotic delivery in pediatric febrile neutropenia: a pilot study. J Crit Care 26:103 e9–e12

Part XVIII
Moving Forward...

Where to Next in Combat Casualty Care Research?

A. M. Pritchard, A. R. Higgs, and M. C. Reade

Introduction

As in previous wars, engagement in the last 13 years of conflict by the armed forces of much of the developed world has produced or benefited from substantial medical advances with direct implications for civilian trauma care. The majority of these advances have been related directly to acute-care surgery and emergency and critical care medicine [1]. For example, the benefit of high ratios of plasma and platelets to red cells; the avoidance of vasopressors in trauma resuscitation; the development of topical hemostatic agents; strategies to prevent and treat invasive mold infection in wounds; the utility of tourniquets for extremity hemorrhage; the value of sending senior emergency physicians, intensivists or anesthetists with suitable equipment to the point of wounding; the utility of a rapid clinical feedback and quality assurance system; and the effectiveness (or lack thereof) of hemostatic drugs, such as factor VIIa and tranexamic acid (TxA). These interventions, along with improvements in trauma systems, have led to the lowest case fatality rate in the history of warfare; a number that continues to decrease despite better pre-hospital care delivering more severely wounded patients to hospital alive (Fig. 1) [2]. A new field of clinical practice and research has been defined, termed "combat casualty care". By convention, this term excludes reconstructive surgery, prosthetic science and rehabilitation, which all typically occur in the country of origin rather than in the theater of operations. In early 2014, it appears likely that the intensity with which western armed forces are engaged with an enemy will diminish, at least in the short term. It is therefore opportune to reflect on the current and likely future research questions that will hopefully build on recent successes, the methods and resources such research will require, and the potential for translation of still more innovations in trauma care into civilian systems.

A. M. Pritchard · A. R. Higgs · M. C. Reade ✉
NATO Role 3 Hospital, Kandahar Airfield, Afghanistan
e-mail: michael.reade@defence.gov.au

J.-L. Vincent (Ed.), *Annual Update in Intensive Care and Emergency Medicine 2014*,   747
DOI 10.1007/978-3-319-03746-2_56, © Springer International Publishing Switzerland
2014

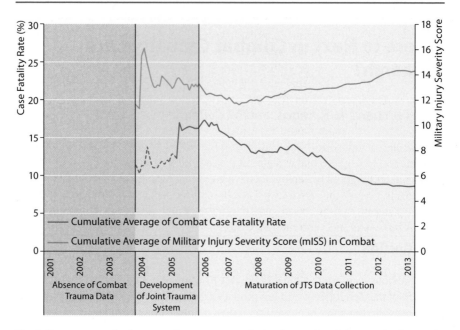

Fig. 1 Improvements in therapy and trauma system design have reduced the case fatality rate in modern combat to 9 %, despite progressively increasing severity of injury. From [2] with permission

Priorities in Future Combat Casualty Care Research

The scope of clinical research relevant to battlefield trauma is broad, encompassing everything from identification of resilient characteristics in recruits to defenses against biological weapons. While no topic is unimportant, priorities should logically be driven by necessity (likelihood of saving the greatest number of lives) and feasibility (likelihood of improving clinical treatment in a useful timeframe). By these characteristics, the following fields are likely to yield the most useful results over the coming decade.

Hemorrhage Control, Fluid Resuscitation, Rapid Diagnostics and Manipulation of Coagulation, Inflammatory-Modulating Resuscitation, and Salvage Techniques for Circulatory Collapse

Hemorrhage accounts for 80–90 % of preventable deaths on the battlefield [3], so clinical interventions addressing hemorrhage offer the greatest potential to save lives. Tourniquets have reduced death from extremity trauma from 9 % in the Vietnam War to 2 % [4], but bleeding from areas not amenable to tourniquets (especially the junctions of the axial and appendicular skeleton) remains the cause of considerable mortality. Up to 25 % of major trauma patients rapidly develop a coagulopathy mediated not by the traditional culprits (hypothermia, acidemia and dilution of clotting factors) but by thrombomodulin expression and activated protein C [5]. Drugs or devices that specifically address junctional bleeding and coagulopathy should logically further reduce death from traumatic hemorrhage. Venous thromboembolic disease is particularly common in combat trauma, occurring in 9 % of patients and appearing more rapidly (within the first 24 hours) than has traditionally been appreciated [6]. This factor must be considered when testing novel interventions for hyperacute coagulopathy. Rapid diagnostic tests that identify the switch between a hypo- and hyper-coagulable state may be useful in addressing this conundrum. Increasing willingness to deploy the most advanced lifesaving technologies to field hospitals has raised the possibility that extracorporeal salvage techniques may also have a place in treating exsanguinating hemorrhage. Evidence supporting these various interventions is currently lacking.

Delivery of Blood Products and Their Derivatives outside Large Hospitals

Many combat hospitals, like smaller civilian hospitals, usually have low blood product usage interspersed with requirements to provide large quantities at short notice. Modern appreciation of the benefit of blood resuscitation rather than crystalloid or non-blood colloid began with combat experience in Iraq. The shelf life of packed red blood cells (PRBC) (42 days) and platelets (5 days) imposes either a large logistic burden and substantial waste, or precludes availability. For example, in the first year after the 2003 invasion of Iraq, 90,000 PRBC units were transported to US field hospitals, but just over 2 % were used [7]. Platelets were unavailable other than in donations of fresh whole blood. Combat hospitals in Afghanistan matured to provide apheresis platelets from local military donors, but this relies on equipment and a stable donor population that may be unavailable in more austere conditions. Alternatives to conventional fractionated blood components would be logistically and clinically highly attractive.

Management of Wounds and Wound Infection

Systemic prevention, identification and treatment of infection
Military ballistic wounds usually result from high energy projectiles and so are typically more often contaminated, have less tissue coverage, and are more prone to infection with multi-drug resistant organisms than civilian wounds. The current military recommended antibiotic infection prophylaxis for extremity wounds is a 1st generation cephalosporin or clindamycin for an initial period of 1–3 days [8]. Further antibiotics are given only in established infection, but early recognition can be difficult. Clinicians must rely on non-specific parameters, such as fever, wound discharge, erythema and white cell count. Traditional inflammatory markers, such

as erythrocyte sedimentation rate (ESR) and C-reactive protein (CRP) have poor specificity, as they remain elevated for at least three weeks post-wounding even in the absence of infection. A more specific diagnostic test to identify infection early should facilitate both better antibiotic stewardship and clinical outcomes.

Local techniques to prevent infection

Longstanding military trauma surgical tradition holds that "the best antibiotic is good surgery". Removal of dead or contaminated material is critically important in primary surgery for all ballistic wounds. The ability to operatively re-inspect wounds at frequent intervals within the first 72 hours is a central feature of modern military surgery. Once only viable tissue is observed within the wound, re-inspections can be reduced in frequency to second-daily or less until a final wound closure strategy is identified. This strategy considerably reduces unnecessary tissue loss compared to early aggressive debridement that might remove tissue that could recover. Irrigation performed before and after adequate debridement is perhaps the most important aspect of primary wound surgery and is known to reduce bacterial load. However, questions (amenable to randomized controlled trials [RCTs]) remain over the optimal nature and method of this technique.

Heterotopic ossification

The incidence of heterotopic ossification in combat-wounded service members is as high as 64.6 %, higher than in civilian trauma patients in whom the rates are 11–50 % in the setting of a significant head injury, and much lower (although less well defined) in others [9]. Amongst military casualties, heterotopic ossification is commonest in those exposed to blast, with traumatic amputations, and with an injury severity score > 16. Civilian risk factors such as head and spinal injury, extent of surgical dissection, systemic inflammation, neoplasm, and genetic predisposition are also likely to be relevant. Heterotopic ossification can cause pain, ulceration, and stiffness, and in amputees this can result in poor prosthesis fitting or compliance. Effective, practical prevention or treatment of heterotopic ossification would be of particular benefit to military casualties.

Compartment syndrome

Compartment syndrome results from an increase in pressure within an osseofascial space. Once pressure increases above the perfusion pressure, tissue anoxia and cell death ensue. Long-term outcomes of compartment syndrome are devastating, particularly in cases where diagnosis has been delayed or missed, resulting in varying degrees of functional limb loss. Compartment syndrome is largely a clinical diagnosis, depending on signs including pain out of proportion to injury and pain upon passive stretch, a palpable tense compartment, pallor, pulselessness, paralysis, and paresthesia. Compartment syndrome is commonest in high energy tibial fractures, crush injury, burns, and when constrictive dressings cause venous outflow obstruction. The leg is the most common region involved, comprising 62 % of cases. Military casualties are particularly at risk due to their high energy wounds and because prolonged evacuation times, usually at altitude in confined spaces with deep sedation, all increase risk. For this reason, military guidelines recommend liberal use of fasciotomy. However, fasciotomy produces substantial morbidity in up to 70 % of cases, including pain, chronic ulceration, delayed union of fractures and sensory changes. Avoiding unnecessary fasciotomy with the aid of intra-compartment pressure monitoring or more novel diagnostic techniques would be a significant advance.

Post-traumatic Stress Disorder and Mild Traumatic Brain Injury

Insurgent preference for improvised explosive devices in Iraq and Afghanistan has produced large numbers of blast-exposed patients. One study found that 12 % of returning combat veterans had features consistent with mild traumatic brain injury (TBI), and a strikingly similar proportion (11 %) had symptoms consistent with post-traumatic stress disorder (PTSD) [10]. The overlap of diagnostic criteria for these two conditions often makes them difficult to tell apart, especially as the features of mild TBI may not occur until some weeks after blast exposure. Ability to predict the long term consequences of mild TBI from features present at the time of initial injury would substantially improve the occupational management of these patients, in addition to better defining a population in which postulated therapies could be subjected to clinical trials. Current practice builds on experience in both warfare and competitive sport, which has identified a 'two-hit' effect in which the second episode of concussion has more profound effects than the first. Particular care is taken with military patients exposed to a second or third concussive force within a 12-month period [8]. Although such approaches are sensible in the absence of better diagnostics, an individualized approach based on objective data logically holds the promise of better care.

Severe Traumatic Brain Injury

Severe wounding of the central nervous system is the commonest cause of death on the modern battlefield [3], with most patients dying of non-survivable wounds before hospital arrival. Although in recent conflicts the number of cases of mild TBI far exceeded those with moderate or severe wounds, survivors of severe TBI are often left with profound disability. US forces members suffered more than 1250 cases of moderate to severe TBI between 2003 and 2010, with penetrating wounds outnumbering non-penetrating by 1.3–2 to 1 [11]. Any treatment that improves function in severe TBI survivors would have tremendous social and economic benefits to military and civilian patients alike.

Training of Healthcare Providers, from Battlefield Medic to Trauma Surgeon

Perhaps surprisingly, evidence has only recently emerged demonstrating the mortality benefit that adequately trained clinicians bring to trauma care. US military patients transported by critical care flight paramedics had a 66 % lower 48-hour mortality than did those transported by army medics with less advanced training and experience [12]. A comparative study of mortality associated with different aeromedical retrieval systems similarly found a significant mortality benefit associated with a team comprising a critical care physician, specialist nurse and two paramedics, in comparison to even well-trained paramedics working without physician support [13]. The question that immediately follows is how to provide the best possible training for medics, nurses and physicians throughout the continuum of trauma management, such that all patients receive the best possible care.

Optimal Design of Trauma Systems

Although not as intuitively appealing as novel drugs and devices, system-level improvements offer the greatest opportunities to improve trauma mortality. For example, after introducing a comprehensive trauma system in Victoria, Australia, trauma mortality halved in the decade 2000–2010 [14]. The US military-led Joint Trauma System has produced similar improvements (Fig. 1) [2]. The particular challenge for the military in any future conflict will be to more rapidly adapt the deployed trauma system to conditions that will almost certainly differ to those in Afghanistan in 2014. Accurate data, insightful epidemiological analysis and intelligent command decisions will be required to mold a system rapidly to clinical need.

Research Programs that will Address Combat Casualty Care Priorities

Hemorrhage Control, Fluid Resuscitation, Rapid Diagnostics and Manipulation of Coagulation, Inflammatory-modulating Resuscitation, and Salvage Techniques for Circulatory Collapse

Hemorrhage control

Modern combat casualty care has replaced the traditional ABC approach with a 'C' ABC model, in which control of catastrophic hemorrhage takes precedence over airway. Novel agents such as the HemCon® Bandage and QuikClot® Combat Gauze have been embraced, albeit with only preclinical supporting evidence. The only device that has been shown to improve survival on the battlefield is the tourniquet, present in either a manufactured or improvised form since ancient Greece. The device issued to all US and Australian service members in Afghanistan is the

C-A-T® (Combat Application Tourniquet), which has 79 % effectiveness when applied to a bleeding limb in the pre-hospital setting, with a low risk of associated morbidity [15]. However, these devices are not effective in controlling junctional or truncal hemorrhage. The Junctional Emergency Treatment Tool (JETT) (North American Rescue, Greer SC USA) gained FDA approval in January 2013 and is currently being evaluated in Afghanistan, albeit not in a comparative trial. The JETT comprises a pelvic sling and bilateral femoral compression pads, and is proposed to be suited to control hemorrhage from both pelvic and femoral vessel injury. The SAM Junctional Tourniquet (SAM Medical Products, Wilsonville OR USA) has a similar action, while simultaneously stabilizing pelvic fractures. Neither of these devices has been the subject of any comparative clinical trials, although preclinical and simulation experiments report both are effective. Clinical trials of such devices are difficult given the heterogeneous patient population and the difficult circumstances in which they are sometimes applied, but at the very least a registry of patient outcomes should be kept to ensure these devices are doing no harm.

Systemic administration of TxA has been shown to reduce blood loss and transfusion requirements when administered for elective surgery, and its use in military trauma is also now widespread following publication of the CRASH-2 [16] and MATTERS [17] studies. Some investigators have pointed to knowledge gaps when patients are treated in modern trauma systems than can deliver TxA and other coagulation-modifying treatments prehospital, and a trial of prehospital TxA is about to commence [18]. Topical TxA may avoid potential systemic adverse effects, and has been shown to reduce blood loss and transfusion requirements in elective surgery [19]. Topical pro-coagulants are not routinely used in the surgical management of military wounds. Currently no trials are being conducted in a military context, but a civilian RCT is currently comparing topical and systemic TxA in total knee arthroplasty (NCT01940523).

Fluid resuscitation

Early crystalloid resuscitation was once a central element of trauma resuscitation. The seemingly self-evident benefit of this practice was disproved by the landmark RCT that found benefit from avoiding all fluid prior to hospital admission [20]. Modern military interpretation of this evidence is more nuanced, with appreciation that with more prolonged hospital times than in urban trauma systems, patients benefit from fluid to maintain consciousness or systolic blood pressure > 90 mmHg [8]. Furthermore, there is emerging evidence that a two-phase approach, providing fluid resuscitation to higher blood pressure targets after an initial period of hypotensive resuscitation, results in better surrogate endpoints in an animal model [21]. The clinical trial to confirm this hypothesis should be possible, but is yet to be planned.

Prehospital administration of blood products appears feasible, and at least one study (NCT01838863) is comparing prehospital resuscitation with either normal saline or fresh frozen plasma (FFP) in severe trauma. Observational studies support a 1:1 PRBC to FFP ratio when a massive transfusion protocol is initiated. Although widely accepted, the optimal PRBC to FFP ratio is unknown. By 2012, 38 studies had compared high versus low PRBC to FFP ratios in massive transfusion. All were observational, so the association between ratio and outcome is potentially confounded, most notably survivor bias [22]. One multicenter RCT, the Pragmatic, Randomized Optimal Platelets and Plasma Ratio study (PROPPR) (NCT01545232) comparing a 1:1:1 ratio of FFP, platelets and PRBC to a 1:1:2 ratio, is likely to complete recruitment by early 2014. Any fixed ratio may be inferior to strategies tailored to individual patients. A preliminary RCT found such an approach feasible, not clearly associated with inferior clinical outcomes and potentially more frugal with valuable blood products [23].

Rapid diagnostics and manipulation of coagulation

Many trauma patients will require little fluid resuscitation and will not develop coagulopathy, whereas others will require massive transfusions and active coagulation management. At extremes, distinguishing these two is straightforward, but this is not true for many patients. The ability to identify patients who will benefit from early blood transfusion using readily available clinical information is improving, for example by noting base deficit, prothrombin time and hemoperitoneum as sensitive and specific predictors [24]. Identifying patients with trauma-induced coagulopathy may facilitate earlier and more targeted treatment. Traditional laboratory coagulation indices usually take too long to be useful. Thromboelastography (TEG) and rotational thromboelastometry (ROTEM) provide rapid information that is more predictive of transfusion requirement than traditional indices [25] and is, at least anecdotally, useful in guiding blood product use. No published RCTs have addressed this question, but the currently recruiting Comparison of Rapid Thrombelastography and Conventional Coagulation Testing for Hemostatic Resuscitation in Trauma trial (NCT01536496) is comparing the utility of TEG to traditional indices in trauma patients requiring blood transfusion. The RETIC (Reversal of Trauma Induced Coagulopathy Using Coagulation Factor Concentrates or Fresh Frozen Plasma) trial (NCT01545635) is using ROTEM to guide the administration of either FFP or fibrinogen, prothrombin, and factor XIII concentrates. The potential to address the specific coagulation defects in individual patients using rapid point-of-care (POC) testing has intuitive appeal that potentially extends to treating the prothrombotic state that frequently follows acute coagulopathy.

Inflammatory-modulating resuscitation fluids

Despite considerable evidence for using predominantly blood product resuscitation in major trauma, pharmacological manipulation of the pro-inflammatory and other systemic effects of trauma remains attractive. Hypertonic saline is the most studied fluid postulated to modulate inflammation (along with other actions) in hemorrhagic shock, potentially by decreasing end-organ damage through suppression of neutrophil and endothelial activation. Unfortunately, clinical trials have been disappointing. The Resuscitation Outcomes Consortium RCT comparing 7.5 % hypertonic saline +/− 6 % dextran with normal saline for resuscitation following traumatic injury [26] terminated at only 23 % of the planned recruitment due to futility and patient safety issues. Large clinical trials of hypertonic saline in TBI with and without hypotension have been similarly disappointing [27, 28]. Numerous inflammatory-modulating additives to resuscitation fluids have been proposed, including ethyl pyruvate, Na^+/H^+ exchange inhibitors (e. g., methanesulfonate), valproic acid, dihydroepiandrosterone, and a mixture of adenosine, magnesium and lidocaine [29], all of which look promising in animal models. However, as the hypertonic saline RCTs demonstrate, large effectiveness trials will be required before such approaches can be recommended. None are currently registered.

Extracorporeal membrane oxygenation

Extracorporeal membrane oxygenation (ECMO) has an established role in trauma patients with severe acute respiratory distress syndrome (ARDS). Single center experience with 52 patients treated with ECMO or pumpless extracorporeal lung assist reported 79 % survival [30]. Patients with traumatic circulatory collapse might also benefit from ECMO, but this has been avoided in trauma due to fear of bleeding with the systemic anticoagulation that is conventionally required. However, six of ten severe trauma patients treated with (initially heparin-free) ECMO survived [31]. A further development of this approach is to use the ECMO circuit to induce profound hypothermia in order to preserve organ function. A multicenter feasibility trial of this 'Emergency Preservation and Resuscitation' approach is about to commence (NCT01042015).

Delivery of Blood Products/Derivatives outside Large Hospitals

Numerous alternatives exist to conventional PRBC, platelets, FFP and cryoprecipitate for the management of traumatic hemorrhage, but (much like those traditional products) few have been evaluated in clinical trials. Considered by regulatory authorities as pharmaceuticals rather than blood, this lack of evidence has prevented approval for widespread use. This situation is now being addressed.

Platelets

Platelets are the most problematic clotting component to supply to remote locations. Dimethylsulphoxide (DMSO)-cryopreserved platelets (with a shelf-life of two years) were assessed in a pilot trail in 1999 [32] and were first used clinically by the Dutch military in 2001, but are only now entering the pilot phase of a definitive clinical trial in comparison to conventional liquid platelets (Cryopreserved vs. Liquid Platelet (CLIP) trial; ACTRN12612001261808). The US Army Medical Research Materiel Command is sponsoring a similar program of research, but currently has no trial registered. Various platelet alternatives are also under investigation. For example, lyophilized platelets/derivatives (Stasix, Entegrion, Inc., NC USA and Thrombosomes, Cellphire Inc., MD USA) show promise in animal models, but are not yet registered in clinical trials.

Plasma and clotting factors

The shelf-life of FFP is two years and cryoprecipitate one year, making supply in smaller hospitals relatively simple. However, these take 30–40 minutes to thaw, and only large trauma hospitals can keep thawed units on hand without unsustainable wastage. A method of delivering concentrated clotting factors that would allow rapid prehospital or early hospital administration would be very useful. Freeze dried plasma is in clinical use in France and Germany, and has been used apparently successfully at the point of wounding by the Israeli military. Having been originally used by the US military in 1941 and then abandoned (because of infection transmission by early preparations), clinical trial evidence is likely to be required before more widespread adoption; no trial is currently registered. Concentrated clotting factors are also appealing for use at point of injury. Fibrinogen concentrate is approved for use in bleeding trauma patients in France and Germany, but elsewhere only for the treatment of congenital fibrinogen deficiency. Although there are several non-randomized studies supporting use in trauma, once again a clinical trial is likely to be required before widespread adoption. Trial feasibility is currently being assessed by at least one group. Prothrombin complex concentrates (containing various quantities of coagulation factors II, VII, IX, and X) are the other commercially available factor concentrates, to date similarly lacking evidence and, therefore, approval for use in trauma.

Red blood cells and their alternatives

DMSO-cryopreserved red cells are registered for limited therapeutic use for patients with rare blood groups. However, it is increasingly appreciated that the effects of PRBC transfusion are not all immediately apparent, requiring very large effectiveness studies such as the TRANSFUSE (5000 patients; ACTRN12612000453886) and ABLE (2510 patients; ISRCTN44878718) studies of the age of PRBC to discern possible adverse effects. It is possible that cryopreserved PRBC may be a superior product to aged liquid-stored PRBC, but testing this theory will need a clinical trial of a similar size. A smaller study (350 patients) is currently underway (NCT01038557) and has published its preliminary, encouraging results [33]. The search for oxygen-carrying red cell substitutes continues. In a trial of 688 patients, hemoglobin based oxygen carrier-201 (HBOC-201)(Hemopure, OPK Biotech LLC, Cambridge, MA, USA) was found to produce more cardiovascular adverse events than conventional red cells [34]. Similarly, human polymerized hemoglobin (Poly-Heme, Northfield Laboratories, Evanston IL, USA) produced a higher incidence of myocardial infarction in a phase III trial in 714 patients [35], and is no longer in production. Arguably, a fairer comparison might have been to crystalloid alone, for situations in which conventional RBC transfusion is unavailable. However, conducting trials in small hospitals without ready PRBC availability is made difficult by the lack of patient volume and research infrastructure. Nonetheless, further trials of HBOC-201 (NCT01881503 and NCT00301483) are registered.

Fresh whole blood

An alternative to fractionated blood products and their derivatives and substitutes is fresh whole blood. Anecdotal experience in the initial stages of the wars in Iraq and Afghanistan was that this was considerably more effective than aged component therapy. However, a large and stable population of donors is required (the health of whom may be compromised), transfusions must be type-specific (there is no universal donor), and there is a greater risk of viral infectious disease transmission and graft versus host disease. These latter two risks might be mitigated by immediate post-transfusion processing, technology that also awaits testing in clinical trials.

Management of Wounds and Wound Infection

Detecting infection
No biomarker is known to be sufficiently sensitive and specific to guide the administration of antibiotics. Procalcitonin (PCT) has been used to reduce seemingly unnecessary antibiotic treatment in pneumonia, and more recently showed promise in the diagnosis of infection after orthopedic surgery in an observational pilot study [36]. A further observational study is planned (NCT01472952). Cell-free DNA is a more novel biomarker that may potentially distinguish infection from trauma. Combined with DNA identification of bacterial species and antibiotic sensitivity, molecular techniques hold currently unproven promise for the better detection of infection in trauma.

Local control of infection
Normal saline is the currently recommended fluid for wound irrigation, but if unavailable, potable water is thought to be acceptable [37]. The added benefit of pulsatile lavage and additives to irrigation fluid is unclear, with contrary arguments in contemporary literature. A contaminated wound model found irrigation with a bulb syringe and normal saline resulted in less rebound and reduced bacterial counts at 48 h vs. pulsatile lavage and various additives [38], but another study found a significant difference in favor of pulse lavage [39]. An RCT comparing pulsed lavage to low pressure lavage after closure of major abdominal wounds is currently underway (ACTRN12612000170820). Another multicenter, blinded, factorial trial (NCT00788398) is comparing alternative irrigating solutions (soap additive vs. standard saline) and pressures (high and low) in patients with open fractures. Military wounds at high risk of infection are usually irrigated with saline before 0.0025 % Dakin's solution (sodium hypochlorite, initially used in the First World War) dressing are applied. While emotively attractive due to its historical precedent in an earlier war, the evidence for this approach is negligible. Currently there are no clinical trials registered. Negative-pressure wound therapy is thought to be a useful but not yet proven clinical adjunct in the management of a wide array of traumatic soft tissue injuries that have a hemostatic wound bed [8].

Heterotopic ossification
Heterotopic ossification prophylaxis is fraught with potential complications, particularly in the blast victim. Traditional treatment in the civilian setting is radiotherapy, which is not recommended. Treatment with non-steroidal anti-inflammatory drugs (NSAIDs) can be effective, although risks gastrointestinal complications and delayed bone healing. The Combat Pill Pack currently issued to US personnel pro-

vides four pills (meloxicam 15 mg, acetaminophen 1000 mg and an antibiotic) to be swallowed in the event of an open combat wound. Neither meloxicam nor any other NSAIDs are routinely continued post-injury in military personnel because of concern over potential adverse effects. This concern is, however, entirely theoretical, and prospective trials of the early introduction of a NSAID vs. placebo for short durations are warranted. Genetic, tissue and serological markers may identify a population group most prone to heterotopic ossification and thus potentially arguing for the continued use of NSAIDs in this patient population. Current research is studying the link between the serological marker, BMP-9, and its receptor, ALK1, and the formation of heterotopic ossification (NCT01433536). Research is also ongoing into alternative forms of prophylaxis including the use of retinoic acid receptor antagonists, as these have been shown to reduce the formation of heterotopic ossification in a murine model [40].

Compartment syndrome

Although intuitively attractive, clinical studies of invasive compartment pressure monitoring to detect compartment syndrome early have shown mixed results. A recent retrospective analysis of 850 cases found a sensitivity of 94 % and specificity of 98 % for the diagnosis of compartment syndrome [41]. This study will reignite interest into the use of pressure monitors as an adjunct for the diagnosis of compartment syndrome in both the civilian and military settings not only for its diagnostic value, but also postoperatively to confirm that an adequate fasciotomy has in fact been performed. Up to 17 % of fasciotomy procedures will require revision because of ineffective fascia release [42]. Revised or delayed fasciotomy procedures are associated with three times the mortality and double the amputation rate of cases where fascitomy was performed adequately. A prospective RCT comparing clinical diagnostic acumen with compartment pressure monitoring would be a tantalizing prospect, though given the often catastrophic outcome that occurs in missed cases clinician equipoise may be lacking. Another diagnostic modality that is gaining momentum for the diagnosis of compartment syndrome is the use of near-infrared spectroscopy (NIRS). This technique utilizes non-invasive passage of light through tissues to measure tissue anoxia, and has been shown to correlate with invasive pressure monitoring in experimentally-induced compartment syndrome [43]. The usefulness of NIRS in a military population is currently under evaluation in a prospective, observational cohort study (NCT01123798) being conducted by the US military at Landstuhl Regional Medical Center.

PTSD and mild TBI

Mild TBI

The US and Australian armed forces use the Military Acute Concussion Evaluation (MACE) in all patients exposed to blast. This tool assesses neurocognitive deficits in orientation, immediate memory, concentration and delayed recall. The MACE is a high-sensitivity, low-specificity method to identify patients at risk for TBI [44], who then undertake more detailed evaluations including computer-based concentration evaluations (such as the CogState [http://www.cogstate.com/go/sport] or Automated Neurological Assessment Metrics [ANAM]), clinical evaluation by a neurologist, and neuroimaging. However, simple automated tests are poorly validated in a combat population. All are affected by other stressors of combat, including fatigue. Deviation from individual baseline is therefore difficult to attribute solely to blast. Even advanced magnetic resonance imaging (MRI) studies have shown a disappointing correlation with mild TBI effects [45], and despite intense effort no serum biomarker has emerged as a useful diagnostic test. Placing blast accelerometer gauges in combatants' helmets is an attempt to correlate exposure with effect, but current devices have limited ability to account for three-dimensional forces. This, along with difficulty in accurately quantifying clinical effects, means that as yet no clear relationship has been established. Fortunately, the opportunity to conduct this research in the combat population may be about to rapidly diminish. The future of this research may lay with studies of athletes involved in sports involving the risk of blunt head trauma.

PTSD
Current treatments for PTSD involve an array of behavioral, cognitive and pharmacologic methods. Newer applications of virtual reality involving Middle East scenario training with PTSD-afflicted veterans of the Iraq and Afghanistan wars have shown potential in reduction of symptoms [46]. Eye movement desensitization and reprocessing is a novel technique with poorly understood mechanisms that has shown promise in smaller studies and is currently the subject of at least two phase III trials (NCT00716638 and NCT01443182). Acknowledging the marked overlap between PTSD and mild TBI, numerous studies are currently examining simultaneous treatment of both. The Mild Traumatic Brain Injury and Post-Traumatic Stress Disorder study is using positron-emission tomography (PET) imaging of the GABAergic receptors to assess the development of PTSD in patients suffering from mild TBI (NCT01547819), and the Brain Indices of Risk for PTSD after mild TBI study will combine MRI results at three and six months post-injury along with neurocognitive testing to evaluate the risk of PTSD development with mild TBI (NCT01625962). Others are considering new pharmacologic options in the prevention of PTSD with prazosin and omega-3 fatty acids (NCT00532493 and NCT00671099, respectively) and a trial of hyperbaric oxygen therapy for both TBI and PTSD is currently recruiting (NCT01105962).

Severe TBI

Several medical therapies for severe TBI have been attempted. For many years corticosteroids were hypothesized to reduce secondary brain injury due to inflammation. The landmark CRASH trial [47] not only showed that, in fact, corticosteroids at inflammatory-modulating doses increase mortality, but demonstrated the peril of widespread adoption of therapy based on pathophysiological theory rather than clinical trials. Erythropoietin, therapeutic hypothermia, progesterone and tranexamic acid all show promise, with large effectiveness trials currently underway (EPO-TBI: 606 patients, NCT00987454; POLAR: 512 patients, NCT00987688; ProTECT III: 1140 patients, NCT00822900; CRASH-3: 10,000 patients, ISRCTN15088122). Various other therapies are in earlier stages of clinical trials, including magnesium, mild hypothermia, and estrogen. The US military has facilitated a collaborative network to conduct multicenter, multispecies preclinical testing of a variety of drugs, including nicotinamide, choline, atorvastatin, and lithium [48]. The surgical management of severe TBI is more difficulty to study, as the DECRA investigators discovered in their trial of decompressive craniectomy for refractory diffuse TBI that took nearly eight years to recruit 155 patients [49]. Although the decompressive craniectomy reduced intracranial pressure (ICP), the poor validity of such a surrogate endpoint was clearly demonstrated, as despite this success, functional outcome at six months was significantly worse in the surgical group. The role of decompressive craniectomy in any form of TBI remains hotly debated.

Training and Clinical Support of Clinicians

Optimal methods of training for clinicians treating trauma patients are difficult to define, as outcome measures are nebulous and situation-dependent. Individual skills, such as intubation, chest tube insertion and cricothyroidotomy, are relatively easily taught, although there is a surprising paucity of evidence supporting the superiority of this approach over a traditional apprenticeship model. Most trauma management is performed by teams, the members of which must integrate their individual skills with those of others. Team training using clinical simulation that incorporates every level of clinician involved in patient care within the pre-hospital environment, trauma bay or operating room is intuitively attractive, but is only starting to be supported by robust evidence. Many studies of simulation record improvements in the simulated behaviors, but until recently there has been little to show this translates into actual practice. A Level 1 trauma center in Roanoke, VA, USA compared the efficiency of residents, attending physicians and nurses during trauma resuscitation before and after a team training session followed by patient simulation exercises. Training resulted in a decrease in emergency department length of stay and time to focused abdominal sonography for trauma (FAST) exam, CT, intubation and transfer to the operating room [50]. Further similar validation of simulation and team training is required before this method can be universally recommended.

Trauma system design

Unlike civilian health administrators, military planners often start with a map devoid of adequate healthcare facilities. This liberates them from constraints imposed by historical precedent, allowing them to deploy assets where they are needed most. Numbers and locations of evacuation assets and hospitals of various sizes are initially determined by logic and military doctrine, but as the conflict evolves the system must be sufficiently flexible to respond to both changing demand and improvements in evidence-based clinical practice. The current conflict has shown how a trauma system constantly informed and able to accommodate these factors will continuously improve its performance [2]. Techniques under development will hopefully assist even more rapid adaptability, such as a continuous analysis of geographical variations in case fatality rate in order to identify outlying areas in need of either better primary prevention or better medical care. As medicine becomes more sub-specialized, the requirement for deployment of certain specialties at particular locations should also be informed by this system. Military doctrine has traditionally held that a patient should arrive at a non-surgical resuscitation facility within the 'golden hour' after wounding, and at a surgical hospital within two hours. The data on which these thresholds are based predate the modern approach to damage control resuscitation and surgery. Retrospective analysis of the natural variation in the Joint Theater Trauma Registry should allow modern time-to-surgery targets to be revised. Only in the closing stages of the current conflict has it been realized that hospital performance has improved to the point of diminishing return, and that the majority of preventable deaths occur pre-hospital. Improvements in pre-hospital care have shown dramatic benefit [12, 13] and so should become the area of greatest research and quality improvement focus. Part of the solution to better pre-hospital care may be technological, with at least one group working on a wireless, video, networked decision support tool for the pre-hospital environment that presents the most important clinical information both to the pre-hospital provider and to a physician in the hospital to which the patient is being taken. The applicability of such approaches to civilian trauma systems should be clear. The US-led Joint Trauma System collects data assessing compliance with various process-level components of its Clinical Practice Guidelines [8]. Improved access to indices of morbidity (mostly assessed on return to country-of-origin) should in future allow this system to determine even better the outcome effects of changes in practice. The anticipated publication of civilian consensus guidelines for process and outcome measures of quality in trauma care should be a valuable tool in this process.

Conclusions

Current operations in Afghanistan by armed forces of the developed world have come to depend on a trauma system that has evolved through time to consist of well-established fixed hospitals with evacuation assets that can rapidly move casualties from the battlefield to initial wound surgery and on to definitive care. The challenge for future combat casualty care will be to produce a similarly low mortality and morbidity in less developed and more austere environments. The keys to meeting this challenge will be to further test and develop clinical interventions, such as those listed in this chapter, and to train the next generation of clinicians in the lessons that have been learnt. If military clinical activity reduces dramatically, in most parts of the world the best means of achieving these objectives will be to partner with civilian hospitals and research institutes. Doing so will benefit civilian and military patients alike. A further task will be to preserve the method of rapidly implementing a trauma system optimally designed for the conditions it must face. The data capture, epidemiological analysis, continuous feedback and institutional buy-in this involves are methods likely to be just as valuable in civilian trauma systems.

Postscript A source of considerable annoyance to English-speaking combatants of many nations is the incorrect use of the term 'injury' for their wounds. At least in military parlance, wounds are deliberately inflicted (and so encompass surgical wounds as well as those caused on the battlefield), whereas injuries are accidental. Although perhaps of little significance to treating clinicians, the distinction is highly valued by our patients – and so we feel should be respected.

References

1. Orman JA, Eastridge BJ, Baer DG, Gerhardt RT, Rasmussen TE, Blackbourne LH (2012) The impact of 10 years of war on combat casualty care research: a citation analysis. J Trauma Acute Care Surg 73:S403–S408
2. Bailey JA, Morrison JJ, Rasmussen TE (2013) Trauma systems development in Afghanistan – lessons for civilian systems? Curr Opin Crit Care 19:569–577
3. Eastridge BJ, Mabry RL, Seguin P et al (2012) Death on the battlefield (2001–2011): implications for the future of combat casualty care. J Trauma Acute Care Surg 73:S431–S437
4. Kragh JF Jr, Littrel ML, Jones JA et al (2011) Battle casualty survival with emergency tourniquet use to stop limb bleeding. J Emerg Med 41:590–597
5. Brohi K, Cohen MJ, Ganter MT et al (2008) Acute coagulopathy of trauma: hypoperfusion induces systemic anticoagulation and hyperfibrinolysis. J Trauma 64:1211–1217
6. Holley AB (2013) Thromboprophylaxis and venous thromboembolism rates in soldiers wounded in Operation Enduring Freedom and Operation Iraqi Freedom. Chest 144:966–973
7. Kauvar DS (2006) Fresh whole blood transfusion: a controversial military practice. J Trauma 61:181–184
8. Joint Trauma System (2013) Clinical Practice Guidelines. Available at: http://www us-aisr.amedd.army.mil/clinical_practice_guidelines html Accessed Nov 2013
9. Potter BK, Fosberg JA (2011) Heterotopic ossification. In: Owens BD, Belmont PJ (eds) Combat Orthopaedic Surgery: lessons Learned In Iraq And Afghanistan. SLACK Books Inc., Thorofare, NJ, USA
10. Schneiderman AI, Braver ER, Kang HK (2008) Understanding sequelae of injury mechanisms and mild traumatic brain injury incurred during the conflicts in Iraq and Afghanistan: persistent postconcussive symptoms and posttraumatic stress disorder. Am J Epidemiol 167:1446–1452
11. Orman JA, Geyer D, Jones J et al (2012) Epidemiology of moderate-to-severe penetrating versus closed traumatic brain injury in the Iraq and Afghanistan wars. J Trauma Acute Care Surg 73:S496–S502
12. Mabry RL, Apodaca A, Penrod J, Orman JA, Gerhardt RT, Dorlac WC (2012) Impact of critical care-trained flight paramedics on casualty survival during helicopter evacuation in the current war in Afghanistan. J Trauma Acute Care Surg 73:S32–S37
13. Morrison JJ, Oh J, DuBose JJ et al (2013) En-route care capability from point of injury impacts mortality after severe wartime injury. Ann Surg 257:330–334

14. Victorian State (2010) Trauma Registry 2008–2009 Summary Report. Victorian Government, Victoria
15. Kragh JF Jr, Walters TJ, Baer DG et al (2008) Practical use of emergency tourniquets to stop bleeding in major limb trauma. J Trauma 64:S38–S49
16. Shakur H, Roberts I, Bautista R et al (2010) Effects of tranexamic acid on death, vascular occlusive events, and blood transfusion in trauma patients with significant haemorrhage (CRASH-2): a randomised, placebo-controlled trial. Lancet 376:23–32
17. Morrison JJ, DuBose JJ, Rasmussen TE, Midwinter MJ (2012) Military Application of Tranexamic Acid in Trauma Emergency Resuscitation (MATTERs) Study. Arch Surg 147:113–119
18. Gruen RL, Jacobs IG, Reade MC (2013) Trauma and tranexamic acid. Med J Aust 199:310–311
19. Georgiadis AG, Muh SJ, Silverton CD, Weir RM, Laker MW (2013) A prospective double-blind placebo controlled trial of topical tranexamic acid in total knee arthroplasty. J Arthroplasty 28(Suppl 8):78–82
20. Bickell WH, Wall MJ Jr, Pepe PE et al (1994) Immediate versus delayed fluid resuscitation for hypotensive patients with penetrating torso injuries. N Engl J Med 331:1105–1109
21. Doran CM, Doran CA, Woolley T et al (2012) Targeted resuscitation improves coagulation and outcome. J Trauma Acute Care Surg 72:835–843
22. Ho AM, Dion PW, Yeung JH et al (2012) Prevalence of survivor bias in observational studies on fresh frozen plasma:erythrocyte ratios in trauma requiring massive transfusion. Anesthesiology 116:716–728
23. Nascimento B, Callum J, Tien H et al (2013) Effect of a fixed-ratio (1:1:1) transfusion protocol versus laboratory-results-guided transfusion in patients with severe trauma: a randomized feasibility trial. CMAJ 185:E583–E589
24. Hsu JM, Hitos K, Fletcher JP (2013) Identifying the bleeding trauma patient: predictive factors for massive transfusion in an Australasian trauma population. J Trauma 75:359–364
25. Holcomb JB (2012) Admission rapid thrombelastography can replace conventional coagulation tests in the emergency department: experience with 1974 consecutive trauma patients. Ann Surg 256:476–486
26. Bulger EM, May S, Kerby JD et al (2011) Out-of-hospital hypertonic resuscitation after traumatic hypovolemic shock: a randomized, placebo controlled trial. Ann Surg 253:431–441
27. Bulger EM, May S, Brasel KJ et al (2010) Out-of-hospital hypertonic resuscitation following severe traumatic brain injury: a randomized controlled trial. JAMA 304:1455–1464
28. Cooper DJ, Myles PS, McDermott FT et al (2004) Prehospital hypertonic saline resuscitation of patients with hypotension and severe traumatic brain injury: a randomized controlled trial. JAMA 291:1350–1357
29. Granfeldt A, Nielsen TK, Solling C et al (2012) Adenocaine and Mg(2+) reduce fluid requirement to maintain hypotensive resuscitation and improve cardiac and renal function in a porcine model of severe hemorrhagic shock. Crit Care Med 40:3013–3025
30. Ried M, Bein T, Philipp A et al (2013) Extracorporeal lung support in trauma patients with severe chest injury and acute lung failure: a 10-year institutional experience. Crit Care 17:R110
31. Arlt M, Philipp A, Voelkel S et al (2010) Extracorporeal membrane oxygenation in severe trauma patients with bleeding shock. Resuscitation 81:804–809
32. Khuri SF, Healey N, MacGregor H et al (1999) Comparison of the effects of transfusions of cryopreserved and liquid-preserved platelets on hemostasis and blood loss after cardiopulmonary bypass. J Thorac Cardiovasc Surg 117:172–183
33. Fabricant L, Kiraly L, Wiles C et al (2013) Cryopreserved deglycerolized blood is safe and achieves superior tissue oxygenation compared with refrigerated red blood cells: a prospective randomized pilot study. J Trauma Acute Care Surg 74:371–376
34. Jahr JS, Mackenzie C, Pearce LB, Pitman A, Greenburg AG (2008) HBOC-201 as an alternative to blood transfusion: efficacy and safety evaluation in a multicenter phase III trial in elective orthopedic surgery. J Trauma 64:1484–1497

35. Moore EE, Moore FA, Fabian TC et al (2009) Human polymerized hemoglobin for the treatment of hemorrhagic shock when blood is unavailable: the USA multicenter trial. J Am Coll Surg 208:1–13
36. Hunziker S, Hugle T, Schuchardt K et al (2010) The value of serum procalcitonin level for differentiation of infectious from noninfectious causes of fever after orthopaedic surgery. J Bone Joint Surg Am 92:138–148
37. Murray CK (2011) Infection in orthopedic extremity injuries. In: Owens BD, Belmont PJ (eds) Combat Orthopaedic Surgery: Lessons Learned In Iraq And Afghanistan. SLACK Books Inc., Thorofare, USA
38. Owens BD, White DW, Wenke JC (2009) Comparison of irrigation solutions and devices in a contaminated musculoskeletal wound survival model. J Bone Joint Surg Am 91:92–98
39. Svoboda SJ, Bice TG, Gooden HA, Brooks DE, Thomas DB, Wenke JC (2006) Comparison of bulb syringe and pulsed lavage irrigation with use of a bioluminescent musculoskeletal wound model. J Bone Joint Surg Am 88:2167–2174
40. Shimono K, Morrison TN, Tung WE et al (2010) Inhibition of ectopic bone formation by a selective retinoic acid receptor alpha-agonist: a new therapy for heterotopic ossification? J Orthop Res 28:271–277
41. McQueen MM, Duckworth AD, Aitken SA, Court-Brown CM (2013) The estimated sensitivity and specificity of compartment pressure monitoring for acute compartment syndrome. J Bone Joint Surg Am 95:673–677
42. Ritenour AE, Dorlac WC, Fang R et al (2008) Complications after fasciotomy revision and delayed compartment release in combat patients. J Trauma 64:S153–S161
43. Gentilello LM, Sanzone A, Wang L, Liu PY, Robinson L (2001) Near-infrared spectroscopy versus compartment pressure for the diagnosis of lower extremity compartmental syndrome using electromyography-determined measurements of neuromuscular function. J Trauma 51:1–8
44. French L, McCrea M, Bagget M (2008) The military acute concussion evaluation. Journal of Special Operations Medicine 8:68–77
45. Mac DCL, Johnson AM, Cooper D et al (2011) Detection of blast-related traumatic brain injury in U.S. military personnel. N Engl J Med 364:2091–2100
46. Cukor J, Spitalnick J, Difede J, Rizzo A, Rothbaum BO (2009) Emerging treatments for PTSD. Clin Psychol Rev 29:715–726
47. Roberts I, Yates D, Sandercock P et al (2004) Effect of intravenous corticosteroids on death within 14 days in 10,008 adults with clinically significant head injury (MRC CRASH trial): randomised placebo-controlled trial. Lancet 364:1321–1328
48. Kochanek PM, Bramlett H, Dietrich WD et al (2011) A novel multicenter preclinical drug screening and biomarker consortium for experimental traumatic brain injury: operation brain trauma therapy. J Trauma 71:S15–S24
49. Cooper DJ, Rosenfeld JV, Murray L et al (2011) Decompressive craniectomy in diffuse traumatic brain injury. N Engl J Med 364:1493–1502
50. Capella J, Smith S, Philp A et al (2010) Teamwork training improves the clinical care of trauma patients. J Surg Educ 67:439–443

Intensive Care "Sans Frontières"

K. Hillman, J. Chen, and J. Braithwaite

Introduction

The specialty of intensive care has made remarkable progress in a relatively short time. Intensive care units (ICUs) now play a crucial role in acute hospitals, supporting patients who have life-threatening conditions, such as trauma and severe infections, as well as maintaining life after major surgery. Since the earliest admissions, there has been a subtle but compelling change in the nature of patients admitted to hospitals and ICUs who are now older with increasing number of co-morbidities and undergo more complex interventions with a higher incidence of complications. This chapter will discuss some of the implications of the changing hospital population.

The specialty of intensive care has had a short but dynamic history of which all of us who have been involved in its development should be proud. Its beginnings were in Copenhagen, Denmark in 1952 in response to the poliomyelitis epidemic [1]. An anesthetist, Bjørn Ibsen, suggested he could support patients' respiration as a result of dysfunctional diaphragms by using positive pressure ventilation. Medical students, working 8-hour shifts, kept the patients alive and reduced mortality from about 80 % to 60 %. Thus, the specialty was born and the learning began. The way we delivered ventilation was refined; the tubes and catheters we inserted became more appropriate; we learnt how to support the circulation with drugs and machines; how to support the kidneys with continuous dialysis; we could feed enterally or parenterally; and use many of the other support therapies, such

K. Hillman ✉ · J. Chen
The Simpson Center for Health Services Research, SWS Clinical School and Liverpool Hospital, affiliated with the Australian Institute of Health Innovation, University of New South Wales, 1871 Liverpool, Australia
e-mail: k.hillman@unsw.edu.au

J. Braithwaite
Center for Clinical Governance Research, Australian Institute of Health Innovation, University of New South Wales, AGSM Building, 2052 Sydney, Australia

J.-L. Vincent (Ed.), *Annual Update in Intensive Care and Emergency Medicine 2014*,   765
DOI 10.1007/978-3-319-03746-2_57, © Springer International Publishing Switzerland 2014

as antimicrobials and drugs to prevent thrombosis and gastric erosions. Another crucial and often under-estimated development in our specialty, was the emergence of intensive care nursing as a separate specialty which, together with other allied health and paramedical services, provides the majority of the 24-hour bedside care.

The specialty of providing care to the seriously ill developed within its own four walls. This enabled the use of the specialized machinery and drugs used to support patients in a practical environment. It also provided territory for the new specialty to develop. Patients could be cared for in this dedicated space. At the same time the skills, knowledge and experience could be learned within a controlled environment and, in doing so, carve out a unique and challenging specialty. The specialty soon became an essential part of modern medicine. The development of intensive care medicine made it possible to continue complex intraoperative care into the postoperative period for areas such as cardiac surgery, neurosurgery and trauma. We were able to prolong the lives of patients while our interventions or nature could restore the body's function. We soon had our own textbooks, journals and conferences.

After such spectacular progress it is probably time to stop and take stock of what our specialty is about and what are its boundaries, both geographically and functionally as well as its relationship with our community. We need to address questions such as where should we be delivering intensive care?; to whom should we be delivering it?; what implications has our specialty for society?; and how does intensive care fit in with the bigger picture of health?

The Changing Nature of Patients in Intensive Care

There have been many impressive developments since Copenhagen in the early 1950 s. But there has also been an imperceptible change in the way we practice intensive care medicine, related largely to the changing nature of our population in both the community and within our hospitals. Our population is aging and living longer [2, 3]. Life-saving interventions which, at one time, we would have only considered using for fit, otherwise well patients are now routinely delivered to older and frailer patients. The changing nature of patients being intensively cared for in hospitals and in our ICUs has important implications for the future of the specialty.

Care of the 'sick elderly' is probably the most common reason for admission to acute hospitals. This factor has subtly and incrementally changed over the last 40 years and almost certainly will increase even more over the next 40 years. The changes have implications for the future of health and intensive care medicine. Hospitalized patients are more vulnerable and, at the same time, are undergoing more complex and potentially dangerous interventions [4–7]. The number of the 'elderly sick' admitted to hospitals and ICUs is also increasing [7, 8–12]. Not surprisingly, the number of patients over the age of 80 is also increasing [13–16].

In attempting to discern what 'sick elderly' means, we need to question the concept of a simple diagnosis. A 20-year old with a urinary tract infection can be treated with oral antibiotics and often continue normal everyday activities. An 80-year old with the same problem may not only require antibiotics but also intravenous fluids, inotropes, ventilation and dialysis. By the time a patient has reached 85 years of age they will often have degrees of hypertension and cognitive dysfunction as well as decreased mobility and associated orthopedic problems. Other age-related co-morbidities are influenced by genetic makeup, the environment and life-style. These include ischemic heart disease, diabetes and strokes. Moreover, organs, such as the kidney, heart, liver and lungs, have a predictable decrease in function as people age. The sum of these underlying so-called co-morbidities and age-related decreases in organ function determines the clinical outcome of the patient as much, if not more than, the acute reason for admission to the ICU.

Medicine is struggling to define what the collective impact of these chronic clinical conditions is. They can easily be listed but this currently does not translate into a concept that informs us about optimal management or prognosis. The closest we have come so far is by exploring the concept of frailty [17–19]. The concept itself is complex with multiple and slippery meanings [20]. It is generally agreed that the term is used for older patients who have decreased general strength and who are unusually susceptible to disease or other infirmities [19]. Other ways of describing it incorporate three qualities: A state of risk or vulnerability; a precarious balance between demands and capacity to cope; and impending or current disability [21]. Although there is little general agreement, scales have been developed in order to quantify frailty [18, 22] (Box 1). Currently in intensive care, there are only limited and crude ways of incorporating a patient's pre-hospital status into our prognostic measures [23–25].

Box 1:
Proposed Clinical definition of the Phenotype of Frailty
Criteria
1. Decreased grip strength
2. Self-reported exhaustion
3. Unintentional weight loss of more than 4.5 kg over the past year
4. Slow walking speed
5. Low physical activity

Definition
Positive for frail phenotype: ≥ 3 criteria present
Intermediate/pre-frail: one or two criteria present
Non-frail: no criteria present
From [17] with permission.

In the past, intensive care has tended to concentrate more on the acute reason for admission to the ICU, such as acute respiratory distress syndrome (ARDS), heart failure, sepsis, renal failure as well as management strategies around these 'diagnoses' such as ventilation, antimicrobials, monitoring and dialysis. Although this is how we developed our skills and knowledge of intensive care, we probably also need to begin to explore the impact of the way failing organs interact as well as the impact of aging and co-morbidities on the clinical state of the patient.

Caring for the Seriously Ill in a Hospital

Before the development of intensive care as a specialty, the seriously ill were cared for in the general wards of a hospital. It is said that as patients became sicker they were moved closer to the nurse's station so that a more careful eye could be kept on them. As the specialty expanded in the 1970 s, an increasing number of hospitals developed ICUs. Some were an extension of existing specialties, such as neurosurgery, cardiothoracic surgery, general medicine, respiratory medicine, trauma and general surgery. Other countries developed a separate specialty of intensive care and established more general ICUs, regardless of the primary specialty under which the patient was admitted to hospital.

At the same time, hospital bed numbers were decreasing and the numbers of admitted elderly and complex patients were increasing [4–7]. Patients were more vulnerable and having more complex interventions with higher rates of complications [4, 5]. Increasing medical specialization was also occurring. There were 41 specialties accredited by the American Medical Association in 1985 and 124 by 200 [26]. By their very nature, specialists became increasingly competent in their own area of expertise and less competent in other specialized areas. Thus, we had the 'perfect storm'. An increasing number of 'sick elderly' patients with multiple problems which crossed many specialist areas were having increasingly complex procedures. The nature of the patient's clinical condition was not matched by the medical expertise necessary to manage them. Some of these patients were cared for in ICU by acute care specialists but their expertise was often not available to seriously ill and at-risk patients on the general floors.

Early research showed what was happening as a result of the perfect storm. Suboptimal care before admission to the ICU on general wards was very common and resulted in potentially avoidable deaths [27]. Up to 80 % of cardiac arrests on the general floor were preceded by a slow deterioration in vital signs [28]. The same slow unrecognized deterioration was also occurring before patients died [29] and before they were admitted to the ICU [30].

As a result, specialists in intensive care developed rapid response systems, which identified seriously ill and at-risk patients early and responded rapidly with staff who had the skills, knowledge and experience essential to managing these patients effectively [31]. The concept was consistent with the way medical care is usually provided in a hospital: When necessary and appropriate, a specialist in one area consults another specialist with expertise in another area. A rapid response call is simply a consultation with another specialist: In this case, an intensive care specialist, or at least a physician specifically trained in acute medicine and resuscitation. Because of the urgent nature of serious illness and the adverse outcomes associated with delay [32], the consultation has to be made consistently and rapidly.

ICUs were initially designed to care for the seriously ill. However, their ability to do that is dependent on factors such as the number of hospital beds; the nature of the severity of illness of patients in those beds; and the capacity of the ICUs to deal with the number of patients requiring its services. As a result, the care of a seriously ill patient in a hospital may be random. If there are many ICU beds in relation to the total number of hospital beds and the general level of illness in the hospital is not high, then all at-risk patients may be in the ICU and rapid response systems may not be as necessary as in a large hospital managing patients with complex problems and which has a relative low ratio of ICU beds to hospital beds. A rapid response system is simply an intervention to care for the seriously ill, the same as an ICU. The difference is geographical, not functional [33]. Both interventions identify and treat patients with serious illness. The level of illness and outcomes of patients who are the subject of rapid response calls is much the same as for patients in the ICU [34, 35]. In the largest study on rapid response calls, only five did not require advanced resuscitation interventions delivered by ICU staff [36].

Mirroring the 'coronary artery syndrome', there is now a 'seriously ill syndrome'. Extending the analogy, cardiologists now work closely with community-based response services and other parts of the hospital in order to rapidly re-establish coronary artery blood flow in blocked vessels. They work outside their coronary care units (CCU) in order to quickly recognize and manage patients' conditions which, in the past, were treated in CCUs after their heart had infarcted. Intensivists are also now realizing the importance of early recognition and treatment of life-threatening diseases [36].

A rapid response system of one sort or another now operates in the majority of hospitals in Australasia, North America, the UK and increasingly in Europe and other parts of the world. Like the concept of an ICU itself, it is difficult to rigorously define how effective rapid response systems are. The latest large trials and meta-analysis suggest that they reduce cardiac arrest rates and mortality by about one-third [37–39]. If this is even close to assessing its impact, the specialty of intensive care is contributing a great deal to hospital care and patient safety.

Other Implications as a Result of the Changing Nature of Patients in Intensive Care

There are other implications for intensivists as the population ages and their clinical condition changes. One of the more important is the increasing demand for ICU beds. With current workforce projections, we will not have staffing levels and capabilities for projected needs [12]. It has been suggested that increasing demand for intensive care has to be met by either increasing capacity [12, 40] or by rationing current services and triaging patients [41]. There is a third option and one that intensivists could play a crucial role in. It is related to the unsustainable cost of health care and the lack of awareness of our society about what modern medicine can, and more importantly, cannot offer.

Around 70 % of our society wants to die in their own home [42]. Approximately the same percentage will die in an institution, often in an acute hospital [42]. How did this paradoxical emerge? Like childbirth in the 1950 s, dying and end-of-life care has been medicalized. There is a conveyor belt taking patients at the end-of-life from the community to the ICU. Starting from the community, when a person deteriorates or has a sudden illness, assistance is summoned, usually in the form of an ambulance. The ambulance has little discretionary power about destination and usually takes the patient to the nearest emergency room (ER). The patients are rapidly assessed in the environment of an ER where there are pressures to admit the patient to hospital, rather than undergo the time-consuming and frustrating process of attempting to secure an appropriate community setting for patients at the end-of-life. Once patients are admitted under a specialist, there are attempts to marginally improve the particular dysfunctional organ responsible for the admission. Other specialists are consulted as the patient has usually been admitted with multiple co-morbidities or, as a result of their frailty, has developed other problems during the course of their admission. Often there is no attempt to look at the patient as a whole in terms of prognosis, personal wishes and potential for reversing any pathology. Hospitals are poor at diagnosing patients at the end-of-life. Approximately 30 % of all rapid response calls are for patients at the end-of-life, in whom it previously had not been considered [43, 44]. Even when a diagnosis has been made, hospitals are also poor at managing end-of-life care [45, 46]. ICUs [42] and rapid response systems often become surrogate ways of managing end-of-life care [45, 47].

While it is tempting to become frustrated with our colleagues for not recognizing patients who are obviously at the end-of-life, a more positive approach may be to acknowledge how our specialty has become the final option of caring for the seriously ill. Our colleagues, locked within their own specialties, often do not have the knowledge of what intensive care can or, more importantly, cannot offer. Out of desperation, they refer many of their patients to intensivists. Some such patients, of course, survive, when many would have thought that they would not. However, our non-intensivist colleagues have little experience or knowledge about prognosis nor of the increasingly complex interventions that are possible in the seriously ill. Rather than make that decision, they increasingly rely on intensivists to provide this expert opinion. Intensivists are no longer simply technicians who accept all admissions to a place surrounded by machines and technologies to support life. We are becoming crucial in the increasingly important role of providing an opinion about the possibilities and limitations of modern medicine.

Our role also becomes crucially important in decisions about resource use and the ethics of the wider society. The costs of hospitals are the largest component of health care costs [4]. The majority of health expenditure is in the last year of life [48]. Critical care currently accounts for 1 % of gross domestic product (GDP) [49, 50], significantly contributing to the unsustainable costs of health care. Moreover, patients do not necessarily want to be admitted to a hospital for end-of-life care; nor do they necessarily want to die surrounded by machines and technology. Intensivists could play a valuable role by beginning discussions with other stakeholders in society, such as politicians, the media and patient groups, about the realistic options that intensive care medicine can offer and being honest and transparent about the limitations of modern medicine as well as discussing the miracles it can sometimes offer.

Conclusions

From modest beginnings, our specialty, in a short time, has contributed enormous value to modern medicine. Our specialty is now involved with many activities outside the four walls of our ICUs. We have been involved in the development of patient retrieval and transportation systems. Intensivists have led in developing systems to rapidly identify and manage seriously ill patients across the entire hospital and, in some cases, in community settings accompanying rapid response ambulances. It is timely that our specialty and our professional and representative bodies also begin to engage our colleagues and society in important issues such as the deployment of resources, the care we can deliver, the limitations of modern medicine and the appropriateness of end-of-life care.

References

1. Lassen HC (1953) A preliminary report on the 1952 epidemic of poliomyelitis in Copenhagen with special reference to the treatment of acute respiratory insufficiency. Lancet 1:37–41
2. Population Division, Department of Economic and Social Affairs. United Nations Secretariat. Long-range world population projections based on 1998 revision. Available at : http://www.un.org/esa/population/publications/longrange/longrange.htm. Accessed Nov 2013
3. World Health Organization. The World Health Report 1998: Life in the 21st century – a vision for all. Available at: http://www.who.int/whr/1998/en/ Accessed Nov 2013
4. Hensher M, Edwards N, Stokes R (1999) The hospital of the future. International trends in the provision and utilization of hospital care. BMJ 219:845–848
5. Hillman K (1999) The changing role of acute-care hospitals. Med J Aust 170:325–328
6. Hillman K (1998) Restructuring hospital services. Med J Aust 169:239
7. Herring AA, Gind AA, Fahimi J et al (2013) Increasing critical care admissions from U.S. emergency departments. Crit Care Med 14:1197–1204
8. Oeppen J, Vaupel JW (2002) Demography. Broken limits to life expectancy. Science 296:1029–1031
9. Fowler RA, Adhikari NH, Bhagwanjee S (2008) Clinical review: critical care in the global context – disparities in burden of illness, access, and economics. Crit Care 12:225
10. Nguyen YL, Angus DC, Boumendil A, Guidet B (2011) The challenge of admitting the very elderly to intensive care. Ann Intensive Care 1:29
11. Bagshaw SM, Webb SA, Delaney A et al (2009) Very old patients admitted to intensive care in Australia and New Zealand: a multi-centre cohort analysis. Crit Care 13:R45
12. Angus DC, Kelley MA, Schmitz RJ, White A, Popovich J Jr, Committee on manpower for Pulmonary and Critical Care Societies (2000) Caring for the critically ill patient. Current and projected workforce requirements for care of the critically ill and patients with pulmonary disease: can we meet the requirements of an aging population? JAMA 284:2762–2770
13. De Rooji SE, Govers A, Korevaar JC, Abu-Hanna A, Levi M, de Jonge E (2006) Short-term and long-term mortality in very elderly patients admitted to an intensive care unit. Intensive Care Med 32:1039–1044

14. Kaarlola A, Tallgren M, Pettila V (2006) Long-term survival, quality of life, and quality-adjusted life-years among critically ill elderly patients. Crit Care Med 34:2120–2126
15. Somme D, Maillet JM, Gisselbrecht M, Novara A, Ract C, Fagon JY (2003) Critically ill old and the oldest-old patients in intensive care: short- and long-term outcomes. Intensive Care Med 29:2137–2143
16. Rooji SE, Abu-Hanna A, Levi M, de Jonge E (2005) Factors that predict outcome of intensive care treatment in very elderly patients: a review. Crit Care 9:R307–R314
17. McDermid RC, Stelfox HT, Bagshaw SM (2011) Frailty in the critically ill: a novel concept. Crit Care 15:301
18. Rockwood K, Song X, MacKnight C et al (2005) A global clinical measure of fitness and frailty in elderly people. Can Med Assoc J 173:489–495
19. Bergman HB, Ferrucci L, Guralnik J et al (2007) Frailty, an emerging research and clinical paradigm: issues and controversies. J Gerontol A Biol Sci Med Sc 62:731–737
20. Kaufman SR (1994) The social construction of frailty: An anthropological perspective. J Aging Stud 8:45–58
21. Kaethler Y, Molnar FJ, Mitchell SL, Soucie P, Man-Son-Hing M (2003) Defining the concept of frailty : a survey of multi-disciplinary health professionals. Geriatr Today 6:26–31
22. Rockwood K, Mitnitski AB, MacKnight C (2002) Some mathematical models of frailty and their clinical implications. Rev Clin Gerontol 12:109–117
23. CSHA Working Group (1994) Canadian Study of Health and Aging: study methods and prevalence of dementia. CMAJ 150:899–913
24. CSHA Working Group (2000) The incidence of dementia in Canada: the Canadian Study of Health and Aging Working Group. Neurology 55:66–73
25. Rockwood K, Wolfson C, McDowell I (2001) The Canadian Study of Health and Aging: organizational lessons from a national, multicenter, epidemiologic study. Int Psychogeriatr 13(Suppl 1):233–7
26. Donini-Lenhoff FG, Hedrick HL (2000) Growth of specialization in graduate medical education. JAMA 284:1284–1289
27. McQuillan P, Pilkington S, Allan A et al (1998) Confidential inquiry into quality of care before admission to intensive care. BMJ 316:1853–1858
28. Schein RMH, Hazday N, Pena M, Ruben BH, Sprung CL (1990) Clinical antecedents to in-hospital cardiopulmonary arrest. Chest 98:1388–1392
29. Hillman KM, Bristow PJ, Chey T et al (2001) Antecedents to hospital deaths. Intern Med J 31:343–348
30. Hillman KM, Bristow PJ, Chey T et al (2002) Duration of life-threatening antecedents prior to intensive care admission. Intensive Care Med 28:1629–1634
31. Hourihan F, Bishop G, Hillman KM, Daffurn K, Lee A (1995) The medical emergency team: a new strategy to identify and intervene in high risk patients. Clin Intensive Care 6:269–272
32. Calzavacca P, Licari E, Tee A et al (2010) The impact of rapid response system on delayed emergency team activation patient characteristics and outcomes – a follow-up study. Resuscitation 81:31–35
33. Hillman K (2002) Critical care without walls. Curr Opin Crit Care 8:594–599
34. Buist M, Bernard S, Nguyen TV, Moore G, Anderson J (2004) Association between clinically abnormal observations and subsequent in-hospital mortality: a prospective study. Resuscitation 62:137–141
35. Jones DA, McIntyre T, Baldwin I, Merder I, Kattula A, Bellomo R (2007) The medical emergency team and end-of-life care: a pilot study. Crit Care Resusc 9:151–156
36. Flabouris A, Chen J, Hillman K et al (2010) Timing and interventions of emergency teams during the MERIT study. Resuscitation 81:25–30
37. Chen J, Bellomo R, Flabouris A et al (2009) The relationship between early emergency team calls and serious adverse events. Crit Care Med 37:148–153
38. Chan PS, Jain R, Nallmothu BK, Berg RA, Sasson C (2010) Rapid response teams. A systematic review and meta-analysis. Arch Intern Med 170:18–26

39. Winters BD, Weaver SJ, Pfoh ER, Yang T, Pham JC, Dy SM (2013) Rapid-response systems as a patient safety strategy. Ann Intern Med 158:417–425
40. Wunsch H, Angus DC, Harrison DA, Linde-Zwirble WT, Rowan KM (2011) Comparison of medical admissions to intensive care units in the united States and United Kingdom. Am J Respir Crit Care Med 183:1666–1673
41. Eastman N, Philips B, Rhodes A (2010) Triaging for adult critical care in the event of over-whelming need. Intensive Care Med 36:1076–1082
42. Angus DC, Barnato AE, Linde-Zwirble WT et al (2004) Use of intensive care at the end of life in the United States: an epidemiologic study. Crit Care Med 32:638–643
43. Parr MJA, Hadfield JH, Flabouris A, Bishop G, Hillman K (2001) The medical emergency team: 12 month analysis of reasons for activation, immediate outcome and not-for-resuscitation orders. Resuscitation 50:39–44
44. Chen J, Flabouris A, Bellomo R et al (2008) The medical emergency team system and not-for-resuscitation orders: results from the MERIT study. Resuscitation 79:391–397
45. Hillman K (2010) Dying safety. Int J Qual Health Care 22:339–340
46. Lorenz KA, Lynn J, Dy SM et al (2008) Improving palliative care at the end of life: a systematic review. Ann Intern Med 148:147–159
47. Jones D, Bagshaw SM, Barrett J et al (2012) The role of the medical emergency team in end-of-life care: a multicentre prospective observational study. Crit Care Med 40:98–103
48. Lubitz J, Cai L, Kramarow E, Lentzner H (2003) Health, life expectancy, and healthcare spending among the elderly. N Engl J Med 349:1048–1055
49. Hapern NA, Pastores SM (2010) Critical care medicine in the United States 2000–2005: an analysis of bed numbers, occupancy rates, payer mix, and costs. Crit Care Med 38:65–71
50. Hapern NA (2009) Can the costs of critical care be controlled? Curr Opin Crit Care 15:591–596

Is Pharmacological, H$_2$S-induced 'Suspended Animation' Feasible in the ICU?

P. Asfar, E. Calzia, and P. Radermacher

Introduction

By definition, 'suspended animation' is a hypometabolic state characterized by the "the slowing of life processes by external means without termination" [1]. Various mammalian species are capable of nearly completely shutting down their vital functions in order to survive otherwise lethal environmental conditions, such as prolonged impairment of O$_2$ supply and/or extreme temperatures. First described and studied in patients as "hibernation artificielle" induced by the so-called "cocktail lytique" during the Indochina war in the early 1950 s, for obvious reasons the concept of inducing such a hypometabolic condition has attracted special interest in intensive care and emergency medicine. Originally, organ-protection, in particular for the central nervous system (CNS), was demonstrated when suspended animation was induced by rapidly cooling experimental animals to core body temperatures of about 10–15 °C using ice-cold infusions and/or cardiopulmonary bypass (CPB). Given the potential undesired adverse effects of hypothermia *per se*, e. g., metabolic acidosis, coagulopathy, prolonged inflammation, and impaired host defense, any pharmacological measure allowing for a therapeutic on-demand induction of suspended animation would be of particular interest. Moreover, more recently, it was suggested that the reduced visceral organ function present in critically ill patients and/or after overwhelming hyperinflammation could be referred to as an adaptive mechanism to maintain ATP-homeostasis due to reduced energy expenditure rather than to irreversible organ failure [2]. A landmark paper by Blackstone et al. produced much excitement among researchers in the field of shock and critical illness:

P. Asfar
Département de Réanimation Médicale et de Médecine Hyperbare, Centre Hospitalier Universitaire, 49933 Angers, France

E. Calzia · P. Radermacher ✉
Sektion Anästhesiologische Pathophysiologie und Verfahrensentwicklung, Klinik für Anästhesiologie, Universitätsklinikum, 89081 Ulm, Germany
e-mail: peter.radermacher@uni-ulm.de

J.-L. Vincent (Ed.), *Annual Update in Intensive Care and Emergency Medicine 2014*,   775
DOI 10.1007/978-3-319-03746-2_58, © Springer International Publishing Switzerland and BioMed Central Ltd. 2014

776 P. Asfar et al.

These authors demonstrated that mice inhaling hydrogen sulfide (H_2S) reversibly decreased their energy expenditure, which was associated with a fall in core temperature [3]. In the meantime, numerous pre-clinical studies have been published on the possible organ-protective effects of H_2S, the available data being equivocal depending on the model used and the type of shock investigated. In this context in particular, the impact of H_2S effects on energy metabolism remains a matter of debate. Therefore, the present chapter reviews the available data on H_2S-induced on-demand hypometabolism, and its relation (directly as well as *via* a possible consecutive drop in body temperature) to organ-protective properties of H_2S.

Rodent Models

In their above-mentioned murine study, Blackstone et al. demonstrated, in awake, spontaneously breathing animals, that exposure to incremental, sub-toxic gaseous H_2S concentrations (20–80 ppm) dose-dependently decreased energy expenditure within a few minutes as assessed by calorimetric measurement of whole-body O_2 uptake and CO_2 production. This fall in metabolic activity was associated with bradypnea and consecutive hypothermia, with core temperature falling to levels close to ambient values [3]. After washout of H_2S, all these metabolic and cardiopulmonary effects were completely reversible, and animals showed no apparent sequelae. Subsequently, Volpato et al. reported that the reduced metabolic activity went along with bradycardia and, consequently, reduced cardiac output, whereas blood pressure and stroke volume remained unaffected [4]. Maintaining normothermia by external warming attenuated the metabolic depressor effect, but did not completely blunt the cardiovascular response [4]. Various other rodent models confirmed these observations: Inhaling gaseous H_2S [5–12] and infusing the soluble sulfide salts, NaSH or Na_2S [6, 13, 14], also induced a reversible reduction in energy expenditure with a subsequent fall in core temperature. Under stress conditions resulting from injurious mechanical ventilation [8, 13], ischemia/reperfusion [7, 9, 12], endotoxin challenge [11], or bacterial sepsis [14], this effect coincided with attenuation of lung [8, 12–14], liver [9], kidney [7] and heart [12] injury. Most importantly, survival was improved after otherwise lethal stress states, e. g., hemorrhagic shock [6] and exposure to hypoxic hypoxia (fraction of inspired O_2 [FiO_2] 5 %) [5]. In addition to anti-oxidant, anti-inflammatory, and anti-apoptotic properties, H_2S was associated with better maintenance of mitochondrial integrity and function [7, 15, 16]: Treatment with either gaseous H_2S treatment or injection of Na_2S prevented mitochondrial swelling, loss of crypts [7, 15], and, at least under hypothermic conditions, outer mitochondrial membrane rupture as documented by the lack of responsiveness of the mitochondrial respiratory chain to stimulation with exogenous cytochrome c [16].

It should be noted that most of the above-mentioned murine data originate from experiments in awake, spontaneously breathing animals. Consequently, the role of anesthesia for a putative H_2S-induced suspended animation remains unclear. Currently, scarce literature is available comparing the effects of anesthesia and H_2S

per se. In spontaneously breathing mice, Li et al. demonstrated that H$_2$S (80 and 250 ppm) produced the same metabolic depression as 0.3 and 0.9 % of isoflurane, respectively, however, without any anesthesia-related muscle atonia. Strikingly, when combining these two interventions, H$_2$S even antagonized the isoflurane-induced metabolic depression [17]. Finally, in mechanically ventilated mice under continuous intravenous (i.v.) anesthesia, the metabolic depressor effect of H$_2$S was completely blunted when normothermia was maintained [16].

Large Animal Species and Humans

Any metabolic depressant property of H$_2$S seems to be dependent on the animal size: In rats the H$_2$S-induced decrease in O$_2$ uptake was several-fold lower than in mice [18]. In larger species (swine, sheep), various authors failed to confirm any H$_2$S-related reduction in metabolic activity at all, regardless of whether inhalation of gaseous H$_2$S or injection of sulfide salts were studied [19–22]. Moreover, in sheep, Derwall et al. [23] demonstrated that during administration of gaseous H$_2$S via an extracorporeal, veno-arterial membrane oxygenator to avoid any airway mucosa damage related to the gas inhalation [24, 25], whole body O$_2$ uptake, CO$_2$ production, and cardiac output remained within the physiological range. At the highest doses administered (300 ppm), H$_2$S did not affect calorimetric energy expenditure either, but caused pulmonary vasoconstriction associated with arterial hypotension and metabolic acidosis [23]. Finally, in human volunteers, inhalation of 10 ppm H$_2$S during exercise decreased O$_2$ uptake, and this effect was referred to a toxic reduction in maximal aerobic capacity rather than to a regulatory effect on mitochondrial respiration, as evidenced by a tendency for muscle lactate to increase and citrate synthase activity to decrease [26]. Consequently, it was questioned whether any therapeutic potential of the H$_2$S-induced "suspended animation"-like hypometabolism observed in mice and rats could be transferred to the clinical setting [27, 28]. On the other hand, when external measures to prevent hypothermia were withheld, Na$_2$S-related organ-protection after kidney ischemia/reperfusion-injury [29] or hemorrhage and resuscitation [30] coincided with a progressive decrease in core temperature (Fig. 1). Moreover, in the latter experiments, immediate post-mortem liver tissue mitochondrial activity showed a tendency towards both reduced oxidative phosphorylation and maximal O$_2$ uptake in the uncoupled state, and, in particular, a significantly decreased "leak respiration", i. e., the respiratory activity necessary to compensate for the proton leakage, slipping, and cation-exchange along the inner mitochondrial membrane (Fig. 2). In other words, H$_2$S supplementation under these conditions provided protective reduction rather than toxic inhibition of cellular respiration.

How can these diverging findings be reconciled? Under stress conditions, e. g., in response to hypoxia or circulatory shock, small rodents can reduce their energy expenditure as a result of decreased 'non-shivering thermogenesis' [31], due to modulation of the uncoupling protein-1, mostly in the brown adipose tissue [32]. In these species, non-shivering thermogenesis represents a large proportion of total

a

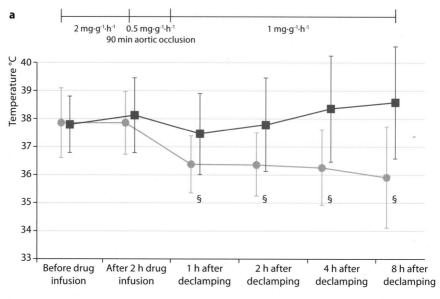

b

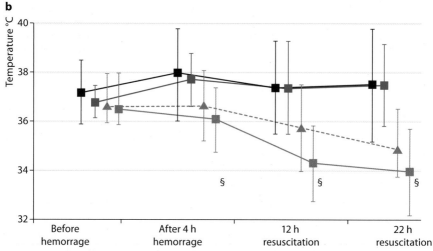

Fig. 1 Time course of body core temperature in swine undergoing (1a) 90 minutes intra-aortic balloon occlusion-induced kidney ischemia/reperfusion-injury (data are adapted from [29]: *Dark blue squares*, vehicle n = 10; *blue circles*, Na$_2$S n = 9; all data are mean ± SD, § designates p < 0.05 between groups); (1b) hemorrhage and resuscitation (data are adapted from [30]: *black squares*, vehicle n = 14; *dark blue squares*, Na$_2$S started two hours before hemorrhage, n = 10; *light blue squares*, Na$_2$S started simultaneously with hemorrhage, n = 11; *blue triangles*, Na$_2$S started immediately after hemorrhage, n = 10; all data are mean ± SD, § designates p < 0.05 'simultaneous' treatment vs. vehicle). Note that in both experimental series at least four hours of drug infusion were necessary to achieve a significant decrease in body temperature

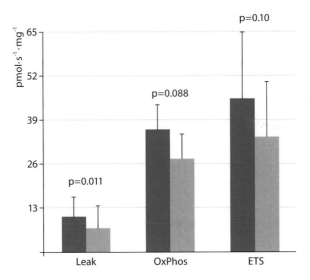

Fig. 2 Leak respiration (Leak), i. e., O_2 consumption necessary to compensate for the proton leakage, slipping, and cation-exchange along the inner mitochondrial membrane; maximal oxidative phosphorylation (OxPhos); and maximal O_2 uptake in the uncoupled state (ETS) in immediate post-mortem liver biopsies of animals undergoing hemorrhage and resuscitation treated with vehicle and Na_2S infusion started simultaneously with the initiation of blood withdrawal. For protocol details, see [30]. All data are mean ± SD of O_2 uptake in pmol/s/mg tissue; *dark blue* columns: vehicle, n = 9; *light blue columns*: Na_2S, n = 10

O_2 uptake, which can be rapidly decreased without affecting ATP formation [31]. This response is independent of any pharmacological intervention, and represents a unique protective adaptation present in numerous mammals [31] and even in humans, e. g., in neonates and during cold acclimatization [32]. However, due to the high area/volume ratio and, consequently, the higher heat dissipation, it is inversely related to body size [31], i. e., to the ratio of O_2 consumption and body weight. Two phenomena support this latter notion: i) No matter the species, newborns present with more pronounced hypoxia-induced hypometabolism than do adults [31]; ii) when the ratio of O_2 consumption and body weight *per se* is low (e. g., in adults of larger species), normoxic O_2 uptake (e. g., during exercise [31]) may be associated with hypoxia-induced hypometabolism. Hence, if possible at all, achieving a suspended animation-like status in larger animals and humans will be more difficult and require much more time because of the small surface area/mass ratio: In fact, in anesthetized and mechanically ventilated swine, after four hours of Na_2S infusion whole body O_2 uptake and CO_2 production started to decrease, subsequently resulting in a moderate decrease in core temperature at ten hours of drug infusion [23] (Fig. 1).

No matter the current debate on the feasibility of pharmacological induction of whole body suspended animation in larger animals, inducing hypometabolism to hibernate isolated organs and, thereby, prolong their tolerance against tissue ischemia or hypoxia remains an attractive option, in particular for organ transplantation. Numerous studies in rodents have demonstrated that H_2S administration improved kidney, liver heart, and lung function and attenuated histological damage after orthotopic organ transplant. This beneficial effect of H_2S administration (NaSH 0.5 mmol/l over 10 minutes before and immediately after initiation of reperfusion) was confirmed in isolated porcine kidneys *ex vivo* undergoing normothermic reperfusion with autologous blood after 25 minutes of warm ischemia and subsequently 18 hours of storage at 4 °C [33].

Hypothermia

Equivocal data are available whether hypothermia, caused by a possible H_2S-related fall in energy expenditure and/or due to external cooling measures, assumes importance for organ protection achieved during H_2S administration. Inhaling H_2S prior to myocardial ischemia at concentrations that had no metabolic depressant effect (10 ppm) attenuated organ damage, but to a lesser degree than concentrations that reduced energy expenditure (100 ppm) [12], suggesting that hypometabolism may indeed enhance the organ-protective properties of H_2S. Of note, in that study as well as in others demonstrating H_2S-related organ production coinciding with reduced metabolic activity, hypothermia was prevented [5, 7, 9, 14,15] in order to elucidate the impact of a simultaneous drop in core temperature. Moreover, organ protection and improved survival were also shown to be in part [12, 13, 15, 34, 35] or even completely [8, 11, 36, 37] independent of any H_2S-induced metabolic depression at all. Finally, data obtained in large animal (swine or sheep) models of shock resulting from ischemia/reperfusion [29, 38–42], hemorrhage and resuscitation [30], or burn injury [36] also suggested that the beneficial effects of infusing Na_2S were at least in part independent of metabolic depression and/or a fall in core temperature. Hence, any moderate hypothermia observed simultaneously with H_2S-induced organ-protection may also be due to attenuation of systemic inflammation rather than to reduced energy expenditure *per se*. In other words, such findings raise a 'chicken and egg' problem, which can be attributed to the so-called $Q10$ effect, i. e., the two to three fold reduction in all chemical reactions and thus metabolism associated with a 10 °C-reduction of body temperature [31]: As an example, during otherwise lethal porcine hemorrhage, therapeutic hypothermia was associated with reduced concentrations of pro-inflammatory cytokines [43]. The potential of H_2S acting as a metabolic depressant in larger species independent of any anti-inflammatory and anti-oxidant property still remains unsettled: In the above-mentioned swine study showing an H_2S-induced drop in O_2 uptake and CO_2 production as well as a consecutive moderate fall in core temperature, animals underwent a short period of aortic occlusion, which did not cause any increase in the blood levels of pro-inflammatory cytokines or markers of oxidative and nitrosative stress [23].

Irrespective of the question as to whether or not there is cause-effect relationship between H_2S-related organ protection and coinciding hypometabolism and/or hypothermia, hypothermia does assume importance for H$_2$S-induced effects on substrate utilization and mitochondrial function. It is well-established that H$_2$S toxicity is due to inhibition of mitochondrial respiration resulting from blockade of the complex IV of the respiratory chain, i.e., cytochrome c oxidase [44]. When compared to normothermia, hypothermia (27 °C) increased the Na$_2$S concentrations necessary to induce inhibition of mitochondrial respiratory activity (from < 1 µM to 2–4 µM), and nearly doubled the Na$_2$S concentrations required for a 50 % reduction in mitochondrial respiratory activity [16, 45]. Hypothermia may also influence the effect of H$_2$S on substrate utilization and, thereby, may even improve the yield of the mitochondrial respiration: In anesthetized and ventilated mice, during normothermia, inhaling 100 ppm H$_2$S did not affect endogenous glucose production (as calculated from the rate of appearance of 1,2,3,4,5,6-^{13}C$_6$-glucose during continuous i.v. isotope infusion), whole body CO$_2$ production, or direct, aerobic glucose oxidation rate (as derived from VCO$_2$ and the expiratory ^{13}CO$_2$/^{12}CO$_2$ ratio) (Fig. 3). However, under hypothermic (core temperature 27 °C) conditions, the rate of direct, aerobic glucose oxidation increased, suggesting a shift toward preferential carbohydrate utilization [16] (Fig. 3). Such a switch in fuel utilization is associated with an improved yield of oxidative phosphorylation: The ATP synthesis/O$_2$ consumption ratio is higher for glycolysis than for β-oxidation, because nicotinamide adenine dinucleotide (NADH) as an electron donor provides three coupling sites rather than just two from FADH$_2$ [46]. During cecal ligation and puncture-induced septic shock, the metabolic effects of inhaled H$_2$S partially disappeared: Inhaled H$_2$S affected neither the sepsis-induced metabolic acidosis [34] nor glucose utilization (Fig. 3), nor the responsiveness to stimulation with exogenous cytochrome c oxidase. Nevertheless, H$_2$S did normalize the sepsis-related increase in "leak respiration" – which was less pronounced during hypothermia – thus allowing for better maintenance of mitochondrial function (Fig. 4). It is unclear whether the lack of effect of H$_2$S on the mitochondrial respiratory chain was due to the septic challenge *per se* and/or to the ongoing treatment: During sepsis, all mice needed continuous i.v. norepinephrine to achieve target hemodynamics characterized by a normotensive and hyperdynamic circulation. In turn, norepinephrine incubation was associated with impairment of tissue mitochondrial respiration.

Timing and Dose

No matter the importance of hypometabolism for the organ-protective properties of H$_2$S administration *per se*, the questions of timing and – due to the potential toxic inhibition of mitochondrial respiration – dosing of H$_2$S remain unsettled. Clearly, there are plenty of data available showing that inhalation of H$_2$S gas and/or the injection of NaSH or Na$_2$S can prevent organ damage when administered prior to or at least simultaneously with the initiation of shock. However, the very few studies comparing a pre- and post-treatment design in mice showed marked reduction [7] or even complete disappearance [37] of the protective potency. In swine undergoing long-term hemorrhage and resuscitation, the results were even more curious [47]:

Fig. 3a, b Whole body CO_2 production (VCO_2) (3a), glycemia (3b), endogenous glucose production (3c), and direct, aerobic whole body glucose oxidation (3d) in anesthetized and mechanically ventilated, normo- (38 °C; *gray* columns) and hypothermic (27 °C; *blue* columns) mice undergoing sham surgery (*light gray* and *light blue* columns) or cecal ligation and puncture (CLP)-induced sepsis (*dark gray* and *dark blue* columns) during inhalation of vehicle (*open columns*) and 100 ppm H_2S (*hatched columns*). Data for sham-surgery are adapted from [16]. All data are mean $\pm$ SD, n = 8–11 per group, # designates $p < 0.05$ vs. normothermia, § designates $p < 0.05$ CLP vs. sham, $ designates $p < 0.05$ H_2S vs. vehicle

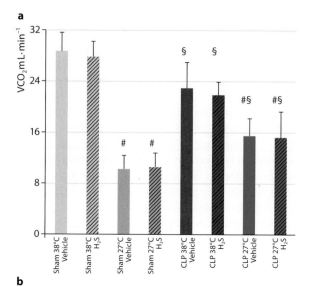

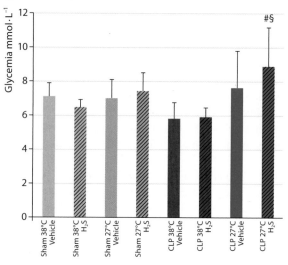

Fig. 3c, d *Continued*

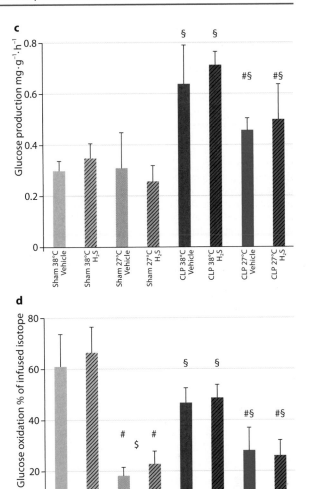

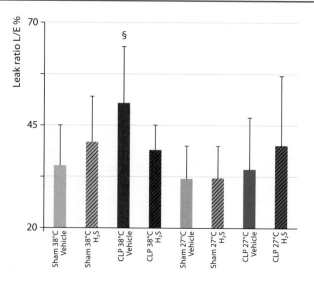

Fig. 4 Leak state O_2 consumption , i. e., the respiratory activity necessary to compensate for the proton leakage, slipping, and cation-exchange along the inner mitochondrial membrane, as a fraction of the maximal O_2 consumption in the uncoupled state, obtained from liver tissue of anesthetized and mechanically ventilated, normo- (38 °C; *gray* columns) and hypothermic (27 °C; *blue* columns) mice undergoing sham surgery (*light gray* and *light blue* columns) or cecal ligation and puncture (CLP)-induced sepsis (*dark gray* and *dark blue* columns) during inhalation of vehicle (*open columns*) and 100 ppm H_2S (*hatched columns*). Data for sham-surgery are adapted from [16]. All data are mean ± SD, $ designates $p < 0.05$ H_2S vs. vehicle

Primed-continuous Na_2S administration (initial bolus of 0.2 mg/kg, followed by 1 mg/kg/h over 12 hours of resuscitation) improved survival when compared to vehicle (survival: 71 %), regardless of whether the Na_2S infusion was started two hours before (pre-treatment: survival 100 %) or simultaneously with (survival 91 %) the initiation of blood withdrawal, or at the start of re-transfusion of shed blood (post-treatment: survival 90 %) [30]. However, a significant decrease in core temperature (Fig. 1b) and organ protection were only present in the group of animals treated simultaneously with the initiation of hemorrhage. Apparently, both the cumulative H_2S dose as well as the rate of its generation assume importance for the effects on metabolism and organ protection, in particular under low flow conditions and/or circulatory shock: In swine undergoing cardiac arrest, primed-continuous Na_2S (0.3 mg/kg followed by 0.3 mg/kg/h over two hours) injected one minute after the start of cardiopulmonary resuscitation (CPR) reduced blood pressure and cardiac output during early resuscitation [21]. Increasing the Na_2S dose (1.0 mg/kg followed by 1.0 mg/kg/h) was associated with impaired neurological recovery. Even injection of comparable total amounts may have markedly different effects due to the different rate of H_2S generation: *In vitro* slow H_2S release from the H_2S donor GYY4137 exerted anti-inflammatory and -apoptotic effects, whereas short-term, high peak free sulfide levels resulting from incubation with NaSH induced the opposite response [48]. *In vivo*, this concept was confirmed in swine undergoing myocardial ischemia/reperfusion injury: A primed-continuous Na$_2$S infusion was superior to bolus injection [39].

Conclusions

The concept of "buying time in suspended animation" [49] has been discussed in the literature for more than a century. Originally induced by rapid external body cooling, any pharmacological measure allowing for a therapeutic, on-demand induction of 'suspended animation' is of particular interest because of the undesired side effects of hypothermia *per se*. Therefore, the landmark paper demonstrating that inhaling H$_2$S could induce a reversible, suspended animation-like hypometabolism [3], produced much excitement among researchers in the field of shock and critical illness. Numerous pre-clinical studies are currently available on H$_2$S-related organ protection, but the effects on energy metabolism remain a matter of debate. In this context, the well-established toxic blockade of cytochrome c oxidase by H$_2$S may assume particular importance. Most studies so far suggest that the beneficial effects of H$_2$S are at least in part independent of an H$_2$S-induced metabolic depression and, in particular, any decrease in core temperature. However, other data suggest that H$_2$S-related hypometabolism may enhance the organ-protective properties. The mechanism behind H$_2$S-induced hypometabolism is still not fully understood, and, moreover, the feasibility of H$_2$S-induced suspended animation in larger animals has been questioned. Clearly, if possible at all, achieving a suspended animation-like status in larger animals and humans will be more difficult and require much more time because of the small surface area/mass ratio. Again the available data are equivocal, suggesting that at least hibernating isolated organs remains an option. Even in larger species, data on the effects of H$_2$S on mitochondrial function and morphology suggest that its supplementation during circulatory shock provides protective reduction rather than toxic inhibition of cellular respiration. Finally, according to the currently available literature, neither inhalation of gaseous H$_2$S nor injection of the soluble sulfide salts, NaSH or Na$_2$S, is likely to become part of clinical practice because of damage to the airway mucosa and possibly toxic peak sulfide concentrations, respectively, but slow H$_2$S-releasing molecules may enable these limitations to be overcome. Hence, there is "nothing rotten about hydrogen sulfide's medical promise" [50], and H$_2$S clearly remains a "hot molecule" [51] in the field of research for a possible pharmacological induction of suspended animation-like hypometabolism.

Acknowledgements

Supported by the Deutsche Forschungsgemeinschaft (KFO 200, DFG RA 396/9-2), the Land Baden-Württemberg (Innovationsfond Medizin), and the Bundesministerium der Verteidigung (Vertragsforschungsvorhaben M/SABX/8A004).

References

1. Suspended animation. Available at: http://en.wikipedia.org/wiki/Suspended_animation. Accessed Nov 2013
2. Singer M, De Santis V, Vitale D, Jeffcoate W (2004) Multiorgan failure is an adaptive, endocrine-mediated, metabolic response to overwhelming systemic inflammation. Lancet 364:545–548
3. Blackstone E, Morrison M, Roth MB (2005) H$_2$S induces a suspended animation-like state in mice. Science 308:518
4. Volpato GP, Searles R, Yu B et al (2008) Inhaled hydrogen sulfide: a rapidly reversible inhibitor of cardiac and metabolic function in the mouse. Anesthesiology 108:659–668
5. Blackstone E, Roth MB (2007) Suspended animation-like state protects mice from lethal hypoxia. Shock 27:370–372
6. Morrison ML, Blackwood JE, Lockett SL, Iwata A, Winn RK, Roth MB (2008) Surviving blood loss using hydrogen sulfide. J Trauma 65:183–188
7. Bos EM, Leuvenink HG, Snijder PM et al (2009) Hydrogen sulfide-induced hypometabolism prevents renal ischemia/reperfusion injury. J Am Soc Nephrol 20:1901–1905
8. Faller S, Ryter SW, Choi AM, Loop T, Schmidt R, Hoetzel A (2010) Inhaled hydrogen sulfide protects against ventilator-induced lung injury. Anesthesiology 113:104–115
9. Bos EM, Snijder PM, Jekel H et al (2012) Beneficial effects of gaseous hydrogen sulfide in hepatic ischemia/reperfusion injury. Transpl Int 25:897–908
10. Seitz DH, Fröba JS, Niesler U et al (2012) Inhaled hydrogen sulfide induces suspended animation, but does not alter the inflammatory response after blunt chest trauma. Shock 37:197–204
11. Tokuda K, Kida K, Marutani E et al (2012) Inhaled hydrogen sulfide prevents endotoxin-induced systemic inflammation and improves survival by altering sulfide metabolism in mice. Antioxid Redox Signal 17:11–21
12. Snijder PM, de Boer RA, Bos EM et al (2013) Gaseous hydrogen sulfide protects against myocardial ischemia-reperfusion injury in mice partially independent from hypometabolism. PLoS One 8:e63291
13. Aslami H, Heinen A, Roelofs JJTH, Zuurbier CJ, Schultz MJ, Juffermans NP (2010) Suspended animation inducer hydrogen sulfide is protective in an in vivo model of ventilator-induced lung injury. Intensive Care Med 36:1946–1952
14. Aslami H, Pulskens WP, Kuipers MT et al (2013) Hydrogen sulfide donor NaHS reduces organ injury in a rat model of pneumococcal pneumosepsis, associated with improved bio-energetic status. PLoS One 8:e63497
15. Elrod JW, Calvert JW, Morrison J et al (2007) Hydrogen sulfide attenuates myocardial ischemia-reperfusion injury by preservation of mitochondrial function. Proc Natl Acad Sci USA 104:15560–15565
16. Baumgart K, Wagner F, Gröger M et al (2010) Cardiac and metabolic effects of hypothermia and inhaled hydrogen sulfide in anesthetized and ventilated mice. Crit Care Med 38:588–595
17. Li RQ, McKinstry AR, Moore JT et al (2012) Is hydrogen sulfide-induced suspended animation general anesthesia? J Pharmacol Exp Ther 341:735–742
18. Haouzi P, Bell HJ, Notet V, Bihain B (2009) Comparison of the metabolic and ventilatory response to hypoxia and H$_2$S in unsedated mice and rats. Respir Physiol Neurobiol 2:316–322
19. Li J, Zhang G, Cai S, Redington AN (2008) Effect of inhaled hydrogen sulfide on metabolic responses in anesthetized, paralyzed, and mechanically ventilated piglets. Pediatr Crit Care Med 9:110–112
20. Haouzi P, Notet V, Chenuel B et al (2008) H$_2$S induced hypometabolism in mice is missing in sedated sheep. Respir Physiol Neurobiol 160:109–115
21. Derwall M, Westerkamp M, Löwer C et al (2010) Hydrogen sulfide does not increase resuscitability in a porcine model of prolonged cardiac arrest. Shock 34:190–195

22. Drabek T, Kochanek PM, Stezoski J et al (2011) Intravenous hydrogen sulfide does not induce hypothermia or improve survival from hemorrhagic shock in pigs. Shock 35:67–73

23. Derwall M, Francis RC, Kida K et al (2011) Administration of hydrogen sulfide via extracorporeal membrane lung ventilation in sheep with partial cardiopulmonary bypass perfusion: a proof of concept study on metabolic and vasomotor effects. Crit Care 15:R51

24. Simon F, Giudici R, Duy CN et al (2008) Hemodynamic and metabolic effects of hydrogen sulfide during porcine ischemia/reperfusion injury. Shock 30:359–364

25. Francis RC, Vaporidi K, Bloch KD, Ichinose F, Zapol WM (2011) Protective and detrimental effects of sodium sulfide and hydrogen sulfide in murine ventilator-induced lung injury. Anesthesiology 115:1012–1021

26. Bhambani Y, Burnham R, Snydmiller G, MacLean IJ (1997) Effects of 10-ppm hydrogen sulfide inhalation in exercising men and women. Cardiovascular, metabolic, and biochemical responses. J Occup Environ Med 39:122–129

27. Tisherman SA, Drabek T (2008) Hydrogen sulfide: metabolic mediator or toxic gas? Pediatr Crit Care Med 9:129–130

28. Haouzi P (2011) Murine models in critical care research. Crit Care Med 39:2290–2293

29. Simon F, Scheuerle A, Gröger M et al (2011) Effects of intravenous sulfide during porcine aortic occlusion-induced kidney ischemia/reperfusion injury. Shock 35:156–163

30. Bracht H, Scheuerle A, Gröger M et al (2012) Effects of intravenous sulfide during resuscitated porcine hemorrhagic shock. Crit Care Med 40:2157–2167

31. Mortola JP (1993) Hypoxic hypometabolism in mammals. News Physiol Scie 8:79–82

32. van Marken Lichtenbelt WD, Schrauwen P (2011) Implications of nonshivering thermogenesis for energy balance regulation in humans. Am J Physiol Regul Integr Comp Physiol 301:R285–R296

33. Hosgood SA, Nicholson ML (2010) Hydrogen sulphide ameliorates ischaemia-reperfusion injury in an experimental model of non-heart-beating donor kidney transplantation. Br J Surg 97:202–209

34. Wagner F, Wagner K, Weber S et al (2011) Inflammatory effects of hypothermia and inhaled H$_2$S during resuscitated, hyperdynamic murine septic shock. Shock 2(35):396–402

35. Wagner F, Scheuerle A, Weber S et al (2011) Cardiopulmonary, histologic, and inflammatory effects of intravenous Na$_2$S after blunt chest trauma-induced lung contusion in mice. J Trauma 71:1659–1667

36. Esechie A, Enkhbaatar P, Traber DL et al (2009) Beneficial effect of a hydrogen sulphide donor (sodium sulphide) in an ovine model of burn- and smoke-induced acute lung injury. Br J Pharmacol 158:1442–1453

37. Minamishima S, Bougaki M, Sips PY et al (2009) Hydrogen sulfide improves survival after cardiac arrest and cardiopulmonary resuscitation via a nitric oxide synthase 3-dependent mechanism in mice. Circulation 120:888–896

38. Sodha NR, Clements RT, Feng J et al (2008) The effects of therapeutic sulfide on myocardial apoptosis in response to ischemia-reperfusion injury. Eur J Cardiothorac Surg 33:906–913

39. Osipov RM, Robich MP, Feng J et al (2009) Effect of hydrogen sulfide in a porcine model of myocardial ischemia-reperfusion: comparison of different administration regimens and characterization of the cellular mechanisms of protection. J Cardiovasc Pharmacol 54:287–297

40. Sodha NR, Clements RT, Feng J et al (2009) Hydrogen sulfide therapy attenuates the inflammatory response in a porcine model of myocardial ischemia/reperfusion injury. J Thorac Cardiovasc Surg 138:977–984

41. Osipov RM, Robich MP, Feng J et al (2010) Effect of hydrogen sulfide on myocardial protection in the setting of cardioplegia and cardiopulmonary bypass. Interact Cardiovasc Thorac Surg 10:506–512

42. Hunter JP, Hosgood SA, Patel M, Rose R, Read K, Nicholson ML (2012) Effects of hydrogen sulphide in an experimental model of renal ischaemia-reperfusion injury. Br J Surg 99:1665–1671

43. Chen Z, Chen H, Rhee P et al (2005) Induction of profound hypothermia modulates the immune/inflammatory response in a swine model of lethal hemorrhage. Resuscitation 66:209–216

44. Cooper CE, Brown GC (2008) The inhibition of mitochondrial cytochrome oxidase by the gases carbon monoxide, nitric oxide, hydrogen cyanide and hydrogen sulfide: chemical mechanism and physiological significance. J Bioenerg Biomembr 40:533–539

45. Gröger M, Matallo J, McCook O et al (2012) Temperature and cell-type dependency of sulfide effects on mitochondrial respiration. Shock 38:367–374

46. Leverve X, Batandier C, Fontaine E (2007) Choosing the right substrate. Novartis Found Symp 280:108–121

47. Drabek T (2012) Hydrogen sulfide-curiouser and curiouser! Crit Care Med 40:2255–2256

48. Whiteman M, Li L, Rose P, Tan C, Parkinson DB, Moore PK (2010) The effect of hydrogen sulfide donors on lipopolysaccharide-induced formation of inflammatory mediators in macrophages. Antioxid Redox Signal 12:1147–1154

49. Roth MB, Nystul T (2005) Buying time in suspended animation. Sci Am 292:48–55

50. Leslie M (2008) Nothing rotten about hydrogen sulfide's medical promise. Science 320:1155–1157

51. Aslami H, Schultz MJ, Juffermans NP (2011) Hydrogen sulfide: a hot molecule. Anesthesiology 115:921–922

Index

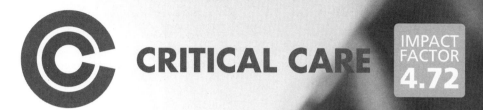

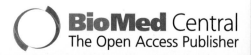

Printing and Binding: Stürtz GmbH, Würzburg